Neuroviral Infections

RNA Viruses and Retroviruses

Neuroviral Infections

RNA Viruses and Retroviruses

Edited by
Sunit K. Singh and Daniel Růžek

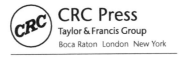

CRC Press
Taylor & Francis Group
Boca Raton London New York

CRC Press is an imprint of the
Taylor & Francis Group, an **informa** business

CRC Press
Taylor & Francis Group
6000 Broken Sound Parkway NW, Suite 300
Boca Raton, FL 33487-2742

First issued in paperback 2020

Version Date: 2012920

ISBN 13: 978-0-367-57653-0 (pbk)
ISBN 13: 978-1-4665-6720-7 (hbk)

Library of Congress Cataloging-in-Publication Data

Neuroviral infections. RNA viruses and retroviruses / editors, Sunit K. Singh, Daniel Ruzek.
    p. ; cm.
RNA viruses and retroviruses
Includes bibliographical references and index.
ISBN 978-1-4665-6720-7 (hardcover : alk. paper)
I. Singh, Sunit K. II. Ruzek, Daniel. III. Title: RNA viruses and retroviruses.
[DNLM: 1. Central Nervous System Viral Diseases. 2. RNA Virus Infections. 3. RNA Viruses--pathogenicity. 4. Retroviridae--pathogenicity. 5. Retroviridae Infections. WC 540]

616.9'18--dc23   2012036938

Visit the Taylor & Francis Web site at
http://www.taylorandfrancis.com

and the CRC Press Web site at
http://www.crcpress.com

Contents

SECTION I RNA Viruses

SECTION II   Retroviruses

Preface

Neurovirology is an interdisciplinary field that represents a melding of virology, clinical neuroscience, molecular biology, and immunology. Apart from clinical neuroscience, neurovirology includes molecular virology, biochemical virology, diagnostic virology, and molecular pathogenesis and is inextricably bound to the field of immunology. Neurovirology became an established field within the past 30 years. Since then, there has been a tremendous explosion of information related to viral infections of the central nervous system, and, also, several new viruses have been discovered. The aim of this book is to present an up-to-date overview on major RNA viruses and retrovirus-mediated neuroviral infections to virologists, specialists in infectious diseases, teachers of virology, and postgraduate students of medicine, virology, neurosciences, or immunology. We hope that it will serve as a useful resource for all others interested in the field of viral infections of the central nervous system.

An inclusive and comprehensive book such as this is clearly beyond the capacity of an individual's effort. Therefore, we are fortunate and honored to have a large panel of internationally renowned virologists as chapter contributors, whose detailed knowledge on viral neuroinfections have greatly enriched this book.

We conceptualized this book in two sections. Section I includes the major RNA virus chapters and Section II concludes with the specific information pertinent to individual major retroviruses and their diseases. Each chapter consists of a review on the classification, epidemiology, clinical features, and diagnostic and therapeutic approaches of one or a group of related viruses.

The professionalism and dedication of executive editor Barbara Norwitz and senior project coordinator Jill Jurgensen at CRC Press greatly contributed to the final presentation of the book. Our appreciations extend to our families for their understanding and support during the compilation of this book.

Sunit K. Singh
Daniel Růžek

Acknowledgement

This book is dedicated to a magnanimous group of virologists, whose willingness to share their in-depth knowledge and expertise has made this extensive overview on viral neuroinfections possible.

Editors

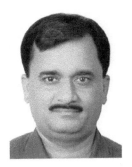

Dr. Sunit Kumar Singh completed his bachelor's degree program from GB Pant University of Agriculture and Technology, Pantnagar, India, and master's degree program from the CIFE, Mumbai, India. After receiving his master's degree, Dr. Singh joined the Department of Paediatric Rheumatology, Immunology, and Infectious Diseases, Children's Hospital, University of Wuerzburg, Wuerzburg, Germany, as a biologist. Dr. Singh completed his PhD degree from the University of Wuerzburg in the area of molecular infection biology. Dr. Singh has completed his postdoctoral trainings at the Department of Internal Medicine, Yale University, School of Medicine, New Haven, Connecticut, USA, and the Department of Neurology, University of California Davis Medical Center, Sacramento, California, USA, in the areas of vector-borne infectious diseases and neuroinflammation, respectively.

He has also worked as visiting scientist at the Department of Pathology, Albert Einstein College of Medicine, New York, USA, Department of Microbiology, College of Veterinary Medicine, Chonbuk National University, Republic of Korea; and the Department of Arbovirology, Institute of Parasitology, Ceske Budejovice, Czech Republic. Presently, he is serving as a scientist and leading a research group in the area of neurovirology and inflammation biology at the prestigious Centre for Cellular and Molecular Biology, Hyderabad, India. His main areas of research interest are Neurovirology and Immunology.

There are several awards to his credit, including the Skinner Memorial Award, Travel Grant Award, NIH-Fogarty Fellowship, and Young Scientist Award. Dr. Singh is associated with several international journals of repute as associate editor and editorial board member.

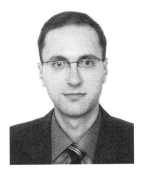

Dr. Daniel Růžek is a research scientist at the Institute of Parasitology, Academy of Sciences of the Czech Republic, and an assistant professor at the Department of Medical Biology, Faculty of Science, University of South Bohemia. He received his PhD in the field of molecular and cellular biology and genetics from the Academy of Sciences of the Czech Republic and the University of South Bohemia. He had postdoctoral training at the Department of Virology and Immunology, Texas Biomedical Research Institute (formerly Southwest Foundation for Biomedical Research), San Antonio, Texas, USA. His primary field is virology with research emphasis on vector-borne viruses, especially tick-borne encephalitis virus, Omsk hemorrhagic fever virus, dengue virus, West Nile virus, and so forth. In 2009, he was awarded with a prestigious international Sinnecker–Kunz Award for young researchers.

Contributors

Anda Baicus
Microbiology Department,
  "Cantacuzino"
University of Medicine and Pharmacy
  "Carol Davila"
Viral Enteric Infections Laboratory
National Institute of Research and
  Development for Microbiology and
  Immunology
Bucharest, Romania

Cristian Baicus
Department of Internal Medicine
Colentina University Hospital
University of Medicine and Pharmacy
  "Carol Davila"
Bucharest, Romania

Ashley C. Banyard
Wildlife Zoonoses and Vector Borne
  Disease Research Group
Department of Virology
Animal Health and Veterinary
  Laboratories Agency
Surrey, United Kingdom

Anirban Basu
Cellular and Molecular Neuroscience
  Division
National Brain Research Centre
Haryana, India

Jennifer M. Best
King's College London
London, United Kingdom

Bartosz Bilski
University of Medical Sciences Poznań
Poznań, Poland

Élodie Brison
Laboratory of Neuroimmunovirology
Institut National de la Recherche
  Scientifique
Université du Québec
Laval, Québec, Canada

Marta S. Contigiani
Laboratorio de Arbovirus
Instituto de Virología "Dr. J. M.
  Vanella"
Universidad Nacional de Córdoba
Córdoba, Argentina

Vlasta Danielová
Centre of Epidemiology and
  Microbiology
National Institute of Public Health
Prague, Czech Republic

Marc Desforges
Laboratory of Neuroimmunovirology
Institut National de la Recherche
  Scientifique
Université du Québec
Laval, Québec, Canada

Jessica Desjardins
Laboratory of Neuroimmunovirology
Institut National de la Recherche
  Scientifique
Université du Québec
Laval, Québec, Canada

Luis Adrián Diaz
Laboratorio de Arbovirus
Instituto de Virología "Dr. J. M.
    Vanella"
Universidad Nacional de Córdoba
and
Instituto de Investigaciones Biológicas y
    Tecnológicas
Consejo Nacional de Investigaciones
    Científicas y Técnicas
Córdoba, Argentina

W. Paul Duprex
Departments of Microbiology and
    Neurology
and
National Emerging Infectious Disease
    Laboratories
Boston University
Boston, Massachusetts

Alan P. Dupuis II
Department of Zoonotic Diseases
New York State Department of Health
Albany, New York

Kallol Dutta
Cellular and Molecular Neuroscience
    Division
National Brain Research Centre
Manesar, Haryana, India

Dominique J. Favreau
Laboratory of Neuroimmunovirology
Institut National de la Recherche
    Scientifique
Université du Québec
Laval, Québec, Canada

Anthony R. Fooks
Wildlife Zoonoses and Vector Borne
    Disease Research Group
Department of Virology
Animal Health and Veterinary
    Laboratories Agency
Surrey, United Kingdom

and
University of Liverpool
National Consortium for Zoonosis
    Research
Neston, United Kingdom

Philippe Gasque
Immunopathology and Infectious
    Disease Research Group
University of la Reunion
St. Denis, Reunion, France

Liliane Grangeot-Keros
Virology Department
Antoine Béclère Hospital
National Reference Laboratory for
    Rubella
Clamart, France

Göran Günther
Department of Medical Sciences
Uppsala University
Uppsala, Sweden

Roy A. Hall
Australian Infectious Diseases Research
    Centre
University of Queensland
St Lucia, Australia

Hideo Hara
Department of Internal Medicine
Saga University
Saga, Japan

Derek M. Healy
Wildlife Zoonoses and Vector Borne
    Disease Research Group
Department of Virology
Animal Health and Veterinary
    Laboratories Agency
Surrey, United Kingdom

Daniel L. Horton
Wildlife Zoonoses and Vector Borne
    Disease Research Group
Department of Virology
Animal Health and Veterinary
    Laboratories Agency
Surrey, United Kingdom

Hélène Jacomy
Laboratory of Neuroimmunovirology
Institut National de la Recherche
    Scientifique
Université du Québec
Laval, Québec, Canada

Marie Christine Jaffar-Bandjee
Immunopathology and Infectious
    Disease Research Group
University of la Reunion
St. Denis, Reunion, France

Claire L. Jeffries
Wildlife Zoonoses and Vector Borne
    Disease Research Group
Department of Virology
Animal Health and Veterinary
    Laboratories Agency
Surrey, United Kingdom

Nicholas Johnson
Wildlife Zoonoses and Vector Borne
    Disease Research Group
Department of Virology
Animal Health and Veterinary
    Laboratories Agency
Surrey, United Kingdom

Patrik Kilian
Institute of Parasitology
Biology Centre of the Academy of
    Sciences of the Czech Republic
and
Faculty of Science
University of South Bohemia
České Budějovice, Czech Republic

Laura D. Kramer
Department of Zoonotic Diseases
New York State Department of Health
and
Department of Biomedical Sciences
State University of New York
Albany, New York

Shiril Kumar
Immunopathology and Infectious
    Disease Research Group
University of la Reunion
St. Denis, Reunion, France

Kang-Sheng Li
Department of Microbiology and
    Immunology
Shantou University Medical College
Shantou, Guangdong, China

Mario Lobigs
Australian Infectious Diseases
    Research Centre
University of Queensland
St Lucia, Australia

Martin Ludlow
Departments of Microbiology and
    Neurology
and
National Emerging Infectious Disease
    Laboratories
Boston University
Boston, Massachusetts

Larry Lutwick
Veterans Affairs New York Harbor
    Health Care Center
and
State University of New York
    Downstate Medical School
Brooklyn, New York

Mathieu Meessen-Pinard
Laboratory of Neuroimmunovirology
Institut National de la Recherche
 Scientifique
Université du Québec
Laval, Québec, Canada

Ritu Mishra
Laboratory of Neurovirology and
 Inflammation Biology
Centre for Cellular and Molecular
 Biology
Council of Scientific and Industrial
 Research
Hyderabad, India

Arshed Nazmi
Cellular and Molecular Neuroscience
 Division
National Brain Research Centre
Manesar, Haryana, India

Mah-Lee Ng
Department of Microbiology
National University of Singapore
Singapore

Slobodan Paessler
Department of Pathology
University of Texas
Galveston, Texas

Jana Preis
Veterans Affairs New York Harbor
 Health Care Center
and
State University of New York
Down State Medical School
Brooklyn, New York

Natalie A. Prow
Australian Infectious Diseases
 Research Centre
University of Queensland
St Lucia, Australia

Duksha Ramful
Immunopathology and Infectious
 Disease Research Group
University of la Reunion
St. Denis, Reunion, France

Susan Reef
Centers for Disease Control and
 Prevention
Atlanta, Georgia

Stephanie Robin
Immunopathology and Infectious
 Disease Research Group
University of la Reunion
St. Denis, Reunion, France

Daniel Růžek
Institute of Parasitology
Biology Centre of the Academy of
 Sciences of the Czech Republic
České Budějovice, Czech Republic

Sunit K. Singh
Laboratory of Neurovirology and
 Inflammation Biology
Centre for Cellular and Molecular
 Biology
Council of Scientific and Industrial
 Research
Hyderabad, India

Lorena I. Spinsanti
Laboratorio de Arbovirus
Laboratorio de Arbovirus
Instituto de Virología "Dr. J.M. Vanella"
Universidad Nacional de Córdoba
Córdoba, Argentina

Pierre J. Talbot
Laboratory of Neuroimmunovirology
Institut National de la Recherche
 Scientifique
Université du Québec
Laval, Québec, Canada

Norma P. Tavakoli
Department of Genetics
New York State Department of Health
and
Department of Biomedical Sciences
State University of New York
Albany, New York

Katherine Taylor
Department of Pathology
University of Texas
Galveston, Texas

Vincent G. Thon-Hon
Immunopathology and Infectious
    Disease Research Group
University of la Reunion
St. Denis, Reunion, France

Aravinthan Varatharaj
Brain Infections Group
Department of Clinical Infection,
    Microbiology and Immunology
University of Liverpool
Liverpool, United Kingdom

Gefei Wang
Department of Microbiology and
    Immunology
Shantou University Medical College
Shantou, Guangdong, China

Michael R. Wilson
Departments of Microbiology and
    Neurology
and
National Emerging Infectious Disease
    Laboratories
Boston University
Boston, Massachusetts

Kim-Long Yeo
Department of Microbiology
National University of Singapore
and
NUS Graduate School for Integrative
    Sciences and Engineering
Centre for Life Sciences
Singapore

Motohiro Yukitake
Division of Neurology
Department of Internal Medicine
Saga University
Saga, Japan

Jun Zeng
Department of Microbiology and
    Immunology
Shantou University Medical College
Shantou, Guangdong, China

Section I

RNA Viruses

1 Alphavirus Neurovirulence

Katherine Taylor and Slobodan Paessler

CONTENTS

1.1 INTRODUCTION

Due to their parasitic, obligate, intracellular nature, evolution favors viruses with the ability to evade the barriers and impediments the host organism utilizes to limit their ability to replicate or cause cellular dysfunction. Avoidance of host defense mechanisms and successful replication often leads to virulence, the ability to cause fatal disease. Neurovirulent viruses alter the highly sensitive nature and critical functioning of the central nervous system (CNS) leading to fatal encephalitis or, in the event of recovery, severe neurological sequelae. With 20 viruses known to cause human encephalitis, arboviruses (arthropod-borne viruses) represent a significant public health threat as emerging infectious diseases both in the United States and worldwide. The focus of this review, arboviruses in the *Alphavirus* genus in the family Togaviridae, contains three viruses capable of causing human encephalitis: Venezuelan equine encephalitis virus (VEEV), eastern equine encephalitis virus (EEEV), and western equine encephalitis virus (WEEV). No specific therapy or vaccine is currently available against these viruses.

For the encephalitic alphaviruses, virulence reflects the severity of neurological disease and is determined by the efficiency of host and viral factors. Peripheral replication, viremia, neuroinvasiveness, and neurotropism combined and interacting together lead to neurovirulence and subsequent disease (Griffin 2007). Each individual component is influenced by the overall molecular character of the infecting

3

virus as well as the subsequent response, genetic background, age, and sex of the infected host (Griffin 2007). The balance of the characteristics of the host and virus ultimately determines outcome to infection, and minor changes in either can drastically impact disease etiology, leading to lethality, persistence, or abortive infection. Thus, each stage or step of viral pathogenesis can be considered a struggle by the virus against host defense to obtain the evolutionary ideal of a relative equilibrium between the host and the virus.

In this context, two experimental paradigms are utilized to determine the components of neurovirulence: (1) the use of mutated viruses to define the molecular changes capable of altering pathogenesis and (2) the study of host variables utilizing analysis of viral pathogenesis in hosts where key immunological components are missing or altered (Fleming 1988). In considering these two experimental approaches, it is important to remember that minor variability and alterations in the viral genome can result in significant changes in neuropathogenesis. Pathogenic alphaviruses can be roughly grouped by a combination of phylogenetics, geographical circulation, and disease manifestation into two groups: Old World and New World viruses. Old World viruses differ significantly from New World viruses in tropism and disease manifestations in humans, causing arthralgia, malaise, or rash, whereas New World alphaviruses result in a flu-like syndrome that may progress to encephalitis. Two Old World viruses, Sindbis and Semliki Forest, have been used extensively in small animal models as prototypical encephalitic alphaviruses through the use of either neuroadapted or the rare naturally encephalitic strains, respectively. Although valuable knowledge regarding neuropathogenesis has been derived from these models, experimental approaches utilizing Old World alphaviruses to represent naturally encephalitic strains need to be confirmed using New World alphaviruses (Atasheva et al. 2008; Charles et al. 2001; Garmashova et al. 2007a,b; Kolokoltsov et al. 2006a,b; Yin et al. 2009). Thus, this review will first seek to understand how changes in viral replication of the primary encephalitic New World viruses, EEE, WEE, and VEE alter pathogenesis followed by analysis of how the host response potentially contributes to the disease.

1.2   ALPHAVIRUS

The encephalitic alphaviruses spread in a biphasic manner through the mammalian host. Viral-host interactions and the viability of the virus as a neurological agent require entry and successful replication at the site of infection. Evidence from experimental models indicates that as the mosquito feeds on the experimental host, virus is deposited from infected saliva extravascularly into the tissues (Turell et al. 1995). Virus then replicates at the site of inoculation, typically skeletal muscle or immune cells such as Langerhan's cells of the skin (Grimley and Friedman 1970; Johnston et al. 2000; Liu et al. 1970; Murphy and Whitfield 1970). As the infected immune cells carry the virus to the draining lymph nodes, the virus is delivered to the vascular system, where it spreads to other target tissues, initiating the secondary phase of infection (Griffin 2007). Griffin (2007), in *Fields Virology*, defines peripheral replication and viremia as key components of neurovirulence. In the initial, peripheral phase, efficient replication at the site of inoculation enhances neuroinvasiveness through viremia although sustained, high levels of blood-borne virus may not be required for neuroinvasion.

Following replication in lymphoid and/or myeloid tissues, the virus enters the CNS, resulting in a second phase of replication in the brain and spinal cord neurons. Entry to the CNS is critical to neurovirulence, but the precise mechanism of entry remains unknown. However, literature supports a model of nasal mucosa infection leading to the infection of the olfactory neurons and neuronal spread to through the CNS (Charles et al. 2001; Steele et al. 1998).

The initiation of inflammation leads to damage to the vascular integrity of the blood–brain barrier (BBB), enabling further entry of the virus to the compromised CNS (Schafer et al. 2009, 2011). The multifocal nature of the infection in the brain by 5 or 6 days postinfection indicates damage to the BBB and free crossing of viral particles across the typically sealed barrier (Charles et al. 2001; Jackson et al. 1991; Roy et al. 2009; Vogel et al. 2005; Zlotnik et al. 1972). Damage to the vascular integrity of the BBB as a result of inflammation has additional support from a range of studies examining viral entry to the CNS (Cook and Griffin 2003; Lossinsky and Shivers 2004; Wang et al. 2004).

Disease symptoms in patients mimic the biphasic nature of both the immune response and viral replication. In patients, as the initial immune response and viral propagation exponentially grow, a fever develops. As the secondary spread of virus begins, patients may develop another fever that coincides with development of neurological symptoms. This phase results in neuropathology and, in some cases, fatal encephalitis. Regardless, in the majority of infected individuals, the host response appears to be sufficient to prevent CNS damage and results in asymptomatic infections. This serves to emphasize how little is known regarding the susceptibility of particular individuals to neurovirulent viruses. For instance, in WEE epidemics, only 1 of 1000 infected individuals actually develop clinical encephalitis with fatality resulting in only 3% of these cases (Rennels 1984). Similar statistics are observed for VEE and EEE, although mortality in these infections is significantly higher. Nevertheless, the question remains why the viruses that are apparently intrinsically of low virulence cause severe disease in some patients and what factors account for occasional severe neurovirulence in some individuals? This is reflected in experimental situations where variability between inbred strains of mice results in alterations in outcomes (Ludwig et al. 2001). In human infections, there is undoubtedly an age-associated susceptibility to the encephalitic alphaviruses, with neurovirulence and associated mortality increasing at the extremes of the age spectrum in pediatric and elderly patients; however, the underlying causes for increased susceptibility in these populations remain poorly defined. The immature CNS may explain the susceptibility in pediatric patients, as WEE is more cytopathic in immature human neuronal cells than mature cells. Additionally, mature neuronal cells are more sensitive to type I IFN requiring less to reduce viral cytopathology and replication (Castorena et al. 2008).

The ability of the immunocompetent host to prevent neuroinvasion is uncertain and viral invasion without associated symptomatic illness has been reported in the literature in experimental models. Indicative of the importance of immune host control at the site of initial replication, intracerebral or intranasal inoculation of many alphaviruses causes fatal disease in experimental models, whereas subcutaneous or intraperitoneal infection results in either asymptomatic disease or a clinical syndrome without lethality or severe neuropathology (Griffin 2007). Although the development of encephalitis and neurological disease in animal models is readily apparent as gauged by seizures or measurable paralysis, the utility of these models in evaluating the human host response is unclear as the disease development may be significantly different. Gaining a clearer understanding of the effects viral infection has on the host is a major component of drug development and vaccine platforms (Holbrook and Gowen 2008).

The two-wave model of infection is supported by a series of studies using VEE viral replicon particles (VRP), which are capable of targeting and infecting the same cells as VEE but unable to propagate beyond the first infected cell, to model early events in neuroinvasion. Direct intracranial infection of VRP resulted in VEE-like encephalitis in mice and was associated with a robust and rapid innate immune response that resulted in compromised BBB integrity. These initial results established a model for the identification of host and viral factors that contribute to the invasion of the brain (Schafer et al. 2009). More recent studies show that replication of the VRP in the nasal mucosa induced the opening of the BBB allowing peripherally administered VRP to enter the brain (Schafer et al. 2009, 2011). Subsequent inhibition of the initial opening of the BBB resulted in a delay in viral neuroinvasion and pathogenesis. Thus, initial entry into the CNS through the olfactory pathways initiates viral replication in the brain, inducing the opening of the BBB and allowing for a secondary wave of virus from the periphery to enter the brain (Schafer et al. 2011). Further supporting initial replication and entry through the olfactory epithelium and neurons, the administration of the toxin tunamycin damages the ultrastructure of the BBB. However, entry to the CNS still appears to occur via the olfactory system despite the prior damage BBB induced by pretreatment with the toxin. An increased viral load in the brain with both virulent and attenuated strains of virus is observed in mice treated with tunamycin to induce artificial BBB breakdown (Steele et al. 2006).

1.3 INTERFERENCE WITH ANTIVIRAL TRANSCRIPTION

All three encephalitic alphaviruses are highly susceptible to the effects of type I IFN (IFN-α and IFN-β), and as such, resistance to type I IFN signaling and production is associated with increasing neurovirulence of the virus (Aguilar et al. 2008a; Armstrong et al. 1971; Jahrling et al. 1976; Jordan 1973; Julander et al. 2007). Closely related virulent and avirulent strains of virus and indeed virulent New World and less virulent Old World alphaviruses demonstrate significant differences in their ability to interfere with gene transcription associated with viral attenuation linked to enhanced susceptibility to the effects of type I IFN. Comparison of IFN-sensitive avirulent strains and IFN-resistant virulent strains has led to comprehensive knowledge of the genes responsible for controlling IFN resistances and subsequent neurovirulence. Research supports the underlying cause of differences in disease presentation and incidence in humans between North and South American isolates of EEE results from alterations to IFN sensitivity. Comparison of replication of NA and SA strains in IFN pretreated Vero cells showed a suppressive effect only on the replication of the less virulent SA strains. However, no differences in induction of IFN *in vivo* were observed (Aguilar et al. 2005). Similar results were found for VEE with attenuation in enzoonotic strains limiting the ability of the virus to interfere with the type I IFN pathways, and this may partially explains the absence of disease symptoms following infection with enzoonotic strains (Anishchenko et al. 2004; Jahrling et al. 1976; Simmons et al. 2009). Conversely, epizootic and epidemic strains are able to limit the host production of type I interferon.

Comparison of both naturally and experimentally attenuated viruses to virulent strains has generated valuable knowledge regarding the basis for IFN resistance and subsequent neurovirulence. Priming neurons with IFN before infection with either VEEV or SINV further demonstrates VEEV's resistance to an established antiviral state compared with SINV as VEEV continues to replicate and produce progeny virion in primed cells in contrast to more sensitive SINV. VEEV resistance was attributed to partial blockade of phosphorylation of IFN signaling pathway molecules, STAT1 and STAT2, mediated by expression of nonstructural proteins. VEEV also inhibits interferon signaling genes (ISG) through structural protein expression (Yin et al. 2009).

Furthermore, comparison of an IFN-sensitive SA EEE strain to a resistant NA EEE strain identified both structural and nonstructural genes as important in IFN sensitivity (Aguilar et al. 2008a,b). Additional data derived from the genetic manipulation of virulent viruses has contributed to the understanding of the mechanisms underlying virulence associated with IFN resistance. Artificial attenuation of virulent EEE results in a marked increased in sensitivity to type I IFN and is associated with decreased virulence of the virus (Aguilar et al. 2008b). Attenuations in WEE and VEE reflect similar results (Anishchenko et al. 2004; Aronson et al. 2000; White et al. 2001). The significant differences in the an antihost response for New World alphaviruses compared with the Old World likely play a role in the increased neurovirulence of the former with the ability to down-regulate the cellular antiviral machinery increases neurovirulence. The recombination events leading to the formation of WEE from SINV and EEV-like ancestors allowed WEEV to acquire capsid protein function to inhibit the transcription of antiviral factors and thereby effectively evade the antiviral effects of type I IFN. Thus, the acquisition of type I IFN evasion led to the emergence of WEEV as a pathogenic virus (Garmashova et al. 2007b; Hahn et al. 1988).

The ability of EEEV and VEEV to interfere with cellular transcription and induce subsequent cytopathic effect is controlled by a N-terminal 35-amino acid long peptide fragment of the capsid protein. One domain is critical in balancing the presence of protein in the cytoplasm and nucleus, and the downstream peptide may contain nuclear localization signals. These domains determine the intracellular distribution of the VEEV capsid and are essential for protein function in the inhibition of transcription. The cytopathologic effects are reduced and infection is attenuated *in vivo* without effecting viral replication by replacing the N-terminal fragment of the VEEV capsid with the Old World alphavirus, SINV (Garmashova et al. 2007a). The pathogenic effect of the capsid protein appears to work via inhibition of multiple receptor-mediated nuclear import pathways leading to down-regulation of the cellular antiviral machinery. Again, the capsid protein of SINV had no effect on nuclear import (Atasheva et al. 2008). Interestingly, the Old World alphaviruses, SINV and SFV, are both able to interfere with cellular transcription. However, different virus-specific proteins are utilized to cause this effect. For the Old World, alphaviruses transcriptional shutoff depends on nsP2, whereas for the New World alphaviruses, it depends on VEEV and EEEV (Garmashova et al. 2007a,b).

Thus, changes to the E2 envelope glycoprotein are significant attenuators of the neurovirulent virus. Early studies comparing TC83 structural proteins to virulent parent strain VEE-TRD found that the two strains differed at 12 nucleotides with no alterations in the nonstructural proteins or the open reading frame coding the viral polyprotein. Only nine of these changes occurred in the dominant population of the RNAs from plaque-purified viruses. Significantly, six of the nine mutations appeared in the E2 surface glycoprotein, and all five of the nucleotide changes producing non-conservative amino acid substitutions were located here (Johnson et al. 1986). Two mutations in E1 were found: one silent and one that did not alter the character of the protein. An additional nucleotide difference was found in the noncoding region preceding the 5′ end of the 26S mRNA. This early publication determined that both E2 and the noncoding regions were candidates for the molecular determinants of VEE neurovirulence. In the early 1990s, the proof of attenuation of VEEV through serial cell-culture passage that resulted in TC83 is encoded in the 5′ noncoding region and the E2 envelope glycoprotein was confirmed. Studies showed E2-120 appears to be the major structural determinant of attenuation, but genetic markers composed of genome nucleotide position 3 in the 5′ noncoding region were also significant to the attenuated phenotype (Kinney et al. 1993). The biological effect of the attenuating mutation in the 5′ untranslated region during murine infection was ultimately traced to increased sensitivity to IFN-α and IFN-β (White et al. 2001).

1.4   CHANGES IN CELLULAR TROPISM

The molecular changes responsible for changes in cellular tropism between the encephalitic alphaviruses are poorly defined; however, viral tropism for the cells of the periphery varies among the three encephalitic alphaviruses. The altered tropism for the cells of the CNS (neurons, oligodendria, microglia, and astrocytes) does not appear to account for the changes in neurovirulence between the closely related strains, as both virulent and avirulent strains are capable of productive infection of neurons. However, the efficiency of replication in neurons differs dramatically without necessarily effecting replication in the cells of the periphery. The molecular basis for enhanced replication appears to be targeted to specific changes in the coding and noncoding regions of the genome, ultimately leading to enhanced neurovirulence (Griffin 2007).

However, altered tropism for other cells may impact the level of peripheral replication, viremia, and subsequent neuroinvasion and virulence. In the case of EEEV and VEEV, such changes are reflected in altered cell tropism. Indeed, the infection of immune cells by viruses may have a significant effect on a pathogenesis as evidenced by differences in tropism between EEE and VEE. In the case of EEEV and VEEV, such changes are reflected in altered cell tropism. Although both viruses cause severe morbidity and mortality in equines and humans, VEEV infects the DCs and macrophages of the lymphoid tissues, whereas EEEV replicates poorly in lymphoid tissues and preferentially infects muscle and fat cells. Both viruses replicate efficiently in mesenchymal cell lineages. The inability of EEEV to replicate in myeloid cell lineages is due to interferon-independent inhibition of EEEV translation. VEEV-infected mice display higher levels of serum IFN and result in IFN up-regulation in more animals compared with EEEV infection. Interestingly, the altered tropism of EEEV may help the virus to evade systemic IFN induction *in vivo* enhancing EEEV neurovirulence and contributing to differences in disease etiology (Gardner et al. 2008).

1.5   HOST-ANTIVIRAL RESPONSE

Viral replication at the site of inoculation, level of viremia, and subsequent spread to secondary sites are controlled by viral clearance after the initiation of the host response. Given the close relation and ability of the innate immune response to modulate the later adaptive immune response needed to effectively clear the virus, an early, robust, and properly directed innate immune response is essential. In the biphasic model of alphavirus infection, as the primary phase of viral replication is initiated, the host begins responding to the pathogenic changes at the site of inoculation by inducing robust production of cytokines, particularly IFN (Griffin 2007). Cytokine production also results in recruitment of other immune effectors capable of generating positive feedback producing an antiviral environment in the host. The infection of immune cells serves to propagate the virus but also results in the infiltration of antigen-presenting cells to the nearest lymph node, introducing antigen to naive B and T cells in the lymph nodes and initiating the adaptive immune response. Given the primary tropism of the encephalitic alphaviruses for dendritic cells, it would be unsurprising if alterations in antigen presentation and subsequent modification of an efficient adaptive immune response occurred; however, little work has been done to determine the effect of such tropism in these infections. These early mechanisms are also required to limit peripheral replication, viremia, and spread to secondary sites of infection before the development of an effective adaptive immune response.

Immunocompentent mice infected with VEEV develop a typical biphasic illness with an early lymphoid phase, characterized by ruffling of fur and progression to hunching, and a later fatal CNS phase, characterized by progression from ataxia to severe paralysis. In the lymphoid phase, peripheral serum viremia and replication in organs is resolved concurrent with production of IgM at 3 days postinfection, which steadily increases to the time of death as well as with rapid, robust production of type I IFN by 18–24 h postinfection that rapidly waned after 24-h postinfection. However, mice still developed fulminate encephalitis, and the mean time to death is 7.8 days (Charles et al. 2001).

In contrast, severely immunocompromised SCID mice fail to develop early signs of disease and symptoms develop at 6–7 days postinfection marked by aggression and agitation with death occurring at 8.9 days postinfection. Animals fail to develop hallmark hind-limb paralysis and become ataxic and progressively less responsive, indicating alterations of the neurological disease in the immunocompromised host. Organ tropism differed in these animals with persistent viral replication at or near peak titer appearing in peripheral organs until the death of the animal without the resolution seen by 120 h after infection in sera and lymphoid tissues in competent animals. Unsurprisingly, patterns of antibody and type I IFN production vary from the immunocompentent host with a complete lack of neutralizing antibody production and lower levels of IFN that increased slowly and were below the limit of detection by 48 h postinfection. The time of death is delayed in these mice, with an average survival time of 8.9 days (Charles et al. 2001).

Given the alteration in clinical symptoms, the pathologies in the brain present as a severe spongiform encephalopathy different from that of the immunocompetent hosts' fulminate encephalitis, indicative of a significant immunological component to CNS pathology. Charles et al. (2011) does not attribute the proximal cause of death to brain lesions in either case. Thus, the establishment of a functional host response in the periphery requires a competent immune system but is unable to prevent death. The changes in peripheral cellular tropism occur more rapidly than can be explained by the adaptive response and likely involve innate nonspecific response to viral pathogens, particularly the lack of IFN in SCID mice, preventing the establishment of the antiviral state (Charles et al. 2001).

Unfortunately, little is known about the specific mechanisms of host defense apart from an early, antiviral role for type I IFN and a correlation of neutralizing antibody production with peripheral clearance.

1.6 INTERFERON

All three of the encephalitic alphaviruses are highly susceptible to the effects of type I IFN and, as mentioned previously, have developed effective evasion tactics to avoid the antiviral effect. In fact, in the absence of type I IFN signaling in receptor knockout mice, even attenuated strains of VEE typically unassociated with illness can cause complete mortality (White et al. 2001). However, prophylactic and, in some cases, early therapeutic treatment with type I IFN or compounds capable of inducing type I IFN provides protection, indicating the importance of the early generation of an immune environment conducive to host protection.

Beginning with the discovery that EEE replication was suppressed in the presence of type I IFN, Wagner (1961, 1963) showed peak viral production and high levels of cytopathogenicity in chick embryos and L-cells correlated with a high-level production of IFN. *In vivo* serum levels of type I IFN are low compared with those of VEE-infected mice and likely reflect the inability of EEE to infect cells of the myeloid lineages because the ability of EEE to antagonize type I IFN induction is cell-dependent (Burke et al. 2009). By artificially increasing the serum type I IFN before infection by administration of a TLR3 agonist, poly-IC, Aguilar et al. (2005) demonstrated a dose-dependent IFN-mediated protection of mice to EEE infection. Similar results are seen for WEE infections, where pretreatment of hamsters with either a consensus type IFN-α or a stimulator of type I IFN signaling, Ampligen, resulted in the complete survival of the animal. The antiviral effect of type I IFN levels was reflected in decreased clinical symptoms and weight loss associated with a significantly lower viral load in the brain at

4 days postinfection (Julander et al. 2007). Complete survival and depression of clinical symptoms is also associated with transiently expressed, artificially high levels of IFN-α in mouse models of WEE infection. Therapeutic treatment up to 7 days before infection provides complete protection. Early prophylactic elevation of IFN-α at 6 h postinfection results in increased survival rates but fails to provide complete protection (Wu et al. 2007a,b). Unsurprisingly, VEE responds similarly to the early induction of type I IFN with artificial induction of signaling through administration of a TLR3 agonist or prophylactic administration of pegylated IFN-α, resulting in delayed time to death and increased survival in mouse models (Julander et al. 2008b). Although the early administration of IFN demonstrates some prophylactic effects in decreasing time to death or disease symptoms, in the case of intranasal or aerosol exposure, the rapid entry of the virus to the CNS may limit or alter the effectiveness of early innate immune mechanisms such as IFN or other unexplored factors. The substantial difference in the effect of therapeutic and prophylactic administration of type I IFN or inducers of IFN production indicates the importance of modulating the specific immune response in the CNS to create a distinct antipathogenic environment after viral spread and replication.

The CNS of immunologically normal mice is still invaded in the presence of very high circulating levels of IFN, indicating that the cells that comprise the CNS may be less sensitive to the presence of IFN or have slower kinetics for the establishment of an effective antiviral state (Charles et al. 2001).

Due to the greater stability of IFN-α, most studies use its modified forms, and to the authors' knowledge, no studies examining the effects of IFN-β have been performed to date. Interestingly, IFN-β treatment of the CNS disorder, multiple sclerosis, helps control the disease in some patients and indicates that mechanisms other than the antiviral effect of the type I interferons may be important in control of CNS damage (Galligan et al. 2010; Plosker 2011).

1.7 INNATE IMMUNE RESPONSE

Pretreatment and, in some cases, therapeutic administration (up to 12 h pi) of cationic-liposome DNA complexes (CDLCs) in mice infected with WEE results in significant protection. This protection was associated with changes in the host immune response due to CDLC administration. Treated mice had significantly increased serum IFN-γ, TNF-α, and IL-12, indicative of a strong TH1-biased antiviral activation of the immune system. In infected animals large increases in IFN-γ, TNF-α, IL-12, MCP-1, and IL-10 in the brain were observed by 72 h pi, as expected, with neuroinvasion and viral replication in the CNS (Schafer et al. 2009). Similar cytokine profiles are found in the brain homogenates of C3H/HeN mice lethally infected with the vaccine strain of VEEV, TC83. In these animals, IL-1a, IL-1b, IL-6, IL-12, MCP-1, IFN-γ, TNF-α, MIP1-α, and RANTES were significantly elevated over time with peak cytokine levels at six to seven days postinfection. Depression in cytokine levels occurs immediately before death around 8 to 10 days postinfection. Interestingly, treatment with IFN-α B/D or TLR3 agonist significantly improved cytokine levels and mean day to death, indicating a connection between mortality and the early host response (Julander et al. 2008a,b). Thus, robust, nonspecific activation of the innate immune response, while necessary to influence the phenotype of the adaptive immune response, requires careful modulation in the CNS to elicit significant protective immunity against rapidly lethal strains of encephalitic alphaviruses (Schafer et al. 2009).

1.8   ADAPTIVE IMMUNE RESPONSE

The second phase of the immune response to alphavirus infection is characterized by the waning of type I IFN and the development of a robust cell-mediated immunity that theoretically limits CNS damage and clears the virus from circulation and sites of replication.

Of the factors in the cell-mediated immune response responsible of resolving infection, the role of B-cells and antibody production is well-defined. The development of antigen specific B-cells capable of antibody production play a key role in reducing peripheral replication and removing virus from the blood stream. Thus, an efficient antibody response is integral to preventing or limiting neurovirulence from the earliest phase. However, the time lag between peripheral infection and antigen-specific antibody production permits spread and replication at secondary sites of infection as mentioned previously, and additional cell-mediated mechanisms may be required to resolve infections once they reach the CNS (Griffin 2007).

In the lymphoid phase of murine infection (CB17), high-titer serum viremia is associated with the production of VEE-specific IgM antibody at 3 days postinfection, with titers increasing until the time of death. Animals failed to develop VEEV-specific IgG or IgA. However, fulminate encephalitis still develops and animals survive only an average of 6.8 days postinfection (Charles et al. 2001). Further reconstitution of SCID mice and depletion of immunologically normal mice identified production of VEE-specific IgM antibody, produced in the absence of T-cell help, as the significant factor determining immune mediated clearance in the periphery. Given the paralysis and death of these animals following infection, it appears that peripheral production of neutralizing antibody does not play a significant role in preventing lethal encephalitis once virus reaches the CNS (Charles et al. 2001).

Once the virus becomes neuroinvasive, the utility of peripherally produced antibody is uncertain, and T cells, particularly CD4$^+$ T cells, are integral in clearance of CNS infection. Indicative of the role of T cells in resolving viral invasion of the CNS, α/β T-cell receptor knockout mice deficient in both CD4$^+$ and CD8$^+$ T cells develop lethal VEE encephalitis following vaccination protective to the wild-type counterpart. Specifically, reconstitution of the CD4$^+$ T cells, but not CD8$^+$ T cells, from vaccinated wild-type donors resulted in recovery following vaccination and challenge in α/β T-cell receptor knockout mice, indicating an integral role for CD4$^+$ T cells in preventing lethal encephalitis (Paessler et al. 2007; Yun et al. 2009). In the absence of a competent T-cell compartment, α/β T-cell receptor knockout mice also have impaired antibody production in the absence of CD4$^+$ T-cell help. However, passive transfer of HIAF antibody failed to induce a protective response in vaccinated animals indicating either a direct role for CD4$^+$ T cells in the CNS or an indirect, B-cell, antibody-independent mechanism of action (Yun et al. 2009). Studies using B-cell-deficient uMT mice infected with an attenuated strain of VEEV resulted in the development of severe, but ultimately, asymptomatic encephalitis. An antibody-independent Th1-biased response characterized by CD4[+] T-cell production of IFN-γ was implicated in the control of viral replication and survival of the animals (Brooke et al. 2010).

Charles et al. (2001) demonstrated that treatment of CD-1 mice with T-cell-depleting factors before infection results in a disease such as that of SCID mice with absent clinical symptoms early in disease and no development of paralysis. However, infection in the absence of T cells had no effect on clearance of virus from the serum and did not prevent production of IgM (Charles et al. 2001). Reconstitution of SCID mice with T cells results in the reversion to fulminant encephalitis seen in wild-type mice, as does the inverse scenario, with the depletion of wild-type Cd-1 in mice leading to spongiosis and vaculation of the neuropil as seen in SCID mice. Analysis of inflammatory infiltrates in the brain indicated that T cells represent the majority of infiltrates and the predominant phenotype was CD8[+] (Charles et al. 2001). Treatment of murine splenocytes with both B- and T-cell mitogens increases the susceptibility of VEE infection and indicates that the activation state of lymphocytes may be critical to lymphoid pathogenesis of VEEV (Charles et al. 2001).

Animal models of infection have provided some insight into the role of IFN-γ in protection. For VEE, the priming of the immune response via the vaccination of mice with a deficiency in the type II IFN (IFN-γ) receptor is only partially protective, unlike the complete protection seen in wild-type animals following vaccination, indicating that type 2 IFN signaling may play some role in preventing the development of encephalitis. However, unlike type I IFN signaling, type 2 IFN signaling is not absolutely required for effective protection (Paessler et al. 2007). Additionally, IFN-γ signaling does not appear to be significant in controlling EEE infection, as IFN-γ-receptor-deficient animals demonstrate equivalent levels of viremia and mortality rates similar to wild-type animals (Aguilar et al. 2008a).

1.9 HOST RESPONSE AND VACCINE DEVELOPMENT

Neurovirulence is considered the standard for vaccine candidates derived from virulent neurotropic viruses (Arya and Agarwal 2008; Fine et al. 2008). Intracranial injection of susceptible mice is routinely used for vaccine safety studies, and the mice are evaluated based on the occurrence of pathological processes in the neurological tissues. Intracranial viral infection causes damage to neuronal and glial cell populations in addition to inducing migration of potentially harmful immunologically active cells in to the perivascular space and brain parenchyma. However, in the case of live vaccine candidates, such as TC83, the current IND vaccine for VEE, these studies fail to take into account the effects of neuroinvasion in the absence of detectable pathologies. The ability of RNA viruses to persist in the CNS and the tropism of live vaccine candidates for the cells of the CNS must also be considered in developing viable vaccines. Arya et al. points out that for practical use of vaccines derived from neurotropic viruses, a close examination of the CNS for subtle lesions is required, particularly neurological developments after vaccination for other such vaccines as seen with poliovirus vaccine lots in the 1960s (Arya and Agarwal 2008; Cristi and Dalbuono 1967). To evaluate potential CNS damage, experimental animals should be observed for much longer periods to examine the occurrence and location of brain lesions after vaccination (Arya and Agarwal 2008).

The current key requirements for the development of a VEEV vaccine are (a) a high level of immunogenic response in mice and hamster, which are both sensitive to infection, and (b) a protective response in the NHP model when challenged with virulent virus (Rao et al. 2006). Unfortunately, the sole parameter for immunogenic response in small animal models is the production of neutralizing antibody that may not necessarily correlate with protection once infection reaches the CNS.

In addition to neurovirulence as a safety parameter, vaccine studies use neutralizing antibody production as a correlate for the efficacy of vaccination. In such cases, antibody is used as a measure of protection; however, the ability of peripherally produced antibody to provide protection and complete clearance of virus once the virus invades the peripheral nervous tissue or the olfactory tissue via olfactory nerve tracts remains poorly determined (Arya and Agarwal 2008; Fine et al. 2008).

Alterations in pathogenesis between closely related strains can be demonstrated from vaccination studies using attenuated strains of virus. These studies also derived important data regarding the host response and indicate that additional parameters to antibody production may be necessary when evaluating safety and efficacy of vaccine or therapeutic candidates.

A series of studies beginning in small animal models and progressing to NHPs compared the current live, attenuated IND vaccine strain, TC83, to candidate V3526, a live attenuated virus derived from an infectious clone of VEEV, TrD. Intracranial inoculation of both TC83 and V3526 results in the replication in the brain, with V3526 replicating at lower levels. Although neither strain was lethal in BALB/c mice, those infected with TC83 developed symptomatic illness, and the infection of C3H/HeN mice resulted in complete lethality, demonstrating the differential susceptibility of different inbred mice strains as shown previously by Steele et al. (Ludwig et al. 2001; Steele et al. 1998). V3526, despite its ability to replicate in the CNS, was "avirulent" in both strains and did not cause symptomatic illness. Interestingly, pathological changes were found in the brains of mice infected with either strain, although, correlating with viral load, changes in V3526 inoculated animals were less severe and of shorter duration than TC83-inoculated animals (Ludwig et al. 2001).

Comparison of wild-type virus to attenuated, vaccine strain TC83 and V3526 showed similar results following aerosol exposure: while the attenuated virus does not necessarily cause symptomatic disease or mortality, they can be neuroinvasive and cause lesions throughout the CNS, which, however, are readily resolved. All three strains infected the brains and induced encephalitis. However, viral spread varied, with a gradient occurring from complete invasion of all regions of the brain with TrD, to sparing the caudal regions with TC83, to the involvement of only the neocortex and diencephalon with V3526. TrD infection resulted in uniform mortality with significant peripheral dissemination between mouse strains. Despite alterations in viral spread through the CNS, TC83 still induced 100% mortality in C3H/HeN animals but not BALB/c mice. Interestingly, significant differences between inbred mouse strains exist, and TC83, which is avirulent, so to speak, in BALB/c mice, causes complete lethality in C3H/HeN animals. V3526 caused no mortality in either strain. Neither attenuated strain extended beyond the infection of the olfactory epithelium (Steele et al. 1998). Thus, viral replication and spread do not necessarily correlate with mortality as seen in the case of the more limited spread of TC83 to caudal regions compared with TRD and equivalent mortality in C3H/ HeN mice.

Manifestations of disease were found in rhesus macaques inoculated intrathalamically/intraspinally with both V3526 and TC83, although a greater percentage of TC83 infected animals developed clinically significant signs. All symptomatic disease resolved by 3 weeks postinfection. Interestingly, one of seven animals infected with attenuated V3526 showed extensive brain lesions similar to all four wild-type animals at D18. Six of seven infected macaques showed scattered lesions throughout the CNS as did four of seven TC83-infected animals at D18. All lesions were resolved by termination of the study at D181. Thus, clinical symptoms do not necessarily correlate with viral invasion, replication, and pathogenesis in the CNS (Atasheva et al. 2008; Fine et al. 2008).

Studies evaluating the propagation-defective VEEV replicon particles in mice resulted in weight loss and inflammatory changes in the brain. However, changes are less severe than those caused by TC83, the current IND vaccine. Peripheral inoculation demonstrated minimal neurovirulence and lack of neuroinvasive potential (Kowalski et al. 2007). Despite the rapid and transient nature of CNS lesions following vaccination, little is known about the degree of magnitude required to induce potentially undetectable but significant pathogenic alterations to the delicate homeostasis of the CNS. Although peripheral inoculation routes with propagation defective particles are likely unable to reach the CNS, this may not be true for live, attenuated vaccine candidates that may in fact reach, replicate, or even persist in the CNS at undetectable levels. The biological relevance of low level replication in the CNS is uncertain, but the immune-privileged nature of the CNS makes any alteration of concern.

Intracranial infection with VRP results in a VEE-like encephalitis. The use of a VRP-mRNP tagging system to distinguish the response of infected cells from bystander cells showed the initiation of a robust and rapid innate inflammatory response in the CNS by both infected neurons and uninfected bystander cells that led to an adaptive immune response characterized by proliferation and activation of microglia and infiltration of inflammatory monocytes as well as CD4[+] and CD8[+] T lymphocytes. Thus, the ability of the naive CNS to induce a robust innate immune response and activate local professional antigen-presenting cells that can, in turn, activate primed cells may be crucial to the outcome of infection by determining the composition and dynamics of the adaptive immune response and ultimate noncytopathic or lethal attempts to clear the virus (Schafer et al. 2009).

A formalin-inactivated form of TC83, C-84, is currently used as a booster if vaccinated individuals fail to develop a response to TC83. The low efficacy and undesirable side effects have led to additional vaccination strategies and vaccine platforms. One such approach utilizes microspheres to encapsulate the vaccine and induce a more robust response. These spheres are composed of DL-lactide-co-glycolide (DL-PLG). Microencapsulating the vaccine increased the primary circulating IgG and resulted in a rapid increase in antibody activity when boosted with a second vaccination. Interestingly, circulating anti-VEE virus antibody response was lower, with nonformalin-fixed virus utilizing this platform. Following systemic challenge with virulent VEE, the microencapsulated virus was more effective at inducing a protective immune response (Greenway et al. 1995).

1.10 CONCLUSION

Alphaviruses represent a significant public health threat. A better understanding of the mechanisms both virus and host use to control infection and prevent neuroinvasion are required for development of safe and effective vaccines and therapeutics.

REFERENCES

Aguilar, P. V., Adams, A. P., Wang, E., Kang, W., Carrara, A.-S., Anishchenko, M., Frolov, I., and Weaver, S. C. (2008a). Structural and nonstructural protein genome regions of eastern equine encephalitis virus are determinants of interferon sensitivity and murine virulence. *J Virol* 82(10), 4920–30.

Aguilar, P. V., Leung, L. W., Wang, E., Weaver, S. C., and Basler, C. F. (2008b). A five-amino-acid deletion of the eastern equine encephalitis virus capsid protein attenuates replication in mammalian systems but not in mosquito cells. *J Virol* 82(14), 6972–83.

Aguilar, P. V., Paessler, S., Carrara, A.-S., Baron, S., Poast, J., Wang, E., Moncayo, A. C., Anishchenko, M., Watts, D., Tesh, R. B., and Weaver, S. C. (2005). Variation in interferon sensitivity and induction among strains of eastern equine encephalitis virus. *J Virol* 79(17), 11300–10.

Anishchenko, M., Paessler, S., Greene, I. P., Aguilar, P. V., Carrara, A. S., and Weaver, S. C. (2004). Generation and characterization of closely related epizootic and enzootic infectious cDNA clones for studying interferon sensitivity and emergence mechanisms of Venezuelan equine encephalitis virus. *J Virol* 78(1), 1–8.

Armstrong, J. A., Freeburg, L. C., and Ho, M. (1971). Effect of interferon on synthesis of Eastern equine encephalitis virus RNA. *Proc Soc Exp Biol Med* 137(1), 13–8.

Aronson, J. F., Grieder, F. B., Davis, N. L., Charles, P. C., Knott, T., Brown, K., and Johnston, R. E. (2000). A single-site mutant and revertants arising *in vivo* define early steps in the pathogenesis of Venezuelan equine encephalitis virus. *Virology* 270(1), 111–23.

Arya, S. C., and Agarwal, N. (2008). Apropos "neurovirulence evaluation of Venezuelan equine encephalitis (VEE) vaccine candidate V3526 in non-human primates." *Vaccine* 26(35), 4413.

Atasheva, S., Garmashova, N., Frolov, I., and Frolova, E. (2008). Venezuelan equine encephalitis virus capsid protein inhibits nuclear import in Mammalian but not in mosquito cells. *J Virol* 82(8), 4028–41.

Bianchi, T. I., Aviles, G., Monath, T. P., and Sabattini, M. S. (1993). Western equine encephalomyelitis: virulence markers and their epidemiologic significance. *Am J Trop Med Hyg* 49(3), 322–8.

Brooke, C. B., Deming, D. J., Whitmore, A. C., White, L. J., and Johnston, R. E. (2010). T cells facilitate recovery from Venezuelan equine encephalitis virus-induced encephalomyelitis in the absence of antibody. *J Virol* 84(9), 4556–68.

Burke, C. W., Gardner, C. L., Steffan, J. J., Ryman, K. D., and Klimstra, W. B. (2009). Characteristics of alpha/beta interferon induction after infection of murine fibroblasts with wild-type and mutant alphaviruses. *Virology* 395(1), 121–32.

Castorena, K. M., Peltier, D. C., Peng, W., and Miller, D. J. (2008). Maturation-dependent responses of human neuronal cells to western equine encephalitis virus infection and type I interferons. *Virology* 372(1), 208–20.

Charles, P. C., Trgovcich, J., Davis, N. L., and Johnston, R. E. (2001). Immunopathogenesis and immune modulation of Venezuelan equine encephalitis virus-induced disease in the mouse. *Virology* 284(2), 190–202.

Cook, S. H., and Griffin, D. E. (2003). Luciferase imaging of a neurotropic viral infection in intact animals. *J Virol* 77(9), 5333–8.

Cristi, G., and Dalbuono, S. (1967). Probable neurological complications caused by the Sabin type of oral antipoliomyelitis vaccine. *Riv Neurol* 37(3), 251–7.

Fine, D. L., Roberts, B. A., Terpening, S. J., Mott, J., Vasconcelos, D., and House, R. V. (2008). Neurovirulence evaluation of Venezuelan equine encephalitis (VEE) vaccine candidate V3526 in nonhuman primates. *Vaccine* 26(27–28), 3497–506.

Fleming, J. O. (1988). Viral neurovirulence. *Lab Invest* 58(5), 481–3.

Galligan, C. L., Pennell, L. M., Murooka, T. T., Baig, E., Majchrzak-Kita, B., Rahbar, R., and Fish, E. N. (2010). Interferon-beta is a key regulator of proinflammatory events in experimental autoimmune encephalomyelitis. *Mult Scler* 16(12), 1458–73.

Gardner, C. L., Burke, C. W., Tesfay, M. Z., Glass, P. J., Klimstra, W. B., and Ryman, K. D. (2008). Eastern and Venezuelan equine encephalitis viruses differ in their ability to infect dendritic cells and macrophages: impact of altered cell tropism on pathogenesis. *J Virol* 82(21), 10634–46.

Gardner, C. L., Yin, J., Burke, C. W., Klimstra, W. B., and Ryman, K. D. (2009). Type I interferon induction is correlated with attenuation of a South American eastern equine encephalitis virus strain in mice. *Virology* 390(2), 338–47.

Garmashova, N., Atasheva, S., Kang, W., Weaver, S. C., Frolova, E., and Frolov, I. (2007a). Analysis of Venezuelan equine encephalitis virus capsid protein function in the inhibition of cellular transcription. *J Virol* 81(24), 13552–65.

Garmashova, N., Gorchakov, R., Volkova, E., Paessler, S., Frolova, E., and Frolov, I. (2007b). The Old World and New World alphaviruses use different virus-specific proteins for induction of transcriptional shutoff. *J Virol* 81(5), 2472–84.

Greenway, T. E., Eldridge, J. H., Ludwig, G., Staas, J. K., Smith, J. F., Gilley, R. M., and Michalek, S. M. (1995). Enhancement of protective immune responses to Venezuelan equine encephalitis (VEE) virus with microencapsulated vaccine. *Vaccine* 13(15), 1411–20.

Griffin, D. E. (2007). Alphaviruses. In: *Fields Virology* (D. M. H. Knipe, P., Ed.), Vol. 1, 5th ed., pp. 1023–54. 2 vols. Wolters Kluwer Health/Lippincott Williams & Wilkins, Philadelphia.

Grimley, P. M., and Friedman, R. M. (1970). Arboviral infection of voluntary striated muscles. *J Infect Dis* 122(1), 45–52.

Hahn, C. S., Lustig, S., Strauss, E. G., and Strauss, J. H. (1988). Western equine encephalitis virus is a recombinant virus. *Proc Natl Acad Sci USA* 85(16), 5997–6001.

Holbrook, M. R., and Gowen, B. B. (2008). Animal models of highly pathogenic RNA viral infections: encephalitis viruses. *Antiviral Res* 78(1), 69–78.

Jackson, A. C., SenGupta, S. K., and Smith, J. F. (1991). Pathogenesis of Venezuelan equine encephalitis virus infection in mice and hamsters. *Vet Pathol* 28(5), 410–8.

Jahrling, P. B., Navarro, E., and Scherer, W. F. (1976). Interferon induction and sensitivity as correlates to virulence of Venezuelan encephalitis viruses for hamsters. *Arch Virol* 51, 23.

Johnson, B. J., Kinney, R. M., Kost, C. L., and Trent, D. W. (1986). Molecular determinants of alphavirus neurovirulence: nucleotide and deduced protein sequence changes during attenuation of Venezuelan equine encephalitis virus. *J Gen Virol* 67(Pt 9), 1951–60.

Johnston, L. J., Halliday, G. M., and King, N. J. (2000). Langerhans cells migrate to local lymph nodes following cutaneous infection with an arbovirus. *J Invest Dermatol* 114(3), 560–8.

Jordan, G. W. (1973). Interferon sensitivity of Venezuelan equine encephalomyelitis virus. *Infect Immun* 7(6), 911–7.

Julander, J. G., Bowen, R. A., Rao, J. R., Day, C., Shafer, K., Smee, D. F., Morrey, J. D., and Chu, C. K. (2008a). Treatment of Venezuelan equine encephalitis virus infection with (–)-carbodine. *Antiviral Res* 80(3), 309–15.

Julander, J. G., Siddharthan, V., Blatt, L. M., Schafer, K., Sidwell, R. W., and Morrey, J. D. (2007). Effect of exogenous interferon and an interferon inducer on western equine encephalitis virus disease in a hamster model. *Virology* 360(2), 454–60.

Julander, J. G., Skirpstunas, R., Siddharthan, V., Shafer, K., Hoopes, J. D., Smee, D. F., and Morrey, J. D. (2008b). C3H/HeN mouse model for the evaluation of antiviral agents for the treatment of Venezuelan equine encephalitis virus infection. *Antiviral Res* 78(3), 230–41.

Kinney, R. M., Chang, G. J., Tsuchiya, K. R., Sneider, J. M., Roehrig, J. T., Woodward, T. M., and Trent, D. W. (1993). Attenuation of Venezuelan equine encephalitis virus strain TC-83 is encoded by the 5′-noncoding region and the E2 envelope glycoprotein. *J Virol* 67(3), 1269–77.

Kolokoltsov, A. A., Fleming, E. H., and Davey, R. A. (2006a). Venezuelan equine encephalitis virus entry mechanism requires late endosome formation and resists cell membrane cholesterol depletion. *Virology* 347(2), 333–42.

Kolokoltsov, A. A., Wang, E., Colpitts, T. M., Weaver, S. C., and Davey, R. A. (2006b). Pseudotyped viruses permit rapid detection of neutralizing antibodies in human and equine serum against Venezuelan equine encephalitis virus. *Am J Trop Med Hyg* 75(4), 702–9.

Kowalski, J., Adkins, K., Gangolli, S., Ren, J., Arendt, H., DeStefano, J., Obregon, J., Tummolo, D., Natuk, R. J., Brown, T. P., Parks, C. L., Udem, S. A., and Long, D. (2007). Evaluation of neurovirulence and biodistribution of Venezuelan equine encephalitis replicon particles expressing herpes simplex virus type 2 glycoprotein D. *Vaccine* 25(12), 2296–305.

Liu, C., Voth, D. W., Rodina, P., Shauf, L. R., and Gonzalez, G. (1970). A comparative study of the pathogenesis of western equine and eastern equine encephalomyelitis viral infections in mice by intracerebral and subcutaneous inoculations. *J Infect Dis* 122(1), 53–63.

Lossinsky, A. S., and Shivers, R. R. (2004). Structural pathways for macromolecular and cellular transport across the blood-brain barrier during inflammatory conditions. Review. *Histol Histopathol* 19(2), 535–64.

Ludwig, G. V., Turell, M. J., Vogel, P., Kondig, J. P., Kell, W. K., Smith, J. F., and Pratt, W. D. (2001). Comparative neurovirulence of attenuated and non-attenuated strains of Venezuelan equine encephalitis virus in mice. *Am J Trop Med Hyg* 64(1–2), 49–55.

Murphy, F. A., and Whitfield, S. G. (1970). Eastern equine encephalitis virus infection: electron microscopic studies of mouse central nervous system. *Exp Mol Pathol* 13(2), 131–46.

Paessler, S., Yun, N. E., Judy, B. M., Dziuba, N., Zacks, M. A., Grund, A. H., Frolov, I., Campbell, G. A., Weaver, S. C., and Estes, D. M. (2007). Alpha-beta T cells provide protection against lethal encephalitis in the murine model of VEEV infection. *Virology* 367(2), 307–23.

Plosker, G. L. (2011). Interferon-beta-1b: a review of its use in multiple sclerosis. *CNS Drugs* 25(1), 67–88.

Rao, V., Hinz, M. E., Roberts, B. A., and Fine, D. (2006). Toxicity assessment of Venezuelan Equine Encephalitis virus vaccine candidate strain V3526. *Vaccine* 24(10), 1710–5.

Rennels, M. B. (1984). Arthropod-borne virus infections of the central nervous system. *Neurol Clin* 2(2), 241–54.

Roy, C. J., Reed, D. S., Wilhelmsen, C. L., Hartings, J., Norris, S., and Steele, K. E. (2009). Pathogenesis of aerosolized Eastern Equine Encephalitis virus infection in guinea pigs. *Virology* 6, 170.

Schafer, A., Brooke, C. B., Whitmore, A. C., and Johnston, R. E. (2011). The role of the blood–brain barrier during Venezuelan equine encephalitis virus infection. *J Virol* 85(20), 10682–90.

Schafer, A., Whitmore, A. C., Konopka, J. L., and Johnston, R. E. (2009). Replicon particles of Venezuelan equine encephalitis virus as a reductionist murine model for encephalitis. *J Virol* 83(9), 4275–86.

Simmons, J. D., White, L. J., Morrison, T. E., Montgomery, S. A., Whitmore, A. C., Johnston, R. E., and Heise, M. T. (2009). Venezuelan equine encephalitis virus disrupts STAT1 signaling by distinct mechanisms independent of host shutoff. *J Virol* 83(20), 10571–81.

Spotts, D. R., Reich, R. M., Kalkhan, M. A., Kinney, R. M., and Roehrig, J. T. (1998). Resistance to alpha/beta interferons correlates with the epizootic and virulence potential of Venezuelan equine encephalitis viruses and is determined by the 5' noncoding region and glycoproteins. *J Virol* 72, 10286.

Steele, K. E., Davis, K. J., Stephan, K., Kell, W., Vogel, P., and Hart, M. K. (1998). Comparative neurovirulence and tissue tropism of wild-type and attenuated strains of Venezuelan equine encephalitis virus administered by aerosol in C3H/HeN and BALB/c mice. *Vet Pathol* 35(5), 386–97.

Steele, K. E., Seth, P., Catlin-Lebaron, K. M., Schoneboom, B. A., Husain, M. M., Grieder, F., and Maheshwari, R. K. (2006). Tunicamycin enhances neuroinvasion and encephalitis in mice infected with Venezuelan equine encephalitis virus. *Vet Pathol* 43(6), 904–13.

Turell, M. J., Tammariello, R. F., and Spielman, A. (1995). Nonvascular delivery of St. Louis encephalitis and Venezuelan equine encephalitis viruses by infected mosquitoes (Diptera: Culicidae) feeding on a vertebrate host. *J Med Entomol* 32(4), 563–8.

Vogel, P., Kell, W. M., Fritz, D. L., Parker, M. D., and Schoepp, R. J. (2005). Early events in the pathogenesis of eastern equine encephalitis virus in mice. *Am J Pathol* 166(1), 159–71.

Wagner, R. R. (1961). Biological studies of interferon. I. Suppression of cellular infection with eastern equine encephalomyelitis virus. *Virology* 13, 323–37.

Wagner, R. R. (1963). Biological studies of interferon. II. Temporal relationships of virus and interferon production by cells infected with Eastern equine encephalomyelitis and influenza viruses. *Virology* 19, 215–24.

Wang, T., Town, T., Alexopoulou, L., Anderson, J. F., Fikrig, E., and Flavell, R. A. (2004). Toll-like receptor 3 mediates West Nile virus entry into the brain causing lethal encephalitis. *Nat Med* 10(12), 1366–73.

White, L. J., Wang, J.-G., Davis, N. L., and Johnston, R. E. (2001). Role of alpha/beta interferon in Venezuelan equine encephalitis virus pathogenesis: effect of an attenuating mutation in the 5' untranslated region. *J Virol* 75(8), 3706–18.

Wu, J. Q., Barabe, N. D., Chau, D., Wong, C., Rayner, G. R., Hu, W. G., and Nagata, L. P. (2007a). Complete protection of mice against a lethal dose challenge of western equine encephalitis virus after immunization with an adenovirus-vectored vaccine. *Vaccine* 25(22), 4368–75.

Wu, J. Q., Barabe, N. D., Huang, Y. M., Rayner, G. A., Christopher, M. E., and Schmaltz, F. L. (2007b). Pre- and post-exposure protection against Western equine encephalitis virus after single inoculation with adenovirus vector expressing interferon alpha. *Virology* 369(1), 206–13.

Yin, J., Gardner, C. L., Burke, C. W., Ryman, K. D., and Klimstra, W. B. (2009). Similarities and differences in antagonism of neuron alpha/beta interferon responses by Venezuelan equine encephalitis and Sindbis alphaviruses. *J Virol* 83(19), 10036–47.

Yun, N. E., Peng, B. H., Bertke, A. S., Borisevich, V., Smith, J. K., Smith, J. N., Poussard, A. L., Salazar, M., Judy, B. M., Zacks, M. A., Estes, D. M., and Paessler, S. (2009). CD4+ T cells provide protection against acute lethal encephalitis caused by Venezuelan equine encephalitis virus. *Vaccine* 27(30), 4064–73.

Zlotnik, I., Peacock, S., Grant, D. P., and Batter-Hatton, D. (1972). The pathogenesis of western equine encephalitis virus (W.E.E.) in adult hamsters with special reference to the long and short term effects on the C.N.S. of the attenuated clone 15 variant. *Br J Exp Pathol* 53(1), 59–77.

2 Neurological Chikungunya

Lessons from Recent Epidemics, Animal Models, and Other Alphavirus Family Members

Vincent G. Thon-Hon, Shiril Kumar, Duksha Ramful, Stephanie Robin, Marie Christine Jaffar-Bandjee, and Philippe Gasque

CONTENTS

2.1 INTRODUCTION: CHIKUNGUNYA, A PARADIGM SHIFT FROM "OLD" TO "NEW" WORLD ALPHAVIRUS?

Infections of the central nervous system (CNS) by viruses are relatively uncommon yet virtually devastating (Bruzzone et al. 2010). Viral invasion and successful infection of the CNS is an important step in the life cycle of many neurotropic viruses such as poliovirus, rabies, and measles (Griffin 2003). Viruses that invade the brain (and peripheral nerve tissues) have been postulated to cause diseases but through very diverse mechanisms with a unique mechanism of entry, replication, defense against the immune system, and dissemination to preferred target cells, and developmental stages of infection (van den Pol 2006). Each of these aspects needs to be carefully addressed to understand the physiopathology of a given virus with neurological complications.

Chikungunya virus (CHIKV) is an alphavirus of the Togaviridae family transmitted by mosquitoes of the *Aedes* (*Ae*) genus (Pialoux et al. 2007; Weaver and Barrett 2004). CHIKV was first isolated in 1952 in Tanganyika now Tanzania (Robinson 1955). Recurrent epidemics have been reported primarily in Africa and Asia (Powers and Logue 2007). The largest epidemic of CHIKV disease ever recorded took place in 2004–2011 and was associated with the emergence of CHIKV that were efficiently transmitted by *Ae. albopictus* a vector that has seen a dramatic global expansion in its geographic distribution (Charrel et al. 2007). The epidemic began in Kenya, spread across the Indian Ocean Islands to India (with an estimated 1.4–6.5 million cases) and South East Asia (Ng and Hapuarachchi 2010). Remarkably, CHIKV has accumulated key mutations (such as E1-A226V and E2-I211T) that probably contributed to the recently changed epidemiology and with possible clinical impacts, yet to be fully ascertained (Schuffenecker et al. 2006). The first autochthonous infections in Europe occurred in Italy in 2007 (less than 250 cases) and few reported cases in France in 2010 (Grandadam et al. 2011; Jaffar-Bandjee et al. 2010; Schwartz and Albert 2010). With increased and faster human transportation in the shrinking world, viruses can potentially move into new geographical locations and expand their geographical range. Thus, imported CHIKV cases have now been reported in nearly 40 countries including the United States, Japan, and several European countries (Powers 2011).

The alphavirus group comprises 29 viruses, six of which are called Old World alphaviruses, and they can cause human joint disorders (arthralgia evolving to arthritis). This is the case for CHIKV, o'nyong-nyong virus (ONNV), Semliki forest virus (SFV), Ross River (RRV), Sindbis virus (SINV), and Mayaro virus (MAYV). The acute phase of the disease with Old World alphaviruses is highly symptomatic (>90%) and is characterized mostly by fever, generalized myalgia, and arthralgia (Borgherini et al. 2008, 2007). Arthralgia and crippling arthritis are symptoms that can persist for years (Simon et al. 2011; Sissoko et al. 2009).

In contrast, the so-called New World alphaviruses such as the eastern equine encephalitis virus (EEEV) and Venezuelan equine encephalitis virus (VEEV) are mostly known for their profound neuropathological activities. These alphaviruses were isolated from diseased horses in California, Virginia, and New Jersey and from humans in Venezuela. Since then, these viruses have been isolated from infected mosquitoes (*Culex*), horses, humans, and other vertebrate species, predominantly birds and rodents.

Due to their worldwide emergence/reemergence as well as potential agents of bioterrorism, EEEV, VEEV, and CHIKV have been declared high priority pathogens by the National Institutes of Health.

Remarkably, it has long been known that CHIKV can contribute to neuropathology but by mechanisms largely ill-characterized (Carey et al. 1969; Chastel 1963; Chatterjee et al. 1965; Hammon et al. 1960; Jadhav et al. 1965; Nimmannitya et al. 1969; Thiruvengadam et al. 1965). The attack rate for CHIKV disease can be

TABLE 2.1
Neurological Chikungunya in Human and Animal Model

Symptoms	Species	Adult	Neonate/ Infant	References
Headache	Human	Yes	–	(Lemant et al. 2008; Lewthwaite et al. 2009; Robin et al. 2008)
Reduced consciousness	Human	Yes	–	(Rampal et al. 2007; Robin et al. 2008)
Febrile seizures	Human	Yes	Yes	(Lewthwaite et al. 2009; Ramful et al. 2007; Robin et al. 2008)
Flaccid paralysis	Human/mouse	Yes	–	(Singh et al. 2008)
Meningeal syndrome	Human	Yes	Yes	(Robin et al. 2008)
Guillain-Barré syndrome	Human	Yes	–	(Economopoulou et al. 2009; Robin et al. 2008; Wielanek et al. 2007)
Epileptic seizures	Human	Yes	Yes	(Economopoulou et al. 2009; Ramful et al. 2007)
Acute encephalopathy	Human	Yes	Yes	(Gerardin et al. 2008; Lemant et al. 2008; Robin et al. 2008)
Neuropathy	Human	Yes	–	(Chandak et al. 2009)
Myeloneuropathy	Human	Yes	–	(Chandak et al. 2009; Kashyap et al. 2010)
Myelomeningoencephalitis	Human	Yes	–	(Economopoulou et al. 2009)
Encephalomyeloradiculitis	Human	Yes	–	(Ganesan et al. 2008)
Meningoencephalitis	Human/macaque	Yes	–	(Economopoulou et al. 2009; Robin et al. 2008)
Optic neuritis	Human	Yes	–	(Rampal et al. 2007)
Encephalomyelitis	Human	Yes	–	(Rampal et al. 2007)
Meningitis	Human	Yes	–	(Lewthwaite et al. 2009)
Encephalitis	Human	Yes	Yes	(Casolari et al. 2008; Chandak et al. 2009; Economopoulou et al. 2009; Kashyap et al. 2010; Rampal et al. 2007; Robin et al. 2008)
Encephalitis	Mouse		Yes	(Wang et al. 2008)

very high; a survey on Grande Comoros Island in 2005 suggested an attack rate of about 50% (Sergon et al. 2007), and in Reunion Island, 266,000 cases were reported (38% of the population) during 2005–2006. Hence, it is certainly the unprecedented incidence rate in the Indian Ocean with efficient clinical facilities that allowed a better description of CHIKV cases with severe encephalitis, meningoencephalitis, peripheral neuropathies, and deaths among neonates (mother-to-child infection), and infants as well as in elderly patients (Economopoulou et al. 2009; Gerardin et al. 2008; Lemant et al. 2008; Lewthwaite et al. 2009; Ramful et al. 2007; Robin et al. 2008; Tandale et al. 2009) (see Table 2.1).

2.2 NEUROLOGICAL CHIKUNGUNYA IN HUMAN NEONATES

Mother-to-child transmission of CHIKV with an estimated prevalence rate of 0.25% was first reported during the 2005–2006 outbreak in La Réunion Island, and this novel mode of transmission occurring during the peripartum maternal infection was responsible for a high rate of neurological morbidity (Gerardin et al. 2008; Ramful et al. 2007). Almost 50% of the neonates were infected from mother with intrapartum viremia. In a population-based series of 47 cases of perinatal mother-to-child CHIKV infection in La Réunion island, neonates developed illness from day 2 to day 10 (mean, 4 days) after birth and 16 (34%) presented severe complications including encephalopathy with seizures in 9 cases in the acute phase of the disease.

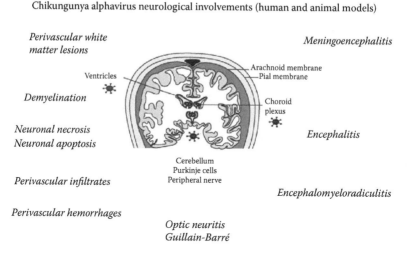

FIGURE 2.1   Chikungunya neuropathology. CHIKV is not classically considered as a true neurotropic virus, but there is substantial recent evidence from neonates and elderly severe CNS cases and together with data from experimental infections (mice and macaque) using different CHIKV strains. CHIKV can infect neurons and cause apoptosis together with mild gliosis (astrocytes and microglia). Activated glial cells may contribute to the inflammatory response potentially contributing to reported demyelination and perivascular white matter lesions. Cells of the adaptive immune response (T and B cells) recruited at the site of injury may have a double-edged sword activity to either protect from infection or promote further neurotoxicity and demyelination. Of critical note, CHIKV and several other alphaviruses can infect the epithelial cells of the choroid plexus and the ependymal cells of the brain ventricles next to the stem cell niche. Peripheral neuropathies have also been reported in acute CHIKV infection in humans.

Mechanical ventilation was needed in 25% of patients due to apneic spells, status epilepticus, or hemodynamic instability, and one neonate died because of necrotizing enterocolitis. Pathological brain MRI was noted in 17 of 30 patients with brain swelling, scattered white matter lesions in the supratentoriel regions, including the corpus callosum and the periventricular and subcortical areas, parenchymal hemorrhages (hematomas and petechias), and early cytotoxic edema on diffusion-weighted sequences evolving toward vasogenic edema in the subsequent course of the disease (Gerardin et al. 2008; Samperiz et al. 2007). Head ultrasound was unspecific with sometimes lenticulothalamostriatal vasculitis. CHIKV RNA was detected in spinal fluid even in apparently uncomplicated cases (23 of the 26 patients tested) even if biochemical and cellular characteristics of the cerebrospinal fluid (CSF) were often unremarkable. Preliminary data concerning long-term clinical follow-up of the infected neonates confirm poor outcome with a mean developmental quotient of 86 (51% of the cases <85) compared with 100 in the control group (p < 0.001) at 2 years old (D. Ramful, personal communication). Gerardin et al. (2008) described persistent disabilities, with cerebral palsy, behavioral deficiencies, epilepsia, and language delay in 4 patients (of 9 with neonatal encephalopathy), where long-term sequelae in imaging studies sometimes included parenchymal cavitations secondary to hematomas and cerebral subcortical atrophy. Conversely, in maternal infection occurring far from delivery, there was no propensity to prematurity, growth restriction, fetal deaths, stillbirths, or congenital anomalies, and newborns seemed to be healthy at birth with no detectable IgM antibody at birth (Fritel et al. 2010) (Figure 2.1).

2.3 NEUROLOGICAL MANIFESTATIONS IN PEDIATRIC PATIENTS

CHIKV fever is usually benign in children and neurological manifestations are rare. However, the two deaths reported in La Réunion Island in children (excluding the neonate mentioned before) were associated with severe neurological presentation of the disease including a case of acute disseminated encephalomyelitis and one case of coma associated with an acute hemorrhagic shock syndrome (Robin et al. 2008). In a hospital-based study in La Réunion Island, Robin et al. (2008) described a case series of 30 pediatric patients with neurological manifestations associated with CHIKV infection ranging from simple (n = 4) and complex febrile seizures (n = 6) to meningeal syndrome (n = 4), acute encephalopathy (n = 4), diplopia, acute disseminated encephalomyelitis (n = 1), and encephalitis (n = 11) with often unremarkable CSF findings and unspecific electroencephalography. Cerebrospinal fluid pleocytosis was found in only 4% of examined cases, although CSF RT-PCR was positive in 61%. Similar findings were subsequently described in infants in India and Mayotte Island (Le Bomin et al. 2008; Lewthwaite et al. 2009).

Risk factors for residual neurological deficit (20% of the patients) in the La Réunion cohort included young age (neonatal infection), severe initial clinical presentation (encephalitis), and initial pathological MRI findings. Neurological clinical manifestations of CHIKV infection in the pediatric population added growing evidence to the potential neurovirulence of this arboviral disease with an age-dependent condition (neonatal infection) and consistent laboratory (CHIKV RNA in CSF of patients) and imaging features (pathological MRI). These findings are consistent with the below mentioned mouse models, where young age is a risk factor for severe disease involving the CNS.

2.4   NEUROLOGICAL CHIKUNGUNYA IN ADULTS

CHIKV is highly symptomatic (arthralgia, myalgia) over a period of days to weeks, and most patients will recover. However, neurological manifestations described in adults requiring hospitalization involved cases of encephalopathy frequently associated with lymphopenia, thrombocytopenia, elevated CRP, and the presence of IgM anti-CHIKV in the CSF (Lemant et al. 2008). It was evident that these patients had severe comorbidities (e.g., diabetes, renal impairment) and with a mortality of almost 50% probably not directly related to CHIKV (Lemant et al. 2008). Similar neurological complications and fatalities were reported by several groups looking at severe hospitalized CHIKV cases from India (Chandak et al. 2009; Rampal et al. 2007; Tandale et al. 2009). Other neurological complications associated with CHIKV were seizures, encephalitis, Guillain-Barré, encephalomyeloradiculitis, and rare deaths (Chandak et al. 2009; Economopoulou et al. 2009; Ganesan et al. 2008; Lebrun et al. 2009; Lemant et al. 2008; Tournebize et al. 2009; Wielanek et al. 2007). Febrile seizures were found to be associated with both adults and neonates (simple febrile seizures) (Lewthwaite et al. 2009; Ramful et al. 2007; Robin et al. 2008), whereas epileptic seizures were observed in 12 of 610 patients (Economopoulou et al. 2009). Three cases of Guillain-Barré syndrome with associated symptoms of facial palsy and weakness in the hand, feet, or both were observed in La Réunion (Wielanek et al. 2007). Encephalomyeloradiculitis was observed after CHIKV infection by neuroimaging data in two patients and brain autopsy in one patient. In both cases, the symptoms were associated with neck rigidity, drowsiness, and extensor plantar response (Ganesan et al. 2008). Of critical note, these reports should not be generalized, given that they are hospital-based studies and were obtained from sick patients with high proportions of complications.

CHIKV infection in adults was also associated to bilateral frontoparietal white matter lesions with restricted diffusion, which are described as an early sign of viral encephalitis (Ganesan et al. 2008). Focal perivascular lymphocytic infiltrates were also present in areas of active demyelination, and some degree of microglial activation was also noted in the gray matter, which may contribute to bystander neuronal loss. Regrettably, this is one of the rare histopathological studies substantiating the contribution of CHIKV to brain damage and most of the evidence comes from *in vitro* studies and animal models (in mice and macaques).

2.5   NEUROLOGICAL CHIKUNGUNYA: ROUTES TO CNS INFECTION AND TISSUE INJURY

Viruses can instigate neurological injuries not only by direct cytolytic actions on neurons or glia (oligodendrocytes, astrocytes) but also by inducing apoptosis, disrupting of the protective blood–brain barrier (BBB), polarizing resident innate immune cells (microglia) to produce proinflammatory cytokines, initiating (auto) immune attack on specific cells, expressing viral genes and inhibiting cellular genes, altering neuronal migration, attenuating neural progenitor replication, and blocking CSF generation and flow. The multiple mechanisms of viral induction of CNS neuroinfection and dysfunction further complicate our understanding of viral agents in brain disease.

Although data are still scarce, the number of recent human cases with CNS involvement appears to support the neurotropic/neuroinfectious activity of CHIKV (Ganesan et al. 2008; Gerardin et al. 2008; Ramful et al. 2007). This unique CNS infection illustrated by subventricular white matter lesions, and intraparenchymal hemorrhages have been described experimentally and in clinical settings for other alphaviruses such as SFV, RRV, EEEV, and SINV (Deresiewicz et al. 1997; Fazakerley et al. 2006; Jackson et al. 1987; Mims et al. 1973) (see Table 2.2).

CHIKV was shown to infect mouse brain and to replicate in primary culture of neurons and glial cells (Chatterjee and Sarkar 1965; Das et al. 2010; Precious et al. 1974). CHIKV can also replicate in a human neuroblastoma cell line, SH-SY5Y, and cause cytopathic activities (Dhanwani et al. 2011; Solignat et al. 2009). Further evidence comes from experimental infections where mice were inoculated with CHIKV (clinical isolates and genetic clones). Interestingly, CNS infection is particularly described in young mice (outbred CD1, ICR) and recapitulating the human clinical disease (Ziegler et al. 2008). Infected mice showed signs of illness suggestive of human clinical pathology such as loss of balance, difficulty of walking, dragging of the hind limbs, skin lesions but with rare mortality. No definite histological evidence of tropism to neurons was reported in these two mouse models, and the CNS infection seemed to be tightly controlled by ill-characterized antiviral mechanisms given that the viral titer was reduced to basal levels at day 10 postinfection. BALB/c mice infected intranasally developed neuronal infection and tissue necrosis in the anterior olfactory lobe (Powers and Logue 2007). Weaver and colleagues also used intranasal injection of CHIKV but the Ross strain selected because of its excessive mouse passage history and which may have increased its neurovirulence (Wang et al. 2008). The 5-week-old *C57BL/6* mice developed encephalitis 7 days postinfection with severe multifocal infection and liquefactive necrosis in the cerebral cortex. Immunohistochemistry techniques revealed that neurons were infected and induced to apoptosis while a prominent microgliosis and perivascular cuffs were distributed throughout the parenchyma. Moreover, the authors reported neuronal degeneration in the hippocampus and multifocal lymphocytic leptomeningitis. In mice deficient in the IFN-α signaling pathway (KO for the IFN-α receptor), CHIKV neuroinfection was particularly severe and targets the leptomeninges, the choroid plexus, and ependymal cells lining the subventricular zone (SVZ) also known as the neural stem cell niche (Hauwel et al. 2005a,b). Of critical note, RRV was also shown to infect ependymal cells and lead to cortical thinning and hydrocephalus (Mims et al. 1973). To what extent CHIKV infection could affect the SVZ niche and subsequently the stem cells is currently unknown. There is also little evidence about the cellular and molecular mechanisms of brain tissue injury, which can be direct (neurotoxicity) or indirect through the mobilization of glial cells. To promote host survival, infected cells may undergo apoptosis, which can be qualified as an "altruistic" suicide in response to viral infections; however, neurons have limited capacity for regeneration.

TABLE 2.2

Cellular Targets, Immune Response, and Long-Term Consequences Following CNS Alphavirus Infection

Alphavirus	CNS Target Cell	CNS Immune Response	Long-Term Consequences
SINV (mice)	*Neurons* (Griffin and Johnson 1977; Johnson 1965) *Purkinje cells* (Johnson 1965) *Meningeal cells* (Johnson 1965) *Ependymal cells* (Jackson et al. 1987; Jackson et al. 1988; Johnson 1965)	*Production of IL-1β, IL-4, IL-6, IL-10, TNF-α, LIF, and TGF-β* (Wesselingh et al. 1994) *Production IFN-γ by CD4+ and CD8+* (Binder and Griffin 2001) *Apoptosis of infected neurons* (Levine et al. 1993; Nava et al. 1998) *Bcl-2 protects against fatal encephalitis* (Levine et al. 1996)	*Hind limb paralysis, death* (Griffin and Johnson 1977; Jackson et al. 1987) *Acute encephalomyelitis* (Jackson et al. 1987), *Kyphoscoliosis* (Jackson et al. 1988) *Swelling of lumbar and thoracic neurons* (Jackson et al. 1988) *Death* (Griffin and Johnson 1977; Jackson et al. 1987)
EEEV (mouse and human)	Neurons (mouse model and human) (Deresiewicz et al. 1997; Griffin 2003)	**Pleocytosis** (Deresiewicz et al. 1997) **In the CSF** (Deresiewicz et al. 1997): - **Elevated protein concentrations** - **Elevated red blood cell counts** **Leukocytosis** (Deresiewicz et al. 1997) **Hyponatremia** (Deresiewicz et al. 1997)	**Large spectrum of general neurological complications (confusion, somnolence, focal weakness, epileptiform discharges, seizures, stupor, altered mental status, paresthesia accompanying paresis, hemiparesis)** (Deresiewicz et al. 1997); **lesions of the basal ganglia and cortex, encephalomalacia, focal intraparenchymal perivascular hemorrhage in the caudate nucleus and putamen, microglial nodules, meningeal enhancement, leptomeningeal vascular congestion, brain hemorrhage, neuronal destruction, neuronophagia, cranial nerve palsies, focal necrosis, spotty demyelination)** (Deresiewicz et al. 1997); **coma and death** (Deresiewicz et al. 1997)

(*continued*)

TABLE 2.2 (Continued)
Cellular Targets, Immune Response, and Long-Term Consequences Following CNS Alphavirus Infection

Alphavirus	CNS Target Cell	CNS Immune Response	Long-Term Consequences
VEEV (human)	*Neurons* (Griffin 2003)	**Meningeal infiltrates composed of lymphocytes, mononuclear cells, and neutrophils** (Steele and Twenhafel 2010)	**General neurological diseases (somnolence, confusion, disorientation, mental depression, convulsions, seizures, ataxia, paralysis)** (Steele and Twenhafel 2010); **predominant CNS pathologies (edema, congestion, hemorrhages, vasculitis, meningitis, encephalitis)** (Zacks and Paessler 2010); **common neurological sequelae** (Zacks and Paessler 2010); **coma and death** (Steele and Twenhafel 2010)
WEEV* (macaque and human)	*In the brain* (Reed et al. 2005) *- Microglia - Purkinje cells In the spinal cord* (Reed et al. 2005) *- α-motor neurons*	*Monocytic inflammation in the CNS expanding perivascular spaces* (Reed et al. 2005) **Occasional infiltrates of lymphocytes, plasma cells, PMN leukocytes surrounding arterioles in the cerebral cortex** (Anderson 1984)	*Demyelination and myelitis in white matter areas* (Reed et al. 2005) **General neurological diseases (partial left seizures, deep consciousness depression, hyperreflexia, bilateral Babinski sign)** (Delfraro et al. 2011) **Severe CNS disorders (multifocal necrosis in the deep gray matter, dilation of the temporal ventricles and compression of the peritroncal and sylvian cisterns)** (Anderson 1984; Delfraro et al. 2011) **Coma and death** (Delfraro et al. 2011)

* Italicized, NHP model; boldface, human studies.

CHIKV can cause programmed cell death through extrinsic apoptosis (death receptor/caspase 8 pathway), intrinsic apoptosis (cytochrome C/caspase 9 pathway) or autophagy of many cell types including neuroblastoma cells (Krejbich-Trotot et al. 2011) and unpublished observations. This will need to be confirmed using primary cultures, but it should be stressed that this is also salutary to the CNS tissue to limit virus spreading.

Astrogliosis and microgliosis have been reported in human and animal models of CHIKV neuroinfection, and these responses may be essential to ward off the infectious challenge through the production of interferon and interferon-stimulated gene (for a review, see Ryman and Klimstra 2008). The immune response to CNS infection has double-edged sword activity, which protects from infections, on the one hand, and promotes further tissue injury if uncontrolled, on the other (Hauwel et al. 2005a). It is essential to have a better understanding of the plausible role of innate immune effectors such as cytokines and complement proteins produced at the site of injury. This is largely unknown in the case of CHIKV neuroinfection, and important information should be obtained from other alphaviruses affecting brain cells and functions.

2.6   NEUROINFECTION BY "OLD WORLD" SINDBIS VIRUS

SINV was named after its first isolation in Sindbis health district near Cairo (Egypt) from a pool of *Culex pipiens* and *Cx univittatus* mosquitoes (Taylor et al. 1955). Other synonyms or subtypes of SINV have been described in Sweden (Ockelbo disease), Finland (Pogosta disease), and Russia (Karelian fever) in the early 1980s, according to the region involved (Brummer-Korvenkontio and Kuusisto 1981; Lvov et al. 1982; Skogh and Espmark 1982). SINV can cause fever, rash, and arthralgia in humans (Turunen et al. 1998) and encephalomyelitis in mice (Jackson et al. 1987). Neuroadapted SINV (NSINV) is a neurovirulent strain that have been developed by serial passage of the original isolate AR339 of SINV from mouse brain (Griffin and Johnson 1977). Infection of weanling mice with NSINV induced an acute encephalomyelitis with high mortality rate, and animals can develop kyphoscoliosis, which is an abnormal curvature of the spine, and hind-limb paralysis (Jackson et al. 1987, 1988). Swelling of lumbar and thoracic neurons has also been documented in NSINV infection (Jackson et al. 1988). SINV is known to infect the Purkinje cells of the cerebellum and meningeal and ependymal cells in mouse (Griffin and Johnson 1977; Jackson et al. 1987, 1988; Johnson 1965). The maturity of infected neurons determines their susceptibility to SINV. Immature neurons replicate SINV to high titers and undergo apoptosis, whereas mature neurons are more resistant to SINV replication and survive viral infection (Binder and Griffin 2001; Burdeinick-Kerr and Griffin 2005). It was shown that infection of neonatal mice with a SINV chimera expressing bcl-2, an anti-apoptotic gene, induced a lower mortality rate (7.5%) (Levine et al. 1996). Hence, controlling neuronal apoptotosis protects mice against fatal SINV encephalitis. After intracerebral inoculation of SINV in mice, transcripts of IL-1β, IL-4, IL-6, IL-10, TNF-α, leukemia inhibitory factor (LIF), and TGF-β were produced by brain cells in response to infection and may contribute to neuronal loss (Wesselingh et al. 1994).

2.7   NEUROINFECTION BY NEW WORLD ALPHAVIRUSES: EEEV, VEEV, WEEV

EEEV, VEEV, and WEEV are New World alphaviruses whose symptoms can be similar to those described for SINV, but as their names suggest, they can frequently cause severe encephalitis in humans and horses (Zacks and Paessler 2010). They are naturally maintained through enzootic cycles involving arthropods as vectors with ensuing amplification in small mammals or birds, and epizootic cycles between bridging mosquitoes vectors and large mammals such as horses and humans, which are dead-end hosts, as they are not viremic enough to infect mosquitoes and propagate the cycle. Among the three, EEEV seems to be the most virulent in humans, causing mortality in approximately 40% of symptomatic cases (Deresiewicz et al. 1997). In survivors, permanent neurological sequelae can occur, and some with severe impairment die within a few days.

EEEV was first isolated in Virginia and New Jersey from infected horses in 1933 (Giltner and Shahan 1933; TenBroeck and Merrill 1933) and was first recognized to infect humans in 1938 after an outbreak in Massachusetts (Feemster 1938). Three children died and two had encephalitis. An interesting coincidence was that those five cases occurred in essentially the same area as the equine disease. The eastern strain of the equine encephalomyelitis virus had next been isolated from human brain tissue of the first case (Feemster 1938). Enzootic transmission cycle of EEEV involves ornithophilic mosquitoes (mainly *Culiseta melanura*) and passerine birds (Komar and Spielman 1994; Scott and Weaver 1989). EEE usually begins abruptly and rapidly instigate fever, chills, myalgia, and arthralgia; after a few days, neurological signs may appear. EEEV has not been as well studied in animals as VEEV; nonetheless, a variety of animal models have been described, such as mice, hamsters, guinea pigs, and non-human primates (NHP), which are the best studied (Zacks and Paessler 2010). In mice and human, EEEV is known to infect neurons (Deresiewicz et al. 1997; Griffin 2003).

VEEV was first isolated in Venezuela from the brain of an encephalitic horse in 1938 (Kubes and Rios 1939) and first recognized to infect humans in 1943 (Casals et al. 1943). VEEV is efficiently amplified during a cycle involving equids and mosquitoes that occurs in an agricultural area (Aguilar et al. 2011). In human, VEEV is usually an acute and often mild systemic disease. Clinical signs can be characterized by fever, chills, generalized malaise, severe headache, photophobia, and myalgia mainly localized in the legs and lumbosacral region. Very young or elderly patients are more likely to develop severe infections. In adults, cases of encephalitis and fatality are scarce (Zacks and Paessler 2010). In mice, neurons are cellular targets for VEEV (Griffin 2003). CNS infection by VEEV has been shown to induce the infiltration of lymphocytes, mononuclear cells, and neutrophils in the meninges. In a minority of cases, these inflammatory cells extended into the Virchow-Robin spaces, which are tiny fluid-filled canals surrounding arteries and veins in brain parenchyma (Steele and Twenhafel 2010). In humans, VEEV-induced fatality can occur in one third of children and 10% in adults of cases. Nevertheless, neurological diseases including disorientation, ataxia, mental depression, and convulsions can reach 14% of cases, mainly in children. The severity of neurological complications can range from somnolence and mild confusion to seizure, ataxia, paralysis, and coma (Steele and Twenhafel 2010). The predominant CNS pathological findings in deadly VEEV human cases comprise edema, congestion, hemorrhages, vasculitis, meningitis, and encephalitis (Zacks and Paessler 2010).

WEEV was first isolated in California from the brain of horses suffering from encephalitis in 1930 (Meyer et al. 1931). In 1938, the virus had been recovered for the first time from the brain of a 20-month-old boy in California (Howitt 1938). WEEV is maintained in an enzootic cycle between passerine birds, which are its natural host and culicine mosquitoes, with a variety of mammals as incidental hosts. WEEV is usually asymptomatic and much milder than EEE. The disease generally appears abruptly and potentially includes fever, chills, headache, nausea, vomiting, anorexia, malaise, and occasional respiratory signs. WEEV appears to be a recombinant virus originated from a recombination between an EEEV-like and an SINV-like ancestor giving rise to a new virus with encephalogenic properties of EEEV and the antigenic specificity of SINV (Hahn et al. 1988). After aerosol exposure to WEEV in the NHP model, abundant microglia and neurons in the cerebral cortex were WEEV-positive. In addition, a low amount of cerebellar Purkinje cells and alpha-motor neurons in the spinal cord gray matter showed WEEV antigens (Reed et al. 2005). From clinical and radiographic data of 38 patients infected by EEEV, Deresiewicz et al. (1997) found biological abnormalities including pleocytosis (97% of cases), elevated protein concentrations and red blood cell counts in CSF (94% and 77%, respectively), leukocytosis (69%), and hyponatremia (60%). They reported a wide spectrum of neurological complications such as confusion, somnolence, focal weakness, epileptiform discharges, seizures, stupor, altered mental status, paresthesia accompanying paresis, and hemiparesis. Lesions of the basal ganglia and cortex were observed in a 14-year-old boy who died from EEE and for whom autopsy revealed a diffuse encephalomalacia, marked perivascular chronic inflammatory changes, and focal intraparenchymal perivascular hemorrhage in the caudate nucleus and putamen. Several microglial nodules were noticed. Deresiewicz et al. (1997) also reported meningeal enhancement, leptomeningeal vascular congestion, brain hemorrhage, neuronal destruction, neuronophagia, cranial nerve parlsies, focal necrosis, spotty demyelination, encephalomalacia, coma, and death.

After aerosol exposure to WEEV of NHP, Reed et al. (2005) demonstrated a pronounced encephalitis characterized by monocytic inflammation expanding in perivascular spaces and infiltrating into the surrounding neutrophils. They found that infection of WEEV in the CNS of NHP resulted in multifocal areas of demyelination in the white matter of the brain and spinal cord, occasionally associated with inflammation. In humans, Anderson (1984) reported a fatal case in a 75-year-old woman infected with WEEV and presenting perivascular infiltrates and multifocal necrosis in the deep gray matter. Recently, a fatal human case was reported in which the 14-year-old boy experienced partial left seizures, consciousness depression, hyperreflexia, and bilateral Babinski sign (Delfraro et al. 2011). Depression of consciousness progressed at a deeper level, and the brain showed dilatation of the temporal ventricles and compression of the peritroncal and sylvian cisterns. The level of coma progressed until the patient died (Delfraro et al. 2011).

2.8 CONCLUSION

As highlighted throughout this review, our understanding of neurological and potentially encephalitic alphavirus is still in its infancy. CHIKV in addition to its profound arthritogenic activity also has encephalitic potential particularly in newborns and elderly patients with severe comorbidities. Moreover, CHIKV is known to persist in tissue sanctuaries (not in the brain as far as we know) and contributes to chronic diseases. Some CHIKV elderly patients can experience rheumatism 5 years postinfection and with long-term brain development defects in neonates. Although cell permissiveness and reactivity has been studied in great depth, the mechanisms of CHIKV persistence and associated tissue injuries remains largely ill-characterized. Therefore, with a proven potential to spread globally, it is now critical to devise strategies to circumvent infection of populations at risk and new epidemics. In the absence of a specific antiviral therapy, treatment remains supportive. Recently, the development of polyvalent immunoglobulins, purified from human plasma samples of convalescent patients that exhibited *in vitro* and *in vivo* neutralizing activities could be of benefit to neonates born from viremic mothers at delivery and to encephalitic patients at the initial stage of the disease (Couderc et al. 2009). Moreover, protection against mosquito bites remains essential in CHIKV prevention. Parental training about prevention of mosquito bites during the perinatal period and distribution of impregnated mosquito nets should be carried out during outbreaks. DEET (*N,N*-diethyl-*m*-toluamide, now called *N,N*-diethyl-3-methylbenzamide) is considered as the most effective insect repellent for personal protection but is not recommended for young children, pregnant, and lactating women due to potential neurotoxic effects.

REFERENCES

Aguilar, P.V., Estrada-Franco, J.G., Navarro-Lopez, R., Ferro, C., Haddow, A.D., Weaver, S.C. 2011. Endemic Venezuelan equine encephalitis in the Americas: hidden under the dengue umbrella. *Future Virol* 6, 721–740.

Anderson, B.A. 1984. Focal neurologic signs in western equine encephalitis. *Can Med Assoc J* 130, 1019–1021.

Binder, G.K., Griffin, D.E. 2001. Interferon-gamma-mediated site-specific clearance of alphavirus from CNS neurons. *Science* 293, 303–306.

Borgherini, G., Poubeau, P., Jossaume, A., Gouix, A., Cotte, L., Michault, A., Arvin-Berod, C., Paganin, F. 2008. Persistent arthralgia associated with chikungunya virus: a study of 88 adult patients on reunion island. *Clin Infect Dis* 47, 469–475.

Borgherini, G., Poubeau, P., Staikowsky, F., Lory, M., Le Moullec, N., Becquart, J.P., Wengling, C., Michault, A., Paganin, F. 2007. Outbreak of chikungunya on Reunion Island: early clinical and laboratory features in 157 adult patients. *Clin Infect Dis* 44, 1401–1407.

Brummer-Korvenkontio, M., Kuusisto, P. 1981. Onko Suomen länsiosa säästynyt 'Pogostalta'? (Has western Finland been spared the 'Pogosta'). *Suom Lääkäril* 32, 2606–2607.

Bruzzone, R., Dubois-Dalcq, M., Kristensson, K. 2010. Neurobiology of infectious diseases: bringing them out of neglect. *Prog Neurobiol* 91, 91–94.

Burdeinick-Kerr, R., Griffin, D.E. 2005. Gamma interferon-dependent, noncytolytic clearance of Sindbis virus infection from neurons *in vitro*. *J Virol* 79, 5374–5385.

Carey, D.E., Myers, R.M., DeRanitz, C.M., Jadhav, M., Reuben, R. 1969. The 1964 chikungunya epidemic at Vellore, South India, including observations on concurrent dengue. *Trans R Soc Trop Med Hyg* 63, 434–445.

Casals, J., Curnen, E.C., Thomas, L. 1943. Venezuelan equine encephalomyelitis in man. *J Exp Med* 77, 521–530.

Casolari, S., Briganti, E., Zanotti, M., Zauli, T., Nicoletti, L., Magurano, F., Fortuna, C., Fiorentini, C., Grazia Ciufolini, M., Rezza, G. 2008. A fatal case of encephalitis associated with Chikungunya virus infection. *Scand J Infect Dis* 40, 995–996.

Chandak, N.H., Kashyap, R.S., Kabra, D., Karandikar, P., Saha, S.S., Morey, S.H., Purohit, H.J., Taori, G.M., Daginawala, H.F. 2009a. Neurological complications of Chikungunya virus infection. *Neurol India* 57, 177–180.

Charrel, R.N., de Lamballerie, X., Raoult, D. 2007. Chikungunya outbreaks—the globalization of vectorborne diseases. *N Engl J Med* 356, 769–771.

Chastel, C. 1963. Human infections in Cambodia by the Chikungunya virus or an apparently closely related agent. II. Experimental pathological anatomy. *Bull Soc Pathol Exot Filiales* 56, 915–924.

Chatterjee, S.N., Chakravarti, S.K., Mitra, A.C., Sarkar, J.K. 1965. Virological investigation of cases with neurological complications during the outbreak of haemorrhagic fever in Calcutta. *J Indian Med Assoc* 45, 314–316.

Chatterjee, S.N., Sarkar, J.K. 1965. Electron microscopic studies of suckling mouse brain cells infected with Chikungunya virus. *Indian J Exp Biol* 3, 227–234.

Couderc, T., Khandoudi, N., Grandadam, M., Visse, C., Gangneux, N., Bagot, S., Prost, J.F., Lecuit, M. 2009. Prophylaxis and therapy for Chikungunya virus infection. *J Infect Dis* 200, 516–523.

Das, T., Jaffar-Bandjee, M.C., Hoarau, J.J., Krejbich Trotot, P., Denizot, M., Lee-Pat-Yuen, G., Sahoo, R., Guiraud, P., Ramful, D., Robin, S., Alessandri, J.L., Gauzere, B.A., Gasque, P. 2010. Chikungunya fever: CNS infection and pathologies of a re-emerging arbovirus. *Prog Neurobiol* 91, 121–129.

Delfraro, A., Burgueno, A., Morel, N., Gonzalez, G., Garcia, A., Morelli, J., Perez, W., Chiparelli, H., Arbiza, J. 2011. Fatal human case of Western equine encephalitis, Uruguay. *Emerg Infect Dis* 17, 952–954.

Deresiewicz, R.L., Thaler, S.J., Hsu, L., Zamani, A.A. 1997. Clinical and neuroradiographic manifestations of eastern equine encephalitis. *N Engl J Med* 336, 1867–1874.

Dhanwani, R., Khan, M., Alam, S.I., Rao, P.V., Parida, M. 2011. Differential proteome analysis of Chikungunya virus-infected new-born mice tissues reveal implication of stress, inflammatory and apoptotic pathways in disease pathogenesis. *Proteomics* 11, 1936–1951.

Economopoulou, A., Dominguez, M., Helynck, B., Sissoko, D., Wichmann, O., Quenel, P., Germonneau, P., Quatresous, I. 2009. Atypical Chikungunya virus infections: clinical manifestations, mortality and risk factors for severe disease during the 2005–2006 outbreak on Reunion. *Epidemiol Infect* 137, 534–541.

Fazakerley, J.K., Cotterill, C.L., Lee, G., Graham, A. 2006. Virus tropism, distribution, persistence and pathology in the corpus callosum of the Semliki Forest virus-infected mouse brain: a novel system to study virus-oligodendrocyte interactions. *Neuropathol Appl Neurobiol* 32, 397–409.

Feemster, R.F. 1938. Outbreak of encephalitis in man due to the eastern virus of equine encephalomyelitis. *Am J Public Health Nations Health* 28, 1403–1410.

Fritel, X., Rollot, O., Gerardin, P., Gauzere, B.A., Bideault, J., Lagarde, L., Dhuime, B., Orvain, E., Cuillier, F., Ramful, D., Samperiz, S., Jaffar-Bandjee, M.C., Michault, A., Cotte, L., Kaminski, M., Fourmaintraux, A. 2010. Chikungunya virus infection during pregnancy, Reunion, France, 2006. *Emerg Infect Dis* 16, 418–425.

Ganesan, K., Diwan, A., Shankar, S.K., Desai, S.B., Sainani, G.S., Katrak, S.M. 2008. Chikungunya encephalomyeloradiculitis: report of 2 cases with neuroimaging and 1 case with autopsy findings. *AJNR Am J Neuroradiol* 29, 1636–1637.

Gerardin, P., Barau, G., Michault, A., Bintner, M., Randrianaivo, H., Choker, G., Lenglet, Y., Touret, Y., Bouveret, A., Grivard, P., Le Roux, K., Blanc, S., Schuffenecker, I., Couderc, T., Arenzana-Seisdedos, F., Lecuit, M., Robillard, P.Y. 2008. Multidisciplinary prospective study of mother-to-child chikungunya virus infections on the island of La Reunion. *PLoS Med* 5, e60.

Giltner, L.T., Shahan, M.S. 1933. The 1933 outbreak of infectious equine encephalomyelitis in the eastern states. *North Am Vet* 14, 25–27.

Grandadam, M., Caro, V., Plumet, S., Thiberge, J.M., Souares, Y., Failloux, A.B., Tolou, H.J., Budelot, M., Cosserat, D., Leparc-Goffart, I., Despres, P. 2011. Chikungunya virus, southeastern France. *Emerg Infect Dis* 17, 910–913.

Griffin, D.E. 2003. Immune responses to RNA-virus infections of the CNS. *Nat Rev Immunol* 3, 493–502.

Griffin, D.E., Johnson, R.T. 1977. Role of the immune response in recovery from Sindbis virus encephalitis in mice. *J Immunol* 118, 1070–1075.

Hahn, C.S., Lustig, S., Strauss, E.G., Strauss, J.H. 1988. Western equine encephalitis virus is a recombinant virus. *Proc Natl Acad Sci U S A* 85, 5997–6001.

Hammon, W.M., Rudnick, A., Sather, G.E. 1960. Viruses associated with epidemic hemorrhagic fevers of the Philippines and Thailand. *Science* 131, 1102–1103.

Hauwel, M., Furon, E., Canova, C., Griffiths, M., Neal, J., Gasque, P. 2005a. Innate (inherent) control of brain infection, brain inflammation and brain repair: the role of microglia, astrocytes, "protective" glial stem cells and stromal ependymal cells. *Brain Res Brain Res Rev* 48, 220–233.

Hauwel, M., Furon, E., Gasque, P. 2005b. Molecular and cellular insights into the coxsackie-adenovirus receptor: role in cellular interactions in the stem cell niche. *Brain Res Brain Res Rev* 48, 265–272.

Howitt, B. 1938. Recovery of the virus of equine encephalomyelitis from the brain of a child. *Science* 88, 455–456.

Jackson, A.C., Moench, T.R., Griffin, D.E., Johnson, R.T. 1987. The pathogenesis of spinal cord involvement in the encephalomyelitis of mice caused by neuroadapted Sindbis virus infection. *Lab Invest* 56, 418–423.

Jackson, A.C., Moench, T.R., Trapp, B.D., Griffin, D.E. 1988. Basis of neurovirulence in Sindbis virus encephalomyelitis of mice. *Lab Invest* 58, 503–509.

Jadhav, M., Namboodripad, M., Carman, R.H., Carey, D.E., Myers, R.M. 1965. Chikungunya disease in infants and children in Vellore: a report of clinical and haematological features of virologically proved cases. *Indian J Med Res* 53, 764–776.

Jaffar-Bandjee, M.C., Ramful, D., Gauzere, B.A., Hoarau, J.J., Krejbich-Trotot, P., Robin, S., Ribera, A., Selambarom, J., Gasque, P. 2010. Emergence and clinical insights into the pathology of Chikungunya virus infection. *Expert Rev Anti Infect Ther* 8, 987–996.

Johnson, R.T. 1965. Virus invasion of the central nervous system: a study of Sindbis virus infection in the mouse using fluorescent antibody. *Am J Pathol* 46, 929–943.

Kashyap, R.S., Morey, S.H., Chandak, N.H., Purohit, H.J., Taori, G.M., Daginawala, H.F. 2010. Detection of viral antigen, IgM and IgG antibodies in cerebrospinal fluid of Chikungunya patients with neurological complications. *Cerebrospinal Fluid Res* 7, 12.

Komar, N., Spielman, A. 1994. Emergence of eastern encephalitis in Massachusetts. *Ann N Y Acad Sci* 740, 157–168.

Krejbich-Trotot, P., Denizot, M., Hoarau, J.J., Jaffar-Bandjee, M.C., Das, T., Gasque, P. 2011. Chikungunya virus mobilizes the apoptotic machinery to invade host cell defenses. *FASEB J* 25, 314–325.

Kubes, V., Rios, F.A. 1939. The causative agent of infectious equine encephalomyelitis in Venezuela. *Science* 90, 20–21.

Le Bomin, A., Hebert, J.C., Marty, P., Delaunay, P. 2008. Confirmed chikungunya in children in Mayotte. Description of 50 patients hospitalized from February to June 2006. *Med Trop (Mars)* 68, 491–495.

Lebrun, G., Chadda, K., Reboux, A.H., Martinet, O., Gauzere, B.A. 2009. Guillain-Barré syndrome after chikungunya infection. *Emerg Infect Dis* 15, 495–496.

Lemant, J., Boisson, V., Winer, A., Thibault, L., Andre, H., Tixier, F., Lemercier, M., Antok, E., Cresta, M.P., Grivard, P., Besnard, M., Rollot, O., Favier, F., Huerre, M., Campinos, J.L., Michault, A. 2008. Serious acute chikungunya virus infection requiring intensive care during the Reunion Island outbreak in 2005–2006. *Crit Care Med* 36, 2536–2541.

Levine, B., Goldman, J.E., Jiang, H.H., Griffin, D.E., Hardwick, J.M. 1996. Bcl–2 protects mice against fatal alphavirus encephalitis. *Proc Natl Acad Sci USA* 93, 4810–4815.

Levine, B., Huang, Q., Isaacs, J.T., Reed, J.C., Griffin, D.E., Hardwick, J.M. 1993. Conversion of lytic to persistent alphavirus infection by the bcl-2 cellular oncogene. *Nature* 361, 739–742.

Lewthwaite, P., Vasanthapuram, R., Osborne, J.C., Begum, A., Plank, J.L., Shankar, M.V., Hewson, R., Desai, A., Beeching, N.J., Ravikumar, R., Solomon, T. 2009. Chikungunya virus and central nervous system infections in children, India. *Emerg Infect Dis* 15, 329–331.

Lvov, D.K., Skvortsova, T.M., Kondrashina, N.G., Vershinsky, B.V., Lesnikov, A.L., Derevyansky, V.S. 1982. Etiology of Karelian fever, a new arbovirus infection. *Vopr Virusol* 6, 690–692.

Meyer, K.F., Haring, C.M., Howitt, B. 1931. The etiology of epizootic encephalomyelitis of horses in the San Joaquin Valley, 1930. *Science* 74, 227–228.

Mims, C.A., Murphy, F.A., Taylor, W.P., Marshall, I.D. 1973. Pathogenesis of Ross River virus infection in mice. I. Ependymal infection, cortical thinning, and hydrocephalus. *J Infect Dis* 127, 121–128.

Nava, V.E., Rosen, A., Veliuona, M.A., Clem, R.J., Levine, B., Hardwick, J.M. 1998. Sindbis virus induces apoptosis through a caspase-dependent, CrmA-sensitive pathway. *J Virol* 72, 452–459.

Ng, L.C., Hapuarachchi, H.C. 2010. Tracing the path of Chikungunya virus—evolution and adaptation. *Infect Genet Evol* 10, 876–885.

Nimmannitya, S., Halstead, S.B., Cohen, S.N., Margiotta, M.R. 1969. Dengue and chikungunya virus infection in man in Thailand, 1962–1964. I. Observations on hospitalized patients with hemorrhagic fever. *Am J Trop Med Hyg* 18, 954–971.

Pialoux, G., Gauzere, B.A., Jaureguiberry, S., Strobel, M. 2007. Chikungunya, an epidemic arbovirosis. *Lancet Infect Dis* 7, 319–327.

Powers, A.M. 2011. Genomic evolution and phenotypic distinctions of Chikungunya viruses causing the Indian Ocean outbreak. *Exp Biol Med (Maywood)* 236, 909–914.

Powers, A.M., Logue, C.H. 2007. Changing patterns of chikungunya virus: re-emergence of a zoonotic arbovirus. *J Gen Virol* 88, 2363–2377.

Precious, S.W., Webb, H.E., Bowen, E.T. 1974. Isolation and persistence of Chikungunya virus in cultures of mouse brain cells. *J Gen Virol* 23, 271–279.

Ramful, D., Carbonnier, M., Pasquet, M., Bouhmani, B., Ghazouani, J., Noormahomed, T., Beullier, G., Attali, T., Samperiz, S., Fourmaintraux, A., Alessandri, J.L. 2007. Mother-to-child transmission of Chikungunya virus infection. *Pediatr Infect Dis J* 26, 811–815.

Rampal, Sharda, M., Meena, H. 2007. Neurological complications in Chikungunya fever. *J Assoc Physicians India* 55, 765–769.

Reed, D.S., Larsen, T., Sullivan, L.J., Lind, C.M., Lackemeyer, M.G., Pratt, W.D., Parker, M.D. 2005. Aerosol exposure to western equine encephalitis virus causes fever and encephalitis in cynomolgus macaques. *J Infect Dis* 192, 1173–1182.

Robin, S., Ramful, D., Le Seach, F., Jaffar-Bandjee, M.C., Rigou, G., Alessandri, J.L. 2008. Neurologic manifestations of pediatric chikungunya infection. *J Child Neurol* 23, 1028–1035.

Robinson, M.C. 1955. An epidemic of virus disease in Southern Province, Tanganyika Territory, in 1952–53. I. Clinical features. *Trans R Soc Trop Med Hyg* 49, 28–32.

Ryman, K.D., Klimstra, W.B. 2008. Host responses to alphavirus infection. *Immunol Rev* 225, 27–45.

Samperiz, E., Gerardin, P., Noormahomed, T., Beullir, G., Boya, I. 2007. Transmission peri-natale du virus chikungunya, à propos de 47 cas à l'île de la Réunion. *Bull Soc Pathol Exot Filiales* 100, 355.

Schuffenecker, I., Iteman, I., Michault, A., Murri, S., Frangeul, L., Vaney, M.C., Lavenir, R., Pardigon, N., Reynes, J.M., Pettinelli, F., Biscornet, L., Diancourt, L., Michel, S., Duquerroy, S., Guigon, G., Frenkiel, M.P., Brehin, A.C., Cubito, N., Despres, P., Kunst, F., Rey, F.A., Zeller, H., Brisse, S. 2006. Genome microevolution of chikungunya viruses causing the Indian Ocean outbreak. *PLoS Med* 3, e263.

Schwartz, O., Albert, M.L. 2010. Biology and pathogenesis of chikungunya virus. *Nature Rev Microbiol* 8, 491–500.

Scott, T.W., Weaver, S.C. 1989. Eastern equine encephalomyelitis virus: epidemiology and evolution of mosquito transmission. *Adv Virus Res* 37, 277–328.

Sergon, K., Yahaya, A.A., Brown, J., Bedja, S.A., Mlindasse, M., Agata, N., Allaranger, Y., Ball, M.D., Powers, A.M., Ofula, V., Onyango, C., Konongoi, L.S., Sang, R., Njenga, M.K., Breiman, R.F. 2007. Seroprevalence of Chikungunya virus infection on Grande Comore Island, union of the Comoros, 2005. *Am J Trop Med Hyg* 76, 1189–1193.

Simon, F., Javelle, E., Oliver, M., Leparc-Goffart, I., Marimoutou, C. 2011. Chikungunya virus infection. *Curr Infect Dis Rep* 13, 218–228.

Singh, S.S., Manimunda, S.P., Sugunan, A.P., Sahina, Vijayachari, P. 2008. Four cases of acute flaccid paralysis associated with chikungunya virus infection. *Epidemiol Infect* 136, 1277–1280.

Sissoko, D., Malvy, D., Ezzedine, K., Renault, P., Moscetti, F., Ledrans, M., Pierre, V. 2009. Post-epidemic Chikungunya disease on Reunion Island: course of rheumatic manifestations and associated factors over a 15-month period. *PLoS Neglect Trop Dis* 3, e389.

Skogh, M., Espmark, A. 1982. Ockelbo-sjukan-ett hud- och ledsyndrom troligen orsakat av myggburet al.fa-arbovirus. *Läkartid* 79, 2379–2380.

Solignat, M., Gay, B., Higgs, S., Briant, L., Devaux, C. 2009. Replication cycle of chikun-gunya: a re-emerging arbovirus. *Virology* 393, 183–197.

Steele, K.E., Twenhafel, N.A. 2010. Review paper: pathology of animal models of alphavirus encephalitis. *Vet Pathol* 47, 790–805.

Tandale, B.V., Sathe, P.S., Arankalle, V.A., Wadia, R.S., Kulkarni, R., Shah, S.V., Shah, S.K., Sheth, J.K., Sudeep, A.B., Tripathy, A.S., Mishra, A.C. 2009. Systemic involve-ments and fatalities during Chikungunya epidemic in India, 2006. *J Clin Virol* 2009 46, 145–149.

Taylor, R.M., Hurlbut, H.S., Work, T.H., Kingston, J.R., Frothingham, T.E. 1955. Sindbis virus: a newly recognized arthropod-transmitted virus. *Am J Trop Med Hyg* 4, 844–862.

TenBroeck, C., Merrill, M.H. 1933. A serological difference between eastern and western equine encephalomyelitis virus. *Proc Soc Exp Biol Med* 31, 217–220.

Thiruvengadam, K.V., Kalyanasundaram, V., Rajgopal, J. 1965. Clinical and pathological studies on chikungunya fever in Madras city. *Indian J Med Res* 53, 729–744.

Tournebize, P., Charlin, C., Lagrange, M. 2009. Neurological manifestations in Chikungunya: about 23 cases collected in Reunion Island. *Rev Neurol (Paris)* 165, 48–51.

Turunen, M., Kuusisto, P., Uggeldahl, P.E., Toivanen, A. 1998. Pogosta disease: clinical obser-vations during an outbreak in the province of North Karelia, Finland. *Br J Rheumatol* 37, 1177–1180.

van den Pol, A.N. 2006. Viral infections in the developing and mature brain. *Trends Neurosci* 29, 398–406.

Wang, E., Volkova, E., Adams, A.P., Forrester, N., Xiao, S.Y., Frolov, I., Weaver, S.C. 2008. Chimeric alphavirus vaccine candidates for chikungunya. *Vaccine* 26, 5030–5039.

Weaver, S.C., Barrett, A.D. 2004. Transmission cycles, host range, evolution and emergence of arboviral disease. *Nat Rev Microbiol* 2, 789–801.

Wesselingh, S.L., Levine, B., Fox, R.J., Choi, S., Griffin, D.E. 1994. Intracerebral cytokine mRNA expression during fatal and nonfatal alphavirus encephalitis suggests a predominant type 2 T cell response. *J Immunol* 152, 1289–1297.

Wielanek, A.C., Monredon, J.D., Amrani, M.E., Roger, J.C., Serveaux, J.P. 2007. Guillain-Barre syndrome complicating a Chikungunya virus infection. *Neurology* 69, 2105–2107.

Zacks, M.A., Paessler, S. 2010. Encephalitic alphaviruses. *Vet Microbiol* 140, 281–286.

Ziegler, S.A., Lu, L., da Rosa, A.P., Xiao, S.Y., Tesh, R.B. 2008. An animal model for studying the pathogenesis of chikungunya virus infection. *Am J Trop Med Hyg* 79, 133–139.

3 Arenaviruses and Neurovirology

Larry Lutwick and Jana Preis

CONTENTS

3.1 INTRODUCTION

The family Arenavirdiae represents a unique genus (Arenavirus) containing more than 30 viruses classified into two groups of agents based on their antigenic properties.

The Old World (Eastern Hemisphere) group also referred to as the Lassa-lymphocytic choriomeningitis (LCM) serocomplex contains viruses indigenous to Africa and LCM (Table 3.1). LCM is the only arenavirus to have a worldwide distribution because of the ubiquitous distribution of its rodent reservoirs (primarily *Mus musculus* and *M. domesticus*), whereas each of the other arenaviruses has a limited geographic distribution directly related to the range of its specific rodent reservoir. The New World (Western Hemisphere) group also called the Tacaribe serocomplex (Table 3.2) is divided into three lineages (clades) designated as A, B, and C.

Representatives of each of the groups are clearly causes of zoonotic infections of man, that is, infections primarily of animals that can be passed directly or indirectly to man. Many of the groups, however, are rare or unproven causes of human infection. In many ways, LCM is one of the ancestors of neurovirology because it was the first clearly documented cause of viral meningitis and much of this chapter will be devoted to the classical agent and the manifestations of disease that it may cause. Human infections caused by other members of Arenaviridae are primarily viral hemorrhagic fevers including Lassa fever in parts of Africa and primarily members of clade B of the New World group including the Guanarito, Junin, Machupo, and Sabia viruses.

TABLE 3.1
Old World Arenaviruses Relevant to Human Infection

Lymphocytic Choriomeningitis Virus

Disease	Lymphocytic choriomeningitis
Location	Wide distribution especially Europe and Americas
Reservoir	*Mus musculus*, *M. domesticus* (house mouse), *Mesocricetus auratos* (Syrian hamster)
Reservoir habitat	Domestically, grasslands
Seasonality	September, October
Human acquisition	Peridomestically

Lassa Virus

Disease	Lassa fever
Location	West Africa, especially Sierra Leone, Nigeria, Liberia, Guinea
Reservoir	*Mastomys natalensis* (multimammate mouse)
Reservoir habitat	Savannah, forest clearings
Seasonality	January to April
Human acquisition	Peridomestically

Note: Other viruses with unclear or little human significance include Mopeia virus (Southern Africa), Mobala virus (Central African Republic), Ippy virus (Central African Republic), Lujo virus (Zambia), Merino Walk virus (South Africa), and Morogoro virus (Guinea).

TABLE 3.2
New World Arenaviruses Relevant to Human Infection

	Guanarito Virus (Clade B)
Disease	Venezuelan hemorrhagic fever
Location	Central Venezuela Portuguesa State and adjacent regions of Barinas state
Reservoir	*Zygodontomys brevicauda* (cane mouse)
Reservoir habitat	Agricultural areas
Seasonality	November to January
Human acquisition	Agriculturally

	Junin Virus (Clade B)
Disease	Argentine hemorrhagic fever
Location	Argentine provinces of Buenos Aires, Córdoba, Santa Fe, and La Pampa
Reservoir	*Calomys musculinus* (corn mouse), *Akondon azalae* (grass field mouse), *Bolomys obscurus* (dark field mouse)
Reservoir habitat	Cultivated fields, grasslands
Seasonality	February to May
Human acquisition	Agriculturally

	Machupo Virus (Clade B)
Disease	Bolivian hemorrhagic fever
Location	Northeastern Bolivia, especially Beni Department
Reservoir	*C. callosus* (vesper mouse)
Reservoir habitat	Brush, peridomestically
Seasonality	April to July
Human acquisition	Peridomestically

Note: The Sabia virus (clade B) from Brazil (Brazilian or Sao Paolo hemorrhagic fever) has caused one natural infection and several laboratory infections. Other virus of unclear or little human relevance, some of which have caused human infection, include the Allpahuayo virus (Peru), Parana virus (Paraguay), and Pinchinde virus (Colombia) in clade A; the Amapari virus (Brazil) and Tacaribe virus (Trinidad) in clade B; and the Latino virus (Bolivia, Brazil), Oliveros virus (Argentina), and others of unclear taxonomic status such as U.S. isolates of Whitewater Arroyo virus, Big Brushy Tank virus, Tonto Creek virus, and Bear Canyon virus in clade C.

3.2 HISTORY

In 1934, reports (Armstrong and Lillie 1934; Armstrong and Wooley 1935) began to appear of a previously undescribed virus causing neurological disease in man. The original isolation was discovered during passage, in monkeys, of an agent from brain tissue of an individual who died in St. Louis, Missouri, during an encephalitis epidemic in 1933. In monkeys and subsequently in mice, the pathology found was a lymphocytic meningitis, most prominent in the choroid plexus structure in the ventricles of the brain where cerebrospinal fluid is produced, consisting of modified ependymal cells. Because of the histopathologic appearance, the agent was called lymphocytic choriomeningitis virus. Although fatal cases of infection were well represented in the initial cases, the most common disease state recognized due to LCM was a benign, self-limited meningitis.

As LCM was the first agent isolated in cases of what became referred to as acute aseptic meningitis in Wallgren's (1925) original description, lymphocytic meningitis (Hughes 1937) or benign lymphocytic meningitis (Dummer 1937), for a substantial amount of time, LCM and aseptic meningitis were regarded as identical (Roebroek et al. 1994). Subsequently, numerous other etiologies of the aseptic meningitis syndrome have been elucidated including many other viruses but LCM will be indelibly associated with the disease.

The Lassa fever virus was first recognized in a nosocomial setting when an American health-care worker, at a mission health care station in the town of Lassa in northeast Nigeria, became sick and precipitated a chain of health-care-associated infections locally and involved laboratory workers in the United States.

3.3 BIOLOGICAL PROPERTIES

Arenaviruses possess negatively stranded RNA genomes with a bisegmental organization (two segments) (Charrel and de Lamballere 2003). The larger genomic segment (referred to as L) consists of about 7200 nucleotides that code for the virus' RNA-dependent RNA polymerase and a small RING finger protein Z. The smaller (S) segment is about 3500 nucleotides in length and codes for two structural proteins, a nucleoprotein (NP), and a glycoprotein precursor (GPC). Each gene on the segments (Emonet et al. 2006) is separated by an intergenic noncoding region (IGR) with a potential to be able to form one or more hairpin configurations, and the gene reading frames are arranged in opposite polarities referred to as ambisense. NP and the polymerase are transcribed into complementary mRNA, whereas GP and Z are from a replicative intermediate (Emonet et al. 2009). The 5′ and 3′ ends of each of the RNA segments possess reasonably well-conserved reversed complementary sequences of 19 nucleotides at each extremity.

GPC is posttranslationally cleaved into the G1 and G2 envelope proteins of the virus as well as a small (58-amino-acid) stable signal peptide (SSP) (Emonet et al. 2009). The cleavage is mediated by the SK1/S1P cellular protease (Kunz et al. 2003). It has been shown that the protease has a strong preference to arenaviral sequences resembling its autoprocessing sites. The Lassa fever virus resembles the protease C-site, whereas the Junin virus has a similarity to the B-site (Pasquato et al. 2011). The authors suggested that arenaviral GP complexes have evolved to mimic the protease's autoprocessing sites to ensure efficient cleavage.

SSP appears to be unique as the protein remains associated with the GP complex after cleavage by the signal protease and helps trafficking of the complex in the cell (Eichler et al. 2003). The surface glycoproteins associate as trimers to form the spikes mediating host cell interactions with GP1 on the distal end of the spike. GP1 contains both the receptor binding and the antibody neutralization sites and remains noncovalently bound to GP2. GP2 contains a transmembrane region that serves to anchor the GP complex to the lipid bilayer of the virus (Burns and Buchmeirer 1991). Both glycoproteins contain N-glycosylations and the pattern of glycosylation is well preserved among arenaviruses. They are important in fusion of the virus to the host cell and also serve as a "cloud" that can mask epitopes on the GP complex from neutralizing antibodies (Bonhomme et al. 2011).

The Z protein is the major factor involved in newly formed viral release from an infected cell (Strecker et al. 2003), which is a process mediated by the areas on the Z protein that are proline-rich, the way many enveloped negative-stranded RNA viruses accomplish with the matrix protein bridging ribonucleoprotein and GP and plays a major role in controlling viral RNA production by locking the viral RNA polymerase in a promoter-bound state and ensuring polymerase packaging during virus maturation (Kranzusch and Whelan 2011).

Arenavirus virions are spherical to pleomorphic in shape with diameters ranging between 50 and 300 nm, with the average diameter of the spherical forms about 120 nm. The virions possess dense lipid-containing viral envelopes that are covered with 8- to 10-nm-long club-like projections of the GP complex. Ribosomes, 20–25 nm (acquired from the host cell and do not appear to be required for viral replication (Leung and Rawls 1977)), are found inside the virions and are the derivation of the name arenavirus, as the structures give the virion a "sandy" appearance. The Latin word *harena* means sand, a sandy place or seashore, or a place of combat, literally "a place strewn with sand." The virions are rapidly inactivated by ultraviolet or gamma wave irradiation and by a pH below 5.5 or above 8.5. Temperatures above 56°C also quickly inactivate the agents.

The diversity and ancestry of LCM, as the prototypic and most widely spread arenavirus, has been studied (Albariño et al. 2010). In analyzing the RNA of 29 strains from a variety of geographic sources (including some of the earliest 1935 isolates), it was found that the strains are highly diverse with several apparent lineages but without correlation with time or place of isolation. Bayesian analysis estimated that the most recent common ancestor was 1000 to 5000 years old, consistent with the complex phylogeographic relationships observed.

As discussed in the sections regarding rodent and human infection, the manifestations of LCM infection can be quite varied, especially in rodents whether self-limited or chronic infection occurs. Quite subtle changes in the glycoprotein of LCM have been shown to be part of the cause of persistence of LCM, as studied in dendritic cells. Dendritic cells are present in tissues in contact with the external environment, such as the skin (where there is a specialized dendritic cell type called Langerhans cells), and the inner lining of the nose, lungs, stomach, and intestines. As an example, LCM clone 13 infection, which results in persistence, and differs from the standard Armstrong strain only by few nucleotides, three of which result in coding changes (Sullivan et al. 2011), two in GP1 and one in the RNA-dependent RNA polymerase. The GP1 changes (especially F260L) mediate exceptionally strong binding affinity to the LCM cellular receptor, alpha-dystroglycan. This effect on dendritic cells results in decreased amounts of costimulatory ligands, an inability to fully prime T cells, up-regulation of T-cell inhibitory receptors, and difficulties in viral clearance of LCM. Alternative receptors have also been described for LCM virus (Kunz et al. 2004), which do not produce immune suppression. A number of the New World arenaviruses can use human transferring receptor 1 as a cellular receptor (Radoshitzky et al. 2007).

LCM entrance into host cells, after receptor binding, appears to be mediated via viropexis in large smooth-walled vesicles followed by a pH-dependent fusion event inside the cell (Borrow and Oldstone 1994). Unlike classical phagocytosis, LCM uptake is a microfilament-independent process, not related to the direct fusion with host cell plasma membrane.

3.4 CLINICAL PRESENTATION

3.4.1 LYMPHOCYTIC CHORIOMENINGITIS VIRUS

3.4.1.1 Rodent Infection

Wild house mice are the natural reservoir for LCM virus. Laboratory or pet rodents such as hamsters and guinea pigs can be infected from exposure to feral mice in a breeding facility, pet store, or home. It is unclear how relevant other rodent species such as chinchillas, dwarf hamsters, and gerbils are in infecting humans with LCM.

3.4.1.2 Human Infection

Transmission of LCM from the rodent reservoirs to man is generally indirect through contact with dried rodent urine or droppings in the environment. The exposure can be related to aerosolization of particles contaminated with rodent urine or saliva, ingestion of contaminated food, or by direct contact with rodent excreta with abraded or broken skin. The kind of incidental contact depends on the habits of both the rodent vehicle and man. As an example, if the infected rodent species is one that prefers a field locale, human infection is associated with agricultural work. Alternatively, if the rodent (like the house mouse) inhabits the urban setting, the arenavirus can be acquired in a domestic setting. Human-to-human transmission of LCM virus does not occur except in intrauterine infection and related to organ transplantation as discussed below.

3.4.1.3 Normal Host

In man, the manifestations of LCM virus infection outside the neonatal period can range from the asymptomatic state (in about a third of cases) to an influenza-like illness without neurological symptomatology (in about half of the cases) to the classical aseptic meningitis, which more rarely can be an overt meningoencephalitis, potentially fatal in outcome.

Initially, LCM manifests with fever and headache that can be also associated with a nonspecific lymphadenopathy (enlarged lymph glands) and a maculopapular rash. The symptom complex can also include malaise, sometimes striking muscle aches, nausea and/or vomiting, and loss of appetite and dysesthesias, particularly hyperesthesias. A history of exposure to rodents or the excreta of these mammals may be elicited to have occurred 1–3 weeks prior to the onset of illness. These initial symptoms may resolve in 3 to 5 days, and in those with subsequent neurological illness, illness recurs after 2 to 4 days with additional illness. The manifestations of the second part of the classical (but not pathognomonic) biphasic or hump-back illness include increasing headache with meningismus (stiff neck), photophobia, and mild-to-moderate lethargy. Persistent lethargy, overt confusion or coma, and seizures indicate the development of meningoencephalitis. Other manifestations that may occur during this second phase of illness include arthralgia/arthritis of the shoulders and particularly the small joints of the hands, parotitis, and unilateral orchitis. The biphasic may not always be recognizable. A similar biphasic illness associated with rodent exposure can occur with leptospirosis, the classical maladie des porchers, a spirochetal illness that also is associated with chronic urinary excretion in some rodents.

The clinical manifestations of LCM virus in man has been clearly documented (Lepine et al. 1937). In a study performed in the prehuman use committee era, investigators inoculated individuals with tertiary syphilis paretic patients with a mouse brain-derived suspension of LCM virus and observed that after an incubation period of 2–3 days, an influenza-like illness developed and was followed by mild, self-limited lymphocytic meningitis without sequelae.

A typical case of LCM aseptic meningitis illness is one described by Roebroek et al. (1994) from the Netherlands. A patient, a previously healthy painter with mice frequently seen in his home, was admitted to the hospital with fever of 38.7°C, malaise, cough, vomiting, a frontally localized throbbing headache, irritability, and cutaneous hyperesthesia for 6 days. Two weeks earlier, he had a nonspecific febrile illness that lasted 5 days. Cerebrospinal fluid examination (Table 3.3) revealed a lymphocytic pleocytosis with a mildly elevated protein and somewhat low glucose (hypoglycorrhachia). Acute and convalescent sera obtained 3 weeks apart revealed a significant rise in LCM virus antibody from 1:8 to 1:32. He slowly recovered over a 4-week period without any sequelae. CSF analysis generally reveals between 100 and 400 cells/mm^3, usually >90% lymphocytes, a protein between 50 and 300 mg/dL (normal, <40 mg/dL), and a normal to slightly low glucose (normal, 50%–70% of blood glucose). Patients tend to have prominent leucopenia and thrombocytopenia in the peripheral blood.

Sporadic cases of LCM infection is generally linked to exposure to mice in the household environment, but outbreaks of the infection tend to be associated with exposure to rodents, especially Syrian hamsters or tissue cell lines derived from them, in a workplace setting such as a laboratory or having hamsters as pets. One of the earliest outbreaks (Lewis et al. 1965; Baum et al. 1966) involved 10 laboratory personnel at the National Institutes of Health in Bethesda, Maryland. The episode

TABLE 3.3
Typical CSF Pattern in LCM Virus Meningitis

	Hospital Day		
	Day 4	Day 13	Day 26
Cells/mm^3	108	63	48
% lymphocytes	95	99	99
CSF glucose	47	49	52
Serum glucose	124	95	63
CSF protein	116	123	76

Source: Roebroek, R.M.J.A. et al., 1994, *Clin. Neurol. Neurosurg.* 96, 178–180. With permission.

was noteworthy in that it was the first hamster-associated epidemic ever reported, and the source was contaminated tumor transplants into hamsters and then transmission among infected to uninfected rodents. All 10 had influenza-like illnesses, and although none developed meningitis, 2 had subsequent arthritis and 3 had orchitis. In 3 cases that occurred following a single exposure to infected material, the incubation periods ranged from 9 to 14 days. A similar outbreak (Hotchin et al. 1974; Hinman et al. 1975) occurred in the early 1970s among staff members of the University of Rochester Medical Center and involved 48 cases with the initial source also was contaminated tumor cells (from a different supplier). Of note, personnel infection occurred not only through direct contact with infected animals but also from the mere presence in the room where the animals were housed. A cluster of LCM infection in researchers was also reported associated with nude (athymic) mice (Dykewicz et al. 1992). The significant risk factors found in the infected workers were cleaning the cages of the nude mice and changing their bedding or water. The source of the virus was also LCM-infected tumor lines. The increased use of nude mice in the laboratory likely precipitated the outbreak as the immunosuppressed rodents shed virus of higher titer especially in their urine.

Pet hamsters are also a clear source for human LCM virus (Deibel et al. 1975; Maetz et al. 1976; Biggar et al. 1975). In a 1975 report from the New York State Department of Health (Deibel et al. 1975), 60 individuals with LCM virus infection were diagnosed, 12 with a physician diagnosis of CNS disease (8 meningitis and 4 meningoencephalitis), and 48 with other illnesses (mostly influenza-like illness). Of the 60, 55 had pet hamsters in their households and 4 were employees of hamster wholesalers or retailers. Infection rates within families with infected pet hamsters varied with the location and type of hamster cage (Biggar et al. 1975). Open cages and cages situated in common living areas were associated with the highest infection rates. Of note in this study, the severity of human illness was not associated with more direct contact with the hamster reservoir.

3.4.1.4   Immunocompromised Host

One of the earliest reports of the manifestations of LCM virus infection in an immunocompromised host was that of Horton et al. (1971) in which MP virus (a strain of LCM) was injected into three far-advanced lymphoma patients under informed consent. Some information had been previously reported (by those who had isolated the strain) (Molomut and Padnos 1965) that the virus might have had some effect in suppressing certain murine tumors. No observable effectiveness occurred, and all three patients subsequently died. Two of the three were persistently viremic and febrile until death, although the role that the virus played in the deaths was unclear. The third patient had 15 days of viremia, which subsequently cleared with the development of antibody to LCM. No changes in the CSF were reported. Much more recently, an adolescent with T-cell lymphoma was found to have LCM virus meningitis by serological testing after presenting with lymphocytic meningitis without encephalopathy or leukemic cells in the CSF in the setting of possible exposure to mice in her home (Al-Zein et al. 2008). She subsequently developed hydrocephalus, requiring CSF shunting but was reported to be infection- and leukemia-free 4 years after the completion of chemotherapy for the leukemia.

LCM infection has also occurred through solid organ transplantation, resulting in rapidly progressive, high-mortality rate disease. Two clusters of cases have been described (Fischer et al. 2006) involving two donors and eight recipients receiving cadaveric kidney, liver, or lung, of which all but one died, between 9 and 76 days after transplantation, despite lowering immunosuppressive therapy in some recipients. The posttransplantation courses were characterized by altered mental status, fever, graft dysfunction, pulmonary infiltrates, and abdominal pain with thrombocytopenia, increased aminotransferase levels, and coagulopathy. Seizures, renal failure, diarrhea, and a peri-incisional rash were also variably noted. Only one of the patients was found to have meningoencephalitis at postmortem examination.

It is important to note that one of the donors had no known history of rodent exposure and no direct evidence of donor infection with LCM virus was found by immunohistochemical analysis, cell culture, RT-PCR, or viral serologies. A member of the second donor's household had adopted a pet hamster 3 weeks prior to the donor's death, but the donor was not the primary caretaker of the hamster and was seronegative for IgM and IgG antibody to LCM virus without any reported symptoms referable to LCM. The viral isolations from the recipients and the hamster were identical. A trace-back analysis of the hamster (Amman et al. 2007) was able to follow the hamster back from a Rhode Island pet store to a distribution center in Ohio to the parent facility in Arkansas. Virus from hamsters at both facilities were discovered to be phylogenetically linked to the index hamster and the transplant recipients.

The organ recipient who survived was treated with ribavirin and decreasing immunosuppressant beginning 26 days after transplantation once the identification of LCM infection in corecipients was made. Treatment resulted in decreasing illness and normalizing laboratory abnormalities, and seroconversion to IgM anti-LCM occurred on day 63 after transplantation. No active infection was found on day 311 with continued immunosuppression. It should be noted that the immunosuppression as reflected by a functional cell-mediated immunity assay remained prominent despite reduction of medication, suggesting an effect caused directly by LCM, which was reconstituted with clearance of the virus (Gautam et al. 2007). Corneas were transplanted from one of the donors to individuals who did not require systemic immunosuppression, and neither patient developed any sign of infection or had graft loss.

Another arenavirus has subsequently been linked to fatal disease in three Australian recipients of organs from a single donor (Palacios et al. 2008). The donor had died 10 days after returning from a 3-month trip to the former Yugoslavia, and all three died within 29 and 36 days after transplantation of illnesses characterized by fever, encephalopathy, and pulmonary infiltrates. Postmortem histopathology of the patients was not elaborated. Arenavirus was identified using high-throughput sequencing identified an Old World arenavirus which was found to be related to LCM virus and specific PCR found presence of the unique virus in blood, liver, and CSF.

3.4.1.5 Congenital Infection

The first report of LCM infection as an intrauterine disease appeared in 1955 in the United Kingdom regarding a neonate who died of meningitis on day 12 of life

(Komrower et al. 1955). It is apparent that fetal infection due to LCM has been an underrecognized event that can present as a spontaneous abortion (Barton and Mets 2001) or with a clinical complex similar to other congenital infections due to organisms such as toxoplasmosis, rubella virus, cytomegalovirus, or syphilis. As urged (Barton and Mets 2001), the public and medical communities need to be aware of the risk that laboratory, pet, and wild rodents can pose to pregnant women.

In a report of 20 children with congenital LCM (Bonthius et al. 2007a), all had chorioretinitis and structural brain abnormalities, but the presenting clinical manifestations including the severity of visual disturbance and the location, character, and severity of the neuropathology varied quite significantly. The combination of microencephaly and periventricular calcifications was the most common finding on imaging, and all these children manifested profound intellectual retardation, cerebral palsy, and seizures. Other imaging findings included hydrocephalus, cerebellar hypoplasia, and porencephalic or periventricular cysts. Isolated cerebellar hypoplasia occurred with jitteriness and ataxia as the only long-term dysfunction. In a companion article, clinical and pathological diversity was assessed in an animal model (Bonthius et al. 2007b). Host age at the time of infection profoundly affected the cellular targets of infection, maximal viral titers, immune response to the viral infection, and the severity, nature, and location of the neuropathology. All of the pathological changes observed in children with congenital LCM infection were reproduced in the rat model by infecting the rat pups at different ages.

In this rat pup model (Bonthius et al. 2007b), host age was clearly an important variable. Infection on postnatal day 1 resulted in prominent infection of astrocytes and neurons, whereas when infection was induced 3 days later, neurons were spared, and if infection was begun on day 21 neither astrocytes nor neurons could be infected. Ependymal cells and the olfactory bulb cells, however, remained susceptible.

Infection on postnatal day 1 (Bonthius et al. 2007b) induced cerebellar hypoplasia manifest by a small but normal cytoarchitectured cerebellum, whereas infection on day 4 or 6 did not cause cerebellar hypoplasia but rather induced a neuronal migration problem (Bonthius et al. 2007c) where cerebellar granular cells did not migrate appropriately into the ventral lobules and encephalomalacia ensued. Furthermore, infection induced on day 21 did not cause any cerebellar pathology but continued the susceptibility of the olfactory bulb and the ventricular lining ependymal cells, resulting in olfactory bulb destruction and hydrocephalus.

Glia, the supportive cells in the central nervous system that do not conduct electric impulses and consist of astrocytes, oligodendrocytes, and microglia, seem to play an important role in LCM virus infection of the developing rat brain. It has been demonstrated (Bonthius et al. 2002) that, in the neonatal rat brain, these cells were the first to be infected and that the spread occurred via glial cells to other glial cells and neurons, specifically neurons in the cerebellum, olfactory bulb, dentate gyrus of the hippocampus, and the periventricular area. The manifestations of neuronal involvement were different based on the location of the neuron involved as shown in Table 3.4. It was thought that the specificity of neuronal involvement may be related to the higher metabolic rate of these neurons (Bonthius et al. 2002).

The neuropathology related to LCM infection in developing rat pup brain is caused by a combination of noncytolytic viral damage and the innate immune

TABLE 3.4

Neuropathology of LCM Virus-Affected Neuronal Regions

Region	Neuropathology
Cerebellum	Dorsal lobules—acute immune-mediated destruction driven by CD8+ lymphocytes
	Ventral lobules—neural migration pathology causing permanently ectopic located cerebellar granular cells within the molecular level
Olfactory bulb	Acute hypoplasia of the bulb due to a reduced production of granule cells. This effect is transient and the bulb can be normal sized by adulthood
Hippocampus	Despite a substantial viral burden, initially the dentate gyrus appears histologically normal but several months later the previously infected cells begin to die resulting in a delayed, prominent loss of dentate granule cells
Periventricular area	No pathological changes despite neuronal infection by LCM virus

Source: Bonthius, D.J. et al., 2002, *J. Virol.* 76, 6618–6635. With permission.

system response. As an example, cerebellar damage appears to be immune-mediated (Bonthius et al. 2002) as shown by the lack of destruction in both the nude (athymic) mouse without a functional cellular immune system and rats treated with antilymphocyte serum.

It is important to note that even if LCM virus has been cleared, progressive deterioration of the previously infected neurons can continue to occur. The mechanism of this effect is not totally clear but may be related to virus-induced hyperexcitability, especially of the GABAergic inhibitory neural circuits (Pearce et al. 1996, 2000).

3.4.2 HEMORRHAGIC FEVER ARENAVIRUSES

3.4.2.1 Rodent Infection

With the exception of the Tacaribe virus that is endemic in fruit-eating bats of the *Artibeus* genus, rodents are the reservoir for these agents. An arenavirus-like virus, the first described in a non-mammal, is noted below. In general, each virus is carried by a single rodent species. Infection rates among the target rodent population are very variable between areas and over time. In the so-called hot spot areas for the Junin virus, the prevalence rate can be 5%–10%, whereas outside these foci, rates are much lower or the virus is completely absent. The viruses can be carried lifelong in seemingly healthy rodents as overt clinical disease is not reported in naturally infected animals.

Laboratory rodents can be infected with the hemorrhagic fever arenaviruses experimentally but have not been found naturally infected. The infections, unlike with LCM, have not been observed in pet rodents, but it is conceivable that exposure to a potentially susceptible rodent may occur if an imported, infected, exotic rodent is exposed in a pet shop, animal "swap meet," or distribution center to other species, as was observed in the monkeypox imported in the United States in the giant pouched Gambian rat and transmitted to American prairie dogs that were subsequently sold as pets (Reed et al. 2004). A non-mammal arenavirus-like pathogen has recently been described in snakes associated with inclusion body disease (Stenglein et al. 2012). This multisystem disease causes behavioral changes in the snakes and, intestingly, has some characteristics of filoviruses as well.

3.4.2.2 Human Viral Hemorrhagic Fever Infection

Human exposure to these pathogens mostly through dried rodent urine can be influenced by the host reservoir's behavior. As an example, the Junin virus rodent hosts tend to aggregate along linear habits such as fence lines and roadsides. Additionally, the Lassa fever reservoir, although found throughout much of sub-Saharan Africa, can exhibit local species population dynamics that can affect the tendency of the rodent to enter houses.

Although uncommon, secondary human-to-human cases of Lassa fever can occur generally related to direct exposure to virus-containing body fluids rather than the aerosol route. As reported (Bausch et al. 2010), at least 25 imported cases of Lassa fever have occurred in the developed world, involving at least 1500 cumulative contacts since 1969 and only a single putative and asymptomatic secondary case occurred. Aerosol transmission may have caused human-to-human cases during a nosocomial outbreak of Machupo virus (Bolivian hemorrhagic fever) in 1971 involving 5 persons (Peters et al. 1974).

3.4.3 Lassa Fever

Following an incubation period of 7–18 days, infected individuals can develop fever, weakness, and malaise that can be associated with cough, severe headache, sore throat, nausea, vomiting, and diarrhea. The spectrum of disease can range from asymptomatic infection to fatal disease with hemorrhage. Severe cases will early on display evidence of increased vascular permeability such as facial edema and pleural effusion. Deterioration may occur quickly, within 6 to 10 days after illness onset, associated with pulmonary edema, respiratory distress, shock, and signs of encephalopathy (Moraz and Kunz 2011). Hepatic disease manifests as multifocal hepatocellular necrosis without cellular infiltration or hepatic failure. Liver failure, however, is not uncommon in the rare cases of Sabia virus infection (Brazilian hemorrhagic fever) and has been described in a few human infections with Whitewater Arroyo virus in the United States (CDC 2000). Signs of bleeding occur in 15%–20% of cases but are not prominent and do not contribute to the hypotension. Disseminated intravascular coagulation is rarely seen.

Neurological signs in Lassa fever (Cummins et al. 1992) include confusion, rapidly followed by tremor, grand mal seizures, abnormal posturing, and coma (Table 3.5). Neither focal neurological signs nor increased intracranial pressure occur. The development of encephalopathy was not found to correlate with the presence of virus or antibody directed at the virus in the CSF. Despite significant encephalopathy, consistent lesions in the brain of fatal cases are not found (Walker et al. 1980).

Sensorineural hearing loss (SNHL) is clearly recognized as a usually late manifestation of Lassa fever. A prospective study of 49 patients with Lassa fever in Sierra

TABLE 3.5
Manifestations of Lassa Fever Encephalopathy, n = 9

Symptom	Number Affected
Confusion	9
Tremor	7
Grand mal seizures	7
Abnormal posturing	3
Coma	8
Death	8

Source: Cummins, D. et al., 1992, *J. Trop. Med. Hyg.* 95, 197–201. With permission.

Leone (Cummins et al. 1990) found 14% of cases developed SNHL with no cases in febrile controls. Additionally, 17.6% (9 of 51) people who had evidence of previous Lassa infection had SNHL, and 26 of 32 locals who had previously developed SNHL had serological evidence of past infection as compared with 6 of 32 controls. Other studies have reported substantially lower risks of SNHL of about 4% (McCormick et al. 1987a).

3.4.4 SOUTH AMERICAN HEMORRHAGIC FEVERS

The South African hemorrhagic fever viruses cause quite similar illnesses, regardless of the specific virus involved. Unlike LCM virus, human-to-human infection can occur with inadequate barrier protection especially with Machupo virus where aerosolization of infectious material can occur (CDC 1994). Such high-dose inocula can decrease the usual incubation period of 5–21 days to as short as 2–3 days.

Presenting with the gradual onset of fever and malaise, these illnesses can also be associated with muscle aches, headache, back pain, and dizziness. Hyperesthesias of the skin similar to LCM virus infection also may occur. Hemorrhagic manifestations include skin petechiae, and gum, vaginal, and gastrointestinal bleeding start at about day 4 of illness and herald the onset of shock. Similar to the process in dengue virus infection, despite some hemorrhage, increasing vascular permeability causes a hemoconcentration state. Disseminated intravascular coagulation can occur with prominent thrombocytopenia.

Neurological manifestations of the South American hemorrhagic fevers may begin with hand tremors and the inability to swallow or speak clearly and can progress to grand mal seizures, coma, and death even without clear-cut signs of vascular leak syndrome or significant bleeding. The mortality rate of these illnesses is 15%–30%, but survival generally occurs without residuae (Emonet et al. 2009). Despite the prominent encephalopathy associated with the South African hemorrhagic fevers, the CSF examination is generally normal. Beginning with moderate to severe confusion, irritability, prominent ataxia, and tremors may progress to delirium, grand mal seizures, and coma. Intercurrent bacterial infections such as pneumonia and bacteremia occur at this time and contribute to the mortality rate.

A convalescence period of several months may occur with substantial irritability, prominent asthenia, and memory loss. Human immune plasma can be used therapeutically, especially in Argentine hemorrhagic fever (Maiztegui et al. 1979; Enria et al. 1984). Increased survival occurs if given at adequate titer, but it is well reported that about 10% of survivors treated in this way, after a period free of symptoms, develop what is referred to as late neurological syndrome (LNS). This syndrome does not seem to occur at all in those who recover in the absence of immune therapy. LNS presents with fever, cerebellar signs, cranial nerve palsies, and an abnormal CSF examination, with a lymphocytic pleocytosis, normal CSF glucose, and a high ratio of CSF/serum anti-Junin virus antibodies. Several animal models have been used to study LNS, including marmosets (Avila et al. 1987) and guinea pigs (Kenyon et al. 1986).

3.5 DIAGNOSIS

These agents can be diagnosed by the use of serologies, detecting antibodies raised against the offending agent. The usual antibody testing using an enzyme-linked immunosorbent assay (ELISA) or indirect fluorescent antibody testing (IFA) can be used. In these assays, a fourfold increase in antibody should be found in assays of acute and convalescent sera run in parallel. Alternatively, a specific IgM can be tested. In these assays, there is substantial cross-reactions between viruses, but with the knowledge of where the index may have been exposed can suggest the arenavirus involved. Virus neutralization testing is highly specific to each virus but requires live virus for testing, creating more laboratory hazard. Unfortunately, in the acute situation where a finite diagnosis is needed, antibody levels may not yet have risen and the neutralizing antibody may not appear into convalescence. A single non-IgM-positive antibody test can also reflect past infection and not be related to the acute illness being evaluated.

Likewise, in the animal reservoir (Charrel and de Lamballerie 2010), finding antibodies specific for an arenavirus in a rodent is a poor indication of active infection because of a poor correlation with whether a live virus is present. In various situations related to the virus and age of the rodent, persistent viral infection can be present with or without detectable antibodies. The presence of antibodies reflects circulation of virus in the rodent cohorts and indicates the need for more specific testing by molecular means.

Measurement of viral antigens is certainly useful in the early detection of arenavirus infection. Jahrling et al. (1985c) found antigens in the first serum available in patients, and antibody positivity did not occur for at least 3 days afterward. The development of antibodies coincided with a declining antigenemia. The antigen testing could be done safely using beta-propiolactone-inactivated sera. Similarly, testing was compared in 305 suspected cases of Lassa fever (Bausch et al. 2000). Using virus isolation with a positive reverse transcriptase-PCR as a gold standard, they found Lassa fever virus antigen and IgM ELISA were 88% sensitive (95% confidence interval 77%–95%) and 90% specific (95% confidence interval 88%–91%) for acute infection. Antigens specific for a virus can also be detected *in situ* by immunoperoxidase staining of surgical or autopsy tissue.

Direct measurement of circulating RNA of the viruses can be done as well. Vieth et al. (2007) developed an assay using the polymerase domain of the L RNA segment that used segments of the Old World arenaviruses and found the assay to be applicable as a complimentary diagnostic test for Lassa virus and LCM virus, to identify new Old World arenaviruses, and to screening potential rodent hosts for Old World arenaviruses. Similar assays have been developed for New World arenaviruses to be used as complementary diagnostic assays for the New World arenaviruses (Lozano et al. 1993; Vieth et al. 2005).

The arenaviruses can be isolated in Vero cells. Attempts at such isolations should be done in an appropriate laboratory, one with biosafety level 4 containment because of the risk of laboratory-acquired infection.

3.6 EPIDEMIOLOGY

Lymphocytic choriomeningitis virus is widely distributed in the Americas and in Europe but has been found in rodents in Asia and Africa as well. The following are examples of seroprevalence of humans and/or rodents and illustrate differences in areas with regard to risk groups.

In Baltimore, Maryland, 4.7% (54/1149) inner-city residents were found to have LCM virus antibodies (Childs et al. 1991). Antibody prevalence increased with age without gender or ethnic differences. Seropositivity was rare as compared with the rates of contact with house mice. The seropositivity of house mice in Baltimore revealed an overall positivity of 9.0% (Childs et al. 1992), with the highest prevalence (13.4%) in the inner-city area where positive mice were identified to be significantly clustered within blocks and households and correlated with mouse density within individual blocks. In Birmingham, Alabama, the overall incidence of antibody was 3.5% (56/1600) (Park et al. 1997), with, as in Baltimore, increased age was significantly correlated with seropositivity (age: <30 years, 0.3%; >30 years, 5.4%) and was negatively linked to socioeconomic status. These authors suggested that, given the age-related data, human LCM infection may be decreasing over the past 30–40 years, presumably related to less rodent contact.

In Nova Scotia, Canada, a seroprevalence of 4% has been reported (Marrie and Saron 1998), with a prominent shift (17 of the 20 seropositives) in females. Few, if any, cases of LCM have been reported from this Canadian province. The rate compared with that of 2.38% in over 7000 males in Santa Fe Province, Argentina (Ambrosio et al. 1994). In and around Madrid, Spain (Liedo et al. 2003), 1.7% of 400 human sera were seropositive with no statistical difference related to age or urban residence; 9% of rodent sera were seropositive.

In nonclassical areas of human LCM infection, no seroprevalence of LCM virus was found in Upper Egypt, but other areas have rodent seropositivity ranging from 1.8% to 11.5% (el Karamany and Imam 1991). Additionally, some mice captured at the Yokohama port in Japan were found to be positive on certain piers but not others and was present in some years and not in others, suggesting introduction from ships without clear persistence (Morita et al. 1991).

Lassa fever is a substantial febrile illness in West Africa that has been estimated to be the cause of as many as 15% of adult admissions to the hospital in adults and as many as 40% of nonsurgical deaths (McCormick et al. 1987a). The annual number of cases ranges from 100,000 to 300,000 with 5000 to 10,000 deaths and 30,000 left with deafness (McCormick et al. 1987; Birmingham and Kenyon 2001). The virus is associated with a high mortality rate during pregnancy as well. The disease has been periodically imported into Europe, North America, and Japan by travelers from the endemic area (CDC 2004; Schmitz et al. 2002). Nosocomial spread in the developed world can occur but is a lower risk than in Africa because of the availability of adequate barrier protection.

Argentine hemorrhagic fever was first recognized in 1943, and the first isolation of the Junin virus was in 1958. A range of 300–600 cases per year are generally reported primarily in individuals involved with agricultural activities in the pampas of the country (Maiztegui et al. 1986). The areas of endemicity have extended, especially northward, but overall, there are hot spots of infection in those areas (Mills et al. 1991).

Bolivian hemorrhagic fever was recognized in 1959 among patients in the town of San Joaquin in the Beni department of northeast Bolivia involving about 1000 cases (Tesh et al. 1999) and the Machupo virus first isolated in 1963. Several outbreaks of the disease occurred in the 1960s, but subsequently, the disease has been recognized only sporadically in the endemic area.

Venezuelan hemorrhagic fever was recognized in the towns of Guanarito and Guanare, Portuguesa State, Venezuela, in 1989 during an outbreak that originally was thought to be dengue (de Manzione et al. 1998). The endemic areas involve the south and southwest parts of the Portuguesa state as well as the adjacent areas of the state of Barinas in the central plains of the country.

3.7 TREATMENT

3.7.1 IMMUNE PLASMA THERAPY

For Argentine hemorrhagic fever (Junin virus), passive transfer of immune plasma can decrease the case fatality rate from 30% to 1% (Enria et al. 1984). Immune plasma may be of benefit in Lassa fever if the plasma has a high titer of neutralizing antibody and is matched to the infecting strain (Jahrling and Peters 1984; Jahrling et al. 1985a). A minimal improvement of case-fatality rates have been found with other arenaviruses, possibly due to the lower titers of antibodies in the preparations.

3.7.2 ANTIVIRAL THERAPY

3.7.2.1 Ribavirin

Ribavirin is a guanosine (1-β-D-ribofuranosyl-1,2,4-triazole-3-carboxamide) that has been used, with variable effectiveness, for Lassa, Junin, and Machupo viruses. In Lassa fever, if intravenous ribavirin is begun within the first 6 days of illness, the mortality rate of severe Lassa fever can be decreased substantially (McCormick et al. 1986). This study identified two distinct risk factors for a high case-fatality rate, elevation of serum aspartate aminotransferase (AST), and significant viremia. Breakdown of the results can be found in Table 3.6. With Lassa fever, the addition

TABLE 3.6
Case-Fatality Rate of Severe Lassa Fever with and without Ribavirin Use

	CFR		
Risk Factor	No Ribavirin	Ribavirin (≤6 days)	Ribavirin (>6 days)
Serum AST >150 IU/L	33/60 (55%)	1/20 (5%)	11/43 (26%)
High viremia	35/46 (76%)	1/11 (9%)	9/19 (47%)

Source: McCormick, J.B. et al., 1986, *N. Engl. J. Med.* 314, 20–26. With permission.

of immune plasma did not reduce case-fatality rates from the levels with or without ribavirin.

Bolivian hemorrhagic fever due to Machupo virus was anecdotally studied due to the less common nature of the infection as compared with Lassa fever. In the report (Kilgore et al. 1997), the two patients treated with immune plasma survived. Likewise, some reports exist that ribavirin may be useful in man with Argentine hemorrhagic fever (Enria and Maiztegui 1994) and is underscored by the effectiveness in primate model (Weissenbacher et al. 1986). Lymphocytic choriomeningitis virus is inhibited *in vitro* by ribavirin, but there are little data to assess its efficacy in substantial LCM disease but it seemed to be effective in LCM-associated organ transplant infection (Fischer et al. 2006).

The substantial toxicity of ribavirin in man is likely tied to its effect on guanosine biosynthesis. Among the side effects found include hemolytic anemia, headache, irritability and anxiety, depression, muscle and joint aches, loss of appetite, and difficulty sleeping as well as being teratogenic for pregnant women.

3.7.2.2 Nonribavirin

T-705 (6-fluoro-3-hydroxy-2-pyrazinecarboxamide, or favipiravir) is a viral RNA-dependent RNA polymerase inhibitor with the likelihood of less toxicity given its mode of action. It has been found to have a broad range of activity among RNA viruses including influenza viruses, flaviviruses, and bunyaviruses. In a cell culture model, it disrupted steps in LCM virus replication that could be rescued by the addition of purine bases or nucleosides (Mendenhall et al. 2011a). In a guinea pig model using an adapted strain of Pichinde virus (Mendenhall et al. 2011b), favipiravir appeared to be highly effective even if begun 1 week after virus challenge when the animals were quite ill. Its effectiveness was also reflected by a more rapid recovery than that of animals treated with ribavirin. Similar data were reported using a hamster model, in which no additional benefit was reported with favipiravir and ribavirin together (Gowen et al. 2008).

The arenavirus Z protein has been studied as an antiviral target. Garcia et al. (2006, 2010) have investigated an aromatic disulfide NSC 20625 that inactivated viral particles. These virions retained GP complex functions for binding and entry into host cells but were unable to replicate viral DNA. NSC 20625-treated virions had abnormal Z protein electrophoretic patterns.

High-throughput screening of small-molecular-weight compounds that inhibit arenavirus entry into cells by blocking binding has been recently reviewed (Lee 2010). Considering that endemic areas of most arenavirus, with the major exception of LCM virus, are in countries with low levels of public health infrastructure, the development of orally dosed, heat-stable, and low-cost compounds is a high priority. A number of compounds have been found that may offer potential using these criteria, which function as inhibitors of arenavirus fusion.

Another target being investigated for anti-arenavirus activity is the cellular protease SKI-1/S1P, which acts on the arenavirus GP precursor protein to a produce fusion-ready GP complex. As a host cell protein, the protease is involved processing a number of host proteins including the sterol regulatory element-binding proteins, activating transcription factor 6, and in parts of lipid metabolism (Lee 2010). Other viral envelopes proteins are processed using SKI-1/S1P include the highly pathogenic, tick-borne bunyavirus Crimean Congo hemorrhagic fever virus (Vincent et al. 2003). Because SKI-S1P performs important host cellular functions, inhibitors need to be found that have high effects in processing arenavirus and as low as possible in its effect upon host cell function. As it is likely that the length of therapy of these inhibitors will be short and the mortality of these viruses is high, compounds such as PF-429242 are being investigated. This aminopyrrolidine amide compound has been able to prevent glycoprotein processing of LCM virus and Lassa fever virus in a cell culture model (Urata et al. 2011).

3.8   PREVENTIVE MEASURES

As LCM is quite widespread in mice, prevention of laboratory-acquired infection involves institution of policies to prevent introduction into the animal population. These policies include seromonitoring of rodents from both commercial suppliers and intramural breeding colonies as well as testing of tumors to be implanted into the mice for virus. Even with these monitoring procedures, introduction of LCM into a laboratory murine facility can occur (Smith et al. 1984). In this introduction, which did not involve human cases, the source was not recognized but may have been from a feral mouse and resulted in depopulation of the facility.

The classical public health principles of infection control should be facilitated in any patient with an illness and appropriate epidemiology compatible with viral hemorrhagic fever. Isolation includes parenteral and droplet precautions, but it is likely that strict universal precautions are likely to be effective (Fisher-Hoch 1993). Small-particle-aerosol precautions using an HEPA filter mask are used in procedures that can generate aerosols, such as endotracheal intubation. Disinfection of items that had direct contact with the patient, including chemical or heat inactivation of human waste, is also suggested.

3.8.1   Vaccines

Despite the ubiquitous distribution of LCM virus and the significant number of arenavirus hemorrhagic fevers, until the late 1990s, no vaccine had truly been successful in preventing these viral infections. In 1998, Maiztegui et al. reported a prospective, randomized, and double-blind, placebo-controlled efficacy study of Candid1, a live, attenuated Junin virus vaccine. In a study involving 6500 male agricultural workers in the disease endemic area, 23 study individuals developed laboratory-confirmed Argentine hemorrhagic fever. Of these, all but one had placebo (protective efficacy 95% with a 95% confidence interval of 82%–99%). Three individuals in each group developed mild infections that did not reach the case definition of hemorrhagic fever. These additional cases produced a protective efficacy for the prevention of any illness linked to Junin virus infection of 84% (95% confidence limits, 60% to 94%). The vaccination was well tolerated, with only 1% reporting adverse effects temporally related to the vaccine administration.

The vaccine strain differed from wild-type by only 6 amino acids, and the attenuation appeared to be related to a single amino acid substitution in the transmembrane domain of the G2 glycoprotein transmembrane domain (Albariño et al. 2011). The mutation (F427I) produces a destabilization of the glycoprotein metastable confirmation. Additionally, the mutation produces an increased dependence on the transferring receptor type 1 for entrance to host cells, affecting the tropism of the vaccine strain (Droniou-Bonzom et al. 2011). Initially produced in the United States, an Argentine-manufactured Candid1 vaccine is now available and appears to be equivalent to the original biologic (Enria et al. 2010).

Several prototypic vaccines have been studied in the search for a vaccine against Lassa fever. These include a recombinant vesicular stomatitis virus vector expressing Lassa viral glycoprotein, which was able to elicit a protective immune response in nonhuman primates (Geisbert et al. 2006); a recombinant yellow fever vaccine virus (the 17D strain) expressing Lassa GP, which protected guinea pigs (Bredenbeek et al. 2006), and an attenuated recombinant Lassa/Mopeia virus, which can protect both guinea pigs and nonhuman primates (Lukashevich et al. 2008).

As reviewed by Shedlock et al. (2011), numerous candidate vaccines have been studied against the LCM virus. These include infectious vaccine platforms including recombinant viruses such as vaccinia, adenovirus, and influenza and recombinant bacterial platforms including *Salmonella* and *Listeria* as well as subunit vaccines involving GP, NP, and virus DNA. Shedlock et al. (2011) reported on a highly optimized DNA vaccine that conferred complete protection against a high-dose lethal LCM virus challenge in mice. The magnitudes of both cellular and humoral immune responses in the mice were robust, approaching that found in natural LCM infection.

Additionally, a multivalent vaccine has been studied against arenaviruses associated with human disease. The technique utilized well-conserved epitopes and a number of epitopes specific for the multiple arenavirus species used combined into a vaccinia virus platform. Mice immunized with this "cocktail" vaccine produced T-cell responses against LCM virus, Lassa, Junin, Guanarito, Machupo, Sabia, and Whitewater Arroyo viruses and protected mice against challenge (Kotturi et al. 2009).

3.9 ANTIVIRAL POSTEXPOSURE PROPHYLAXIS

Suggested postexposure prophylaxis (PEP) for arenaviruses aims primarily for Lassa fever although can be applied to the other hemorrhagic fever viruses empirically. Bausch et al. (2010) recommends using ribavirin only in the event of a real high-risk exposure (Table 3.7), especially in the setting of exposure to patients with

TABLE 3.7
Definitive High-Risk Exposures to High Viremic Lassa Fever Infection

1. Prolonged (for hours) and continuous contact in an enclosed space to a patient with Lassa fever without the use of personal protective equipment (PPE).
2. Participation in emergency procedures such as suctioning, intubation, and resuscitation after cardiac arrest without the use of appropriate PPE.
3. Penetration of skin by a contaminated sharp instrument such as a blood-contaminated needle.
4. Contamination of mucosal surfaces or broken skin with blood or body fluids such as a blood splash in the eyes or mouth.

Source: Bausch, D.G. et al., 2010, *Clin. Infect. Dis.* 51, 1435–1441. With permission.

severe symptomatology that occurs late in the disease with the highest levels of viremia. There are no suggestions of using PEP during the incubation period or after recovery. The only exception to late PEP use is in the setting of sexual transmission as significantly delayed times of viral eradication (although no more than 3 months) can occur in the gonads (WHO 2000). An oral regimen of a 35-mg/kg loading dose (maximum dose 2500 mg) is given to be followed with 15 mg/kg (maximum dose 1000 mg) 3 times daily for 10 days. A usual adult dose is 2400 mg followed by 1000 mg three times daily. The general form of oral ribavirin consists of a 200-mg tablet. Even if not totally effective, oral PEP should substantially decrease viremia and, as a consequence, lower morbidity and mortality. Dosing requires downward adjustment in persons with creatinine clearances of less than 50 mL/min.

3.10 FUTURE PERSPECTIVES

New arenaviruses continue to be recognized with a rate of one every 1–2 years. A majority of the isolates are from rodents without known human infection. Many other arenaviruses remain unrecognized, and especially as mankind invades areas where some of these agents are endemic, the distinct possibility of new zoonotic infections exists either in sporadic or outbreak form. Human behavior such as deforestation replacing wooded lands with agricultural fields and pastures with adjacent human habitats is a classical scenario for the type of ecology change to produce such infections. As stated by Tesh (2002), "The arenaviruses are very old and probably evolved with their rodent hosts; but when people change the ecology, allowing an increase in the abundance of the rodent hosts, the risk of human–virus contact increases."

Additionally, it is well recognized that, as occurs with influenza viruses, genetic reassortments of arenaviruses can occur with the two single-stranded RNAs. Rivere and Oldstone (1986) studied this process in LCM virus and found that reassortants can cause lethal infection in mice, whereas neither the parent strains nor the reciprocal reassortants did. The authors suggest that such alterations could account for unanticipated outbreaks of virulence by an arenavirus. This seems to have occurred in the natural outbreak of Lassa fever with reassortment *in vivo* of different isolates of the virus (Jahrling et al. 1985b). Whether reassortment can occur between arenaviruses is not as clear. It is important to note that depending upon the diagnostic assay used, such viruses may not be easily differentiated from the wild type strains.

Finally, on a darker aspect, certain arenavirus hemorrhagic fever (Junin, Machupo, and Lassa) agents have been deemed category A bioterrorism pathogens. As discussed by Bausch and Peters (2009), although there is no record of deployment of a hemorrhagic fever virus as a weapon, research and development aimed to weaponize these agents is reported to have taken place in the former Soviet Union and the United States prior to the abolition of these activities. It is not known that any country is covertly developing these agents as weapons, but real concerns persist regarding clandestine activity using stocks produced during the Soviet era that may not have been destroyed with the fall of the former Soviet Union. Additionally, the Japanese cult group that successfully released neurotoxic gas on the Tokyo subway and attempted to release aerosols of anthrax spores attempted to acquire Ebola virus, a filovirus causing hemorrhagic fever. Possible scenarios for the dissemination of these agents, either singly or in combination, include (Bausch and Peters 2009) implantation of infected humans in the community or hospitals to initiate person-to-person transmission, release of an infected reservoir into a "virgin" environment, and direct dissemination of the virus through artificially produced aerosols or fomites.

REFERENCES

Al-Zein, N., Boyce, T.G., Correa, A.G., Rodriguez, V. 2008. Meningitis caused by lymphocytic choriomeningitis virus in a patient with leukemia. *J. Pediatr. Hematol. Oncol.* 30, 781–784.

Albariño, C.G., Bird, B.H., Chakrabarti, A.K., Dodd, K.A., Flint, M., Bergeron, E., White, D.M., Nichol, S.T. 2011. The major determinant of attenuation in mice of the Candid1 vaccine for Argentine hemorrhagic fever is located in the G2 glycoprotein transmembrane domain. *J. Virol.* 85, 10404–10408.

Albariño, C.G., Palacios, G., Khristova, M.L., Erickson, B.R., Carroll, S.A., Comer, J.A., Hui, J., Briese, T., St. George, K., Ksiazek, T.G., Lipkin, W.I., Nichol, S.T. 2010. High diversity and ancient common ancestry of lymphocytic choriomeningitis virus. *Emerg. Infect. Dis.* 16, 1093–1100.

Ambrosio, A.M., Feuillade, M.R., Gamboa, G.S., Maiztegui, J.I. 1994. Prevalence of lymphocytic choriomeningitis virus infection in a human population of Argentina. *Am. J. Trop. Med. Hyg.* 50, 381–386.

Amman, B.R., Pavlin, B.I., Albariño, C.G., Comer, J.A., Erickson, B.R., Oliver, J.B., Sealy, T.K., Vincent, M.J., Nichol, S.T., Paddock, C.D., Tumpey, A.J., Wagoner, K.D., Glauer, R.D., Smith, K.A., Winpisinger, K.A., Parsely, M.S., Wyrick, P., Hannafin, C.H., Bandy, U., Zaki, S., Rollin, P.E., Ksiazek, T.G. 2007. Pet rodents and fatal lymphocytic choriomeningitis in transplant patients. *Emerg. Infect. Dis.* 13, 719–725.

Armstrong, C., Lillie, R.D. 1934. Experimental lymphocytic choriomeningitis of monkeys and mice produced by a virus encountered in studies of the 1933 St. Louis encephalitis epidemic. *Pub. Health. Rep.* 49, 1019–1027.

Armstrong, C., Wooley, J.G. 1935. Studies on the origin of a newly discovered virus which causes lymphocytic choriomeningitis in experimental animals. *Pub. Health. Rep.* 50, 537–541.

Avila, M.M., Samoilovich, S.R., Laguens, R.P., Merani, M.S., Weissenbacher, M.C. 1987. Protection of Junin virus-infected marmosets by passive administration of immune serum: association with late neurologic signs. *J. Med. Virol.* 21, 67–74.

Barton, L.L., Mets, M.B. 2001. Congenital lymphocytic choriomeningitis virus infection: decade of rediscovery. *Clin. Infect. Dis.* 33, 370–374.

Bausch, D.G., Hadi, C.M., Khan, S.H., Lertora, J.J. 2010. Review of the literature and proposed guidelines for the use of oral ribavirin as postexposure prophylaxis for Lassa fever. *Clin. Infect. Dis.* 51, 1435–1441.

Baum, S., Lewis, A.M., Jr., Rowe, W.P., Huebner, R.J. 1966. Epidemic nonmeningitis lymphocytic choriomeningitis-virus infection: an outbreak in a population of laboratory personnel. *N. Engl. J. Med.* 274, 934–936.

Bausch, D.G., Rollin, P.E., Demby, A.H., Coulibaly, M., Kanu, J., Conteh, A.S., Wagoner, K.D., McMullan, L.K., Bowen, M.D., Peters, C.J., Ksiazek, T.G. 2000. Diagnosis and clinical virology of Lassa fever as evaluated by enzyme-linked immunosorbent assay, indirect fluorescent-antibody test, and virus isolation. *J. Clin. Microbiol.* 38, 2670–2677.

Bausch, D.G., Peters, C.J. 2009. The viral hemorrhagic fevers. In: *Beyond Anthrax: The Weaponization of Infectious Diseases.* Lutwick L.I., Lutwick S.M. (Eds). Humana Press: New York, pp. 107–144.

Biggar, R.J., Woodall, J.P., Walter, P.D., Haughie, G.E. 1975. Lymphocytic choriomeningitis outbreak associated with pet hamsters. Fifty-seven cases from New York State. *JAMA* 232, 494–500.

Birmingham, K., Kenyon, G. 2001. Lassa fever is unheralded problem in West Africa. *Nature Med.* 7, 878.

Bonhomme, C.J., Capul, A.A., Lauron, E.J., Bederka, L.H., Knopp, K.A., Buchmeier, M.J. 2011. Glycosylation modulates arenavirus glycoprotein expression and function. *Virology* 409, 223–232.

Bonthius, D.J., Mahoney, J., Buchmeier, M.J., Karacay, B., Taggard, D. 2002. Critical role for glial cells in the propagation and spread of lymphocytic choriomeningitis virus in the developing rat brain. *J. Virol.* 76, 6618–6635.

Bonthius, D.J., Nichols, B., Harb, H., Mahoney, J., Karacay, B. 2007b. Lymphocytic choriomeningitis virus infection of the developing brain: critical role of host age. *Ann. Neurol.* 62, 356–374.

Bonthius, D.J., Perlman, S. 2007. Congenital viral infections of the brain: lessons learned from lymphocytic choriomeningitis virus in the neonatal rat. *PLoS Pathogens* 3, e149. Doi:10.1371/journal.ppat.0030149.

Bonthius, D.J., Wright, R., Tseng, B., Barton, L., Marco, E., Karacay, B., Larsen, P.D. 2007a. Congenital lymphocytic choriomeningitis virus infection: spectrum of disease. *Ann. Neurol.* 62, 347–355.

Borrow, P., Oldstone, M.B.A. 1994. Mechanism of lymphocytic choriomeningitis virus entry into cells. *Virology* 198, 1–9.

Bredenbeek, P.J., Molenkamp, R., Spaan, W.J., Deubel, V., Marianneau, P., Salvato, M.S., Moshkoff, D., Zapata, J., Tikhonov, I., Patterson, J., Carrion, R., Ticer, A., Brasky, K., Lukashevich, I.S. 2006. A recombinant yellow fever 17D vaccine expressing Lassa virus glycoproteins. *Virology* 345, 299–304.

Burns, J.W., Buchmeier, M.J. 1991. Protein-protein interactions in lymphocytic choriomeningitis virus. *Virology* 183, 620–629.

Centers for Disease Control and Prevention. 1994. Bolivian hemorrhagic fever—El Beni Department, Bolivia, 1994. *Morbid. Mortal. Week. Rep.* 43, 443–446.

Centers for Disease Control and Prevention. 2000. Fatal illnesses associated with a new world arenavirus—California, 1999–2000. *Morbid. Mortal. Week. Rep.* 49, 709–711.

Centers for Disease Control and Prevention. 2004. Imported Lassa fever—New Jersey, 2004. *Morbid. Mortal. Week. Rep.* 53, 894–897

Charrel, R.N., de Lamballerie, X. 2003. Arenaviruses other than Lassa virus. *Antiviral Res.* 57, 89–100.

Charrel, R.N., de Lamballerie, X. 2010. Zoonotic aspects of arenavirus infections. *Vet. Microbiol.* 140, 213–220.

Childs, J.E., Glass, G.E., Korch, G.W., Ksiazek, T.G., Leduc, J.W. 1992. Lymphocytic choriomeningitis virus infection and house mouse (*Mus musculus*) distribution in urban Baltimore. *Am. J. Trop. Med. Hyg.* 47, 27–34.

Childs, J.E., Glass, G.E., Ksiazek, T.G., Rossi, C.A., Oro, J.G., Leduc, J.W. 1991. Human-rodent contact and infection with lymphocytic choriomeningitis and Seoul viruses in an inner-city population. *Am. J. Trop. Med. Hyg.* 44, 117–121.

Cummins, D., Bennett, D., Fisher-Hoch, S.P., Farrar, B., Machin, S.J., McCormick, J.B. 1992. Lassa fever encephalopathy: clinical and laboratory features. *J. Trop. Med. Hyg.* 95, 197–201.

Cummins, D., McCormick, J.B., Bennett, D., Samba, J.A., Farrar, B., Machin, S.J., Fisher-Hoch, S.P. 1990. Acute sensorineural deafness in Lassa fever. *JAMA* 264, 2093–2096.

de Manzione, N., Salas, R.A., Paredes, H, Godoy, O., Rojas, L., Araoz, F., Fulhorst, C.F., Ksiazek, T.G., Mills, J.N., Ellis, B.A., Peters, C.J., Tesh, R.B. 1998. Venezuelan hemorrhagic fever: clinical and epidemiological studies of 165 cases. *Clin. Infect. Dis.* 26, 308–313.

Deibel, R., Woodall, J.P., Decher, W.J., Schryver, G.D. 1975. Lymphocytic choriomeningitis virus in man. Serologic evidence of association with pet hamsters. *JAMA* 232, 501–504.

Droniou-Bonzom, M.E., Reignier, T., Oldenburg, J.E., Cox, A.U., Exline, C.M., Rathbun, J.Y., Cannon, P.M. 2011. Substitutions in the glycoprotein (GP) of the Candid#1 vaccine strain of Junin virus increase dependence on human transferring receptor 1 and destabilize the metastable conformation of GP. *J. Virol.* 85, 13457–13462.

Dummer, C.M. 1937. Benign lymphocytic meningitis. *JAMA* 108, 633–636.

Dykewicz, C.A., Dato, V.M., Fisher-Hoch, S.P., Howarth, M.V., Perez-Oronoz, G.I., Ostroff, S.M., Gary, H., Jr., Schonberger, L.B., McCormick, J.B. 1992. Lymphocytic choriomeningitis outbreak associated with nude mice in a research institute. *JAMA* 267, 1349–1353.

Eichler, R., Lenz, O., Strecker, T., Eickmann, M., Klenk, H.D., Garten, W. 2003. Identification of Lassa virus glycoprotein signal peptide as a trans-acting maturation factor. *EMBO Rep.* 4, 1084–1088.

el Karamany, R.M., Imam, I.Z. 1991. Antibodies to lymphocytic choriomeningitis virus in wild rodent sera in Egypt. *J. Hyg. Epidemiol. Microbiol. Immunol.* 35, 97–103.

Emonet, S.F., de la Torre, J.C., Domingo, E., Sevilla, N. 2009. Arenavirus genetic diversity and its biological implications. *Infect. Genet. Evol.* 9, 417–429.

Emonet, S., Lemasson, J.J., Gonzalez, J.P., de Lamballerie, X., Charrel, R.N. 2006. Phylogeny and evolution of old world arenaviruses. *Virology* 350, 251–257.

Enria, D.A., Ambrosio, A.M., Briggiler, A.M., Feuillade, M.R., Crivelli, E., Study Group on Argentine Hemorrhagic Fever. 2010. Candid#1 vaccine against Argentine hemorrhagic fever produced in Argentina: immunogenicity and safety. *Medicina—Buenos Aires* 70, 215–222.

Enria, D.A., Briggiler, A.M., Fernandez, N.J., Levis, S.C., Maiztegui, J.I. 1984. Importance of dose of neutralising antibodies in treatment of Argentine haemorrhagic fever with immune plasma. *Lancet* 324, 255–256.

Enria, D.A., Maiztegui, J.I. 1994. Antiviral treatment of Argentine hemorrhagic fever. *Antiviral Res.* 23, 23–31.

Fischer, S.A., Graham, M.B., Kuehnert, M.J., Kotton, C.N., Srinivasan, A., Marty, F.M., Comer, J.A., Guarner, J., Paddock, C.D., DeMeo, D.L., Shieh, W.J., Erickson, B.R., Bandy, U., DeMaria, A., Jr., Davis, J.P., Delmonico, F.L., Pavlin, B., Likos, A., Vincent, M.J., Sealy, T.K., Goldsmith, C.S., Jernigan, D.B., Rollin, P.E., Packard, M.M., Patel, M., Rowland, C., Helfand, R.F., Nichol, S.T., Fishman, J.A., Ksiazek, T., Zaki, S.R. 2006. Transmission of lymphocytic choriomeningitis virus by organ transplantation. *N. Engl. J. Med.* 354, 2235–2249.

Fisher-Hoch, S. 1993. Stringent precautions are not advisable when caring for patients with viral hemorrhagic fevers. *Med. Virol.* 3, 7–13.

Garcia, C.C., Djavani, M., Topisirovic, I., Borden, K.L., Salvato, M.S., Damonte, E.B. 2006. Arenavirus Z protein as an antiviral target: virus inactivation and protein oligomerization by zinc finger-reactive compounds. *J. Gen. Virol.* 87, 1217–1228.

Garcia, C.C., Topisirovic, I., Djavani, M., Borden, K.L., Damonte, E.B., Salvato, M.S. 2010, An antiviral disulfide compound blocks interactions between arenavirus Z protein and cellular promyelocytic leukemia protein. *Acta Biochem. Biophys. Res. Commun.* 393, 625–630.

Gautam, A., Fischer, S.A., Yango, A.F., Gohh, R.Y., Morrissey, P.E., Monaco, A.P. 2007. Suppression of cell-mediated immunity by a donor-transmitted lymphocytic choriomeningitis virus in a kidney transplant recipient. *Transplant. Infect. Dis.* 9, 339–342.

Geisbert, T.W., Jones, S., Fritz, E.A., Shurtleff, A.C., Geisbert, J.B., Liebscher, R., Grolla, A., Ströher, U., Fernando, L., Daddario, K.M., Guttieri, M.C., Mothé, B.R., Larsen, T., Hensley, L.E., Jahrling, P.B., Feldmann, H. 2006. Development of a new vaccine for the prevention of Lassa fever. *PLoS Med.* 2, e183.

Gowen, B.B., Smee, D.F., Wong, M.H., Hall, J.O., Jung, K.H., Bailey, K.W., Stevens, J.R., Furuta, Y., Morrey, J.D. 2008. Treatment of late stage disease in a model of arenaviral hemorrhagic fever: T-705 efficacy and reduced toxicity suggests an alternative to ribavirin. *PLoS One* 11, e3725.

Hinman, A.R., Sikora, E., Kinch, W., Hinman, A., Woodall, J. 1975. Outbreak of lymphocytic choriomeningitis virus infections in medical center personnel. *Am. J. Epidemiol.* 101, 103–110.

Horton, J., Hotchin, J.E., Olson, K.B., Davies, J.N. 1971. The effects of MP virus infection in lymphoma. *Cancer Res.* 31, 1066–1068.

Hotchin, J., Sikora, E., Kinch, W., Hinman, A., Woodall, J. 1974. Lymphocytic choriomeningitis in a hamster colony causes infection of hospital personnel. *Science* 185, 1173–1174.

Hughes, W. 1937. Acute lymphocytic meningitis. *Br. Med. J.* 1, 1063–1065.

Jahrling, P.B., Frame, J.D., Rhoderick, J.B., Monson, M.H. 1985a. Endemic Lassa fever in Liberia. IV. Selection of optimally effective plasma for treatment by passive immunization. *Trans. R. Soc. Trop. Med. Hyg.* 79, 380–384.

Jahrling, P.B., Frame, J.D., Smith, S.B., Monson, M.H. 1985b. Endemic Lassa fever in Liberia, III. Characterization of Lassa virus isolates. *Trans. R. Soc. Trop. Med. Hyg.* 79, 374–377.

Jahrling, P.B., Niklasson, B.S., McCormick, J.B. 1985c. Early diagnosis of human Lassa fever by ELISA detection of antigen and antibody. *Lancet* 325, 250–252.

Jahrling, P.B., Peters, C.J. 1984. Passive antibody therapy of Lassa fever in cynomolgus monkeys: importance of neutralizing antibody and Lassa virus strain. *Infect. Immun.* 44, 528–533.

Kenyon, R.H., Green, D.E., Eddy, G.A., Peters, C.J. 1986. Treatment of Junin virus-infected guinea pigs with immune serum: development of late neurological disease. *J. Med. Virol.* 20, 207–218.

Kilgore, P.E., Ksiazek, T.G., Rollin, P.E., Mills, J.N., Villagra, M.R., Montenegro, M.J., Costales, M.A., Paredes, L.C., Peters, C.J. 1997. Treatment of Bolivian hemorrhagic fever with intravenous ribavirin. *Clin. Infect. Dis.* 24, 718–722.

Komrower, G., Williams, B.L., Stones, P.B. 1955. Lymphocytic choriomeningitis in the newborn. *Lancet* 1, 697–698.

Kotturi, M.F., Botten, J., Sidney, J., Bui, H.H., Giancola, L., Maybeno, M., Babin, J., Oseroff, C., Pasquetto, V., Greenbaum, J.A., Peters, B., Ting, J., Do, D., Vang, L, Alexander, J., Grey, H., Buchmeier, M.J., Sette, A. 2009. A multivalent and cross-protective vaccine strategy against arenaviruses associated with human disease. *PLoS Pathog.* 5, e1000695.

Kranzusch, P.J., Whelan, S.P.J. 2011. Arenavirus Z protein controls viral RNA synthesis by locking a polymerase-promoter complex. *Proc. Natl. Acad. Sci. USA* 108, 19743–19748.

Kunz, S., Edelmann, K.H., de la Torre, J.C., Gorney, R., Oldstone, M.B. 2003. Mechanisms for lymphocytic choriomeningitis virus glycoprotein cleavage, transport, and incorporation into virions. *Virology* 314, 178–183.

Kunz, S., Sevilla, N., Rojek, J.M., Oldstone, M.B. 2004. Use of alternative receptors different than alpha-dystroglycan by selected isolates of lymphocytic choriomeningitis virus. *Virology* 325, 432–445.

Lee, A.M. 2010. Novel approaches in anti-arenaviral drug development. *Virology* 411, 163–169.

Lepine, P., Mollaret, P., Kreis, B. 1937. Réceptivité de l'homme au virus murin de la chorioméningite lymphocytaire. Reproduction expérimentale de la méningite lymphocytaire benigne. *Compt. Rend. Soc. Biol.* 204, 1846–1850.

Leung, W.-C., Rawls, W.E. 1977. Virion-associated ribosomes are not required for the replication of Pichinde virus. *Virology* 81, 174–176.

Lewis, A.M., Jr., Rowe, W.P., Turner, H.C., Huebner, R.J. 1965. Lymphocytic choriomeningitis virus in hamster tumor: spread to hamsters and humans. *Science* 150, 363–364.

Lledó, L., Gegúndez, M.I., Saz, J.V., Bahamontes, N., Beltrán, M. 2003. Lymphocytic choriomeningitis virus infection in a province of Spain: analysis of sera from the general population and wild rodents. *J. Med. Virol.* 70, 273–275.

Lozano, M.E., Ghiringhelli, P.D., Romanowski, V., Grau, O. 1993. A simple nucleic acid amplification for the rapid detection of Junin virus in whole blood samples. *Virus Res.* 27, 37–53.

Lukashevich, I.S., Carrion, R., Jr., Salvato, M.S., Mansfield, K., Brasky, K., Zapata, J., Cairo, C., Goicochea, M., Hoosien, G.E., Ticer, A., Bryant, J., Davis, H., Hammamieh, R., Mayda, M., Jett, M., Patterson, J. 2008. Safety, immunogenicity and efficacy of the ML29 reassortment vaccine for Lassa fever in small non-human primates. *Vaccine* 26, 5246–5254.

Maetz, H.M., Sellers, C.A., Bailey, W.C., Hardy, G.E., Jr. 1976. Lymphocytic choriomeningitis from pet hamster exposure: a local public health experience. *Am. J. Publ. Health* 66, 1082–1085.

Maiztegui, J., Fernandez, N.J., de Damilano, A.J. 1979. Efficacy of immune plasma in treatment of Argentine haemorrhagic fever and association between treatment and a late neurological syndrome. *Lancet* 314, 1216–1217.

Maiztegui, J., Feuillade, M., Briggiler, A. 1986. Progressive extension of the endemic area and changing incidence of Argentine hemorrhagic fever. *Med. Microbiol. Immunol.* 175, 149–152.

Maiztegui, J.I., McKee, K.T., Jr., Barrera Oro, J.G., Harrison, L.H., Gibbs, P.H., Feuillade, M.R., Enria, D.A., Briggiler, A.M., Levis, S.C., Ambrosio, A.M., Halsey, N.A., Peters, C.J. 1998. Protective efficacy of a live attenuated vaccine against Argentine hemorrhagic fever. *J. Infect. Dis.* 177, 277–83.

Marrie, T.J., Saron, M.-F. 1998. Seroprevalence of lymphocytic choriomeningitis virus in Nova Scotia. *Am. J. Trop. Med. Hyg.* 58, 47–49.

McCormick, J.B., King, I.J., Webb, P.A., Scribner, C.L., Craven, R.B., Johnson, K.M., Elliott, L.H., Belmont-Williams, R. 1986. Lassa fever: effective therapy with ribavirin. *N. Engl. J. Med.* 314, 20–26.

McCormick, J.B., King, I.J., Webb, P.A., Johnson, K.M., O'Sullivan, R., Smith, E.S., Trippel, S., Tong, T.C. 1987a. A case-control study of the clinical diagnosis and course of Lassa fever. *J. Infect. Dis.* 155, 445–455.

McCormick, J.B., Webb, P.A., Krebs, J.W., Johnson, K.M., Smith, E.S. 1987b. A prospective study of the epidemiology and ecology of Lassa fever. *J. Infect. Dis.* 155, 437–444.

Mendenhall, M., Russell, A., Juelich, T., Messina, E.L., Smee, D.F., Freiberg, A.N., Holbrook, M.R., Furuta, Y., de la Torre, J.C., Nunberg, J.H., Gowen, B.B. 2011a. T-705 (favipiravir) inhibition of arenavirus replication in cell culture. *Antimicrob. Agents Chemother.* 55, 782–787.

Mendenhall, M., Russell, A., Smee, D.F., Hall, J.O., Skirpstunas, R., Furuta, Y., Gowen, B.B. 2001b. Effective oral favipiravir (T-705) therapy initiated after the onset of clinical disease in a model of arenavirus hemorrhagic fever. *PLoS Negl. Trop. Dis.* 5, e1342.

Mills, J.N., Ellis, B.A., McKee, K.T., Jr., Ksiazek, T.G., Oro, J.G., Maiztegui, J.I., Calderon, G.E., Peters, C.J., Childs, J.E. 1991. Junin virus activity in rodents from endemic and nonendemic loci in central Argentina. *Am. J. Trop. Med. Hyg.* 44, 589–597.

Molomut, N., Padnos, M. 1965. Inhibition of transplantable and spontaneous murine tumors by the MP virus. *Nature* 208, 948–950.

Moraz, M.-L., Kunz, S. 2011. Pathogenesis of arenavirus hemorrhagic fever. *Expert Rev. Anti-Infect. Ther.* 9, 49–59.

Morita, C., Matsuura, Y., Kawashima, E., Takahashi, S., Kawaguchi, J., Iida, S., Yamanaka, T., Jitsukawa, W. 1991. Seroepidemiological survey of lymphocytic choriomeningitis in wild house mouse (*Mus musculus*) in Yokohama port, Japan. *J. Vet. Med. Sci.* 53, 219–222.

Palacios, G., Druce, J., Du, L., Tran, T., Birch, C., Briese, T., Conlan, S., Quan, P.L., Hui, J., Marshall, J., Simons, J.F., Egholm, M., Paddock, C.D., Shieh, W.J., Goldsmith, C.S., Zaki, S.R., Catton, M., Lipkin, W.I. 2008. A new arenavirus in a cluster of fatal transplant-associated diseases. *N. Engl. J. Med.* 358, 990–998.

Park, J.Y., Peters, C.J., Rollin, P.E., Ksiazek, T.G., Katholi, C.R., Waites, K.B., Gray, B., Maetz, H.M., Stephensen, C.B. 1997. Age distribution of lymphocytic choriomeningitis virus serum antibody in Birmingham, Alabama: evidence of a decreased risk of infection. *Am. J. Trop. Med. Hyg.* 57, 37–41.

Pasquato, A., Burri, D.J., Traba, E.G., Hanna-El-Daher, L., Seidah, N.G., Kunz, S. 2011. Arenavirus envelope glycoproteins mimic autoprocessing sites of the cellular convertase subtilisin kexin isozyme-1/site-1 protease. *Virology* 417, 18–26.

Pearce, B.P., Steffensen, S.C., Paoletti, A.D., Henriksen, S.J., Buchmeier, M.J. 1996. Persistent dentate granule cell hyperexcitability after neonatal infection with lymphocytic choriomeningitis virus. *J. Neurosci.* 16, 220–228.

Pearce, B.P., Valadi, N.M., Po, C.L., Miller, A.H. 2000. Viral infection of developing GABAergic neurons in a model of hippocampal distribution. *Neuroreport* 11, 2433–2438.

Peters, C.J., Kuehne, R.W., Mercado, R.R., Le Bow, R.H., Spertzel, R.O., Webb, P.A. 1974. Hemorrhagic fever in Cochabamba, Bolivia. *Am. J. Epidemiol.* 99, 425–433.

Radoshitzky, S.R., Abraham, J., Spiropoulou, C.F., Kuhn, J.H., Nguyen, D., Li, W., Nagel, J., Schmidt, P.J., Nunberg, J.H., Andrews, N.C., Farzan, M., Choe, H. 2007. Transferrin receptor 1 is a cellular receptor for New World haemorrhagic fever arenaviruses. *Nature* 446, 92–96.

Reed, K.D., Melski, J.W., Graham, M.B., Regnery, R.L., Sotir, M.J., Wegner, M.V., Kazmierczak, J.J., Stratman, E.J., Li, Y., Fairley, J.A., Swain, G.R., Olson, V.A., Sargent, E.K., Kehl, S.C., Frace, M.A., Kline, R., Foldy, S.L., Davis, J.P., Damon, I.K. 2004. The detection of monkeypox in humans in the Western Hemisphere. *N. Engl. J. Med.* 350, 342–350.

Riviere, Y., Oldstone, M.B.A. 1986. Genetic reassortants of lymphocytic choriomeninigitis: unexpected disease and mechanism of pathogenesis. *J. Virol.* 59, 363–368.

Roebroek, R.M.J.A., Postma, B.H., Dijkstra, U.J. 1994. Aseptic meningitis caused by lymphocytic choriomeningitis virus. *Clin. Neurol. Neurosurg.* 96, 178–180.

Schmitz, H., Köhler, B., Laue, T., Drosten, C., Veldkamp, P.J., Günther, S., Emmerich, P., Geisen, H.P., Fleischer, K., Beersma, M.F., Hoerauf, A. 2002. Monitoring of clinical and laboratory data in two cases of imported Lassa fever. *Microbes Infect.* 4, 43–50.

Shedlock, D.J., Talbott, K.T., Cress, C., Ferraro, B., Tuyishme, S., Mallilankaraman, K., Cisper, N.J., Morrow, M.P., Wu, S.J., Kawalekar, O.U., Khan, A.S., Sardesai, N.Y., Muthumani, K., Shen, H., Weiner, D.B. 2011. A highly optimized DNA vaccine confers complete protective immunity against high-dose lethal lymphocytic choriomeningitis virus challenge. *Vaccine* 29, 6755–6762.

Smith, A.L., Paturzo, F.X., Gardner, E.P., Morgenstern, S., Cameron, G., Wadley, H. 1984. Two epizootics of lymphocytic choriomeningitis virus occurring in laboratory mice despite intensive monitoring programs. *Can. J. Comp. Med.* 48, 335–337.

Strecker, T., Eichler, R., Meulen, J., Weissenhorn, W., Klenk, H.D., Garten, W., Lenz, O. 2003. Lassa virus Z protein is a metrix protein and sufficient for the release of virus-like particles. *J. Virol.* 77, 10700–10705.

Stenglein, M.D., Sanders, C., Kistner, A.L., Ruby, J.G., Franco, J.Y., Reavill, D.R., Dunker, F., DeRisi, J.L. 2012. Identification, characterization, and *in vitro* culture of highly divergent arenaviruses from boa constrictors and annulated tree boas: candidate etiological agents for snake inclusion body disease. *mBio* 3(4):doi:10.1128/mBio.00180-12.

Sullivan, B.M., Emonet, S.F., Welch, M.J., Lee, A.M., Campbell, K.P., de la Torre, J.C., Oldstone, M.B. 2011. Point mutation in the glycoprotein of lymphocytic choriomeningitis virus is necessary for receptor binding, dendritic cell infection, and long-term persistence. *Proc. Natl. Acad. Sci. U S A* 108, 2969–2974.

Tesh, R.B. 1999. Epidemiology of arenaviruses in the Americas. In: Saluzzo, J.F., Dodet B. (Eds). *Emergence and Control of Rodent-Borne Viral Diseases.* Elsevier, Paris, pp. 213–224.

Tesh, R.B. 2002. Viral hemorrhagic fevers of South America. *Biomedica* 22, 287–295.

Urata, S., Yun, N., Pasquato, A., Paessler, S., Kunz, S., de la Torre, J.C. 2011. Antiviral activity of a small-molecule of arenavirus glycoprotein processing by a cellular site 1 protease. *J. Virol.* 85, 795–803.

Vieth, S., Drosten, C., Charrel, R., Feldmann, H., Günther, S. 2005. Establishment of conventional and fluorescence energy transfer-based real-time assays for the detection of pathogenic New World viruses. *J. Clin. Microbiol.* 32, 229–235.

Vieth, S., Drosten, C., Lenz, O., Vincent, M., Omilabu, S., Hass, M., Becker-Ziaja, B., ter Meulen, J., Nichol, S.T., Schmitz, H., Günther, S. 2007. RT-PCR assay of Lassa virus and related Old World arenaviruses targeting the L gene. *Trans. R. Soc. Trop. Med. Hyg.* 101, 1253–1264.

Vincent, M.J., Sanchez, A.J., Erickson, B.R., Basak, A., Chretien, M., Seidah, N.G., Nichol, S.T. 2003. Crimean-Congo hemorrhagic fever virus glycoprotein proteolytic processing by subtilase SKI-1. *J. Virol.* 77, 8640–8649.

Wallgren, A. 1925. Une nouvelle maladie infectieuse du système nerveux central? *Acta Paediatr.* 4, 158–163.

Walker, D.H., McCormick, J.B., Johnson, K.M., Webb, P.A., Komba-Kono, G., Elliott, L.H., Gardner, J.J. 1980. Pathologic and virologic study of fatal Lassa fever in man. *Am. J. Pathol.* 107, 349–356.

Weissenbacher, M.C., Calello, M.A., Merani, M.S., McCormick, J.B., Rodriguez, M. 1986. Therapeutic effect of the antiviral agent ribavirin in Junin virus infection of primates. *J. Med. Virol.* 20, 261–267.

World Health Organization. 2000. *WHO Lassa fever fact sheet No. 179*, Geneva: WHO.

4 Bunyaviruses

Patrik Kilian, Vlasta Danielová, and Daniel Růžek

CONTENTS

4.1 INTRODUCTION

The family Bunyaviridae is one of the largest viral families. At present, more than 350 different bunyaviruses are known to infect animals. Members of the Bunyaviridae family are divided into five genera. Viruses belonging to the Orthobunyavirus, Nairovirus, and Phlebovirus genera are typical arboviruses (i.e., viruses transmitted by arthropods), whereas members of the Hantavirus genus are so-called roboviruses (rodent-borne viruses, since they are transmitted through rodent excrement). The last genus in the Bunyaviridae family, Tospovirus, includes viruses that infect plants and these are transmitted mainly by thrips. The family also includes 41 unassigned viruses with an unclear taxonomic classification. Uukuvirus, which was previously assigned to a separate genus, is now included in the Phlebovirus genus. Although there are several bunyaviruses that can infect humans, only a few of them are associated with infections of the central nervous system (CNS). This chapter mainly focuses on members of the Orthobunyavirus genus and to a lesser extent the Phlebovirus genus, which are both known to cause human neuroinfections.

4.2   GENERAL PROPERTIES OF BUNYAVIRUSES

4.2.1   STRUCTURE OF THE VIRAL PARTICLE

The structure of the viral particle is analogous across the genera of the Bunyaviridae family. The majority of the data that are available focuses on the virus Bunyamwera (BUNV), a prototype virus of the Bunyaviridae family. The virions have a spherical shape and a diameter that is approximately 100 nm in length (Figure 4.1) (Obijeski et al. 1977). Under the electron microscope, typical spikes of approximately 10 nm in size can be seen; these are formed by two viral glycoproteins, Gn and Gc (formerly G2 and G1 according to their migration in acrylamide gel). The viral genome consists of three segments of single-stranded RNA of negative polarity. Thus, the viral RNA cannot be directly translated into proteins and is not infectious. Each genomic segment is named according to its size: S (small), M (medium), and L (large). The sizes of the segments differ between genera (Table 4.1). The 5′ and 3′ termini of each segment consist of noncoding sequences (NCR; noncoding region) of various lengths. Approximately 11 terminal bases from both ends are highly conserved and

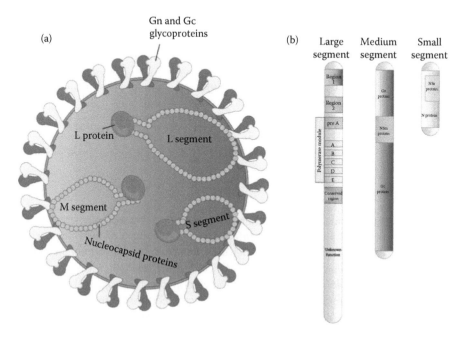

FIGURE 4.1   (a) Schematic drawing of bunyavirus particle; (b) coding region of each genomic segment with regard to the genus Orthobunyavirus.

TABLE 4.1
Differences in Length of Genomic Segments

Genus	Segment	Approximate Length (Bases)
Orthobunyavirus	S	960
	M	4460
	L	6875
Nairovirus	S	1712
	M	4890
	L	12,230
Hantavirus	S	1690
	M	3920
	L	6530
Phlebovirus	S	1720
	M	3230
	L	6430
Tospovirus	S	2915
	M	4820
	L	6890

complementary to each other (Elliott 1990). These complementary sequences allow for the formation of the characteristic panhandle structures shown by the individual genomic segments. These structures can be observed by electron microscopy (Obijeski et al. 1976). In addition, the genomic segments are closely associated with molecules of the structural protein N, and together with the RNA-dependent RNA polymerase (RdRp; called also L protein) they form ribonucleoprotein particles (RNP) (Elliott 1990). The segmented form of the genome facilitates the rapid evolutionary change shown by bunyaviruses due to genomic reassortment.

4.2.2 LARGE GENOMIC SEGMENT

The large genomic segment contains one long open reading frame that encodes one protein (L protein; RdRp). The molecular weight of the L protein is about 259 kDa (in phleboviruses, 241 kDa). The enzyme activity is multifunctional and crucial for the life cycle of the virus. Endonuclease function and possible RNA helicase activity have been revealed. However, most of the active sites on this protein have not been identified so far. Several structural motifs in the RdRp sequence have been identified using in silico methods. The first motifs to be identified, A, B, C, and D (Poch et al. 1989), were thought to represent the core of the polymerase active site. This role was subsequently confirmed experimentally (Jin and Elliott 1992). Two other structural motifs were identified in close proximity to the N terminus of the L protein by Müller et al. (1994). Two additional polymerase module motifs, preA and E, were also identified (Figure 4.1). The function of the conserved region close to the middle of the L protein is unknown (Aquino et al. 2003), and the endonuclease domain was identified within Region 1 (Reguera et al. 2010). The endonuclease activity is dependent on metal ions (especially manganese) and on catalytic lysine 95. No other conserved regions or potential functional domains were described in the second part of the L protein near its C terminus. However, mutants containing a tag in the C terminus of the L protein exhibit restricted growth kinetics in Vero cells and are producers of smaller plaques when compared with the wild type (Shi and Elliott 2009). Recently, it was revealed that the L protein of BUNV is able to repair single nucleotide deletions or insertions in the 5′ and 3′ NCRs (Walter and Barr 2010).

In comparison to other genera of the Bunyaviridae family, nairoviruses have a much larger L genomic segment and have a different composition. The L protein of nairoviruses is almost twice as large, reaching 459 kDa when compared with other bunyaviruses, and exhibits a wide range of enzymatic activity. Interestingly, the amino terminus is predicted to harbor a conserved ovarian tumor (OTU-like) protease, which shows autoproteolytical activity. The major function of the OTU-like domain seems to be autoproteolytical cleaving of the L protein to yield a polymerase and a helicase. Other activities such as deubiquitation have also been proposed (Honig et al. 2004).

4.2.3 MEDIUM GENOMIC SEGMENT

The size of the medium (M) genomic segment varies between genera of the Bunyaviridae family (Table 4.1). The segment has a single open reading frame, which encodes a polyprotein, and is contranslationally cleaved into two structural proteins Gn and Gc. Orthobunyaviruses and tospoviruses encode one additional nonstructural protein, NSm. In orthobunyaviruses, the sequence for NSm is located between the Gn and the Gc genes, whereas in tospoviruses the NSm sequence is encoded in the antisense form (Nichol et al. 2005). A short signal sequence precedes the sequences of each of the proteins. The signal sequence is recognized and cleaved by a host protease (Elliott 1990).

Gc and Gn proteins are type I transmembrane proteins. The N termini of the Gc and Gn proteins are projected onto the surface of the viral particle and the C terminus is integrated into the viral envelope. After translation, both proteins undergo several modifications and accumulate in the membrane of the Golgi apparatus (GA) where virus assembly occurs. The bunyavirus particle does not contain a matrix protein joining RNP with a lipid envelope, but instead a 78-aa-long cytoplasmic tail (CT) of Gn protein that is considered to be crucial for interaction with RNP and further packaging (Överby et al. 2007). The CT plays an important role (probably together with the CT of the Gc protein) during membrane fusion between the host endosome and the viral envelope (Shi et al. 2007). The transmembrane domain (TMD) of the Gn protein is shorter and contains about 18 aa. The TMD contains a signal sequence for the targeting and retention of the Gc–Gn heterodimer in the GA (Shi et al. 2004). Using a reverse genetics approach, the N terminal half of the Gc protein was shown to be dispensable (Shi et al. 2009). Both Gn and Gc proteins are modified by N-linked glycosylations. Deletion of the glycosylation sites in the Gn protein completely alters its folding and transportation to the GA. Glycans attached to the Gc protein play an enhancement role during virus replication (Shi et al. 2005).

The nonstructural protein NSm is a transmembrane protein of approximately 11 kDa and is translocated together with Gc and Gn into the membrane of the GA (Fuller and Bishop 1982; Nakitare and Elliott 1993). Using a hydrophobicity profile prediction, three hydrophobic (I, III, V) and two hydrophilic (II, IV) domains were identified. Although the internal part of the molecule (mainly domain III, but also part of domains II and IV) is dispensable for the viral life cycle, domain I is important for virus maturation. In infected cells, the NSm is found inside unusual tubes associated with the GA (Shi et al. 2006). Members of Tospovirus genus use the NSm to facilitate cell-to-cell transport of the virus through plasmodesmata (Storms et al. 1995).

4.2.4 SMALL GENOMIC SEGMENT

The small (S) genomic segment encodes the structural nucleocapsid protein N. In the case of Orthobunyavirus, Phlebovirus, Tospovirus, and Hantavirus genera, the S segment also encodes one additional protein: the nonstructural protein NSs (Elliott 1990; Jääskeläinen et al. 2007). However, the ORF for this protein is not present in the S segment of Anopheles A, Anopheles B, or the Tete group of the Orthobunyavirus genus (Mohamed et al. 2009).

Nucleocapsid protein N contains approximately 235 aa. The primary function of this protein is to encapsidate both viral RNA (vRNA) and complementary RNA (cRNA) to protect their secondary structure and promote transcription by the L protein. The N protein binds to the RNA on the 5′ end but also binds nonspecifically to other parts of the RNA. The N protein forms long multimers and in this way encapsulates the entire RNA molecule (Leonard et al. 2005; Osbourne and Elliott 2000). In addition to protecting RNA molecules, the N protein also facilitates the formation of the panhandle structure of the RNA and is considered to be an RNA chaperone (Mir and Panganiban 2006). The N protein also interacts with other structural proteins (L, Gc, and Gn) and enables the formation of the ribonucleoprotein and assembly of the viral particle.

The function of the nonstructural protein NSs (12 kDa) is not completely understood. Although NSs is not encoded by all members of the Bunyaviridae family and is not important for virus viability, it can play an important role during the pathogenesis of the infection (Janssen et al. 1986; Bridgen et al. 2001). Sequence homology between the N terminus of NSs and the proapoptotic protein Reaper from *Drosophila* has been reported (Colón-Ramos et al. 2003). *In vitro* experiments showed that NSs induces the release of cytochrome C from the mitochondria of the host cells through binding to the Scythe protein; this triggers caspase activation and ultimately leads to cell apoptosis. Moreover, both NSs protein and Reaper block translation of the cell proteins. *In vivo* experiments with the recombinant Sindbis virus (Togaviridae, Alphavirus) that was modified to express NSs showed induction of neuronal apoptosis when inoculated intracerebrally into suckling mice. However, other experiments with the Bunyamwera virus and La Crosse Virus (LACV) suggested that the NSs protein had an antiapoptotic effect (Kohl et al. 2003; Blaquori et al. 2007). There is evidence to suggest that the NSs protein serves as an important inhibitor of both interferon α and β in infected cells rather than as a modulator of apoptosis (Bridgen et al. 2001; Blaquori et al. 2007).

4.3 REPLICATION IN THE HOST

As is typical for most RNA viruses, the replication of bunyaviruses takes place in the cytoplasm of the host cell (Figure 4.2). The exact manner that is used for bunyavirus cell entry is still not fully understood. Nevertheless, basic similarities to other enveloped viruses can be found. The first step requires the virus particle to attach itself to a specific receptor on the surface of the host cell. Orthobunyaviruses are thought to use protein Gc for this step in both mammalian and insect cells (Hacker et al. 1995), although there are some data to suggest that the Gn protein is involved as a receptor ligand in insect cells (Ludwig et al. 1991). Based on experiments with the Uukuniemi virus, it is known that viral binding to the cell surface is specific but quite inefficient. Receptors on either insect or mammalian cells remain completely unknown. After the virus attaches to the receptor, endocytosis occurs very rapidly (Lozach et al. 2010). The Uukuniemi phlebovirus is internalized by clathrin independent endocytosis, but orthobunyaviruses are internalized by clathrin-coated vesicles (Santos et al. 2008; Lozach et al. 2010). After endocytosis, the virus quickly reaches the endosome. As a consequence of the acidification inside the endosome, Gn and Gc proteins change their conformation and trigger the fusion of the viral envelope with the endosomal membrane, then RNP is released into the cytoplasm of the host cell (Hacker and Hardy 1997). During the membrane fusion, a dominant role is played by the Gc protein, although the interaction with the Gn protein is also important (Jacoby et al. 1993; Plassmeyer et al. 2007; Shi et al. 2007).

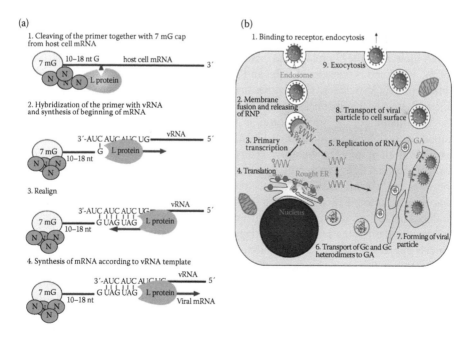

FIGURE 4.2 (a) Basic steps in the initiation of transcription; (b) general overview of bunyavirus replication (in black: replication steps; in gray: cell organelles: ER, endoplasmic reticulum; GA, Golgi apparatus).

Once RNP is released into the cytoplasm, the panhandle structure of the RNA is relaxed and the N proteins dissociate from the 3′ terminus of the RNA. Primary transcription of the vRNA to mRNA occurs in the cytoplasm through the cap-snatch mechanism. The endonuclease activity of the L protein is responsible for cleavage of the 5′ cap together with several nucleotides from selected host mRNAs (Figure 4.2b). The cleaved cap subsequently associates with the vRNA, and this initiates synthesis of the complementary strand. The viral protein N plays an important role in this process as it serves as a cap binding protein (similar to the eukaryotic eIF4E), and helps the L protein to cleave host mRNA (Panganiban and Mir 2009). Some specific host mRNAs are cleaved preferentially; for instance, LACV in mosquito cells utilizes preferable mRNA coding for proteins that are similar to apoptosis inhibitors from *Drosophila* (Borucki et al. 2002). To provide sufficient mRNAs for cleavage, hantaviruses have developed effective strategies for their storage in the cell. After the binding of N protein to the 5′ cap, the mRNAs are translocated to the so-called P-bodies where the mRNA is protected from degradation by binding to a viral nucleocapsid protein (Mir et al. 2008). At the 3′ end of the synthesized RNA, a couple of nucleotides are missed. These missed nucleotides are added by a mechanism called realign, when the L protein slides back to the start of the template vRNA after transcribing several nucleotides (Figure 4.2b) (Jin and Elliott 1993; Garcin et al. 1995). Only vRNA that is associated with an N protein can serve as a template for mRNA transcription (Dunn et al. 1995).

Transcription of the S and L genomic segments is terminated by at least two terminating sequences, which are localized in the 5′ NCR. However, no analogous sequences were found in the M segment (Barr et al. 2006). Immediately after transcription, the translation of viral proteins begins. The translation starts when the N protein associates with the 5′ cap of the mRNA. The N protein mimics the activity of eIF4G (eukaryotic translation initiation factor 4 gamma), which activates the host cell's 43S preinitiation complex and thus facilitates translation (Panganiban and Mir 2009). Replication of the viral genome is started upon primary transcription and occurs through a cRNA intermediate with a positive polarity. Nevertheless, cRNA lacks the 5′ cap and its transcription is primer independent. The mechanism by which the L protein starts the primer independent transcription is poorly understood. It may have some association with the attachment of the N protein (Schmaljohn and Nichol 2007). Viral replication is a complex process and takes place in so-called viral factories. The viral factory is formed by the GA, mitochondria, and rough endoplasmatic reticulum. The key part of the viral factory is an unusual tubular structure that consists of the viral NSm and actin from the host cell that form a connection between the different parts of the replicating complex. Both viral L protein and N protein are held in a globular domain that provides protection to the newly synthesized RNAs, and allows for the formation of RNPs. The RNPs are then transported to the GA along the fibrous structures (Fontana et al. 2008). The glycoproteins Gc and Gn form heterodimers, which are transported via vesicles to the GA, where they wait for the RNPs. After the interaction between the N protein (RNPs) and the glycoproteins, the complex buds into the GA and forms an immature viral particle called an intracellular annular virus. The glycans that are attached to Gc and Gn proteins are further modified during the passage through GA. The first maturation step takes place in the *trans*-GA and produces a dense, intracellular particle. The particles are then transported in vesicles toward the host cell membrane where they undergo a second maturation step that results in the formation of extracellular dense virus particles. After that, the particles are released from the host cell by exocytosis (Salanueva et al. 2003). Interestingly, the lipid envelope of plant tospoviruses is formed by wrapping Golgi membranes around RNPs (Kikkert et al. 1999).

4.3.1 ANTIVIRAL RESPONSE OF INFECTED CELLS

Bunyaviruses have successfully adapted to counteract cell immunity; this is mainly due to the viral NSs protein, which acts as an inhibitor of the interferon (INF) response. In BUNV infected cells, NSs interacts with part of the cell mediator protein, MED8. As a basic component of RNA polymerase II machinery (RNAP II), the mediator protein plays a key role in all transcriptional processes that are performed by RNAP II. The interaction between the C-terminus of the NSs and MED8 inhibits the phosphorylation of serine 2 within RNAP II, which is crucial for mRNA elongation. This mechanism inhibits mRNA transcription in the host cell, including synthesis of INF (Thomas et al. 2004; Leonard et al. 2006). However, different mechanisms of INF response inhibition have been observed in bunyaviruses. The NSs protein of the LACV directly causes RNAP II degradation in a proteasome-dependent manner (Verbruggen et al. 2011). Rift Valley fever virus (RVFV) inhibits the INF response by direct interaction of NSs protein with the host cell transcription factor TFIIH, and this decreases the amount required for mRNA transcription.

The accumulation of viral proteins, maturation and budding of viral particles leads to Golgi apparatus fragmentation and a breakdown of the cell secretory pathway (Salanueva et al. 2003). These processes result in cell death. However, in mosquito cells the situation is completely different. Here, the massive synthesis of viral proteins in the primary phase is followed by a recession, and the infection goes into a persistent phase (Scallan and Elliott 1992). During the primary phase of the infection in mosquito cells *in vitro*, the cells become highly mobile and form projections that connect to other cells. Structures such as microtubules, mitochondria, GA, and lysozymes can be seen in the projections. The viral nonstructural protein NSm was also observed inside these structures. However, it seems that NSm does not enter uninfected cells via the projections. The most probable function of the structures is to deliver warning signals to uninfected cells. Generally, the formation of complexes consisting of N and L viral proteins is considered to be the first phase of persistent infection (López-Montero and Risco 2011). A similar situation can be observed in mammalian cells when the interferon-induced antiviral protein MxA combines with viral protein N and formed complexes are accumulated in the perinuclear area. Since N protein is required for viral replication, its aggregation limits its utilization for viral multiplication (Kochs et al. 2002). Nevertheless, similar proteins that are responsible for the aggregation of L and N proteins in mosquito cells have not yet been identified.

4.3.2 REPLICATION IN MOSQUITO VECTOR

Perhaps, all of the encephalitis bunyaviruses are transmitted by mosquitoes. The mechanism by which viruses multiply in the mosquito body is well understood thanks to studies performed by Dr. Danielová on the Ťahyňa virus (Danielová 1962, 1968). It is important that the virus not only persists in the mosquito but that it replicates without affecting its vector (Elliott and Wilkie 1986; Scallan and Elliott 1992).

Approximately 24 h after the ingestion of an infectious blood meal by the mosquito, the titer of the virus dramatically decreases and the minimum level is reached about 3 or 4 days postfeeding. During this so-called eclipse phase, the titer of the virus is at the minimal level and it is not possible to transmit the infection to the host. Subsequently, the virus starts to multiply in mosquito midgut cells but is still detectable only in the abdomen. After multiplying in the midgut cells, the virus spreads into the hemocoel and is delivered via the hemolymph to other organs including the salivary glands, legs, ovaries, and Malpighian tubes. In these organs, the virus is detectable after 7 days after feeding. In case of the Ťahyňa virus, the mosquito is able to transmit the virus about 1 week after the infection. The highest viral titer in the mosquito is seen around 14 days after infection, and the titer is stable (after a slight decrease) for at least 30 days. In the *Aedes aegypti* mosquito, infection was observed 51 days postfeeding and is considered to be lifelong.

However, not all of the mosquitoes that ingest infectious blood became infected. The ability of the vector to biologically transmit the virus is called vector competence and is dependent on several factors on both sides: mosquito and virus. From the mosquito side, there are many barriers that the virus needs to overcome before reaching the salivary glands for horizontal transfer or ovaries for vertical transmission (Figure 4.3). The permeability of individual barriers varies between mosquito species and may be connected to different enzymes that are present in the mosquito midgut or the presence of specific cell receptors. The basal lamina of the mosquito midgut represents an important barrier. The pores in this noncellular structure are just 10 nm in diameter, but it is not clear how viral particles are able to cross it (Mellor 2000). From the side of the virus, especially products of the M genomic segment (Gn, Gc, and NSm) determine successful *per os* infection of the mosquito (Beaty et al. 1982).

Interestingly, it has been shown that infection with the LACV affects the behavior of infected mosquitoes. In a laboratory experiment, infected females were able to mate earlier and more frequently than uninfected ones (Gabitszch et al. 2006; Reese et al. 2009).

4.3.3 Pathogenesis of Orthobunyavirus Infection

Most of the studies on the pathogenesis of orthobunyavirus infection have been done using the LACV in laboratory mice. Mice are considered to be a good laboratory animal model, mimicking the course of the infection in humans. There are variations in the disease outcome that depend on a number of factors, including the viral dose inoculated, the virulence of the virus strain, genetic background, or the age of the infected individual. In the case of California encephalitis infections, young individuals have a higher risk of contracting the severe form of the disease than older people. On the other hand, in the case of the Jamestown Canyon virus, older individuals are more susceptible than younger ones (Rust et al. 1999). Suckling mice are highly susceptible to subcutaneous infection, whereas adult individuals do not develop high viremia but are susceptible to intracerebral inoculation. Thus, suckling mice are more useful models for studies that focus on the extraneural phase of the disease, and adults for the neural phase of infection (Janssen

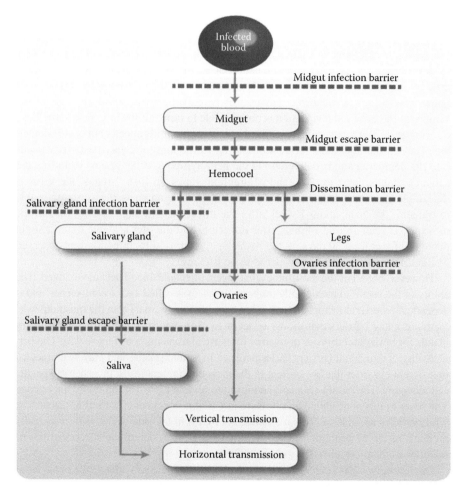

FIGURE 4.3 Barriers that the virus needs to overcome for the infection of the mosquito vector, and successful transmission.

et al. 1984). Mosquito saliva is important for a successful infection because it promotes virus transmission, probably via the inhibition of an early interferon response at the mosquito feeding site (Borucki et al. 2002).

During the extraneural phase of the infection, the virus primarily replicates in striated muscles and to a lesser extent in smooth or heart muscles. The virus is then thought to penetrate the lymphatic system and access the blood, then viremia appears. During the viremic phase, the virus crosses the blood–brain barrier and invades the CNS. Replication in the CNS is highly age-dependent. In suckling mice, there is a pancellular infection, whereas in adult mice the virus primarily replicates in neurons (Griot et al. 1993). The LACV also induces apoptosis of the neurons (Pekosz et al. 1996). Death occurs approximately 3–4 days after infection. However, most of the infections do not progress to the CNS phase. The basic steps taken by California encephalitis viruses are depicted in Figure 4.4. An alternative model of

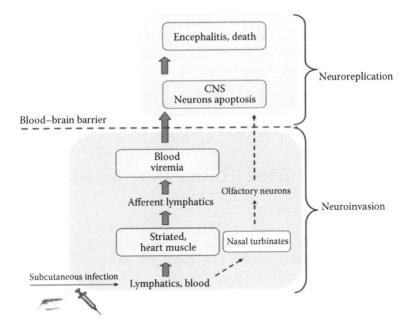

FIGURE 4.4 Classical (bold arrows) and alternative (dashed arrows) steps of pathogenesis for the California serogroup virus infection.

orthobunyavirus pathogenesis has been published by Bennett et al. (2008). In this case, i.e. an intraperitoneal infection of a weanling Swiss Webster mouse with the LACV, the virus initially replicated in tissues near the site of inoculation and then unidentified cells in nasal turbinates became infected via the blood stream. In this case, olfactory neurons facilitated virus entry into the CNS. Together with the previous observation, it seems that the virus can use more than one method for entry into the CNS. The observed differences in the course of the infection may be due to the use of different strains of mice or virus used in each study or due to different sites of inoculation.

4.3.3.1 Genetic Determinants of Virulence and Infectivity

Bunyaviruses, like other animal viruses, can differ in virulence in experimental animals. From experiments with laboratory mice, several determinants of virulence have been identified. As suckling mice are highly susceptible, they are the perfect model for studying neuroinvasiveness, whereas adults are used for neurovirulence experiments. These tests suggest that major determinants of the neuroinvasiveness, i.e., the ability to replicate in peripheral tissues and reach the CNS, are probably located in the M genomic segment, which encodes viral glycoproteins. Thus, peripheral attenuation is possibly related to the interaction of the viral glycoproteins with the host cell receptors and also to fusion activity. However, in the case of neurovirulence, it seems that major determinants are encoded in the L genomic segment and this is linked to the virus' ability to replicate in neurons in the adult mice. Although genetic determinants of neurovirulence and neuroinvasiveness are mapped to the L and M segments, respectively, it is possible that the products of the S genomic segment influence virulence as well (Janssen et al. 1986; Endres et al. 1991; Griot et al. 1993). A recent study that compared the sequences of the M and S segments of the biologically different strain of Ťahyňa virus did not identify unambiguous mutations, which can alter virulence after subcutaneous or intracerebral inoculation (Kilian et al. 2010). It is likely that the biological properties of the virus are determined by several accidental mutations or by several substitutions that occur independently in all three genomic segments.

4.4   ORTHOBUNYAVIRUS: ECOLOGY AND EPIDEMIOLOGY

4.4.1   ECOLOGY

Orthobunyaviruses are arboviruses that are distributed throughout the world. There are more than 150 viruses belonging to this genus, and all of those that affect humans are transmitted by mosquitoes. Only viruses from the Simbu serogroup, including the epidemiologically notable Oropouche virus, are transmitted by *Ceratopogonidae*. Viruses circulate between their vectors and natural hosts, mostly mammals and birds, quite independently of the presence of humans. Although the viral infection of vectors and natural hosts do not reveal any apparent symptoms, human infection can range from an unapparent infection to a very severe disease. In most cases humans are dead-end hosts without the possibility of further virus transmission; there is only one exception, i.e., the urban cycle of the Oropouche virus. A high level of virus–vector specificity is often developed, but on occasion, a wide range of susceptible mosquito species are available. Nevertheless, their vector competence highly differs and is virus-specific.

4.4.1.1   Serogroup California

Viruses of this serogroup, named after the California virus, the first isolated virus from this group, were isolated in North and South America, Asia, Africa, and Europe. Because of its association with a severe human disease, the ecology of the LACV, isolated in the United States, has been studied more extensively than other members of the California serogroup in North America. The primary vector of this virus, *Aedes triseriatus*, is a mosquito that uses tree-hole breeding and can be found in woodland. Nevertheless, this mosquito species can also be found in suburban locations where discarded containers (tires, cans, etc.) are used as a substitute for natural breeding places. This way, the virus can invade distant localities. LACV is transmitted by this mosquito transovarially (Watts et al. 1973), which allows hibernation of the virus in its eggs. It can also be transmitted venereally from an infected male mosquito to a female; this is another way to horizontally transmit the virus (Thompson and Beaty 1977, 1978). Transovarial transmission has been demonstrated in eight California serogroup viruses; this probably serves as the primary method of viral maintenance during periods of vector inactivity. As demonstrated experimentally, transovarial transmission of the California virus in *Aedes dorsalis* can provide a stable infection in a mosquito population for several consecutive generations and maintains the virus during unfavorable conditions (Turell and Le Duc 1983). This suggests that vertical transmission is more important for maintenance of a virus focus than it is for amplification through horizontal transmission. In the horizontal transmission cycle, chipmunks, tree squirrels, cottontail rabbits, and foxes have been found as principal natural hosts, providing high viremia that lasts 2–5 days and thus enables mosquito infection. Some other susceptible hosts were found by serological surveys (white-tailed deer, woodchuck, etc.) (Yuill 1983).

The California encephalitis virus was primarily isolated from *Aedes melanimon*, but *Aedes dorsalis* appears to be the principal vector (Crane et al. 1977). The primary vector of the Jamestown Canyon virus is *Culiseta inornata*, although *Aedes triseriatus* also plays an important role. *Culiseta inornata* also appears to be the principal vector of the Snowshoe hare virus together with several *Aedes* species (Turell and Le Duc 1983). In addition to North America, this virus has been found in northern and Asian Russia.

It is an epidemiological question, whether *Aedes albopictus*, a synanthropic species, which spread from Asia to other continents including North America in half of the 1980s and which is susceptible to the California group viruses, will be integrated into their circulation cycle. Under laboratory conditions, a stable infection of the San Angelo virus (California group) in *Aedes albopictus* has been demonstrated (Turell and Le Duc 1983).

Ťahyňa virus (TAHV), the first arbovirus isolated from mosquitoes in Europe, was recovered in the former Czechoslovakia in 1958 (Bárdoš and Danielová 1959). Later, it was isolated in many European countries including European and Asian Russia, Middle Asian republics, China, Turkey, Northern and northeastern Africa and as a Lumbo variety also in Central, West, and South Africa (Hubálek and Halouzka 1996; Zhi Lu 2009). Its ecology was studied very extensively. *Aedes vexans* appears to be the primary vector for TAHV. Virus isolations from mosquitoes collected in the field and laboratory experiments have shown other species that can serve as vectors: *Aedes cantans, Aedes caspius, Aedes dorsalis, Aedes cinereus, Aedes sticticus*, and *Culiseta annulata*. Nevertheless, most of the TAHV isolated strains originated from *Aedes vexans* (Danielová 1992). Moreover, its infection threshold is the lowest of all other examined species (Danielová 1966, 1972b), and it can transmit TAHV transovarially (Danielová and Ryba 1979) enabling virus hibernation. Virus hibernation has also been shown in hibernating females of *Culiseta annulata* (Danielová and Minář 1969). However, it has been shown that active virus circulation is associated with the breeding wave of *Aedes vexans* following late spring or summer flooding, although other species susceptible to TAHV infection may already be active (Danielová 1972a). Hares, rabbits, hedgehogs, and pigs are considered to be primary hosts (Málková 1980). It was found that hedgehogs, which are heterotherm animals, can play a role in virus hibernation shortly before their overwintering. The viremia then persists for up to a couple of days after their awakening (Málková et al., unpublished data).

The Inkoo virus, first isolated in Finland, is another member of the California serogroup in Europe (Brummer-Korvenkontio et al. 1973). It is distributed mainly in northern Europe and Russia, transmitted by *Aedes communis* and *Aedes punctor* in Scandinavia; in Russia it was also isolated from *Aedes hexodontus* and *Aedes punctor* (Mitchell et al. 1993).

4.4.1.2 Serogroup Simbu

Viruses from this serogroup are distributed globally and are transmitted by culi-
coids. From the epidemiological aspect, the Oropouche virus is the most important
member of this serogroup. although it was first isolated in Trinidad, it is most widely
distributed in Brazil and Peru, predominantly in the Amazon basin regions (Pinheiro
et al. 1981). This virus reveals the distinctiveness of its ecology. It circulates and
perpetuates in a sylvatic cycle among forest primates, sloths, birds, and an unidentified vector, but it can be introduced into urban settings by infected people or by
Culicoides paraensis, which initiates an urban ecological cycle. In the urban cycle,
Culicoides paraensis plays the role of vector, and humans serve as amplifier hosts.
Unlike most other arboviruses, the anthropophilic *Culicoides paraensis* can transmit the virus to the human population without a wild animal host, as humans develop
a high enough viremia for the infection of the vector. Although the infection rate of
Culicoides paraensis is rather low, vast amounts can be found in rural regions where
it breeds in decaying waste from agricultural products. Outbreaks occur when there
is a large concentration of both vectors and susceptible humans (Pinheiro et al. 1981).

4.4.2 Epidemiology

The Orthobunyavirus genus includes more than 150 viruses, which have been
divided into 18 antigenic groups. Currently, 48 virus species are known. However,
serogroups are still frequently used as taxonomical units. As is commonly seen with
other arboviral infections, the unapparent forms of the disease predominate and their
presence can be revealed by serological surveys only. Most of these viruses cause
febrile illness or influenza-like symptoms, but some of them have the ability to cause
a severe disease. Neither a vaccine nor a specific treatment is yet known and therefore the treatment is only symptomatological. Unless there has been an outbreak, the
actual number of people who have contracted the disease is mostly underreported.

From an epidemiological point of view, the most important serogroups are the
California group found in North and South America, Europe, Africa, and Asia; the
Simbu group, found in South and Central America, Africa, Asia, and Australia;
group C occurring in South and Central America and the Bunyamwera group distributed predominantly in Africa but also in Europe, Asia, and North America.

4.4.2.1 Serogroup California

The California encephalitis virus is the prototype member of this serogroup. The
virus was isolated in 1941 and is thought to be a cause of human encephalitis in
California (Hammon and Reeves 1952). Later, it was discovered that the LACV,
isolated from the brain of a 4-year-old girl in 1964 (Thompson et al. 1965), is responsible for severe disease, predominantly in children younger than 16 years of age, and
that it appears more frequently. The incidence of LACV infection can be up to 20–30
cases per 100,000 inhabitants in endemic areas.

Like the two mentioned above, the Jamestown Canyon virus occurs in North
America. Unlike the LACV, the Jamestown Canyon virus was shown to be a cause
of human encephalitis that is predominant and more severe in adults (Grimstad et
al. 1986). These three viruses all cause similar encephalitic diseases that differ with

respect to age dependence and severity of symptoms. It seems that the LACV and the Jamestown Canyon virus cause encephalitis more frequently than the California encephalitis virus (Campbell et al. 1992).

The Snowshoe hare virus is another virus within the California serogroup found in North America that causes meningitis and encephalitis in humans. This virus is distributed across the northern United States, Canada, and Alaska as far as the arctic (Fauvel et al. 1980). Many cases of clinical illness caused by the Snowshoe hare virus frequently go unrecognized.

In terms of causing human disease, the LACV is the most significant member of this serogroup. According to the CDC, approximately 80–100 LACV neuroinvasive disease cases are reported each year in the United States, less severe cases being significantly underdiagnosed and underreported. In the past, most cases of LACV neuroinvasive disease have been reported in the upper Midwestern states. Recently however, more cases have been reported from the mid-Atlantic and southeastern states. Most of the cases appear between July and September, but in subtropical endemic areas (e.g., the Gulf States), rare cases can occur in winter as well. People living in or visiting woodland habitats and those who work outside or participate in outdoor recreational activities in areas where the disease is common are at risk of infection from the LACV (thus the higher frequency in men 1:1.5 is explained).

After a 5- to 15-day incubation period, 2–3 days of fever follow (temperature ranges from 38°C to 41°C). Other symptoms include headaches, nausea, vomiting, fatigue, and lethargy. Severe neuroinvasive disease occurs most frequently in children under the age of 16. Although seizures are common, fatal cases are rare (<1%) and most patients recover completely. In some cases neurologic sequelae (recurrent seizures, hemiparesis, and neurobehavioral abnormalities) of varying duration have been reported. In addition, approximately 10% of children develop epilepsy, and less than 2% could have some learning dysfunction or cognitive disorder (Soldan and Gonzáles-Scarano 2005). A temporal lobe abnormality similar to that seen in herpes simplex encephalitis was observed in a 10-year-old child (Sokol et al. 2001). As there is no specific antiviral treatment for clinical LACV infection available, symptomatological treatment is used. No vaccine against the LACV yet exists.

Diagnosis of a LACV infection is performed serologically by the detection of LACV-specific IgM antibodies in serum or by CSF IgG seroconversion. Positive tests should be confirmed by neutralizing antibody testing of acute- and convalescent-phase serum specimens. As cross-reactivity between California serogroup viruses occurs sympatrically, a less specific diagnostic method could lead to misleading results. At present, molecular biology techniques (RT-PCR, SSCP) are available for accurate diagnosis.

As the primary vector of the Ťahyňa virus is thought to be *Aedes vexans*, which breeds rapidly after floods and is able to seek hosts from a long distance, high numbers of humans are seropositive, mostly after an unapparent infection. The seroprevalence reaches up to more than 50% of inhabitants in endemic areas. Clinical manifestation of the Ťahyňa virus infection was serologically diagnosed in many cases; in several of them, the virus was isolated from the viremic blood of an infected individual. The incubation period is short, only 1–2 days. After that, the majority of apparent clinical cases of Ťahyňa virus infection manifest as a sudden febrile onset associated with a headache and a combination of mostly catarrhal symptoms in the pharynx and respiratory tract, conjunctivitis, sore throat, anorexia, gastrointestinal disorders, weakness, malaise, myalgia, arthralgia, and sometimes bronchopneumonia. The disease usually lasts from 3 to 8 days, but rarely longer. Aseptic meningitis and other neurological symptoms including coma have been observed, predominantly in children. Every seventh influenza-like disease and every fifth case with neurological symptoms in children is thought to be caused by the Ťahyňa virus in South Moravia (the Czech Republic) during the summer season. Fatal cases were not reported (Šimková 1980; Bárdoš et al. 1975, 1980). Besides Czechoslovakia, the infections caused by the Ťahyňa virus have been observed in other European and Asian countries (Janbon et al. 1974; Kolobukhina et al. 1990; Lvov et al. 1977; Zhi Lu 2009).

Clinical manifestation of the Inkoo virus is similar to that of the Ťahyňa virus, including the neurological symptoms (Kolobukhina et al. 1990; Lvov et al. 1996).

4.4.2.2 Serogroup Simbu

Unlike other orthobunyaviruses, humans infected with the Oropouche virus develop viremia levels capable of infecting *Culicoides paraensis*, which serves as a vector for this virus. It has been demonstrated that the urban cycle of the Oropouche virus involves a man-to-man cycle maintained by *Culicoides paraensis*. Thus, humans appear to serve as amplifier hosts in the urban cycle. This fact, together with the high abundance of the anthropophilic *Culicoides paraensis* promotes epidemic situations. Over the past 45 years, many outbreaks of Oropouche fever have been reported, with approximately 500,000 of these cases in the Americas. Oropouche virus has been isolated in Trinidad, Panama, Peru, and Brazil. During the past 40 years, Oropouche fever has emerged as a public health problem in tropical areas of Central and South America (Azevedo et al. 2007). Clinical manifestation appears after a 4- to 8-day incubation period with a sudden onset of fever, chills, headache, myalgia, arthralgia, sometimes rash, meningitis or encephalitis, but no fatal cases or permanent sequelae have been reported. On the other hand, prostration is common (Le Duc and Pinheiro 1988).

4.4.2.3 Serogroup C

Several viruses (Apeu, Caraparu, Ossa, Madrid, Marituba, Murutucu, Restan, Nepuyo, Itaqui, Oriboca) associated predominantly with the tropical forests in Central and South America have been isolated from febrile humans, monkeys, rodents, marsupials, fruit bats, and mosquitoes. No large epidemics have been recorded. Sporadic infections of people are characterized by fever, rigors, photophobia, conjunctivitis, tachycardia, myalgia, arthralgia, prostration, leucopenia, and occasionally jaundice (Swanepoel 2004).

4.5 PHLEBOVIRUSES: ECOLOGY AND EPIDEMIOLOGY

Although members of the Phlebovirus genus are not typical representatives of neurovirulent viruses, there are at least two viruses that should be mentioned. The first is Toscana virus which affects mainly inhabitants and travellers in the Mediterranean region. The second is RVFV, which circulates mainly on the African continent and can also cause encephalitis in humans.

4.5.1 Toscana Virus

Like most bunyaviruses, Toscana (TOSV) is an arthropod-borne virus. The first isolation of the virus was reported in 1971 in Tuscany, Italy, from the mosquito *Phlebotomus perniciosus*. The main vector for this virus is the sand fly belonging to the Phlebotominae family, mainly the *Phlebotomus*, *Lutzomyia*, and *Sergentomyia* genera that colonize humid habitats in the Mediterranean region (Verani et al. 1988). TOSV is circulating in Algeria, Spain, Portugal, Cyprus, Greece, and Turkey (Valassina et al. 2003; Depaquit et al. 2010). Very little is known about the vertebrate host of TOSV because serological studies revealed no antibody prevalence among domestic and wild animals. However, isolation of TOSV from the brain of a bat (*Pipistrellus kuhli*) indicates some possible ecological importance to these vertebrates (Verani et al. 1988). However, no conclusive evidence has been reported. Nevertheless, it has been proposed that transmission in nature is possible in the absence of a vertebrate host. In this case, the vector itself can be considered as a reservoir. Subsequently, TOSV is transmitted transovarialy and even venerealy from an infected male to an uninfected female during copulation. In winter, the virus may persist in diapausing phlebotomus larvae (Tesh et al. 1992).

TOSV causes a predominantly influenza-like infection but during the summer months it is frequently associated with encephalitis and meningitidis (Braito et al. 1998). During a three year investigation, it was shown that 81% of aseptic meningitides in summer are caused by TOSV (Valassina et al. 2000). In another study, seroprevalence of anti-TOSV antibodies in a high risk group, such as forestry workers in Italy, reached more than 72% (Valassina et al. 2003). Among other residents, seroprevalence ranges from 3% to 22% in Italy, 5% to 26% in Spain, and about 12% in France (Depaquit et al. 2010). TOSV infection can affect both children and adults, and the highest number of reported cases is in August. As mentioned previously, TOSV infections are mainly asymptomatic or influenza-like. However, some neurological symptoms can occur. A typical TOSV infection manifests as high fever, headache, sore eyes, and photophobia. Rarely, aseptic meningitides can be present. The disease is often milder in children. Laboratory diagnosis is based primarily on detection of the viral nucleic acid by RT-PCR or by isolating the virus from the blood of an infected individual. Detection of rising IgM antibodies may also help.

4.5.2 Rift Valley Fever Virus: Ecology and Epidemiology

Since its first isolation in 1930 in Kenya, East Africa, the RVFV has been found in many countries on the African continent and even in Madagascar and Saudi Arabia (Daubney et al. 1931; Andriamandimby et al. 2010). RVFV mainly affects livestock such as goats, camels, or sheep. Although RVFV infections in animals are mainly mild or unapparent, large outbreaks periodically emerge and cause heavy mortality among newborn animals or abortion in pregnant females, which is associated with high economic losses. For humans who have been infected because they work with sick animals or have been bitten by an infected mosquito, disease is mainly associated with acute febrile illness, hepatitis, retinitis, renal failure, hemorrhagic fever and rarely encephalitis or meningoencephalitis (Bouloy and Weber 2010).

RVFV can be transmitted by a variety of mosquitoes including those of the *Aedes*, *Anopheles*, *Culex*, *Mansonia*, and *Eretmapoites* genera. Two different types of viral circulation in nature can be distinguished: the epizootic and the interepizootic cycles. The epizootic cycle mainly prevails during the heavy rain season when the mosquito population is increasing and the virus can be transmitted from mosquitoes to mammals and then to the uninfected vector. The interepizootic (or survival) cycle relies on transovarial transmission of the virus, so it must survive in mosquito eggs until the next rainfall occurs and a sizeable amount of infected mosquitoes hatch. Newborn mosquitoes infect new animals and trigger the start of a new epizootic cycle. Infected livestock develop a high viremia, which allows infection of other mosquitoes. Depending on a number of factors such as the availability of susceptible hosts and abundance of efficient vectors, large outbreaks can occur (Sall et al. 1998). Additionally, the virus can be transmitted in the eggs of mosquitoes "by contaminated wind" to a new region (Sellers et al. 1982). The main mode of transmission to humans is by close contact with infected animal body fluids during slaughter or handling of aborted animals. Humans can also be infected after a mosquito bite or drinking raw milk.

The infection in humans is mainly asymptomatic or manifests as common flu-like symptoms. The incubation period is very short; approximately 2–5 days. After that, patients develop moderate fever, headaches, weakness, nausea, and muscle pain. The fever usually lasts for one week and most patients recover completely. Further complications have been observed in less than 5% of cases and are associated with CNS manifestation such as confusion, lethargy, convulsion, or coma. Encephalitis symptoms may last for about 4 weeks and most patients recover completely. The others can suffer from neurologic sequelae such as hemiparesis. In less than 1% of affected people, the infection can lead to highly lethal hemorrhagic fever. An increased fatality rate reaching almost 14% was observed during an outbreak in Saudi Arabia (Pepin et al. 2010). The infection in animals takes a similar course to that in humans; however, mortality is much higher, reaching up to 30% in adult animals and even 100% among newborn individuals. The infection often leads to abortion or a decrease in milk production (Balkhy and Memish 2003; LeBeaud et al. 2010).

The laboratory diagnosis of an RVFV infection relies on the detection of IgM antibodies in a single specimen or on increasing tendencies of IgG antibodies. In a patient with the developed encephalitis form, IgM antibodies can also be detected in cerebrospinal fluid. In an appropriately equipped BSL-3 or BSL-3+/4 laboratory, isolation of the virus from the blood of patients in the acute phase can be performed. Further, molecular biology techniques such as PCR or qPCR are also available (Garcia et al. 2001; Sall et al. 2001).

The treatment of diseases caused by RVFV is symptomatic only, and no specific treatment is known. Thus, prevention programs are highly encouraged. To date, both live attenuated and inactivated vaccines are available. However, both of these are only for veterinary use; no vaccines for human use have been registered. Several new generation vaccines such as recombinant viral vectors or DNA vaccines are also under development (Ikegami and Makino 2009; Boshra et al. 2011).

4.6   CONCLUSIONS

Bunyaviruses represent a unique group of viruses that can infect vertebrates, invertebrates or plants. Only a few of the Orthobunyavirus and Phlebovirus genus are, however, associated with neuroinfections in humans. Although diseases caused by bunyaviruses are often mild, their importance should not be underestimated. Vector-borne diseases, including those caused by bunyaviruses, are being studied by scientists all over the world. Climate change, together with changes in land usage, increase vector populations and allow them to spread to new areas. Together with their vector, bunyaviruses can be introduced to an immunologically naive population and cause severe outbreaks, e.g., as shown by RVFV, which was introduced to Saudi Arabia. However, bunyaviruses possess another feature that provides them with some epidemiological advantages: genomic segment reassortment. Thanks to this mechanism, bunyaviruses can change their properties very rapidly. Ngari virus is an example of an orthobunyavirus that has caused outbreaks in Somalia and Kenya. Ngari genomic segments originated from the Bunyamwera and Batai orthobunyaviruses. Although considerable progress has been made in bunyavirus research over recent years, there is no vaccine or specific treatment as yet. This, combined with their global distribution, means that bunyaviruses present a considerable worldwide public health challenge.

REFERENCES

Andriamandimby, S. F., Randrianarivo-Solofoniaina, A. E., Jeanmaire, E. M., Ravololomanana, L., Razafimanantsoa, L. T., Rakotojoelinandrasana, T., Razainirina, J., Hoffmann, J., Ravalohery, J. P., Rafisandratantsoa, J. T., Rollin, P. E., and Reynes, J. M. 2010. Rift Valley fever during rainy seasons, Madagascar, 2008 and 2009. *Emerg. Infect. Dis.* 16:963–70.

Aquino, V. H., Moreli, M. L., and Moraes Figueiredo, L. T. 2003. Analysis of oropouche virus L protein amino acid sequence showed the presence of an additional conserved region that could harbour an important role for the polymerase activity. *Arch. Virol.* 148:19–28.

Azevedo, R. S. S., Nunes, M. R. T., Chiang, J. O., Bensabath, G., Vasconcelos, H. B., Pinto, A. Y. N., Martins, L. C., Monteiro, H. A. O., Rodrigues, S. G., and Vasconcelos, P. F. C. 2007. Reemergence of Oropouche Fever, Northern Brazil. *Emerg. Infect. Dis.* 13: 912–5.

Balkhy, H. H., and Memish, Z. A. 2003. Rift Valley fever: an uninvited zoonosis in the Arabian peninsula. *Int. J. Antimicrob. Agents.* 21:153–7.

Bárdoš, V., and Danielová, V. 1959. The Ťahyňa virus—a virus isolated from mosquitoes in Czechoslovakia. *J. Hyg. Epidemiol. (Praha)* 3:264–276.

Bárdoš, V., Medek, M., Kania, V., and Hubálek, Z. 1975. Isolation of Ťahyňa virus from the blood of sick children. *Acta Virol.* 19:447.

Bárdoš, V., Medek, M., Kania, V., Hubálek, Z., and Juřicová, Z. 1980. Das klinisch Bild der Ťahyňa–Virus (California Gruppe)-Infektionen bei Kindern. *Pediat. Grenzgeb.* 19:11–23.

Barr, J. N., Rodgers, J. W., and Wertz, G. W. 2006. Identification of the Bunyamwera bunyavirus transcription termination signal. *J. Gen. Virol.* 87:189–98.

Beaty, B. J., Miller, B. R., Shope, R. E., Rozhon, E. J., and Bishop, D. H. 1982. Molecular basis of bunyavirus per os infection of mosquitoes: role of the middle-sized RNA segment. *Proc. Natl. Acad. Sci. U S A* 79:1295–7.

Bennett, R. S., Cress, C. M., Ward, J. M., Firestone, C. Y., Murphy, B. R., and Whitehead, S. S. 2008. La Crosse virus infectivity, pathogenesis, and immunogenicity in mice and monkeys. *Virol. J.* 11:5–25.

Blakqori, G., Delhaye, S., Habjan, M., Blair, C. D., Sánchez-Vargas, I., Olson, K. E., Attarzadeh-Yazdi, G., Fragkoudis, R., Kohl, A., Kalinke, U., Weiss, S., Michiels, T., Staeheli, P., and Weber, F. 2007. La Crosse bunyavirus nonstructural protein NSs serves to suppress the type I interferon system of mammalian hosts. *J. Virol.* 81:4991–9.

Borucki, M. K., Kempf, B. J., Blitvich, B. J., Blair, C. D., and Beaty, B. J. 2002. La Crosse virus: replication in vertebrate and invertebrate hosts. *Microbes. Infect.* 4:341–50.

Boshra, H., Lorenzo, G., Busquets, N., and Brun, A. 2011. Rift Valley fever: recent insights into pathogenesis and prevention. *J. Virol.* 85:6098–105.

Braito, A., Ciufolini, M. G., Pippi, L., Corbisiero, R., Fiorentini, C., Gistri, A., and Toscano, L. 1998. Phlebotomus-transmitted toscana virus infections of the central nervous system: a seven-year experience in Tuscany. *Scand. J. Infect. Dis.* 30:505–8.

Bridgen, A., and Elliott, R. M. 1996. Rescue of a segmented negative-strand RNA virus entirely from cloned complementary DNAs. *Proc. Natl. Acad. Sci. U S A* 93:15400–4.

Brummer-Korvenkontio, M., Sikku, P., Korhonen, P., Ulmanen, I., Reunala, T., and Karvonen, J. 1973. Arboviruses in Finland IV. Isolation and characterization of Inkoo virus, a Finnish representative of the California group. *Amer. J. Trop. Med. Hyg.* 22:404–13.

Campbell, G. L., Reeves, W. C., and Hardy, J. L. 1992. Seroepidemiology of California and Bunyamvera serogroup bunyavirus infections in humans in California. *Am. J. Epidemiol.* 136:308–19.

Colón-Ramos, D. A., Irusta, P. M., Gan, E. C., Olson, M. R., Song, J., Morimoto, R. I., Elliott, R. M., Lombard, M., Hollingsworth, R., Hardwick, J. M., Smith, G. K., and Kornbluth, S. 2003. Inhibition of translation and induction of apoptosis by Bunyaviral nonstructural proteins bearing sequence similarity to reaper. *Mol. Biol. Cell.* 14:4162–72.

Crane, G. T., Elbel, R. E., and Calisher, C. H. 1977. Transovarial transmission of California encephalitis virus in the mosquito *Aedes dorsalis* at Blue Lake, Utah. *Mosq. News.* 36:63.

Danielová, V. 1962. Multiplication dynamics of Ťahyňa virus in different body parts of *Aedes vexans* mosquito. *Acta Virol.* 6:227–30.

Danielová, V. 1966. Quantitative relationships of Ťahyňa virus and the mosquito *Aedes vexans.* *Acta Virol.* 10:62–5.

Danielová, V. 1968. Penetration of the Ťahyňa virus to various organs of the *Aedes vexans* mosquito. *Folia. Parasitol.* 15:87–91.

Danielová, V. 1972a. The seasonal occurrence of the virus Ťahyňa. *Folia Parasitol. (Praha).* 19:1898–192.

Danielová, V. 1972b. The vector efficiency of *Culiseta annulata* in relation to Ťahyňa virus. *Folia Parasitol. (Praha).* 19:259–62.

Danielová, V. 1992. Relationships of mosquitoes to Ťahyňa virus as determinant factors of its circulation in nature, *Studie ČSAV 3*, Academia, Prague, 102 pgs.

Danielová, V., and Minář, J. 1969. Experimental overwintering of the virus Ťahyňa in mosquitoes *Culiseta annulata* (Schrk.) (Diptera, Culicidae). *Folia Parasitol. (Praha).* 15:183–7.

Danielová, V., and Ryba, J. 1979. Laboratory demonstration of transovarial transmission of Ťahyňa virus *Aedes vexans* and the role of this mechanism in overwintering of this arbovirus. *Folia Parasitol (Praha).* 26:361–6.

Daubney, R., Hudson, J. R., and Gamham, P. C. 1931. Enzootic hepatitis of Rift Valley fever: an undescribed virus disease of sheep, cattle and man from East Africa. *J. Pathol. Bacteriol.* 34:545–9.

Depaquit, J., Grandadam, M., Fouque, F., Andry, P. E., and Peyrefitte, C. 2010. Arthropod-borne viruses transmitted by Phlebotomine sandflies in Europe: a review. *Euro. Surveill.* 15:19507.

Dunn, E. F., Pritlove, D. C., Jin, H., and Elliott, R. M. 1995. Transcription of a recombinant bunyavirus RNA template by transiently expressed bunyavirus proteins. *Virology* 211:133–43.

Elliott, R. M., and Wilkie, M. L. 1986. Persistent infection of Aedes albopictus C6/36 cells by Bunyamwera virus. *Virology* 150:21–32.

Elliott, R. M. 1990. Molecular biology of the Bunyaviridae. *J. Gen. Virol.* 71:501–22.

Endres, M. J., Jacoby, D. R., Janssen, R. S., Gonzalez-Scarano, F., and Nathanson, N. 1989. The large viral RNA segment of California serogroup bunyaviruses encodes the large viral protein. *J. Gen. Virol.* 70:223–8.

Fauvel, M., Arsob, H., Calisher, C. H., Davignon, L., Chagnon, A., Skvorc-Ranko, R., and Belloncik, S. 1980. California group encephalitis in three children from Quebec: clinical and serological findings. *CMA J.* 122:60–4.

Fontana, J., López-Montero, N., Elliott, R. M., Fernández, J. J., and Risco, C. 2008. The unique architecture of Bunyamwera virus factories around the Golgi complex. *Cell Microbiol.* 10:2012–28.

Fuller, F., and Bishop, D. H. 1982. Identification of virus-coded nonstructural polypeptides in bunyavirus-infected cells. *J. Virol.* 41:643–8.

Gabitzsch, E. S., Blair, C. D., and Beaty, B. J. 2006. Effect of La Crosse virus infection on insemination rates in female Aedes triseriatus (Diptera:Culicidae). *J. Med. Entomol.* 43:850–2.

Garcia, S., Crance, J. M., Billecocq, A., Peinnequin, A., Jouan, A., Bouloy, M., and Garin, D. 2001. Quantitative real-time PCR detection of Rift Valley fever virus and its application to evaluation of antiviral compounds. *J. Clin. Microbiol.* 39:4456–61.

Garcin, D., Lezzi, M., Dobbs, M., Elliott, R. M., Schmaljohn, C., Kang, C. Y., and Kolakofsky, D. 1995. The 5′ ends of Hantaan virus (Bunyaviridae) RNAs suggest a prime-and-realign mechanism for the initiation of RNA synthesis. *J. Virol.* 69:5754–62.

Grimstad, P. R., Calisher, C. H., Harroff, N. N., and Wentworth, B. B. 1986. Jamestown Canyon virus (California serogroup) is the etiologic agent of widespread infection of Michigan humans. *Am. J. Trop. Med. Hyg.* 35:376–86.

Griot, C., Gonzalez-Scarano, F., and Nathanson, N. 1993. Molecular determinants of the virulence and infectivity of California serogroup bunyaviruses. *Annu. Rev. Microbiol.* 47:117–38.

Hacker, J. K., and Hardy, J. L. 1997. Adsorptive endocytosis of California encephalitis virus into mosquito and mammalian cells: a role for G1. *Virology* 235:40–7.

Hacker, J. K., Volkman, L. E., and Hardy, J. L. 1995. Requirement for the G1 protein of California encephalitis virus in infection *in vitro* and *in vivo*. *Virology* 206:945–53.

Hammon, W. M., and Reeves, R. W. 1952. California encephalitis virus, a newly described agent, *Calif. Med.* 77:303–309.

Honig, J. E., Osborne, J. C., and Nichol, S. T. 2004. Crimean-Congo hemorrhagic fever virus genome L RNA segment and encoded protein. *Virology* 321:29–35.

Hubálek, Z., and Halouzka, J. 1996. Arthropod-borne viruses vertebrates in Europe, *Acta Sci. Nat. Acad. Sci. Bohemicae (Brno).* 30(4–5):95 pgs.

Ikegami, T., and Makino, S. 2009. Rift Valley fever vaccines. *Vaccine* 27(Suppl 4):D69–72.

Jääskeläinen, K. M., Kaukinen, P., Minskaya, E. S., Plyusnina, A., Vapalahti, O., Elliott, R. M., Weber, F., Vaheri, A., and Plyusnin, A. 2007. Tula and Puumala hantavirus NSs ORFs are functional and the products inhibit activation of the interferon-beta promoter. *J. Med. Virol.* 79:1527–36.

Jacoby, D. R., Cooke, C., Prabakaran, I., Boland, J., Nathanson, N., and Gonzalez-Scarano, F. 1993. Expression of the La Crosse M segment proteins in a recombinant vaccinia expression system mediates pH-dependent cellular fusion. *Virology* 193:993–6.

Janbon, M., Bertrand, A., Hannoun, C., Mandin, J., Janbon, F., and Jourdan, J. 1974. Méningoencéfalite à virus Tahyna. *J. Med. Montpellier.* 9:7–10.

Janssen, R. S., Nathanson, N., Endres, M. J., and Gonzalez-Scarano, F. 1986. Virulence of La Crosse virus is under polygenic control. *J. Virol.* 59:1–7.

Janssen, R., Gonzalez-Scarano, F., and Nathanson, N. 1984. Mechanisms of bunyavirus virulence. Comparative pathogenesis of a virulent strain of La Crosse and an avirulent strain of Tahyna virus. *Lab. Invest.* 50:447–55.

Jin, H., and Elliott, R. M. 1992. Mutagenesis of the L protein encoded by Bunyamwera virus and production of monospecific antibodies. *J. Gen. Virol.* 73:2235–44.

Jin, H., and Elliott, R. M. 1993. Non-viral sequences at the 5' ends of Dugbe nairovirus S mRNAs. *J. Gen. Virol.* 74:2293–7.

Kikkert, M., Van Lent, J., Storms, M., Bodegom, P., Kormelink, R., and Goldbach, R. 1999. Tomato spotted wilt virus particle morphogenesis in plant cells. *J. Virol.* 73:2288–97.

Kilian, P., Růzek, D., Danielová, V., Hypsa, V., and Grubhoffer, L. 2010. Nucleotide variability of Tahyna virus (Bunyaviridae, Orthobunyavirus) small (S) and medium (M) genomic segments in field strains differing in biological properties. *Virus Res.* 149:119–23.

Kochs, G., Janzen, C., Hohenberg, H., and Haller, O. 2002. Antivirally active MxA protein sequesters La Crosse virus nucleocapsid protein into perinuclear complexes. *Proc. Natl. Acad. Sci. U S A* 99:3153–8.

Kohl, A., Clayton, R. F., Weber, F., Bridgen, A., Randall, R. E., and Elliott, R. M. 2003. Bunyamwera virus nonstructural protein NSs counteracts interferon regulatory factor 3-mediated induction of early cell death. *J. Virol.* 77:7999–8008.

Kolobukhina, L. V., Lvov, D. K., Butenko, A. M., Nedyalkova, M. S., Kuznetsov, A. A., and Galkina, I. V. 1990. Signs and symptoms of infections caused by California serogroup viruses in humans in the U.S.S.R. *Arch. Virol.* Suppl I:243–7.

LaBeaud, A. D., Kazura, J. W., and King, C. H. 2010. Advances in Rift Valley fever research: insights for disease prevention. *Curr. Opin. Infect. Dis.* 23:403–8.

Le Duc, J. W., and Pinheiro, F. P. 1988. *The Arboviruses Epidemiology and Ecology*, CRC Press, Boca Raton, FL.

Leonard, V. H., Kohl, A., Hart, T. J., and Elliott, R. M. 2006. Interaction of Bunyamwera Orthobunyavirus NSs protein with mediator protein MED8: a mechanism for inhibiting the interferon response. *J. Virol.* 80:9667–75.

Leonard, V. H., Kohl, A., Osborne, J. C., McLees, A., and Elliott, R. M. 2005. Homotypic interaction of Bunyamwera virus nucleocapsid protein. *J. Virol.* 79:13166–72.

López-Montero, N., and Risco, C. 2011. Self-protection and survival of arbovirus-infected mosquito cells. *Cell Microbiol.* 13:300–15.

Lozach, P. Y., Mancini, R., Bitto, D., Meier, R., Oestereich, L., Overby, A. K., Pettersson, R. F., and Helenius, A. 2010. Entry of bunyaviruses into mammalian cells. *Cell Host Microbe.* 7:488–99.

Lu, Z., Lu, X. J., Fu, S. H., Zhang, S., Li, Z. X., Yao, X. H., Feng, Y. P., Lambert, A. J., Ni da, X., Wang, F. T., Tong, S. X., Nasci, R. S., Feng, Y., Dong, Q., Zhai, Y. G., Gao, X. Y., Wang, H. Y., Tang, Q., and Liang, G. D. 2009. Tahyna virus and human infection, China. *Emerg. Infect. Dis.* 15:306–9.

Ludwig, G. V., Israel, B. A., Christensen, B. M., Yuill, T. M., and Schultz, K. T. 1991. Role of La Crosse virus glycoproteins in attachment of virus to host cells. *Virology* 181:564–71.

Lvov, D. K., Kolobukhina, L. V., Gromashevsky, V. L., Skvortsova, T. M., Morozova, T. N., Galkina, I. V., and Nedyalkova, M. S. 1996. Isolation of California antigenic group (CAL) from patients with acute neuroinfection syndrome. *Arbovirus Inf. Exch.* June:16–18.

Lvov, D. K., Kostyukov, M. A., Pak, T. P., Gordeeva, Z. E., Bunietbekov, A. A., and Gulyamov, Y. G. 1977. Isolation of Tahyna virus (California group, Bunyaviridae) from the blood of febrile patients in the Taadjik SSR. *Vop. Virusol.* 22:682–5 (in Russian).

Málková, D. 1980. Hosts of the virus. In: *Ťahyňa Virus Natural Focus in Southern Moravia*, Rosický, B., and Málková, D. (eds.), Transactions of ČSAV, Math and Nat Sci Ser, 88, Academia Prague: 54–72.

Mellor, P. S. 2000. Replication of arboviruses in insect vectors. *J. Comp. Pathol.* 123:231–47.

Mir, M. A., and Panganiban, A. T. 2006. The bunyavirus nucleocapsid protein is an RNA chaperone: possible roles in viral RNA panhandle formation and genome replication. *RNA* 12:272–82.

Mir, M. A., Duran, W. A., Hjelle, B. L., Ye, C., and Panganiban, A. T. 2008. Storage of cellular 5′ mRNA caps in P bodies for viral cap-snatching. *Proc. Natl. Acad. Sci. U S A* 105:19294–9.

Mitchel, C. J., Lvov, S. D., and Savage, H. M. 1993. Vector and host relationships of California serogroup viruses in Western Siberia. *Am. J. Trop. Med. Hyg.* 49:53–62.

Mohamed, M., McLees, A., and Elliott, R. M. 2009. Viruses in the Anopheles A, Anopheles B, and Tete serogroups in the Orthobunyavirus genus (family Bunyaviridae) do not encode an NSs protein. *J. Virol.* 83:7612–8.

Müller, R., Poch, O., Delarue, M., Bishop, D. H., and Bouloy, M. 1994. Rift Valley fever virus L segment: correction of the sequence and possible functional role of newly identified regions conserved in RNA-dependent polymerases. *J. Gen. Virol.* 75:1345–52.

Nakitare, G. W., and Elliott, R. M. 1993. Expression of the Bunyamwera virus M genome segment and intracellular localization of NSm. *Virology* 195:511–20.

Nichol, S. T., Beaty, B. J., Elliott, R. M., Goldbach, R., Plyusnin, A., Schmaljohn, C. S., and Tesh, R. B. 2005. Bunyaviridae. In: *Virus Taxonomy Classification and Nomenclature of Viruses Eighth Report of the International Committee on the Taxonomy of Viruses*, Fauquet, C. M., Mayo, M. A., Maniloff, J., Desselberger, U., and Ball, L. A. (eds.), Elsevier Academic Press. str. 695–716. ISBN 0–12–249951–4.

Obijeski, J. F., and Murphy, F. A. 1977. Bunyaviridae: recent biochemical developments. *J. Gen. Virol.* 37:1–14.

Obijeski, J. F., Bishop, D. H., Palmer, E. L., and Murphy, F. A. 1976. Segmented genome and nucleocapsid of La Crosse virus. *J. Virol.* 20:664–75.

Osborne, J. C., and Elliott, R. M. 2000. RNA binding properties of bunyamwera virus nucleocapsid protein and selective binding to an element in the 5′ terminus of the negative-sense S segment. *J. Virol.* 74:9946–52.

Överby, A. K., Pettersson, R. F., and Neve, E. P. 2007. The glycoprotein cytoplasmic tail of Uukuniemi virus (Bunyaviridae) interacts with ribonucleoproteins and is critical for genome packaging. *J. Virol.* 81:3198–205.

Panganiban, A. T., and Mir, M. A. 2009. Bunyavirus N: eIF4F surrogate and cap-guardian. *Cell Cycle.* 8:1332–7.

Pekosz, A., Phillips, J., Pleasure, D., Merry, D., and Gonzalez-Scarano, F. 1996. Induction of apoptosis by La Crosse virus infection and role of neuronal differentiation and human bcl-2 expression in its prevention. *J. Virol.* 70:5329–35.

Pepin, M., Bouloy, M., Bird, B. H., Kemp, A., and Paweska, J. 2010. Rift Valley fever virus (Bunyaviridae: Phlebovirus): an update on pathogenesis, molecular epidemiology, vectors, diagnostics and prevention. *Vet. Res.* 41:61.

Pinheiro, F. P., Travassos da Rosa, A. P., and Gomes, M. I. 1982. Trasmission of Oropouche virus from man to hamster by the midge *Culicoides paraensis. Science* 215:1251–3.

Plassmeyer, M. L., Soldan, S. S., Stachelek, K. M., Roth, S. M., Martín-García, J., and González-Scarano, F. 2007. Mutagenesis of the La Crosse Virus glycoprotein supports a role for Gc (1066–1087) as the fusion peptide. *Virology* 358:273–82.

Poch, O., Sauvaget, I., Delarue, M., and Tordo, N. 1989. Identification of four conserved motifs among the RNA-dependent polymerase encoding elements. *EMBO J.* 8:3867–74.

Reese, S. M., Beaty, M. K., Gabitzsch, E. S., Blair, C. D., and Beaty, B. J. 2009. Aedes triseriatus females transovarially infected with La Crosse virus mate more efficiently than uninfected mosquitoes. *J. Med. Entomol.* 46:1152–8.

Reguera, J., Weber, F., and Cusack, S. 2010. Bunyaviridae RNA polymerases (L-protein) have an N-terminal, influenza-like endonuclease domain, essential for viral cap-dependent transcription. *PLoS Pathog.* 6pii: e1001101.

Rust, R. S., Thompson, W. H., Matthews, C. G., Beaty, B. J., and Chun, R. W. 1999. La Crosse and other forms of California encephalitis. *J. Child. Neurol.* 14:1–14.

Salanueva, I. J., Novoa, R. R., Cabezas, P., López-Iglesias, C., Carrascosa, J. L., Elliott, R. M., and Risco, C. 2003. Polymorphism and structural maturation of bunyamwera virus in Golgi and post-Golgi compartments. *J. Virol.* 77:1368–81.

Sall, A. A., Thonnon, J., Sene, O. K., Fall, A., Ndiaye, M., Baudez, B., Mathiot, C., and Bouloy, M. 2001. Single-tube and nested reverse transcriptase-polymerase chain reaction for detection of Rift Valley fever virus in human and animal sera. *J. Virol. Methods.* 91:85–92.

Sall, A. A., Zanotto, P. M., Vialat, P., Sène, O. K., and Bouloy, M. 1998. Molecular epidemiology and emergence of Rift Valley fever. *Mem. Inst. Oswaldo Cruz* 93:609–14.

Santos, R. I., Rodrigues, A. H., Silva, M. L., Mortara, R. A., Rossi, M. A., Jamur, M. C., Oliver, C., and Arruda, E. 2008. Oropouche virus entry into HeLa cells involves clathrin and requires endosomal acidification. *Virus Res.* 138:139–43.

Scallan, M. F., and Elliott, R. M. 1992. Defective RNAs in mosquito cells persistently infected with Bunyamwera virus. *J. Gen. Virol.* 73:53–60.

Schmaljohn, C. S., and Nichol, S. T. 2007. Bunyaviridae. In: *Fields Virology*, Knipe, D. M., and Howley, P. M. (eds.), 5th Ed. Lippincott Williams & Wilkins, str. 1741–1789.

Sellers, R. F., Pedgley, D. E., and Tucker, M. R. 1982. Rift Valley fever, Egypt 1977: disease spread by windborne insect vectors? *Vet. Rec.* 110:73–7.

Shi, X., and Elliott, R. M. 2009. Generation and analysis of recombinant Bunyamwera orthobunyaviruses expressing V5 epitope-tagged L proteins. *J. Gen. Virol.* 90:297–306.

Shi, X., Brauburger, K., and Elliott, R. M. 2005. Role of N-linked glycans on bunyamwera virus glycoproteins in intracellular trafficking, protein folding, and virus infectivity. *J. Virol.* 79:13725–34.

Shi, X., Kohl, A., Léonard, V. H., Li, P., McLees, A., and Elliott, R. M. 2006. Requirement of the N-terminal region of orthobunyavirus nonstructural protein NSm for virus assembly and morphogenesis. *J. Virol.* 80:8089–99.

Shi, X., Kohl, A., Li, P., and Elliott, R. M. 2007. Role of the cytoplasmic tail domains of Bunyamwera orthobunyavirus glycoproteins Gn and Gc in virus assembly and morphogenesis. *J. Virol.* 81:10151–60.

Shi, X., Lappin, D. F., and Elliott, R. M. 2004. Mapping the Golgi targeting and retention signal of Bunyamwera virus glycoproteins. *J. Virol.* 78:10793–802.

Šimková, A. 1980. Man in the natural focus of the virus. In: *Ťahyňa Virus Natural Focus in Southern Moravia*, Rosický, B., and Málková, D. (eds.), Transactions of ČSAV, Math and Nat Sci Ser, 88, Academia Prague: 72–90.

Sokol, D. K., Kleiman, M. B., and Garg, B. P. 2001. LaCrosse viral encephalitis mimics herpes simplex viral encephalitis. *Pediatr. Neurol.* 25:413–5.

Soldan, S. S., and González-Scarano, F. 2005. Emerging infectious diseases: the Bunyaviridae. *J. Neurovirol.* 11:412–23.

Storms, M. M., Kormelink, R., Peters, D., Van Lent, J. W., and Goldbach, R. W. 1995. The nonstructural NSm protein of tomato spotted wilt virus induces tubular structures in plant and insect cells. *Virology* 214:485–93.

Swanepoel, R. 2004. Bunyaviridae. In: *Principles and Practice of Clinical Virology*, Zuckermann, A. J., Banatvala, J. E., Pattison, J. R., Griffiths, J. R., and Schoub, B. D., (eds.), 5th ed. J Wiley and Sons, Ltd. 555–588.

Tesh, R. B., Lubroth, J., and Guzman, H. 1992. Simulation of arbovirus overwintering: survival of Toscana virus (Bunyaviridae: Phlebovirus) in its natural sand fly vector Phlebotomus perniciosus. *Am. J. Trop. Med. Hyg.* 47:574–81.

Thomas, D., Blakqori, G., Wagner, V., Banholzer, M., Kessler, N., Elliott, R. M., Haller, O., and Weber, F. 2004. Inhibition of RNA polymerase II phosphorylation by a viral interferon antagonist. *J. Biol. Chem.* 279:31471–7.

Thompson, W. H., and Beaty, B. J. 1977. Venereal transmission of La Crosse (California encephalitis) arbovirus in *Aedes triseriatus* mosquitoes. *Science* 196:530.

Thompson, W. H., and Beaty, B. J. 1978. Venereal transmission of La Crosse virus from male to female. *Am. J. Trop. Med. Hyg.* 27:187–95.

Thompson, W. H., Kalfayan, B., and Anslow, R. O. 1965. Isolation of California group virus from a fatal human illness. *Am. J. Epidemiol.* 81:245–53.

Turell, M. J., and LeDuc, J. W. 1983. The role of mosquitoes in the natural history of California serogroup viruses. In: *California Serogroup Viruses*, Calisher, C. H., and Thompson, W. H. (eds.), AR Liss, Inc, New York: 43–55.

Valassina, M., Cusi, M. G., and Valensin, P. E. 2003. A Mediterranean arbovirus: the Toscana virus. *J. Neurovirol.* 9:577–83.

Valassina, M., Meacci, F., Valensin, P. E., and Cusi, M. G. 2000. Detection of neurotropic viruses circulating in Tuscany: the incisive role of Toscana virus. *J. Med. Virol.* 60:86–90.

Verani, P., Ciufolini, M. G., Caciolli, S., Renzi, A., Nicoletti, L., Sabatinelli, G., Bartolozzi, D., Volpi, G., Amaducci, L., and Coluzzi, M. 1988. Ecology of viruses isolated from sand flies in Italy and characterized of a new Phlebovirus (Arabia virus). *Am. J. Trop. Med. Hyg.* 38:433–9.

Verbruggen, P., Ruf, M., Blakqori, G., Överby, A. K., Heidemann, M., Eick, D., and Weber, F. 2011. Interferon antagonist NSs of La Crosse virus triggers a DNA damage response-like degradation of transcribing RNA polymerase II. *J. Biol. Chem.* 286:3681–92.

Walter, C. T., and Barr, J. N. 2010. Bunyamwera virus can repair both insertions and deletions during RNA replication. *RNA* 16:1138–45.

Watts, D. M., Pantuwatana, S., DeFoliart, G. R., Yuill, T. M., and Thompson, W. H. 1973. Transovarial transmission of La Crosse virus (California encephalitis group) in the mosquito, *Aedes triseriatus*. *Science* 182:1140–1.

Yuill, T. M. 1983. The role of mammals in the maintenance and dissemination of La Crosse virus. In: *California Serogroup Viruses*, Calisher, C. H., and Thompson, W. H., (eds.), AR Liss, Inc, New York: 77–87.

5 Human Coronaviruses

Respiratory Pathogens Revisited as Infectious Neuroinvasive, Neurotropic, and Neurovirulent Agents

*Marc Desforges, Dominique J. Favreau,
Élodie Brison, Jessica Desjardins,
Mathieu Meessen-Pinard,
Hélène Jacomy, and Pierre J. Talbot*

CONTENTS

5.1   INTRODUCTION

The central nervous system (CNS) is a highly complex biological system that maintains life, and insures its quality. However, like the rest of the organism, it is not immune to microbial infection in general and viral infection in particular. The viruses that penetrate the CNS therefore possess neuroinvasive properties and are usually also neurotropic, meaning that they infect neural cells (neurons and glial cells) and by doing so may also become neurovirulent as they can participate in the development of neurological diseases.

Neurological diseases are diverse and often remain not well understood, but one constant fact is that they usually end up in loss of neuronal cells because a portion of these precious cells will eventually die by different mechanisms. These pathologies may be genetically determined or caused by environmental factors or be provoked or perpetuated through a combination of both genes and environment. Among the several environmental factors presumed or known to be involved are the viruses, which possess potential neuropathogenic properties. Indeed, a viral origin of neurological diseases is often suspected, but causes of neurological syndromes of viral origin have often been difficult to identify, since CNS viral infections are often thought to represent complications of systemic viral illnesses. Some of these neurovirulent viruses are able to infect neurons and/or glial cells, causing either an acute disease (e.g., rabies-induced death; reviewed by Hankins and Rosekrans 2004) or chronic disease (e.g., measles virus-associated subacute sclerosing panencephalitis; SSPE; reviewed by Young and Rall 2009). Several diseases once described as degenerative, such as SSPE, are actually slow viral infections with long asymptomatic incubation periods and prolonged durations of overt clinical illness. Neuropathology can be a direct result of the infection, which will alter cell functions or an indirect consequence of the infection, for example through the action of proinflammatory mediators (neuroinflammation) that have direct detrimental effects on neural cells or attract inflammatory leukocytes to the site of infection or both.

Neurodegenerative diseases such as Parkinson's disease (PD), Alzheimer's disease (AD), amyotrophic lateral sclerosis (ALS), or multiple sclerosis (MS) have all been postulated to have an infectious origin and described to comprise an inflammatory component that could be triggered or enhanced by a viral infection. Among these different neurological diseases, MS represents the archetype of scientific uncertainties toward a CNS affliction of unknown etiology: both genes and environment have been suspected, and several genes as well as several environmental factors may contribute to neuropathogenesis. Several viruses have been implicated in MS etiology or propagation in the last five decades, although not one has so far withstood the test of time or closer scrutiny, perhaps because several different viruses may be involved (Cook and Dowling 1980; Gilden 2005; Kakalacheva et al. 2011; Talbot et al. 2001). However, the idea that ubiquitous viruses to which a genetically determined aberrant response is made and leads to relatively rare neurological diseases has garnered increasing support.

In the long list of viruses that are neuroinvasive, neurotropic, and potentially neurovirulent, the coronaviruses, from the order Nidovirales (reviewed by Siddell and Snijder 2008), are prevalent and have been occasionally associated with neuro-degenerative diseases of the CNS including MS, PD, and even AD. In humans, these viruses are recognized respiratory pathogens involved in upper respiratory tract infection in the population in general and in lower respiratory tract infection associated with pneumonia and asthma exacerbation in more vulnerable populations such as infant, elderly, and immunocompromised persons. Human coronaviruses (HCoVs) other than SARS-CoV co-circulate during seasonal outbreaks, and they are distributed worldwide, whereas SARS-CoV has not been detected in humans since 2003 (Vabret et al. 2009). Over the years, some coronaviruses have been associated with neurological diseases in animals and among the five different coronaviruses able to infect humans, at least three strains are neuroinvasive and neurotropic (Xu et al. 2005; Gu et al. 2005; Arbour et al. 2000).

5.2   VIRUSES AND HUMAN NEUROLOGICAL DISEASES

Viral infection of the human CNS does occur and often induces acute encepha-litis, which can even lead to death depending on the tropism of the different viruses involved (Whitley and Gnann 2002). Rabies virus (Hankins and Rosekrans 2004), herpes simplex virus (HSV) (Aurelian 2005), as well as arthropod-borne flaviviruses, including West Nile virus (WNV), Japanese encephalitis virus (JEV), and dengue virus (Mackenzie et al. 2004), all represent well characterized viral agents that can induce encephalitis in humans.

Long-term human neurological diseases may also be linked to viral infection. In HIV dementia, the human immunodeficiency virus (HIV) induces the degeneration of neurons in the hippocampus (reviewed by Mattson et al. 2005) with such neuro-degeneration resulting in motor dysfunction and possibly cognitive impairment (Nath and Berger 2004; Berger and Arendt 2000). Progressive multifocal leuko-encephalopathy (PML) represents a human demyelinating disease where severe and prolonged immunosuppression leads to the reactivation of the latent polyoma JC virus (JCV; reviewed by Weissert 2011; Roberts 2005). Subacute panencephalitis sclerosis (SSPE), a progressive fatal neurological disease, is also clearly linked to a viral cause: the persistence of measles virus within the CNS (Rima and Duprex 2005).

However, in several long-term human neurological diseases, it is very hard to ascertain a role of any given virus, due to the difficulty of establishing the time point at which this (or these) virus(es) become(s) involved. In this regard, Giovannoni et al. (2006) have elaborated a series of new criteria, adapted from Sir Austin Bradford Hill's for causation (Hill 1965). According to these authors, these "new" criteria should replace Koch's postulate when one wants to evaluate the relevance of any given virus in relation to multiple sclerosis etiology (Giovannoni et al. 2006). It is obvious that these criteria could also more efficiently fulfill the requirements for other long-term human neurological diseases potentially related to a viral infection as well. The HSV-1 and HHV-6 viruses were proposed as poten-tial infectious agents causing or exacerbating AD (Itzhaki et al. 2004). Influenza A was described as a factor that may increase the risk of PD (Takahashi and Yamada

1999) and viral respiratory infections in general were also described as a possible risk factor in the development of PD (Tsui et al. 1999). Epidemiological studies have also revealed an association between the risk of ALS and herpesviruses and echoviruses infection (Cermelli et al. 2003). Finally, psychiatric disorders were also investigated as a possible consequence of Borna disease virus (BDV) infection (Waltrip et al. 1995).

5.3 THE CORONAVIRUSES: AN OVERVIEW

The Coronaviruses are members of the family Coronaviridae within the order Nidovirales. They are classified in three different genera, namely α-, β-, and γ-coronaviruses (de Groot et al. 2012) and are ubiquitous mainly respiratory and enteric pathogens, with neurotropic and neuroinvasive properties in various hosts including humans, cats, pigs, and rodents. Coronaviruses form a group of enveloped viruses that have the largest genome among RNA viruses. This 30-kb positive single-stranded polyadenylated RNA possesses 4 or 5 genes encoding structural proteins (S, E, M, N; HE for the genus β-coronavirus) and several genes encoding nonstructural proteins (Figure 5.1).

The spike protein (S) is a large type 1 transmembrane glycosylated protein responsible for the recognition of the cellular receptor used by the virus to infect a susceptible cell (Cavanagh 1995). The larger portion of the S protein is exposed outside the surface of the viral envelope where it forms a homotrimer (Delmas and Laude 1990), visible by electron microscopy, and which gives the virus its "crown-like" (*corona* in Latin) morphology from what its name is derived (Figure 5.1a). The envelope (E) protein is a small structural protein anchored in the viral envelope, which has a role in the assembly of the virion and which appears responsible for the adequate curving of the viral envelope (Liu et al. 2007). The membrane (M) protein possesses three transmembrane domains and interacts with all the other structural proteins of the virus and therefore helps to shape and maintain the structure of the virion (Hogue and Machamer 2008). The nucleocapsid (N) protein associates with the viral genome and plays an essential role in encapsidating it in a helical nucleocapsid within the viral particle (Hogue and Machamer 2008; Macneughton and Davies 1978). The hemagglutinin-esterase (HE) is only present in most species of the β-coronavirus genus. Like the S protein, it is a type 1 transmembrane protein that forms homodimers (Hogue and Machamer 2008) and that interacts with different types of sialic acid associated with an apparent role in hemagglutination. It also possesses an acetyl-esterase function, which may be important early during infection or during the release of viral particles from the infected cells at the end of the replication cycle of the β-coronaviruses (Rottier 1990). The larger part of the genome, the ORF1a and 1b, encode two polyproteins (pp1a and pp1ab) which are cleaved by two viral proteases to yield 15 to 16 nonstructural proteins (nsp), which all play a role in the replication of the virus (Gorbalenya et al. 2006; Lai and Cavanagh 1997). The other nonstructural (ns) proteins are accessory and appear to mainly play a role in pathogenesis and in the virus–host interaction (Narayanan et al. 2008).

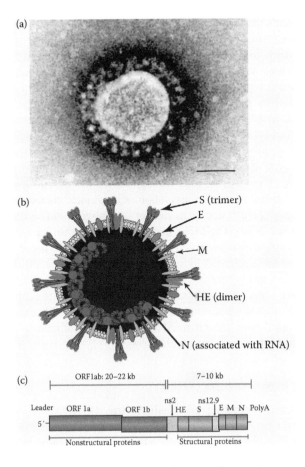

FIGURE 5.1 Overview of the coronaviruses: electron microscopic appearance (a; bar = 100 nm) and schematic diagram of the viral particle (b) and of the 30-kb RNA genome (c). The viral particle and the genome of the β-coronavirus HCoV-OC43 are represented as an example, but the overall organization of all the coronaviruses is the same, with the exception of the HE gene, which encodes a hemagglutinin-esterase protein, only present as a fifth structural protein in the viral envelope of some coronaviruses. The nonstructural (ns) proteins are specific to each genus and their number varies between the different coronaviruses. ORF1 encodes two large polyproteins designated pp1a and pp1ab, which are cleaved by viral proteases to yield 15 to 16 nonstructural proteins (nsp).

5.4 NONHUMAN CORONAVIRUSES INFECTING THE CNS

5.4.1 MOUSE HEPATITIS VIRUS

The first coronavirus shown to be neurotropic was the mouse hepatitis virus (MHV), a member of the β-coronavirus genus, as early as 1949 when the JHM strain was isolated from mice with disseminated encephalomyelitis and extensive demyelination (Cheever et al. 1949; Bailey et al. 1949).

MHV represents the best characterized coronavirus. It infects mice and rats and some strains are neurotropic and neuroinvasive, causing a large spectrum of diseases from hepatitis to encephalitis and chronic demyelination. It is the subject of several good reviews, which describe every aspects of its implication in neurological diseases and which highlight the importance of both viral and host factors in the process (reviewed by Bender and Weiss 2010; Cowley and Weiss 2010; Hosking and Lane 2010). Briefly, MHV can invade the CNS using the transneuronal route through the olfactory nerve (Barnett and Perlman 1993; Lavi et al. 1988). During the acute phase of infection of the CNS, MHV induces encephalitis and appears to infect different type of cells, which appear to vary for the different strains (Bender and Weiss 2010). The virus spreads throughout the brain and rapidly reaches the spinal cord, and an important up-regulation of cytokines, chemokines, and matrix metalloproteinases (MMP) occurs as part of the antiviral innate immune response (Hosking and Lane 2010). The MHV can also persist within the CNS and induce a chronic demyelinating disease, which is partially immune-mediated, similar to what is observed in multiple sclerosis in humans (Hosking and Lane 2010). Furthermore, using the C57BL/6 murine model, it was shown that the moderately neurovirulent MHV-A59 strain induced a modulation in expression of different types of genes within the CNS, including several immunity-related, and that this modulation in transcriptomic profile was accompanied by the activation of autoreactive T cells specific to myelin basic protein (Gruslin et al. 2005).

5.4.2 SWINE CORONAVIRUSES (PHEV)

The porcine hemagglutinating encephalitis virus (PHEV) was demonstrated to induce disease ranging from gastroenteritis to encephalomyelitis in piglets (Siddell et al. 1983; Andries and Pensaert 1980). The virus was isolated from the brains of suckling pigs suffering from encephalomyelitis several years ago (Greig et al. 1962), and the disease could be experimentally reproduced in piglets following intranasal inoculation (Alexander 1962). Moreover, using murine models, the neuroinvasiveness and neurotropism of the virus were demonstrated (Hirano et al. 2004; Yagami et al. 1986). PHEV induced a poor inflammatory reaction in CNS and infected cells showed no cytopathological changes (Hirano et al. 2004).

5.4.3 FELINE CORONAVIRUSES (FCoV)

Feline infectious peritonitis (FIP) is a common cause of death in cats, caused by a highly virulent variant of the feline coronavirus (FCoV), called FIPV, which either represents a naturally distinct circulating virulent form of FCoV (Brown et al. 2009) or which emerges from the less virulent virus feline enteric coronavirus (FECV) after acquiring mutations (Rottier et al. 2005; Vennema et al. 1998). The intestine was identified as the major site of persistence (Meli et al. 2004; Foley et al. 1997), but the virus also persists in macrophages of healthy cats (Kipar et al. 2010). These infected macrophages disseminate systemically and trigger immunological responses, which result in microgranuloma formation, vasculitis, organ failure, and death (Vennema et al. 1998; Poland et al. 1996; Pedersen and Boyle 1980). Neurological FIP may occur in about one cat out of three with FIP disease (Foley et al. 1998; Kline et al. 1994).

The neurological FIP appears partially immune-mediated and may result in uncontrolled inflammation in different parts of the brain that leads to diverse pathological manifestations including meningitis (Slauson and Finn 1972) and even spinal cord involvement (Legendre and Whitenack 1975). During neurological FIP, there is often a small amount of virus present in FIP-affected brain tissue (Foley et al. 1998), but inflammatory cells are nevertheless recruited to the brain and appear to contribute to disease, in part, through uncontrolled secretion of cytokines (Foley et al. 2003).

5.5 HUMAN CORONAVIRUSES INFECTING THE CNS

Coronaviruses are all molecularly related in structure and mode of replication (Brian and Baric 2005; Lai and Holmes 2001). Therefore, historically, the close structural and biological relatedness of HCoV to the neurotropic animal coronaviruses has led to speculation about the possible involvement of HCoV in neurological diseases. Up until today, no clear specific association was made with any known human neuropathology. However, HCoV-229E and HCoV-OC43 (Arbour et al. 2000; Arbour et al. 1999a,b; Bonavia et al. 1997), as well as SARS-CoV (Xu et al. 2005; Gu et al. 2005), were shown to be neuroinvasive and neurotropic. The significance of the presence of HCoVs in the human CNS and the related possible implications for neurological diseases is discussed in the next sections.

5.6 HUMAN CORONAVIRUSES: EPIDEMIOLOGY OF RESPIRATORY PATHOGENS

HCoV were first isolated in the mid-1960s from patients with upper respiratory tract disease (McIntosh et al. 1967; Hamre and Procknow 1966; Tyrrell and Bynoe 1965), and up until the fall of 2002, the only two known serological groups were represented by strains OC43 and 229E, which are respiratory pathogens responsible for 10 to 35% of common colds (Myint 1995). Over the last decade, several new coronaviruses were identified, including the human HCoV-NL63 (van der Hoek et al. 2004), HKU1 (Woo et al. 2005a), and the SARS-CoV, the causative agent of the severe acute respiratory syndrome (SARS) (Drosten et al. 2003; Fouchier et al. 2003).

Therefore, HCoVs are now represented by five different strains; HCoV-229E, -OC43, -NL63, -HKU1, and SARS-CoV. HCoV other than SARS-CoV are primarily associated with upper and lower respiratory tract disease worldwide (Vabret et al. 2009). However, even before the SARS epidemic of 2002, the HCoV were regularly associated with severe respiratory distress in newborns (Gagneur et al. 2002; Sizun et al. 1993) and as important trigger of acute asthma exacerbations (El-Sahly et al. 2000; Johnston et al. 1995; Nicholson et al. 1993). More recently, HCoVs were associated with acute lower respiratory tract infection, including pneumonia, in both infants and immunocompromised patients (Gerna et al. 2006; Woo et al. 2005b). As summarized by Vabret and collaborators, two epidemiologic pictures of

HCoV infections have to be distinguished today. HCoVs other than SARS-CoV co-circulate during seasonal outbreaks, and they are distributed worldwide, even though a "regional" distribution may vary according to the geographic area and season. On the other hand, the SARS-CoV, which was responsible for the first emerging infectious disease pandemic of the 21st century, 8096 probable cases of SARS were reported with a fatality of about 10% between the fall of 2002 and summer of 2003, has stopped circulating in July of 2003 with the help of drastic public health policy around the world (Vabret et al. 2009). Only a few additional sporadic cases were reported between the fall of 2003 and the spring of 2004 in China and Singapore, most of them being laboratory-related infections (Gu and Korteweg 2007; http://www.who.int/csr/don/archive/disease/severe_acute_respiratory_syndrome/en/index.html). Since the end of the SARS outbreak, it has been confirmed that bats are the natural reservoir of the SARS-CoV (Li et al. 2005).

Among the five HCoV strains, at least HCoV-229E and HCoV-OC43, as well as SARS-CoV, possess neuroinvasive properties as viral RNA can be detected in the human brain (Xu et al. 2005; Gu et al. 2005; Arbour et al. 2000).

5.7 RESPIRATORY HUMAN CORONAVIRUSES INVADING THE CNS

As reviewed by Talbot and collaborators for HCoVs other than SARS-CoV (Talbot et al. 2008) and for SARS-CoV (Nicholls et al. 2008; Gu and Korteweg 2007), coronaviruses that infect humans are primarily respiratory pathogens and they usually target first epithelial cells from the respiratory tract (Miura and Holmes 2009).

One factor that influences a virus-induced pathogenesis is the type of cell susceptible to this virus in a tissue or a specific organ. Binding of the virus to its target cell through a receptor is a critical early step in infection. HCoV-229E uses aminopeptidase N (APN), also called CD13 (Yeager et al. 1992). SARS-CoV (Li et al. 2003) and HCoV-NL63 (Hofmann et al. 2005) use angiotensin-converting enzyme 2 (ACE2); SARS-CoV can also use L-SIGN (CD209L) (Jeffers et al. 2004). However, the cellular receptor for HCoV-HKU1 and HCoV-OC43 remains to be identified. Sialic acid in the form of N-acetyl-9-O-acetylneuraminic acid was identified as a ligand for the S protein of HCoV-OC43 (Kunkel and Herrler 1993) and as a receptor determinant during infection (Krempl et al. 1995), and it is now known that this particular sialic acid is essential for infection of susceptible human epithelial and neuronal cells (Desforges 2011). The major histocompatibility complex (MHC) class I C molecule (HLA-C) was recently identified as an attachment factor that facilitates the infection of susceptible cells by HCoV-HKU1 (Chan et al. 2009). All of the known receptors mentioned above have been shown to be expressed in different cell types within the respiratory tract and other tissues, including the CNS.

HCoVs are recognized respiratory pathogens, however, infectious particles, antigens or RNA, were detected in tissues other than the respiratory tract, including the CNS. To be neuroinvasive, viruses such as HCoV-229E and -OC43 and SARS-CoV may use two different routes from the periphery. The first, called the hematogenous route, involves the presence of a given virus in the blood where it can either remain free for a period of time before it can infect the endothelial cells of the blood–brain barrier (BBB) or infect leukocytes that will become some sort of viral reservoir.

Both situations occur during HIV infection of the CNS. Indeed, HIV-infected leukocytes migrating through the BBB (called the Trojan horse hypothesis; reviewed by Kim et al. 2003) is one of the routes, and direct infection of the endothelial cells from the BBB is also possible even though the viral replication is low (Argyris et al. 2007). A second form of any viral spread toward the CNS is through neuronal dissemination, where a given virus infects neurons in periphery and uses the machinery of transportation within those cells in order to gain access to the CNS.

Infection of human leukocytic cell lines and of monocytes/macrophages by HCoV-229E and HCoV-OC43 was reported (Desforges et al. 2007; Collins 2002), and infection by HCoV-229E of peritoneal macrophages (Patterson and Macnaughton 1982) and murine dendritic cells expressing the human APN (Wentworth et al. 2005) suggests that HCoVs may use these cells to disseminate to other tissues, where they could be associated with other types of pathologies. SARS-CoV was also shown to be able to infect human monocytes/macrophages (Nicholls et al. 2006; Gu et al. 2005), which produced a small amount of infectious particles (Yilla et al. 2005). Moreover, monocyte-derived dendritic cells are also susceptible to a low-level productive infection by SARS-CoV (Spiegel et al. 2006).

Both the human monocytic cell line THP-1 and human primary monocytes are activated to produce TNF-α and MMP-9 following infection by HCoV-229E in cell culture (Desforges et al. 2007). As activated monocytes eventually become macrophages as they invade tissues, this activation suggests that HCoV-229E-infected monocytes would become activated *in vivo*, thus facilitating their passage toward other tissues, especially in immunocompromised individuals, as this was observed for murine cytomegalovirus (MCMV) (Reuter et al. 2004). The fact that HCoV-229E could only infect partially immunocompromised transgenic mice (Lassnig et al. 2005) suggests that HCoV-229E could take advantage of an immunosuppressed environment and disseminate to different organs within susceptible individuals. The establishment of a persistent infection in a human leukocytic cell line (Desforges et al. 2007) is also consistent with the possibility that monocytes/macrophages serve as a reservoir and vector for HCoV-229E toward other tissues, including the CNS for this neuroinvasive HCoV (Arbour et al. 2000). The same situation may occur for SARS-CoV, which infects monocytes-macrophages (Nicholls et al. 2006; Gu et al. 2005) as a study with a mouse model suggests that after an intranasal infection, the virus primarily replicate in the lungs before going into the brain (McCray et al. 2007). Furthermore, considering the fact that SARS-CoV is able to modulate the innate immunity in dendritic cells (Spiegel et al. 2006), one can also speculate that these cells could also serve as an eventual reservoir for this virus in order to reach and maintain itself in the CNS. Our results indicate that HCoVs were also shown to infect human endothelial cells of the BBB in culture (unpublished data), and it has been speculated that SARS-CoV could do the same after viremia (Guo et al. 2008), as both ACE-2 and CD209L are expressed on the endothelial cells of the human BBB (Li et al. 2007). Therefore, the neuroinvasive HCoVs could use the hematogenous route to penetrate the CNS as illustrated in Figure 5.2.

On the other hand, after an intranasal infection, both HCoV-OC43 (Jacomy and Talbot 2003) and SARS-CoV (McCray et al. 2007) were shown to infect the lungs in mice and to be neuroinvasive as HCoV-OC43 (Butler et al. 2006; St-Jean et al.

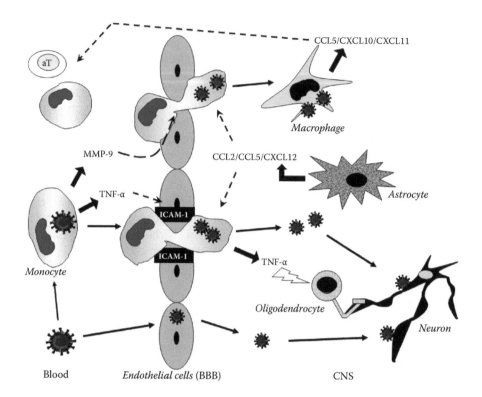

FIGURE 5.2 Hematogenous route of neuroinvasion and possible mechanism of neuroviru-lence of HCoV. Human monocytes are susceptible to infection by HCoVs including SARS-CoV and are activated after infection. This activation involves, among other factors, the production of MMP-9, which increases the permeability of the BBB, and of TNF-α, which up-regulates the adhesion molecule ICAM-1 on endothelial cells of the BBB, facilitating the passage of infected monocytes into the central nervous system (CNS). Viruses may also directly infect endothelial cells to gain access to the CNS, where they can infect neurons. Once in the CNS, the infected and activated monocytes produce proinflammatory cytokines, such as TNF-α that can damage the myelin-synthesizing oligodendrocytes and/or neurons. Infected monocyte-derived macrophages that entered the CNS (or microglia) may produce chemokines, such as CCL5, CXCL10, or CXCL11, which will chemoattract activated T cells and/or other monocytes into the CNS. These cells may then mediate an immune-mediated pathogenesis after infection. Moreover, after sensing the infection, astrocytes may produce chemokines, such as CCL2, CCL5, and CXCL12, that will also participate in the recruitment of more infected leukocytes. Thus, coronaviruses can initiate a neuroinflammatory loop lead-ing to neuropathology.

2004) and SARS-CoV (Netland et al. 2008) were detected in the CNS of susceptible mice. Therefore, these two coronaviruses may use both the hematogenous and the transneuronal route through the olfactory nerve toward the CNS. Furthermore, as shown here in Figure 5.3, once in the brain, HCoV-OC43 is able to disseminate in the cortex and medulla but the cerebellum remains uninfected. The hippocampus represents another specific structure infected by HCoV-OC43 in the brain. Once in

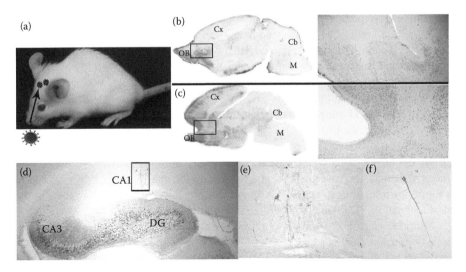

FIGURE 5.3 Transneuronal route of neuroinvasion through the olfactory nerve and spread into the CNS of HCoV. (a) After intranasal infection of susceptible mice, HCoV-OC43 is able to get into the brain through the olfactory nerve and replicate in the CNS. (b) At 3 days postinfection, viral antigens are detected in neuronal cells in the olfactory bulb (OB). The right panel presents a higher magnification of the insert on the left panel. (c) At 7 days postinfection, virus is still present in the OB, and spread is observed into the cortical area (Cx) and the medulla (M). The cerebellum (Cb) is spared from infection. The right panel presents a higher magnification of the insert on the left panel. (d) The hippocampus is infected by HCoV-OC43 as shown by the presence of viral antigens in numerous neurons of the dentate gyrus (DG) and in CA3 pyramidal neurons. The low number of infected neurons in the CA1 pyramidal layer (insert magnified in e) suggests that the virus uses the Schaffer's collaterals from CA3 cells before spreading to CA1 cells. This illustrates the transneuronal spread of HCoV. (f) Hippocampal neuron infected by HCoV-OC43 illustrating that infection occurs in the whole dendritic tree and axonal extension.

this region of the brain, the virus appears to propagate by a transneuronal route as also illustrated and described in Figure 5.3.

5.7.1 Human Coronaviruses Other than SARS-CoV: Possible Association with Neurological Diseases in Humans

Traditionally, the four Koch's postulates have been applied to establish whether a particular infectious agent causes a specific disease (Koch 1942). However, as beautifully presented by Fredericks and Relman (1996), there are situations where Koch's postulates have to be reconsidered. Several viral infections, and especially the slow viral infections related to diseases that are rare manifestations of a particular infection, represent this kind of situation where Koch's postulate should be replaced. Two well-known examples of the latter situation are related to Epstein-Barr virus (EBV), where only a minority of individuals will develop Burkitt's lymphoma and to the human T-cell lymphotrophic virus (HTLV-1), which will cause the progressive tropical spastic paraparesis/HTLV-1-associated myelopathy (PTSP/HAM) in only 1% of infected individuals (reviewed by Giovannoni et al. 2006).

The presence of HCoV-229E and HCoV-OC43 has been detected in different neurological diseases in humans. An association that was made with PD stems from a report of antiviral antibodies (Fazzini et al. 1992) and HCoV RNAs (Cristallo et al. 1997) in the cerebrospinal fluid (CSF) of PD patients. Moreover, detection of viral RNA in human PD brains revealed that three out of three patients were positive for HCoV-229E and one of them also for HCoV-OC43 (Arbour et al. 2000). Like many neurodegenerative diseases, genetic and environmental factors seem to be involved in the etiology of PD (Olanow and Tatton 1999). Influenza A was described as a factor that may increase the risk of PD (Takahashi and Yamada 1999), and viral respiratory infections in general were also described as a possible risk factor in the development of PD (Tsui et al. 1999).

Multiple sclerosis (MS) represents another human neurological disease where an infectious agent or agents may play a triggering role, with viruses the most likely culprit in genetically predisposed individuals (Kurtzke 1993). There is a presumption that several neurotropic viruses could be involved in MS pathogenesis but that they may do so through similar direct and/or indirect mechanisms (reviewed by Kakalacheva et al. 2011; Gilden 2005; Talbot et al. 2001; Johnson 1985; Cook and Dowling 1980). However, research has not isolated or directly linked any specific virus with MS. Association of coronaviruses with MS was suggested by their isolation from the CNS of two patients (Burks et al. 1980). Other reports include intrathecal antibody synthesis (Salmi et al. 1982) and ultrastructural observation (Tanaka et al. 1976). One report demonstrated a significant association of colds with MS exacerbation and a significant association of HCoV-229E infection in MS patients (Hovanec and Flanagan 1983) and another report on the association of viral infections and MS (Sibley et al. 1985) commented that seasonal HCoV infection patterns do fit the observed occurrence of MS exacerbations. Acute disseminated encephalomyelitis (ADEM) is a neurological disorder characterized by inflammation of the brain and spinal cord caused by damage to the myelin and is seen most frequently after nonspecific upper respiratory tract infections. Even though the etiological agent remains unknown, HCoV-OC43 was detected in the CNS of a child with ADEM (Yeh et al. 2004).

As previously stated, although any direct correlation between HCoV-229E and HCoV-OC43 and neuropathology in humans remains to be investigated, the detection of RNA in human brains does confirm that they are truly neuroinvasive (Arbour et al. 2000). Furthermore, the case of these HCoVs in the CNS may represent a new example where the traditional Koch's postulate should be replaced by the previously cited adapted Hill's criteria (Giovannoni et al. 2006).

Even though HCoV-NL63 and HKU1 have never been detected in human CNS, a recent report suggests that they may represent a comorbid risk factor in individuals with serious mental disorders. The authors of this report are careful in the conclusions they draw, as they are aware of the highly circumstantial nature of this association of HCoV with recent psychotic symptoms, which is based on high titers of IgG specific to these viruses in the serum of patients (Severance et al. 2011). Nevertheless, studies to evaluate the extent that HCoV-NL63 and HKU1 can be neuroinvasive are warranted.

5.7.2 SARS-CoV: Possible Association with Neurological Diseases in Humans

The neuroinvasive properties of SARS-CoV were first suspected when viral RNA was detected in the CSF of a 32-year-old female patient in Hong Kong in 2004 (Lau et al. 2004). The year after, SARS-CoV neuroinvasive properties were indeed demonstrated. The virus was isolated from brain tissue of a SARS patient who presented neurological symptoms and a neuropathology associated with necrosis of neuronal cells and glial cell activation. Moreover, the chemokine CXCL9/Mig (monokine induced by γ-interferon) was expressed by glial cells in association with infiltration of T cells and macrophages (Xu et al. 2005). The same year, another report indicated that SARS-CoV RNA was also detected in the brain of eight different patients who died from SARS, as the presence of the genomic RNA was detected in the cytoplasm of numerous hypothalamic and cortical neurons. Furthermore, edema and scattered red degeneration were observed in the brain of six out of the eight autopsied brains (Gu et al. 2005). Therefore, SARS-CoV is neuroinvasive, neurotropic, and could be associated with the development of a neurological disease. Furthermore, the involvement of SARS-CoV in CNS infections was underscored by the findings that made use of transgenic mouse models expressing the human angiotensin-converting enzyme 2 (ACE-2), which is the cellular receptor used by the SARS-CoV to infect susceptible cells. Indeed, using these mice, it was shown that the SARS-CoV could invade the CNS after an intranasal infection primarily through the olfactory bulb (Netland et al. 2008) or even after an intraperitoneal infection (Tseng et al. 2007), with concomitant neuronal loss (Netland et al. 2008; Tseng et al. 2007).

5.8 POSSIBLE MECHANISMS OF HUMAN CORONAVIRUS-INDUCED NEUROPATHOGENESIS

Viral infection of oligodendrocytes could lead to demyelinating disease through the alteration of their normal function or cytolysis as is the case for reactivated JCV, which induces the progressive lysis of oligodendrocytes during PML (Roberts 2005; Sweet et al. 2002). The release of myelin components could also provide targets for autoimmune attack. Infection or activation of astrocytes and microglia could lead to release of inflammatory mediators that could damage oligodendrocytes (Hovelmeyer et al. 2005; Gonzalez-Scarano and Baltuch 1999; Miller et al. 1997; McLarnon et al. 1993).

Several years ago, HCoV-OC43 was shown to productively infect cultured mouse CNS cells and human fetal glial cells were also susceptible to HCoV-OC43 infection, although no infectious virus was detected (Pearson and Mims 1985). Over the years, our own studies have shown that cell lines representative of the human CNS are susceptible to productive infection by HCoV-229E and HCoV-OC43, including long-term viral persistence (Arbour et al. 1999a,b), and that primary cultures of fetal and adult human astrocytes and adult microglia are susceptible to infection by both HCoV strains (Bonavia et al. 1997) with preliminary results consistent with infection of adult oligodendrocytes and human brain endothelial cells (unpublished data).

Furthermore, making use of a different mouse model, we also showed that HCoV-OC43 induces an acute vacuolating encephalitis (Jacomy and Talbot 2003) and viral persistence in the CNS associated with motor disabilities (Jacomy et al. 2006), suggesting that respiratory pathogens, like neurotropic and neuroinvasive HCoVs, could be associated with neurodegenerative disease in susceptible individuals. Like the mouse coronavirus MHV (the murine counterpart of HCoV-OC43), which is able to induce a chronic white matter pathology characterized by focal demyelinating lesions in brain and spinal cord in mice that survived acute encephalitis (Weiner 1973; Lampert et al. 1973) associated with immunopathological mechanism (Houtman and Fleming 1996; Wang et al. 1990), the HCoV-OC43 appears to be able to establish itself in the CNS where it could eventually participate in the development of a chronic demyelinating disease resembling MS. Furthermore, we have demonstrated that MHV activates myelin basic protein-reactive T-cells (Gruslin et al. 2005) and identified HCoV-myelin T-cell cross-reactivity in MS patients (Boucher et al. 2007; Talbot et al. 1996). Moreover, variants of HCoV-OC43 harboring mutations in the Spike protein (S), acquired after a persistent infection in human neural cells, are able to induce a long-term demyelination in the spinal cord of susceptible mice (Jacomy et al. 2010) resembling the lesions observed in MS patients. This suggests that persistence in neural cells has allowed HCoV-OC43 to acquire mutations that may modify the capacity of the virus to spread in the CNS correlating with demyelination in the spinal cord, which ends up in a modification in the resulting neuropathology it causes in susceptible hosts.

We have shown that HCoV-OC43-infected astrocytes and microglia are activated to produce proinflammatory mediators (Edwards et al. 2000). Activation of CNS glial cells, astrocytes, and especially microglia is now recognized as a hallmark of neurological disorders (reviewed by Raivich and Banati 2004; Nelson et al. 2002), including MS (Sriram and Rodriguez 1997) and AD (Barger and Harmon 1997). Viruses that enter the CNS, such as HCoV (Arbour et al. 2000; Bonavia et al. 1997) are thus prime candidate mediators of some of this neuropathologically relevant activation involving release of proinflammatory molecules such as cytokines, chemokines, nitric oxide (NO), and reactive oxygen intermediates (ROS; reviewed by Bilzer and Stitz 1996), as well as local antigen presentation to infiltrating T lymphocytes (Aloisi et al. 2000). Studies of the interaction of viruses with microglial cells may hold keys to understanding some neuropathogenic mechanisms. Even though HIV appears to be able to infect neurons in very young children (Canto-Nogues et al. 2005), in the adult CNS, HIV does not infect neurons, and it is therefore believed that, the damage induced to neurons in HIV dementia is initiated by either cellular soluble mediators such as MMP released from infected infiltrating macrophages (Zhang et al. 2003) or by HIV proteins released from infected glial cells (Mattson et al. 2005). Our results showing that HCoV-OC43 induces neuronal apoptosis in murine primary cultures and *in vivo* (murine model), with apoptotic cells being infected or not, suggests that, like it is the case for HIV, soluble mediators released by glial cells surrounding neurons may be involved in the neuronal degeneration that leads to neuropathology (Jacomy et al. 2006). As stated above, HCoV-229E and HCoV-OC43 have the potential to infect different cells in the CNS. However, we have shown that the neurons are the main target cell of HCoV-OC43 in the CNS of susceptible mice (Jacomy and Talbot 2003) and in mixed primary cultures from the murine CNS (Jacomy et al. 2006) (Figure 5.4a) and in co-cultures of human neurons and astrocytes (Figure 5.4b) obtained from the

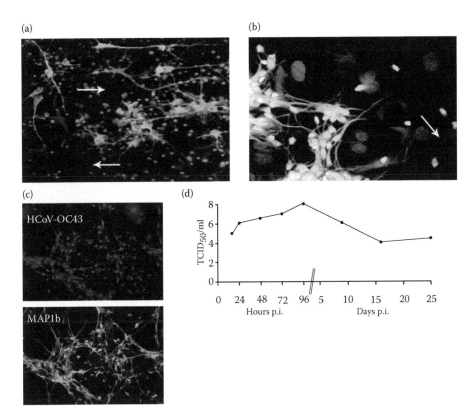

FIGURE 5.4   (See color insert.) The main target of HCoV-OC43 infection is the neuron in mouse and human cell cultures. (a) Mixed primary cultures from the murine CNS. (b) Cocultures of human neurons and astrocytes obtained from differentiated human NT2 cell line using a protocol, which gives rise to a mixture of neurons and astrocytes. In both type of cultures, HCoV-OC43 primarily targets the neuron for infection leading to axonal beading (white arrows in a and b). The +viral S protein is in green in infected neurons and red represents the glial fibrillary acidic protein (GFAP) in activated astrocytes. The blue signal is the nucleus detected by the DNA-specific dye DAPI. (c) NT2-N cells (95% pure human neuronal culture) infected by HCoV-OC43. The viral S protein is in red in infected neurons and green represents the microtubule associated protein 1b (MAP1b) expression in differentiated neurons. (d) HCoV-OC43 can establish a long term infection of the NT2-N cells for up to 25 days postinfection even though cell death occurred in a portion of the NT2-N cells after acute infection.

differentiation of the human NT2 cell line using a modified protocol that give rises to a mixture of neurons and astrocytes (Sandhu et al. 2003).

The NT2 cell line may also be differentiated as a 95% pure neuronal culture named NT2-N, which expresses different markers of human neuronal cells (Pleasure et al. 1992). Even though cell death was induced in a portion of the NT2-N cells after infection by HCoV-OC43, these cells were able to sustain a long time productive infection by HCoV-OC43 for at least 25 days (Figure 5.4d). When analyzing this transcriptome modulation of the infected NT2-N cells (Figure 5.5) and by confirming the results by RT-PCR, it became clear that, like other coronaviruses

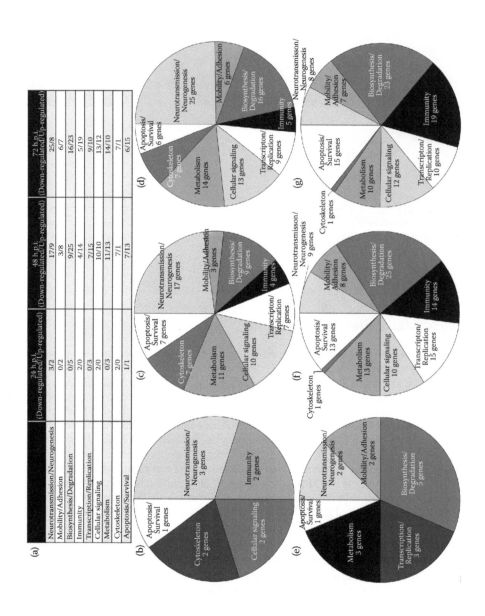

(a)	24 h.p.i. (Down-regulated/Up-regulated)	48 h.p.i. (Down-regulated/Up-regulated)	72 h.p.i. (Down-regulated/Up-regulated)
Neurotransmission/Neurogenesis	3/2	17/9	25/8
Mobility/Adhesion	0/2	3/8	6/7
Biosynthesis/Degradation	0/5	9/25	16/23
Immunity	2/0	4/14	5/19
Transcription/Replication	0/3	7/15	9/10
Cellular signaling	2/0	10/10	13/12
Metabolism	0/3	11/13	14/10
Cytoskeleton	2/0	7/1	7/1
Apoptosis/Survival	1/1	7/13	6/15

(Bechill et al. 2008; Chan et al. 2006) in different cell types, HCoV-OC43 induces the modulation of expression of several genes related to the unfolded protein response (UPR) in infected human NT2-N and LA-N-5 neuronal cell lines (Favreau et al. 2009). The UPR is associated with the induction of ER (endoplasmic reticulum) stress and represents a process that serves in cell homeostasis but which can become deleterious to the cell when the stimulus is too strong or when it remains for a long period of time (Ron and Walter 2007). Moreover, ER stress and impaired UPR has been associated with human neurological diseases (Lindholm et al. 2006; Paschen 2003). Using two different variants of HCoV-OC43, we were able to relate the level and duration of the UPR induction in neuronal cells with the S protein. Indeed, compared to the wild type HCoV-OC43 virus, a variant harboring two-point mutations in the putative receptor binding domain of the S protein, acquired during a persistent infection of human neural cells, induced a stronger UPR, which eventually led to more activation of caspase 3 and neuronal cell-death (Favreau et al. 2009). This is of particular interest as we previously showed that caspase 3 activation and apparent apoptosis was induced in the brain of infected mice and in mixed primary cultures from the murine CNS (Jacomy et al. 2006).

The analysis of the transcriptomic modulation in the NT2-N neuronal cells infected by the HCoV-OC43 also indicates that the level of expression of different families of genes that can be related to diverse metabolic pathways is either up- or down-regulated after the infection (Figure 5.5). For instance, the genes related to the induction of the UPR are compromised in the "biosynthesis and degradation" family. The modulation of expression of several genes in this family was directly correlated with an ER stress and effective UPR in HCoV-OC43-infected neuronal cells (Favreau et al. 2009). Therefore, one can argue that evaluating the complete transcriptome of infected cells will certainly help to decipher the more complete neuronal cell response after infection. In this regard, recent results from our laboratory clearly indicate that the "apoptosis/cell survival" (Favreau et al. 2012) and the "neurotransmission/neurogenesis" family (Brison et al. 2011) identified in Figure 5.5 represent important pathways in the neuron response to HCoV-OC43 infection.

Neurotransmission between adjacent neurons is an essential process in the CNS where glutamate is the major excitatory neurotransmitter involved in several functions. In physiological conditions, glutamate is synthesized by neurons and released in the synaptic cleft. Two types of ionotropic transmembrane receptors for glutamate that mediates synaptic transmission exist in the central nervous sytem (CNS). The

---

FIGURE 5.5 Virus-induced modulation of the neuronal transcriptome in the NT2-N model of human neurons. Infection of NT2-N cells by HCoV-OC43 induces a modulation of the whole neuronal transcriptome. Exhaustive analysis on a genome-wide scale revealed that the level of expression of several different genes encoding cellular proteins involved in diverse metabolic pathways was significantly modulated. The genes were classified within nine different functional families, as shown in panel a, where the number indicates the number of genes that are either down- or up-regulated at 24, 48, and 72 h postinfection (hpi). The relative proportion of the different gene families that are down-regulated are represented in pie charts: (b) 24, (c) 48, and (d) 72 hpi, and the relative proportion of the different gene families that are up-regulated are represented in pie charts: (e) 24, (f) 48, and (g) 72 hpi.

first is named the α-amino-3-hydroxy-5-methyl-4-isoxazolepropionic acid receptor (also known as AMPAr) and the second N-methyl-D-aspartate receptor (NMDAr) (reviewed by Watkins and Jane 2006). Activation of the downstream AMPA receptor allows the entry of sodium ions in the postsynaptic neuron in order to mediate the neuronal membrane depolarization. Using another type of glutamate receptor, called the glutamate-transporter 1 (GLT-1), astrocytic cells clear the excess of extracellular glutamate in the synaptic cleft by uptake through special receptors that are high-affinity tansporters of glutamate (reviewed by Kuzmiski and Bains 2010). A disruption of glutamate homeostasis may induce neuronal degeneration and eventual cell death by an excitotoxic process (Mark et al. 2001), which is an excessive stimulation by the neurotransmitter glutamate on its specific receptors (AMPAr and NMDAr) (Olney 1969; Figure 5.6), This is of particular interest considering that since then,

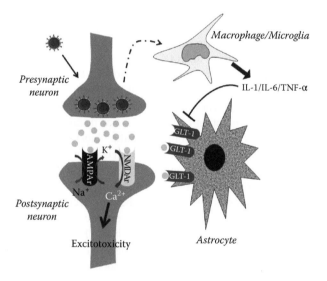

FIGURE 5.6   HCoV infection induces neuronal death by excitotoxicity. Glutamate serves as the primary excitatory neurotransmitter in the mammalian CNS. In physiological conditions, glutamate is mainly synthesized by neurons and released into the synaptic cleft. Activation of AMPA receptors (AMPAr) allows entry of sodium ions into the postsynaptic neuron, which is responsible for depolarization of the neuronal membrane. This leads to activation of NMDA receptors (NMDAr) that allow an entry of calcium ions into the postsynaptic neuron. Over-stimulation of glutamate receptors (AMPAr and NMDAr) leads to neuronal injury by excito-toxicity. In pathological conditions, regulation of glutamate release and uptake may be altered by HCoV-OC43 infection, which induces an overwhelming stress in infected neurons of the spinal cord that may lead to an increased synthesis/release of glutamate into the synaptic cleft, leading to high level of calcium influx and excitotoxicity where neurons could be dam-aged and die following excessive stimulation of glutamate on its specific receptors. In this model, virus infection of neurons is detected by macrophage/microglia, which produce high level of pro-inflammatory cytokines, which will in turn down-regulate the expression of the glutamate receptor GLT-1 on astrocytes, which is responsible for the uptake of glutamate. Therefore, these astrocytes will no longer be able to recapture the excess of glutamate and neuronal cells will undergo excitotoxicity and eventual degeneration and death.

glutamate excitotoxicity was shown to be involved in several viral infections such as WNV, Sindbis virus, JEV, HIV and HSV (Blakely et al. 2009; Carmen et al. 2009; Golembewski et al. 2007; Mishra et al. 2007; Haughey et al. 2001). The loss of neuronal subpopulations in the brain during HIV dementia was also related to an indirect mechanism conjugating glial activation, cytokines released and excitotoxic transmission (Alirezaei et al. 2008; Masliah et al. 1996). Using a mouse model, we recently showed that during infection by HCoV-OC43, hippocampal neurons died in part by this glutamate excitotoxicity as they were partially protected from degeneration in mice that were treated with the AMPA receptor antagonist (GYKI-52466) (Brison et al. 2011). Therefore, HCoV infection of the CNS may also involve excitotoxicity, which could account for the neurological disease associated with the infection. From a scientific point of view, it is interesting to note that this process has over the years been associated with diverse human neurological diseases such as Huntington's disease, AD, PD, and ALS, as well as MS (Lau and Tymianski 2010; Haeberlein and Lipton 2009).

Less work has been done in relation to the potential neurovirulence of the other coronaviruses that can infect humans. However, some very interesting and relevant data have been gathered on the underlying possible mechanisms related to the SARS-CoV. Following infection of the mouse CNS, SARS-CoV was detected in a large number of neurons in the cerebrum, thalamus, and brain stem although the olfactory bulb and the cerebellum appeared relatively spared. Death of mice occurred before significant infiltration of immune cells in the CNS, suggesting that the rapid infection of neurons was the cause of death in the absence of encephalitis (McCray et al. 2007). Moreover, it was shown only the year after that SARS-CoV could enter the brain via the olfactory bulb and that it was able to spread very fast by a transneuronal route to connected areas of the brain. Moreover, mice infected by SARS-CoV likely died from death or dysfunction of infected neurons in particular regions of the brain, including the cardiorespiratory centers of the medulla (Netland et al. 2008). This fact is of high interest as SARS-CoV can be neuroinvasive in humans and that in those cases, infected neurons underwent necrosis (Xu et al. 2005).

5.9   CONCLUSION AND SIGNIFICANCE

The presence of coronaviruses in the human CNS is now a recognized fact. Indeed, they appear to be part of a viral flora of the brain, with potential neuropathological consequences in genetically susceptible individuals with or without additional environmental insults. Even though these respiratory pathogens could induce an acute encephalitis as established using a murine model, they may also be associated with the induction or exacerbation of other types of neurological diseases for which it is very hard to ascertain a role to any given virus due to the difficulty of establishing the time point at which this virus becomes involved.

In that regard, the "new" Hill's criteria elaborated by Giovannoni and collaborators may represent a highly relevant tool in order to evaluate the relevance of these recognized human respiratory pathogens as a factor that will influence the development or the exacerbation of a long-term human neurological disease potentially related to a viral infection. The examples of neurological diseases once described as degenerative and which are slow viral infections with long-term asymptomatic incubation periods related to different human viruses are potent indicators that it may be relevant to associate the recognized presence of HCoVs in the CNS with human neurological diseases. Therefore, more in-depth studies on neuroinvasive, neurotropic, and potentially neurovirulent HCoVs are warranted in order to better understand how they influence the neural cell functions and eventual destiny in conjunction with genetic factors of the host.

ACKNOWLEDGEMENT

Work from our laboratory was supported by Operating Grant No. MT-9203 from the Institute of Infection and Immunity (III) of the Canadian Institutes of Health Research (CIHR) and Discovery Grant No. 42619-2009 from the Natural Sciences and Engineering Research Council of Canada (NSERC) to P.J.T., who is the holder of the Tier-1 (Senior) Canada Research Chair in Neuroimmunovirology award. E.B. acknowledges a graduate studentship from the Multiple Sclerosis Society of Canada. J.D. acknowledges a graduate studentship from NSERC. M.M.-P. acknowledges a doctoral studentship from the *Fondation Armand-Frappier.* D.J.F. acknowledges a doctoral studentship from the *Fonds de la recherche en santé du Québec* (FRSQ).

REFERENCES

Alexander, T. J. (1962). Viral encephalomyelitis of swine in Ontario—experimental and natural transmission. *American Journal of Veterinary Research* 23, 756–62.

Alirezaei, M., Kiosses, W. B., Flynn, C. T., Brady, N. R., and Fox, H. S. (2008). Disruption of neuronal autophagy by infected microglia results in neurodegeneration. *PLoS One* 3(8), e2906.

Aloisi, F., Serafini, B., and Adorini, L. (2000). Glia-T cell dialogue. *Journal of Neuroimmunology* 107(2), 111–7.

Andries, K., and Pensaert, M. B. (1980). Virus isolated and immunofluorescence in different organs of pigs infected with hemagglutinating encephalomyelitis virus. *American Journal of Veterinary Research* 41(2), 215–8.

Arbour, N., Cote, G., Lachance, C., Tardieu, M., Cashman, N. R., and Talbot, P. J. (1999a). Acute and persistent infection of human neural cell lines by human coronavirus OC43. *Journal of Virology* 73(4), 3338–50.

Arbour, N., Day, R., Newcombe, J., and Talbot, P. J. (2000). Neuroinvasion by human respiratory coronaviruses. *Journal of Virology* 74(19), 8913–21.

Arbour, N., Ekande, S., Cote, G., Lachance, C., Chagnon, F., Tardieu, M., Cashman, N. R., and Talbot, P. J. (1999b). Persistent infection of human oligodendrocytic and neuroglial cell lines by human coronavirus 229E. *Journal of Virology* 73(4), 3326–37.

Argyris, E. G., Acheampong, E., Wang, F., Huang, J., Chen, K., Mukhtar, M., and Zhang, H. (2007). The interferon-induced expression of APOBEC3G in human blood-brain barrier exerts a potent intrinsic immunity to block HIV-1 entry to central nervous system. *Virology* 367(2), 440–51.

Aurelian, L. (2005). HSV-induced apoptosis in herpes encephalitis. *Current Topics in Microbiology and Immunology* 289, 79–111.

Bailey, O. T., Pappenheimer, A. M., Cheever, F. S., and Daniels, J. B. (1949). A murine virus (Jhm) causing disseminated encephalomyelitis with extensive destruction of myelin: II. PATHOLOGY. *Journal of Experimental Medicine* 90(3), 195–212.

Barger, S. W., and Harmon, A. D. (1997). Microglial activation by Alzheimer amyloid precursor protein and modulation by apolipoprotein E. *Nature* 388(6645), 878–81.

Barnett, E. M., and Perlman, S. (1993). The olfactory nerve and not the trigeminal nerve is the major site of CNS entry for mouse hepatitis virus, strain JHM. *Virology* 194(1), 185–91.

Bechill, J., Chen, Z., Brewer, J. W., and Baker, S. C. (2008). Coronavirus infection modulates the unfolded protein response and mediates sustained translational repression. *Journal of Virology* 82(9), 4492–501.

Bender, S. J., and Weiss, S. R. (2010). Pathogenesis of murine coronavirus in the central nervous system. *Journal of Neuroimmune Pharmacology* 5(3), 336–54.

Berger, J. R., and Arendt, G. (2000). HIV dementia: the role of the basal ganglia and dopaminergic systems. *Journal of Psychopharmacology* 14(3), 214–21.

Bilzer, T., and Stitz, L. (1996). Immunopathogenesis of virus diseases affecting the central nervous system. *Critical Reviews in Immunology* 16(2), 145–222.

Blakely, P. K., Kleinschmidt-DeMasters, B. K., Tyler, K. L., and Irani, D. N. (2009). Disrupted glutamate transporter expression in the spinal cord with acute flaccid paralysis caused by West Nile virus infection. *Journal of Neuropathology and Experimental Neurology* 68(10), 1061–72.

Bonavia, A., Arbour, N., Yong, V. W., and Talbot, P. J. (1997). Infection of primary cultures of human neural cells by human coronaviruses 229E and OC43. *Journal of Virology* 71(1), 800–6.

Boucher, A., Desforges, M., Duquette, P., and Talbot, P. J. (2007). Long-term human coronavirus-myelin cross-reactive T-cell clones derived from multiple sclerosis patients. *Clinical Immunology* 123(3), 258–67.

Brian, D. A., and Baric, R. S. (2005). Coronavirus genome structure and replication. *Current Topics in Microbiology and Immunology* 287, 1–30.

Brison, E., Jacomy, H., Desforges, M., and Talbot, P. J. (2011). Glutamate excitotoxicity is involved in the induction of paralysis in mice after infection by a human coronavirus with a single point mutation in its spike protein. *Journal of Virology* 85(23), 12464–73.

Brown, M. A., Troyer, J. L., Pecon-Slattery, J., Roelke, M. E., and O'Brien, S. J. (2009). Genetics and pathogenesis of feline infectious peritonitis virus. *Emerging Infectious Diseases* 15(9), 1445–52.

Burks, J. S., DeVald, B. L., Jankovsky, L. D., and Gerdes, J. C. (1980). Two coronaviruses isolated from central nervous system tissue of two multiple sclerosis patients. *Science* 209(4459), 933–4.

Butler, N., Pewe, L., Trandem, K., and Perlman, S. (2006). Murine encephalitis caused by HCoV-OC43, a human coronavirus with broad species specificity, is partly immune-mediated. *Virology* 347(2), 410–21.

Canto-Nogues, C., Sanchez-Ramon, S., Alvarez, S., Lacruz, C., and Munoz-Fernandez, M. A. (2005). HIV-1 infection of neurons might account for progressive HIV-1-associated encephalopathy in children. *Journal of Molecular Neuroscience* 27(1), 79–89.

Carmen, J., Rothstein, J. D., and Kerr, D. A. (2009). Tumor necrosis factor-alpha modulates glutamate transport in the CNS and is a critical determinant of outcome from viral encephalomyelitis. *Brain Research* 1263, 143–54.

Cavanagh, D. (1995). The coronavirus surface glycoprotein. In *The Coronaviridae* (S. G. Siddell, Ed.), pp. 73–113. Plenum Press, New York.

Cermelli, C., Vinceti, M., Beretti, F., Pietrini, V., Nacci, G., Pietrosemoli, P., Bartoletti, A., Guidetti, D., Sola, P., Bergomi, M., Vivoli, G., and Portolani, M. (2003). Risk of sporadic amyotrophic lateral sclerosis associated with seropositivity for herpesviruses and echovirus-7. *European Journal of Epidemiology* 18(2), 123–7.

Chan, C. M., Lau, S. K., Woo, P. C., Tse, H., Zheng, B. J., Chen, L., Huang, J. D., and Yuen, K. Y. (2009). Identification of major histocompatibility complex class I C molecule as an attachment factor that facilitates coronavirus HKU1 spike-mediated infection. *Journal of Virology* 83(2), 1026–35.

Chan, C. P., Siu, K. L., Chin, K. T., Yuen, K. Y., Zheng, B., and Jin, D. Y. (2006). Modulation of the unfolded protein response by the severe acute respiratory syndrome coronavirus spike protein. *Journal of Virology* 80(18), 9279–87.

Cheever, F. S., Daniels, J. B., and et al. (1949). A murine virus (JHM) causing disseminated encephalomyelitis with extensive destruction of myelin. *Journal of Experimental Medicine* 90(3), 181–210.

Collins, A. R. (2002). *In vitro* detection of apoptosis in monocytes/macrophages infected with human coronavirus. *Clinical and Diagnostic Laboratory Immunology* 9(6), 1392–5.

Cook, S. D., and Dowling, P. C. (1980). Multiple sclerosis and viruses: an overview. *Neurology* 30(7 Pt 2), 80–91.

Cowley, T. J., and Weiss, S. R. (2010). Murine coronavirus neuropathogenesis: determinants of virulence. *Journal of Neurovirology* 16(6), 427–34.

Cristallo, A., Gambaro, F., Biamonti, G., Ferrante, P., Battaglia, M., and Cereda, P. M. (1997). Human coronavirus polyadenylated RNA sequences in cerebrospinal fluid from multiple sclerosis patients. *New Microbiologica* 20(2), 105–14.

de Groot, R. J., Baker, S. C., Baric, R., Enjuanes, L., Gorbalenya, A. E., Holmes, K. V., Perlman, S. Poon, L., Rottier, P. J. M., Talbot, P. J., Woo, P. C. Y., and Ziebuhr, J., Ed. (2012). Family Coronaviridae. Virus Taxonomy: Ninth report of the International Committee on Taxonomy of Viruses. Edited by A. M. Q. King, Adams, M. J., Carsten, E. B., and Lefkowitz, E. J. New York: Elsevier.

Delmas, B., and Laude, H. (1990). Assembly of coronavirus spike protein into trimers and its role in epitope expression. *Journal of Virology* 64(11), 5367–75.

Desforges, M. (2011). *Paper presented at the XIIth International symposium on Nidoviruses, Traverse City, USA.*

Desforges, M., Miletti, T. C., Gagnon, M., and Talbot, P. J. (2007). Activation of human monocytes after infection by human coronavirus 229E. *Virus Research* 130(1–2), 228–40.

Drosten, C., Gunther, S., Preiser, W., van der Werf, S., Brodt, H. R., Becker, S., Rabenau, H., Panning, M., Kolesnikova, L., Fouchier, R. A., Berger, A., Burguiere, A. M., Cinatl, J., Eickmann, M., Escriou, N., Grywna, K., Kramme, S., Manuguerra, J. C., Muller, S., Rickerts, V., Sturmer, M., Vieth, S., Klenk, H. D., Osterhaus, A. D., Schmitz, H., and Doerr, H. W. (2003). Identification of a novel coronavirus in patients with severe acute respiratory syndrome. *New England Journal of Medicine* 348(20) 1967–76.

Edwards, J. A., Denis, F., and Talbot, P. J. (2000). Activation of glial cells by human coronavirus OC43 infection. *Journal of Neuroimmunology* 108(1–2), 73–81.

El-Sahly, H. M., Atmar, R. L., Glezen, W. P., and Greenberg, S. B. (2000). Spectrum of clinical illness in hospitalized patients with "common cold" virus infections. *Clinical Infectious Diseases* 31(1), 96–100.

Favreau, D. J., Desforges, M., St-Jean, J. R., and Talbot, P. J. (2009). A human coronavirus OC43 variant harboring persistence-associated mutations in the S glycoprotein differentially induces the unfolded protein response in human neurons as compared to wild-type virus. *Virology* 395(2), 255–67.

Favreau, D. J., Meessen-Pinard, M., Desforges, M., and Talbot, P. J. (2012). Human coronavirus-induced neuronal programmed cell death is cyclophilin d dependent and potentially caspase dispensable. *Journal of Virology* 86(1), 81–93.

Fazzini, E., Fleming, J., and Fahn, S. (1992). Cerebrospinal fluid antibodies to coronavirus in patients with Parkinson's disease. *Movement Disorders* 7(2), 153–8.

Foley, J. E., Lapointe, J. M., Koblik, P., Poland, A., and Pedersen, N. C. (1998). Diagnostic features of clinical neurologic feline infectious peritonitis. *Journal of Veterinary Internal Medicine/American College of Veterinary Internal Medicine* 12(6), 415–23.

Foley, J. E., Poland, A., Carlson, J., and Pedersen, N. C. (1997). Patterns of feline corona-virus infection and fecal shedding from cats in multiple-cat environments. *Journal of the American Veterinary Medical Association* 210(9), 1307–12.

Foley, J. E., Rand, C., and Leutenegger, C. (2003). Inflammation and changes in cytokine lev-els in neurological feline infectious peritonitis. *Journal of Feline Medicine and Surgery* 5(6), 313–22.

Fouchier, R. A., Kuiken, T., Schutten, M., van Amerongen, G., van Doornum, G. J., van den Hoogen, B. G., Peiris, M., Lim, W., Stohr, K., and Osterhaus, A. D. (2003). Aetiology: Koch's postulates fulfilled for SARS virus. *Nature* 423(6937), 240.

Fredericks, D. N., and Relman, D. A. (1996). Sequence-based identification of microbial pathogens: a reconsideration of Koch's postulates. *Clinical Microbiology Reviews* 9(1), 18–33.

Gagneur, A., Sizun, J., Vallet, S., Legr, M. C., Picard, B., and Talbot, P. J. (2002). Coronavirus-related nosocomial viral respiratory infections in a neonatal and paediatric intensive care unit: a prospective study. *Journal of Hospital Infection* 51(1), 59–64.

Gerna, G., Campanini, G., Rovida, F., Percivalle, E., Sarasini, A., Marchi, A., and Baldanti, F. (2006). Genetic variability of human coronavirus OC43-, 229E-, and NL63-like strains and their association with lower respiratory tract infections of hospitalized infants and immunocompromised patients. *Journal of Medical Virology* 78(7), 938–49.

Gilden, D. H. (2005). Infectious causes of multiple sclerosis. *Lancet Neurology* 4(3), 195–202.

Giovannoni, G., Cutter, G. R., Lunemann, J., Martin, R., Munz, C., Sriram, S., Steiner, I., Hammerschlag, M. R., and Gaydos, C. A. (2006). Infectious causes of multiple sclero-sis. *Lancet Neurology* 5(10), 887–94.

Golembewski, E. K., Wales, S. Q., Aurelian, L., and Yarowsky, P. J. (2007). The HSV-2 pro-tein ICP10PK prevents neuronal apoptosis and loss of function in an *in vivo* model of neurodegeneration associated with glutamate excitotoxicity. *Experimental Neurology* 203(2), 381–93.

Gonzalez-Scarano, F., and Baltuch, G. (1999). Microglia as mediators of inflammatory and degenerative diseases. *Annual Review of Neuroscience* 22, 219–40.

Gorbalenya, A. E., Enjuanes, L., Ziebuhr, J., and Snijder, E. J. (2006). Nidovirales: evolving the largest RNA virus genome. *Virus Research* 117(1), 17–37.

Greig, A. S., Mitchell, D., Corner, A. H., Bannister, G. L., Meads, E. B., and Julian, R. J. (1962). A Hemagglutinating Virus Producing Encephalomyelitis in Baby Pigs. *Canadian Journal of Comparative Medicine and Veterinary Science* 26(3), 49–56.

Gruslin, E., Moisan, S., St-Pierre, Y., Desforges, M., and Talbot, P. J. (2005). Transcriptome profile within the mouse central nervous system and activation of myelin-reactive T cells following murine coronavirus infection. *Journal of Neuroimmunology* 162(1–2), 60–70.

Gu, J., Gong, E., Zhang, B., Zheng, J., Gao, Z., Zhong, Y., Zou, W., Zhan, J., Wang, S., Xie, Z., Zhuang, H., Wu, B., Zhong, H., Shao, H., Fang, W., Gao, D., Pei, F., Li, X., He, Z., Xu, D., Shi, X., Anderson, V. M., and Leong, A. S. (2005). Multiple organ infection and the pathogenesis of SARS. *Journal of Experimental Medicine* 202(3), 415–24.

Gu, J., and Korteweg, C. (2007). Pathology and pathogenesis of severe acute respiratory syn-drome. *American Journal of Pathology* 170(4), 1136–47.

Guo, Y., Korteweg, C., McNutt, M. A., and Gu, J. (2008). Pathogenetic mechanisms of severe acute respiratory syndrome. *Virus Research* 133(1), 4–12.

Haeberlein, S. L. B., and Lipton, S. A. (2009). Excitotoxicity in neurodegenerative disease. In *Encyclopedia of Neurosciences* (A. J. Harmar, R. A. Hills, and E. M. Rosser, Eds.), Vol. 4, pp. 77–86. Elsevier.

Hamre, D., and Procknow, J. J. (1966). A new virus isolated from the human respiratory tract. *Proceedings of the Society for Experimental Biology and Medicine. Society for Experimental Biology and Medicine* 121(1), 190–3.

Hankins, D. G., and Rosekrans, J. A. (2004). Overview, prevention, and treatment of rabies. *Mayo Clinic Proceedings. Mayo Clinic* 79(5), 671–6.

Haughey, N. J., Nath, A., Mattson, M. P., Slevin, J. T., and Geiger, J. D. (2001). HIV-1 Tat through phosphorylation of NMDA receptors potentiates glutamate excitotoxicity. *Journal of Neurochemistry* 78(3), 457–67.

Hill, A. B. (1965). The environment and disease: association or causation? *Proceedings of the Royal Society of Medicine* 58, 295–300.

Hirano, N., Nomura, R., Tawara, T., and Tohyama, K. (2004). Neurotropism of swine haemagglutinating encephalomyelitis virus (coronavirus) in mice depending upon host age and route of infection. *Journal of Comparative Pathology* 130(1), 58–65.

Hofmann, H., Pyrc, K., van der Hoek, L., Geier, M., Berkhout, B., and Pohlmann, S. (2005). Human coronavirus NL63 employs the severe acute respiratory syndrome coronavirus receptor for cellular entry. *Proceedings of the National Academy of Sciences of the United States of America* 102(22), 7988–93.

Hogue, B. G., and Machamer, C. E. (2008). Coronavirus structural proteins and virus assembly. In *Nidoviruses* (S. Perlman, T. Gallagher, and E. J. Snijder, Eds.), pp. 179–200. ASM Press, Washington.

Hosking, M. P., and Lane, T. E. (2010). The pathogenesis of murine coronavirus infection of the central nervous system. *Critical Reviews in Immunology* 30(2), 119–30.

Houtman, J. J., and Fleming, J. O. (1996). Pathogenesis of mouse hepatitis virus-induced demyelination. *Journal of Neurovirology* 2(6), 361–76.

Hovanec, D. L., and Flanagan, T. D. (1983). Detection of antibodies to human coronaviruses 229E and OC43 in the sera of multiple sclerosis patients and normal subjects. *Infection and Immunity* 41(1), 426–9.

Hovelmeyer, N., Hao, Z., Kranidioti, K., Kassiotis, G., Buch, T., Frommer, F., von Hoch, L., Kramer, D., Minichiello, L., Kollias, G., Lassmann, H., and Waisman, A. (2005). Apoptosis of oligodendrocytes via Fas and TNF-R1 is a key event in the induction of experimental autoimmune encephalomyelitis. *Journal of Immunology* 175(9), 5875–84.

Itzhaki, R. F., Wozniak, M. A., Appelt, D. M., and Balin, B. J. (2004). Infiltration of the brain by pathogens causes Alzheimer's disease. *Neurobiology of Aging* 25(5), 619–27.

Jacomy, H., Fragoso, G., Almazan, G., Mushynski, W. E., and Talbot, P. J. (2006). Human coronavirus OC43 infection induces chronic encephalitis leading to disabilities in BALB/C mice. *Virology* 349(2), 335–46.

Jacomy, H., St-Jean, J. R., Brison, E., Marceau, G., Desforges, M., and Talbot, P. J. (2010). Mutations in the spike glycoprotein of human coronavirus OC43 modulate disease in BALB/c mice from encephalitis to flaccid paralysis and demyelination. *Journal of Neurovirology* 16(4), 279–93.

Jacomy, H., and Talbot, P. J. (2003). Vacuolating encephalitis in mice infected by human coronavirus OC43. *Virology* 315(1), 20–33.

Jeffers, S. A., Tusell, S. M., Gillim-Ross, L., Hemmila, E. M., Achenbach, J. E., Babcock, G. J., Thomas, W. D., Jr., Thackray, L. B., Young, M. D., Mason, R. J., Ambrosino, D. M., Wentworth, D. E., Demartini, J. C., and Holmes, K. V. (2004). CD209L (L-SIGN) is a receptor for severe acute respiratory syndrome coronavirus. *Proceedings of the National Academy of Sciences of the United States of America* 101(44), 15748–53.

Johnson, R. T. (1985). Viral aspects of multiple sclerosis. *In Handbook of Clinical Neurology Demyelinating Diseases* (J. C. Koetsier, Ed.), pp. 319–36. Elsevier, Amsterdam.

Johnston, S. L., Pattemore, P. K., Sanderson, G., Smith, S., Lampe, F., Josephs, L., Symington, P., O'Toole, S., Myint, S. H., Tyrrell, D. A. et al. (1995). Community study of role of viral infections in exacerbations of asthma in 9–11 year old children. *BMJ* 310(6989), 1225–9.

Kakalacheva, K., Munz, C., and Lunemann, J. D. (2011). Viral triggers of multiple sclerosis. *Biochimica et Biophysica Acta* 1812(2), 132–40.

Kim, W. K., Corey, S., Alvarez, X., and Williams, K. (2003). Monocyte/macrophage traffic in HIV and SIV encephalitis. *Journal of Leukocyte Biology* 74(5), 650–6.

Kipar, A., Meli, M. L., Baptiste, K. E., Bowker, L. J., and Lutz, H. (2010). Sites of feline coronavirus persistence in healthy cats. *Journal of General Virology* 91(Pt 7), 1698–707.

Kline, K., Joseph, R., and Averill, D. A. J. (1994). Feline infectious peritonitis with neurological z *Journal of American Animal Hospital Association*. 30, 111–18.

Koch, R. (1942). *The aetiology of tuberculosis* (translation of *Die Aetiologie der Tuberculose (1882)*. Dover Publications, New York.

Krempl, C., Schultze, B., and Herrler, G. (1995). Analysis of cellular receptors for human coronavirus OC43. *Advances in Experimental Medicine and Biology* 380, 371–4.

Kunkel, F., and Herrler, G. (1993). Structural and functional analysis of the surface protein of human coronavirus OC43. *Virology* 195(1), 195–202.

Kurtzke, J. F. (1993). Epidemiologic evidence for multiple sclerosis as an infection. *Clinical Microbiology Reviews* 6(4), 382–427.

Kuzmiski, J. B., and Bains, J. S. (2010). Metabotropic glutamate receptors: gatekeepers of homeostasis. *Journal of Neuroendocrinology* 22(7), 785–92.

Lai, M. M., and Cavanagh, D. (1997). The molecular biology of coronaviruses. *Advances in Virus Research* 48, 1–100.

Lai, M. M., and Holmes, K. V. (2001). Coronaviridae: the viruses and their replication. 4th ed. In *Fields Virology* (B. N. Fields, D. M. Knipe, P. M. Howley, and D. E. Griffin, Eds.), Vol. 1, pp. 1163–1185. Lippincott Williams & Wilkins, Philadelphia.

Lampert, P. W., Sims, J. K., and Kniazeff, A. J. (1973). Mechanism of demyelination in JHM virus encephalomyelitis. Electron microscopic studies. *Acta Neuropathologica* 24(1), 76–85.

Lassnig, C., Sanchez, C. M., Egerbacher, M., Walter, I., Majer, S., Kolbe, T., Pallares, P., Enjuanes, L., and Muller, M. (2005). Development of a transgenic mouse model susceptible to human coronavirus 229E. *Proceedings of the National Academy of Sciences of the United States of America* 102(23), 8275–80.

Lau, A., and Tymianski, M. (2010). Glutamate receptors, neurotoxicity and neurodegeneration. *Pflugers Archiv: European Journal of Physiology* 460(2), 525–42.

Lau, K. K., Yu, W. C., Chu, C. M., Lau, S. T., Sheng, B., and Yuen, K. Y. (2004). Possible central nervous system infection by SARS coronavirus. *Emerging Infectious Diseases* 10(2), 342–4.

Lavi, E., Fishman, P. S., Highkin, M. K., and Weiss, S. R. (1988). Limbic encephalitis after inhalation of a murine coronavirus. *Laboratory Investigation* 58(1), 31–6.

Legendre, A. M., and Whitenack, D. L. (1975). Feline infectious peritonitis with spinal cord involvement in two cats. *Journal of the American Veterinary Medical Association* 167(10), 31–2.

Li, J., Gao, J., Xu, Y. P., Zhou, T. L., Jin, Y. Y., and Lou, J. N. (2007). Expression of severe acute respiratory syndrome coronavirus receptors, ACE2 and CD209L in different organ derived microvascular endothelial cells. *Zhonghua Yi Xue Za Zhi* 87(12), 833–7.

Li, W., Moore, M. J., Vasilieva, N., Sui, J., Wong, S. K., Berne, M. A., Somasundaran, M., Sullivan, J. L., Luzuriaga, K., Greenough, T. C., Choe, H., and Farzan, M. (2003). Angiotensin-converting enzyme 2 is a functional receptor for the SARS coronavirus. *Nature* 426(6965), 450–4.

Li, W., Shi, Z., Yu, M., Ren, W., Smith, C., Epstein, J. H., Wang, H., Crameri, G., Hu, Z., Zhang, H., Zhang, J., McEachern, J., Field, H., Daszak, P., Eaton, B. T., Zhang, S., and Wang, L. F. (2005). Bats are natural reservoirs of SARS-like coronaviruses. *Science* 310(5748), 676–9.

Lindholm, D., Wootz, H., and Korhonen, L. (2006). ER stress and neurodegenerative diseases. *Cell Death and Differentiation* 13(3), 385–92.

Liu, D. X., Yuan, Q., and Liao, Y. (2007). Coronavirus envelope protein: a small membrane protein with multiple functions. *Cellular and Molecular Life Sciences CMLS* 64(16) 2043–8.

Mackenzie, J. S., Gubler, D. J., and Petersen, L. R. (2004). Emerging flaviviruses: the spread and resurgence of Japanese encephalitis, West Nile and dengue viruses. *Nature Medicine* 10(12 Suppl), S98–S109.

Macneughton, M. R., and Davies, H. A. (1978). Ribonucleoprotein-like structures from coronavirus particles. *Journal of General Virology* 39(3), 545–9.

Mark, L. P., Prost, R. W., Ulmer, J. L., Smith, M. M., Daniels, D. L., Strottmann, J. M., Brown, W. D., and Hacein-Bey, L. (2001). Pictorial review of glutamate excitotoxicity: fundamental concepts for neuroimaging. *AJNR. American Journal of Neuroradiology* 22(10), 1813–24.

Masliah, E., Ge, N., and Mucke, L. (1996). Pathogenesis of HIV-1 associated neurodegeneration. *Critical Reviews in Neurobiology* 10(1), 57–67.

Mattson, M. P., Haughey, N. J., and Nath, A. (2005). Cell death in HIV dementia. *Cell Death and Differentiation* 12 Suppl 1, 893–904.

McCray, P. B., Jr., Pewe, L., Wohlford-Lenane, C., Hickey, M., Manzel, L., Shi, L., Netland, J., Jia, H. P., Halabi, C., Sigmund, C. D., Meyerholz, D. K., Kirby, P., Look, D. C., and Perlman, S. (2007). Lethal infection of K18-hACE2 mice infected with severe acute respiratory syndrome coronavirus. *Journal of Virology* 81(2), 813–21.

McIntosh, K., Becker, W. B., and Chanock, R. M. (1967). Growth in suckling-mouse brain of "IBV-like" viruses from patients with upper respiratory tract disease. *Proceedings of the National Academy of Sciences of the United States of America* 58(6), 2268–73.

McLarnon, J. G., Michikawa, M., and Kim, S. U. (1993). Effects of tumor necrosis factor on inward potassium current and cell morphology in cultured human oligodendrocytes. *Glia* 9(2), 120–6.

Meli, M., Kipar, A., Muller, C., Jenal, K., Gonczi, E., Borel, N., Gunn-Moore, D., Chalmers, S., Lin, F., Reinacher, M., and Lutz, H. (2004). High viral loads despite absence of clinical and pathological findings in cats experimentally infected with feline coronavirus (FCoV) type I and in naturally FCoV-infected cats. *Journal of Feline Medicine and Surgery* 6(2), 69–81.

Miller, S. D., Vanderlugt, C. L., Begolka, W. S., Pao, W., Neville, K. L., Yauch, R. L., and Kim, B. S. (1997). Epitope spreading leads to myelin-specific autoimmune responses in SJL mice chronically infected with Theiler's virus. *Journal of Neurovirology* 3 Suppl 1, S62–S65.

Mishra, M. K., Koli, P., Bhowmick, S., and Basu, A. (2007). Neuroprotection conferred by astrocytes is insufficient to protect animals from succumbing to Japanese encephalitis. *Neurochemistry International* 50(5), 764–73.

Miura, T. A., and Holmes, K. V. (2009). Host-pathogen interactions during coronavirus infection of primary alveolar epithelial cells. *Journal of Leukocyte Biology* 86(5), 1145–51.

Myint, S. H. (1995). Human coronavirus infections. In *The Coronaviridae* (S. G. Siddell, Ed.), pp. 389–401. Plenum Press, New York.

Narayanan, K., Huang, C., and Makino, S. (2008). Coronavirus accessory proteins. In *Nidoviruses* (S. Perlman, T. Gallagher, and E. J. Snijder, Eds.). ASM Press, Washington, DC.

Nath, A., and Berger, J. (2004). HIV Dementia. *Current Treatment Options in Neurology* 6(2), 139–151.

Nelson, P. T., Soma, L. A., and Lavi, E. (2002). Microglia in diseases of the central nervous system. *Annals of Medicine* 34(7–8), 491–500.

Netland, J., Meyerholz, D. K., Moore, S., Cassell, M., and Perlman, S. (2008). Severe acute respiratory syndrome coronavirus infection causes neuronal death in the absence of encephalitis in mice transgenic for human ACE2. *Journal of Virology* 82(15), 7264–75.

Nicholls, J., Peiris, J. S. M., and Perlman, S. (2008). Severe acute respiratory syndrome: epidemiology, pathogenesis, and animal models. In *Nidoviruses* (S. Perlman, T. Gallagher, and E. J. Snijder, Eds.), pp. 299–311. ASM Press, Washington, DC.

Nicholls, J. M., Butany, J., Poon, L. L., Chan, K. H., Beh, S. L., Poutanen, S., Peiris, J. S., and Wong, M. (2006). Time course and cellular localization of SARS-CoV nucleoprotein and RNA in lungs from fatal cases of SARS. *PLoS Medicine* 3(2), e27.

Nicholson, K. G., Kent, J., and Ireland, D. C. (1993). Respiratory viruses and exacerbations of asthma in adults. *British Medical Journal* 307(6910), 982–6.

Olanow, C. W., and Tatton, W. G. (1999). Etiology and pathogenesis of Parkinson's disease. *Annual Review of Neuroscience* 22, 123–44.

Olney, J. W. (1969). Brain lesions, obesity, and other disturbances in mice treated with monosodium glutamate. *Science* 164(880), 719–21.

Paschen, W. (2003). Endoplasmic reticulum: a primary target in various acute disorders and degenerative diseases of the brain. *Cell Calcium* 34(4–5), 365–83.

Patterson, S., and Macnaughton, M. R. (1982). Replication of human respiratory coronavirus strain 229E in human macrophages. *Journal of General Virology* 60(Pt 2), 307–14.

Pearson, J., and Mims, C. A. (1985). Differential susceptibility of cultured neural cells to the human coronavirus OC43. *Journal of Virology* 53(3), 1016–9.

Pedersen, N. C., and Boyle, J. F. (1980). Immunologic phenomena in the effusive form of feline infectious peritonitis. *American Journal of Veterinary Research* 41(6), 868–76.

Pleasure, S. J., Page, C., and Lee, V. M. (1992). Pure, postmitotic, polarized human neurons derived from NTera 2 cells provide a system for expressing exogenous proteins in terminally differentiated neurons. *Journal of Neuroscience* 12(5), 1802–15.

Poland, A. M., Vennema, H., Foley, J. E., and Pedersen, N. C. (1996). Two related strains of feline infectious peritonitis virus isolated from immunocompromised cats infected with a feline enteric coronavirus. *Journal of Clinical Microbiology* 34(12), 3180–4.

Raivich, G., and Banati, R. (2004). Brain microglia and blood-derived macrophages: molecular profiles and functional roles in multiple sclerosis and animal models of autoimmune demyelinating disease. *Brain Research. Brain Research Reviews* 46(3), 261–81.

Reuter, J. D., Gomez, D. L., Wilson, J. H., and Van Den Pol, A. N. (2004). Systemic immune deficiency necessary for cytomegalovirus invasion of the mature brain. *Journal of Virology* 78(3), 1473–87.

Rima, B. K., and Duprex, W. P. (2005). Molecular mechanisms of measles virus persistence. *Virus Research* 111(2), 132–47.

Roberts, M. T. (2005). AIDS-associated progressive multifocal leukoencephalopathy: current management strategies. *CNS Drugs* 19(8), 671–82.

Ron, D., and Walter, P. (2007). Signal integration in the endoplasmic reticulum unfolded protein response. *Nature Reviews. Molecular Cell Biology* 8(7), 519–29.

Rottier, P. J. (1990). Background paper. Coronavirus M and HE: two peculiar glycoproteins. *Advances in Experimental Medicine and Biology* 276, 91–4.

Rottier, P. J., Nakamura, K., Schellen, P., Volders, H., and Haijema, B. J. (2005). Acquisition of macrophage tropism during the pathogenesis of feline infectious peritonitis is determined by mutations in the feline coronavirus spike protein. *Journal of Virology* 79(22), 14122–30.

Salmi, A., Ziola, B., Hovi, T., and Reunanen, M. (1982). Antibodies to coronaviruses OC43 and 229E in multiple sclerosis patients. *Neurology* 32(3), 292–5.

Sandhu, J. K., Pandey, S., Ribecco-Lutkiewicz, M., Monette, R., Borowy-Borowski, H., Walker, P. R., and Sikorska, M. (2003). Molecular mechanisms of glutamate neurotoxicity in mixed cultures of NT2-derived neurons and astrocytes: protective effects of coenzyme Q10. *Journal of Neuroscience Research* 72(6), 691–703.

Severance, E. G., Dickerson, F. B., Viscidi, R. P., Bossis, I., Stallings, C. R., Origoni, A. E., Sullens, A., and Yolken, R. H. (2011). Coronavirus immunoreactivity in individuals with a recent onset of psychotic symptoms. *Schizophrenia Bulletin* 37(1), 101–7.

Sibley, W. A., Bamford, C. R., and Clark, K. (1985). Clinical viral infections and multiple sclerosis. *Lancet* 1(8441), 1313–5.

Siddell, S. G., Anderson, R., Cavanagh, D., Fujiwara, K., Klenk, H. D., Macnaughton, M. R., Pensaert, M., Stohlman, S. A., Sturman, L., and van der Zeijst, B. A. (1983). Coronaviridae. *Intervirology* 20(4), 181–9.

Siddell, S. G., and Snijder, E. J. (2008). An introduction to nidoviruses. In *Nidoviruses* (S. Perlman, T. Gallagher, and E. J. Snijder, Eds.), pp. 1–14. ASM Press, Washington.

Sizun, J., Soupre, D., Giroux, J. D., Alix, D., De, P., Legrand, M. C., Demazure, M., and Chastel, C. (1993). Nasal colonization with coronavirus and apnea of the premature newborn. *Acta Paediatrica* 82(3), 238.

Slauson, D. O., and Finn, J. P. (1972). Meningoencephalitis and panophthalmitis in feline infectious peritonitis. *Journal of the American Veterinary Medical Association* 160(5), 729–34.

Spiegel, M., Schneider, K., Weber, F., Weidmann, M., and Hufert, F. T. (2006). Interaction of severe acute respiratory syndrome-associated coronavirus with dendritic cells. *Journal of General Virology* 87(Pt 7), 1953–60.

Sriram, S., and Rodriguez, M. (1997). Indictment of the microglia as the villain in multiple sclerosis. *Neurology* 48(2), 464–70.

St-Jean, J. R., Jacomy, H., Desforges, M., Vabret, A., Freymuth, F., and Talbot, P. J. (2004). Human respiratory coronavirus OC43: genetic stability and neuroinvasion. *Journal of Virology* 78(16), 8824–34.

Sweet, T. M., Del Valle, L., and Khalili, K. (2002). Molecular biology and immunoregulation of human neurotropic JC virus in CNS. *Journal of Cellular Physiology* 191(3), 249–56.

Takahashi, M., and Yamada, T. (1999). Viral etiology for Parkinson's disease—a possible role of influenza A virus infection. *Japanese Journal of Infectious Diseases* 52(3), 89–98.

Talbot, P. J., Arnold, D., and Antel, J. P. (2001). Virus-induced autoimmune reactions in the CNS. *Current Topics in Microbiology and Immunology* 253, 247–71.

Talbot, P. J., Jacomy, H., and Desforges, M. (2008). Pathogenesis of human coronaviruses other than severe acute respiratory syndrome coronavirus. In *Nidoviruses* (S. Perlman, T. Gallagher, and E. J. Snijder, Eds.), pp. 313–324. ASM Press, Washington, DC.

Talbot, P. J., Paquette, J. S., Ciurli, C., Antel, J. P., and Ouellet, F. (1996). Myelin basic protein and human coronavirus 229E cross-reactive T cells in multiple sclerosis. *Annals of Neurology* 39(2), 233–40.

Tanaka, R., Iwasaki, Y., and Koprowski, H. (1976). Intracisternal virus-like particles in brain of a multiple sclerosis patient. *Journal of the Neurological Sciences* 28(1), 121–6.

Tseng, C. T., Huang, C., Newman, P., Wang, N., Narayanan, K., Watts, D. M., Makino, S., Packard, M. M., Zaki, S. R., Chan, T. S., and Peters, C. J. (2007). Severe acute respiratory syndrome coronavirus infection of mice transgenic for the human Angiotensin-converting enzyme 2 virus receptor. *Journal of Virology* 81(3), 1162–73.

Tsui, J. K., Calne, D. B., Wang, Y., Schulzer, M., and Marion, S. A. (1999). Occupational risk factors in Parkinson's disease. *Canadian Journal of Public Health* 90(5), 334–7.

Tyrrell, D. A., and Bynoe, M. L. (1965). Cultivation of a novel type of common-cold virus in organ cultures. *British Medical Journal* 1(5448), 1467–70.

Vabret, A., Dina, J., Brison, E., Brouard, J., and Freymuth, F. (2009). [Human coronaviruses]. *Pathologie-Biologie* 57(2), 149–60.

van der Hoek, L., Pyrc, K., Jebbink, M. F., Vermeulen-Oost, W., Berkhout, R. J., Wolthers, K. C., Wertheim-van Dillen, P. M., Kaandorp, J., Spaargaren, J., and Berkhout, B. (2004). Identification of a new human coronavirus. *Nature Medicine* 10(4), 368–73.

Vennema, H., Poland, A., Foley, J., and Pedersen, N. C. (1998). Feline infectious peritonitis viruses arise by mutation from endemic feline enteric coronaviruses. *Virology* 243(1), 150–7.

Waltrip, R. W., 2nd, Buchanan, R. W., Summerfelt, A., Breier, A., Carpenter, W. T., Jr., Bryant, N. L., Rubin, S. A., and Carbone, K. M. (1995). Borna disease virus and schizophrenia. *Psychiatry Research* 56(1), 33–44.

Wang, F. I., Stohlman, S. A., and Fleming, J. O. (1990). Demyelination induced by murine hepatitis virus JHM strain (MHV-4) is immunologically mediated. *Journal of Neuroimmunology* 30(1), 31–41.

Watkins, J. C., and Jane, D. E. (2006). The glutamate story. *British Journal of Pharmacology* 147 Suppl 1, S100–8.

Weiner, L. P. (1973). Pathogenesis of demyelination induced by a mouse hepatitis. *Archives of Neurology* 28(5), 298–303.

Weissert, R. (2011). Progressive multifocal leukoencephalopathy. *Journal of Neuroimmunology* 231(1–2), 73–7.

Wentworth, D. E., Tresnan, D. B., Turner, B. C., Lerman, I. R., Bullis, B., Hemmila, E. M., Levis, R., Shapiro, L. H., and Holmes, K. V. (2005). Cells of human aminopeptidase N (CD13) transgenic mice are infected by human coronavirus-229E *in vitro*, but not *in vivo*. *Virology* 335(2), 185–97.

Whitley, R. J., and Gnann, J. W. (2002). Viral encephalitis: familiar infections and emerging pathogens. *Lancet* 359(9305), 507–13.

Woo, P. C., Lau, S. K., Chu, C. M., Chan, K. H., Tsoi, H. W., Huang, Y., Wong, B. H., Poon, R. W., Cai, J. J., Luk, W. K., Poon, L. L., Wong, S. S., Guan, Y., Peiris, J. S., and Yuen, K. Y. (2005a). Characterization and complete genome sequence of a novel coronavirus, coronavirus HKU1, from patients with pneumonia. *Journal of Virology* 79(2), 884–95.

Woo, P. C., Lau, S. K., Tsoi, H. W., Huang, Y., Poon, R. W., Chu, C. M., Lee, R. A., Luk, W. K., Wong, G. K., Wong, B. H., Cheng, V. C., Tang, B. S., Wu, A. K., Yung, R. W., Chen, H., Guan, Y., Chan, K. H., and Yuen, K. Y. (2005b). Clinical and molecular epidemiological features of coronavirus HKU1-associated community-acquired pneumonia. *Journal of Infectious Diseases* 192(11), 1898–907.

Xu, J., Zhong, S., Liu, J., Li, L., Li, Y., Wu, X., Li, Z., Deng, P., Zhang, J., Zhong, N., Ding, Y., and Jiang, Y. (2005). Detection of severe acute respiratory syndrome coronavirus in the brain: potential role of the chemokine mig in pathogenesis. *Clinical infectious diseases: an official publication of the Infectious Diseases Society of America* 41(8), 1089–96.

Yagami, K., Hirai, K., and Hirano, N. (1986). Pathogenesis of haemagglutinating encephalomyelitis virus (HEV) in mice experimentally infected by different routes. *Journal of Comparative Pathology* 96(6), 645–57.

Yeager, C. L., Ashmun, R. A., Williams, R. K., Cardellichio, C. B., Shapiro, L. H., Look, A. T., and Holmes, K. V. (1992). Human aminopeptidase N is a receptor for human coronavirus 229E. *Nature* 357(6377), 420–2.

Yeh, E. A., Collins, A., Cohen, M. E., Duffner, P. K., and Faden, H. (2004). Detection of coronavirus in the central nervous system of a child with acute disseminated encephalomyelitis. *Pediatrics* 113(1 Pt 1), e73–6.

Yilla, M., Harcourt, B. H., Hickman, C. J., McGrew, M., Tamin, A., Goldsmith, C. S., Bellini, W. J., and Anderson, L. J. (2005). SARS-coronavirus replication in human peripheral monocytes/macrophages. *Virus Research* 107(1), 93–101.

Young, V. A., and Rall, G. F. (2009). Making it to the synapse: measles virus spread in and among neurons. *Current Topics in Microbiology and Immunology* 330, 3–30.

Zhang, K., McQuibban, G. A., Silva, C., Butler, G. S., Johnston, J. B., Holden, J., Clark-Lewis, I., Overall, C. M., and Power, C. (2003). HIV-induced metalloproteinase processing of the chemokine stromal cell derived factor-1 causes neurodegeneration. *Nature Neuroscience* 6(10), 1064–71.

6 Nonpolio Enteroviruses, Polioviruses, and Human CNS Infections

Anda Baicus and Cristian Baicus

CONTENTS

6.1 INTRODUCTION

Human enteroviruses (HEVs) are members of the Enterovirus genus in the Picornaviridae family. This family consists of the following genera: Aphthovirus, Cardiovirus, Enterovirus, Hepatovirus, Parechovirus, Erbovirus, Kobuvirus, and Teschovirus (Carsten and Ball 2009).

Poliovirus, the prototype strain of the Enterovirus genus, is the etiological agent of an acute paralytic disease, poliomyelitis. The studies on poliovirus began in 1908, when Landsteiner and Popper transmitted the disease to monkeys (Landsteiner and Popper 1908). Flexner supposed that poliovirus was strictly neurotropic, in 1910 (Flexner and Lewis 1910), and Enders et al., in 1949, cultured poliovirus strains in nonneuronal tissue culture, opening the way for the production of viral vaccines (Enders et al. 1949).

In 1948, the large group of viruses to which the polioviruses belong was discovered. The pathogenesis of the infection in human and in experimental suckling mice was at the origin of the classification of human enteroviruses (HEV) into four clusters: (i) polioviruses (PV), which cause acute flaccid paralysis (AFP) (poliomyelitis) in humans but not in mice; (ii) coxsackieviruses A (CVA), which cause myositis, diseases of the central nervous system (CNS), exanthems and herpangina in humans, and acute flaccid paralysis and myositis in mice; (iii) coxsackieviruses B (CVB), which cause myocarditis and dilated cardiomyopathy, muscle disorders in humans, and spastic paralysis and focal and limited myositis in striated muscles, in mice (Godman et al. 1952); (iv) enteric cytopathogenic human orphan (ECHO) viruses, which were not associated at the beginning with human or mice diseases.

Traditionally the enteroviruses are divided into five clusters, based on the differences in host range and pathogenic potential: poliovirus, human enterovirus A (HEV-A), human enterovirus B (HEV-B), human enterovirus C (HEV-C), and human enterovirus D (HEV-D). Different viral serotypes were included within each of these clusters on the basis of their antigenicity. The recent isolates of HEVs received consecutive numbers starting with HEV68. On the basis of phylogenetic analyses, HEVs are classified into four species of enteroviruses (HEV-A, HEV-B, HEV-C and HEV-D), and three species of rhinoviruses. The three poliovirus serotypes belong to the human enterovirus C species (Brown et al. 2003). HEV isolates should be classified as the same serotype if they diverge in the VP1 region less than 25%, and 12% within corresponding nucleotide and amino acid sequences (Oberste et al. 1999; Caro et al. 2001). The species HEV-A consists of coxsackieviruses CVA2–8, 10, 12, 14, 16, human enteroviruses HEV71, 76, 89–92, 114; the species HEV-B consists of coxsackieviruses CVA9, CVB1–6, echoviruses (ECHO) (1–7, 9, 11–21, 24–27, 29–33), HEV69, 73–75, 77–88, 93, 97, 98, 100, 101, 106, 107, the species HEV-C consists of PV1–3, coxsackieviruses A1, 11, 13, 17, 19, 20, 21, 24, Human enteroviruses HEV95, 96, 99, 102, 104, 105, 109, 113, and the species HEV-D consists of human enteroviruses HEV68, 70, 94, 111.

6.1.1 CLASSIFICATION, MORPHOLOGY, GENOME STRUCTURE, ORGANIZATION, AND PROTEIN FUNCTIONS

6.1.1.1 Biological Properties

Enteroviruses are small particles, about 30 nm in diameter, with a positive sense, single stranded RNA within a nonenveloped icosahedral symmetric protein capsid. The genome is approximately 30% of the virion mass. Enteroviruses are resistant to alcohol, phenol, quaternary ammonium ether, chloroform, and sodium deoxycholate, detergents that destroy other viruses (e.g., orthomyxoviruses) and are acid stable. All enteroviruses have a density of about 1.34 g/mL in caesium chloride, and a sedimentation coefficient of about 156S. The viral particle is inactivated by drying, ultraviolet light, treatment with 0.3% formaldehyde, 0.1 N HCl, or free residual chlorine at a level of 0.3–0.5 ppm, and heating at 50°C for 30 min. Their inactivation at all temperatures tested is inhibited by magnesium chloride (a concentration of 1 mol/L hinders inactivation). This property has led to the use of $MgCl_2$ as a stabilizer of oral polio vaccine (WHO 1997/2004).

6.1.1.2 Morphology

The viral capsid is formed of 60 identical units, protomers, and copies of the four capsid proteins VP1, VP2, VP3, and VP4. The surface of the virion is formed by the viral proteins, VP1, VP2, VP3, each containing about 250 amino acids. The inner surface is formed by the smaller and relatively unstructured viral protein VP4 (70 amino acids), in conjunction with the amino (N-) terminal extension of VP1 and VP2. The core structures of the proteins VP1–VP3 are the same topologically, each consisting of eight-strand antiparallel β barrel. The aspect of β barrel is wedge-shaped, and the β strands are joined at one end by four short loops. The major structural differences among VP1, VP2, and VP3 are in the conformation and size of the loops and in the sequences of N- and C-terminal extensions. The antigenic sites of the virus are determined by these loops, and the N-terminal extensions contribute to its stability. The three-dimensional structures of the capsid proteins of some enteroviruses have been determined by X-ray crystallography and cryoelectron microscopy (Hendry et al. 1999; Hogle et al. 1985; Hogle and Filman 1989; Muckelbauer et al. 1995). It has been shown that the surface of enterovirus has a star shaped peak at the five fold axis of symmetry, surrounded by a channel of 2.4 nm deep and 1.2 to 3.0 nm wide (the canyon), and another protrusion at the three fold axis of symmetry. The canyon is the attachment site for the enterovirus receptor. A lipid factor is located in a hydrophobic pocket, beneath the floor of the canyon. By interaction of the virus with the receptor, this lipidic factor must be displaced before the conformational changes in the capsid. This pocket has been used as a target for antiviral compounds that filled it and prevented conformational rearrangements associated with uncoating and releasing of RNA (Rossmann et al. 2002).

6.1.1.3 Genome Structure, Organization, and Protein Functions

The enterovirus genome is a positive sense, single stranded RNA of about 7500 nt in size. It is infectious because it functions as mRNA, and is directly translated into a polyprotein in a cap-independent manner by the host cell ribosomes. The RNA genome is covalently linked at its 5′ end to a virus encoded proteine Vpg (22-amino acid long), and has a polyadenylated 3′ end (poly A). The genome is monocistronic, with a 5′ untranslated region (UTR) (about 10% of the genome, ranging between 742 and 750 nt), followed by the single open reading frame (ORF), which encodes a polyprotein of about 250 kDa, and by a 3′UTR (about 1% of the genome, ranging between 70 and 100 nt).

The secondary structure of the 5′UTR genome looks like a tRNA-like structure. It contains a cloverleaf structure playing a role in the initiation of negative strand

RNA synthesis, and an internal ribosomal entry site (IRES), which mediates the cap independent translation of the viral RNA. The 3′UTR has a secondary structure (pseudoknot) involved in RNA replication, and it is highly conserved among the enteroviruses. The 3′ poly A end has a role in infectivity (Hellen and Wimmer 1995).

6.1.2   Cell Biology of Enterovirus Infection

Enterovirus replication takes place in the cell cytoplasm. The enterovirus infection begins with the attachment of the virus to a specific receptor on the surface of the host cell membrane. Many picornaviruses have receptor molecules belonging to the integrin (e.g., $\alpha_v\beta_3$, $\alpha_v\beta_6$), SCR (Short Consensus Repeat) like (e.g., DAF [decay accelerating factor], CD 55) and the immunoglobulin superfamilies (e.g., CD155, ICAM-1 intercellular adhesion molecule-1). The poliovirus uses only one receptor (CD155) for attachment and entry into the cell (He et al. 2000), but some enteroviruses (CAV 21) have been shown to use a cellular receptor (DAF, CD 55) for attachment, and a coreceptor (ICAM-1) for entry into the cell (Shafren et al. 1997). Coxsackievirus B3 (CVB3) recruits CAR (coxsackievirus adenovirus receptor) to the site of infection by binding to a second receptor DAF that is expressed in the epithelial cells (Coyne and Bergelson 2006). The extracellular region of the receptors from the immunoglobulin superfamily comprises 2 to 5 amino-terminal immunoglobulin-like domains. The amino-terminal domain (D1) of these molecules is involved in the binding with the conserved amino acid residues of the picornavirus canyon, which can trigger viral instability and uncoating.

After binding to the receptor, the virus protein shell is removed and its genome enters the cytoplasm. The interaction between the cell receptor sequences and the residues of the canyon floor displaces residues at the protomer interface and below the canyon floor. This conformational change results in externalization of myristoylated capsid protein VP4 and the N-terminus of the capsid protein VP1. An altered A viral particle (135S) results, with a higher affinity for lipid membranes than native particles. The insertion of the externalized proteins into membrane binds the virus particle to the cellular membrane in a receptor-independent manner. Thus, the pores and channels are created in the cell membrane through which the viral RNA may enter the cytoplasm. By using a combination between the imaging of fluorescent PV in live cells and biochemical assays, it was demonstrated that PV enters the cell by independent classical clathrin- and caveolin-mediated pathways, sense an energy-, actin-, and tyrosine kinase dependent endocytic mechanism. This process is followed by low pH-mediated exposure of hydrophobic residues in an early endocytic vesicle (Thorley et al. 2010).

In the cytoplasm of the infected cell, a cellular phosphodiesterase removes the Vpg prior to RNA translation. The cellular enzymes are responsable for RNA translation to polyprotein. The 40S ribosomal subunit associates with the IRES and scans the RNA to the initiation codon AUG, where a 60 S ribosomal subunit joins the complex, and elongation of translatation polyprotein occurs. The cleaveage of the eukaryotic translation initiation factor (eIF4G), which is a factor of the initiation complex (eIF4F) by the viral 2A protease, is responsible for the inhibition of cap-dependent initiation of translation. The viral polyprotein is clevead by virus-encoded proteases (2A, 3C, 3CD) into 3 intermediate proteins, P1, P2, and P3. Protease 2A separates the structural protein P1 from the nonstructural proteins P2 and P3. Protease 3CD cleaves P1 into VP0, VP3, and VP1. The cleavage of VP0 into VP4 and VP2 proteins occurs during viral maturation, and it may be linked to the encapsidation of the RNA. The nonstructural proteins precursors P2 and P3 are separated by 3C/3CD protease into 2A, 2B, 2C, 3A, 3B (Vpg), 3C, and 3D. The viral 2A and 3C proteases mediate the inhibition of cellular RNA synthesis. 3D is an RNA-dependent RNA polymerase necessary for viral RNA synthesis and 2B-C, 3A-B proteins play different roles in viral multiplication.

The replication involves transcription of the positive stranded RNA into a complementary negative stranded RNA that is used as a template for many new single positive strands. The process begins with a VPg uridylation and synthesis of complementary negative-strand RNA molecules via the transcription of poly(A) by the RNA dependent RNA polymerase 3D. The replication takes place in the cytoplasm of host cell endoplasmic reticulum-derived rosette-like membranous structures that act as scaffold for assembly of the replication complex and protect the RNA from nucleases. Other cellular and viral factors are involved in RNA synthesis, cellular RNA binding proteins, viral proteins 2A, 2B, 2C, 3AB, 3C, and 3CD. The RNA-dependent RNA polymerase lacks proofreading activities, and this results in rapid accumulation of mutations upon replication. The new positive RNA strand synthesis is linked to the encapsidation or it could be a template for translation. The time required for a simple replication cycle ranges from 5 to 10 h and it depends on the serotype, multiplicity of infection, pH, and temperature. In the enterovirus assembly, the earliest component is the 5S protomer, which consists of one copy of each of VP0, VP3, and VP1. The protomer is the precursor of the 14S pentamer, with the composition (VP0-VP3-VP1)$_5$. 12 pentamers form, by self association, 75S procapsids (empty capsids) (VP0-VP3-VP1)$_{60}$. By insertion of the newly synthesized RNA into the procapsid is formed the provirion 150S, that is not infectious. The cleavage of VP0 into VP4 and VP2 is responsible for conversion of the provirion into the virion, making the viral assembly irreversible. In the infected cells, the positive stranded genome is amplified through a negative stranded intermediary to about 50000 copies /cell, but only 0.1%–2% of them are infectious. The progeny viruses are released from the cell by cell lysis. The morphological changes developed by the cells infected with HEV strains include cytopathic effects, condensation of chromatin, nuclear blebbing, proliferation of membranous vesicles, changes in membrane permeability, leakage of intracellular components, and shrivelling of the entire cell (Racaniello 2006).

6.2 CLINICAL PRESENTATIONS

The clinical manifestations in enterovirus infections are determined by factors such as viral serotype, infecting dose, tissue tropism, portal of entry, patient's age, gender, and immune status. The ability of these viruses to multiply in the gastrointestinal tract gave their name, even if they are not responsible for enteric disease. Most enteroviral infections are asymptomatic or are associated with undifferentiated febrile illness, associated with milder respiratory illness or a rashes disease. The nonspecific lower respiratory illnesses caused by the HEVs can results in bronchitis, bronchiolitis, and pneumonia. HEV strains including HEV68, 71, coxsackieviruses A9, A21, B2, B4, and echovirus 9, 11, 22 have been isolated from samples of the patients with severe or fatal viral bronchopneumonia (Chang et al. 1999; Jacques et al. 2008; Oberste et al. 2004). Less commonly, some infections cause severe illness such as viral meningitis, encephalitis, acute flaccid paralysis, acute hemorrhagic conjunctivitis (AHC), neonatal sepsis-like disease, myocarditis, and pleurodynia. Severe chronic diseases such as dilated cardiomyopathy, neuromuscular diseases, and type 1 diabetes could be associated with enterovirus infections. The rates of these infections are higher in infants, compared with adults.

6.2.1 NEUROLOGICAL DISEASES

Viral infection of the CNS can involve the meninges (meningitis), the brain (encephalitis), the spinal cord (myelitis), spinal roots (radiculitis), or a combination of sites (meningoencephalitis, encephalomyelitis, or myeloradiculitis). HEV infections are more frequently associated with viral meningitis, but infrequently associated with encephalitis. In aseptic meningitis, there is clinical and laboratory evidence for meningeal inflammation, with negative bacterial culture. The etiologies of aseptic meningitis include viruses (enteroviruses, herpes simplex virus, human immunodeficiency virus, West Nile virus, varicella-zoster virus, mumps, and lymphocytic choriomeningitis virus), bacterial infections (mycobacteria, spirochetes), parameningeal infections, brain abscess, medications, and malignancy. The clinical symptoms of aseptic meningitis are similar to those of bacterial meningitis: fever that ranges from 38°C to 40°C, headache, no change in mental status, no seizures, stiff neck, photophobia, occasionally anorexia, nausea, and vomiting. Over 90% of aseptic meningitis cases in infants are due to HEV, and the most common symptoms are fever and irritability. The outbreaks of meningitis are caused by certain serotypes of HEV-B species: coxsackievirus B5, echoviruses 6, 9, 30, whereas coxsackievirus A9, B3, and B4 are mostly endemic (Lee and Davies 2007). The children recover completely within 3 to 7 days of onset, but symptoms often persist in adults for longer (Rotbart et al. 1998).

In acute viral encephalitis, direct invasion of the brain occurs as an extension of viral meningitis or via retrograde spread through the peripheral nerves. In this disease, an altered level of consciousness, often with seizure, and focal neurological signs, occur. In pure encephalitis, photophobia and nuchal rigidity are usually absent, but they often occur in meningoencephalitis. 11% to 22% of all cases of viral encephalitis are caused by HEV strains, most often coxsackievirus types A9, B2, B5, and echovirus types 6 and 9.

HEV71 has been recognized as a highly neurotropic virus. Aseptic meningitis, encephalitis, flaccid paralysis, and rhombencephalitis occur as complications in children younger than 5 years. The necessity to improve surveillance for HEV71-associated HFMD (hand, foot, and mouth disease) outbreaks, even for adults, has been demonstrated by several studies (Chan et al. 2003; Hamaguchi et al. 2008; Ooi et al. 2010). The distribution of viral lesions in the HEV71 infections involves the pyramidal and extrapyramidal tracts of the CNS. The neurological recovery is poor, and the risk of mortality is increased for the patients with diffuse cerebral edema or intractable seizures. The recovery is rapid for the patients with self-limited seizure activity (Fowlkes et al. 2008).

Poliomyelitis is an acute flaccid paralysis (AFP) caused by three poliovirus (PV) serotypes. Most of poliovirus infections are asymptomatic (90%) or are associated with minor illness (abortive poliomyelitis, 4%–8%) characterized by fever, headache, sore throat, malaise, listlessness, nausea, and vomiting. In patients with persistent viremia (1%–2%), the virus enters the nervous system by crossing the blood–brain barrier or by axonal transportation from a peripheral nerve and attacks the anterior horn of the spinal cord, leading to inflammation and possible cell death. About one third of cases with CNS infections are limited to aseptic meningitis. In 0.1%–1% of cases, poliovirus infection is associated with paralytic poliomyelitis. The persisting asymmetric weakness (flaccid paralysis), which results from lower motor neuron damage is the characteristic sign of poliomyelitis. The severity of this disease ranges from flaccid paralysis of a single extremity to tetraplegia, with development of the paralysis over 2 to 3 days. In the affected extremities, decreased or absent tendon reflexes without sensory loss occur. The proximal limb muscle is more involved than the distal, and the legs are more involved than the arms. Most recoveries occur within 6 months, but a long time (2 years) may be required for complete remission. The involvement of the motor cranial nerves (most common the VIIth, IXth, and Xth) occurs in bulbar poliomyelitis, which is characterized by dysphagia, dysarthria, difficulty in handling secretions, respiratory compromise, and cardiovascular dysfunction. During the 1950s, before vaccination programs, iron lungs were used to assist the breathing of patients with such polio disease (Melnick 1996).

In the differential diagnosis enters the polio-like illnesses, which can be caused by nonpolio enteroviruses (CVA7, HEV70, 71), West Nile Virus, and *Borrelia burgdorferi*. Other diseases produce acute paralysis associated with other clinical features, such as spinal cord disorders (transverse myelitis, infarction, compression), peripheral neuropathy (Guillain-Barré syndrome, acute intermittent porphyria, infectious, and toxic neuropathies), disorders of the neuromuscular transmission (myasthenia gravis, botulism, tick paralysis), and disorders of the muscles (inflammatory myopathy and rhabdomyolysis) (Simmons 2010).

Postpoliomyelitis syndrome (PPS) is a neurological disorder that occurs in persons who had a period of partial or complete functional recovery after acute paralytic poliomyelitis, followed by an interval (usually 15 years or more) of stable neurological function. The symptoms are new or increased muscle weakness and/or atrophy, muscle and joint pain, increased muscular fatigability, fasciculations, cramps, general fatigue, and cold intolerance (Farbu et al. 2006). The distal degeneration of the enlarged postpoliomyelitis motor units is the most likely cause (Grimby et al. 1998; Lin and Lim 2005). Contributing factors to PPS may be aging with motor unit loss, overuse, and disuse. The excessive metabolic effort on remaining motor neurons over years leads to atrophy of the orphaned muscle fibers, with progressive weakness in the previously affected muscles, followed by fatigue and pain.

6.2.2 Skin and Eye Diseases

The hand, foot, and mouth disease (HFMD) is a self-limiting childhood disease characterized by fever, vesicular lesions on the buccal mucosa and tongue, and small, tender cutaneous lesions on the hands, feet, and buttocks. Herpangina is a disease characterized by an onset with fever and odynophagia associated with vesicular or ulcerative lesions of the tonsils, uvula, and soft palate (Keels 2010). HEV71, CVA16, CVA10 cause HFMD and herpangina. The illness usually resolves in 2 to 3 days without complications (Pallansch and Ross 2001). The main complications of HFMD are encephalitis and a polio-like disease. The infection with CVA16 is not associated with neurological disease, but the rash it causes is indistinguishable from that caused by HEV71. In children younger than 5 years, the exanthem caused by enteroviruses manifest as rubelliform or roseola-like rashes on the face, neck, and trunk. The petechial and purpuric rash caused by infection with echovirus 9 or CVA9 could create a confusion with meningococcemia if aseptic meningitis occurs simultaneously. A highly contagious acute hemorrhagic conjunctivitis (AHC) is commonly caused by HEV70 and a new antigenic variant CVA24v and adenovirus (Leveque et al. 2010; Sane et al. 2008). This ocular infection is characterized by pain, periorbital swelling, red eyes with conjunctival hemorrhage and excessive tearing, usually with involvement of the second eye within 24 to 48 h. The illness is self-limited and resolves within 10 days without complications. When AHC is caused by HEV70, the CNS diseases can occur.

6.2.3 FETAL AND NEONATAL INFECTIONS

Maternal enteroviral infection during pregnancy can have a transplacental spread to the fetus, increasing the risk of early spontaneous abortions or in rare cases of intrauterine fetal death (Johansson et al. 1992). Most neonates of infected mothers are unaffected, because the transplacental passage of virus does not occur easily (Amstey et al. 1988). Clinical presentations of the neonate infections that occur in the perinatal period vary from nonspecific febrile illness, to severe life-threatening disease. The severe enteroviral infections in neonates are caused by echovirus 6, 11, 20, 21, 31, and CVB types 2 and 5. Coxsackieviruses B1 and A9 have been reported to occur, but very rarely (Lu et al. 2005). Approximately 50% of severe cases have meningoencephalitis, 25% have myocarditis, and 25% have a sepsis-like disease. Neonatal myocarditis due to coxsackievirus infection is often accompanied by encephalitis, and sometimes by hepatitis (Lin 2003). The rate of mortality is low (10%) for the group with meningoencephalitis and high (100%) for the group with sepsis-like disease (most deaths occur within 1 week of onset) (Burchett and Dalgic 2008).

6.2.4 INFECTIONS IN IMMUNOCOMPROMISED PATIENTS

In patients with acquired or hereditary defects in B lymphocytes, enterovirus infections result in chronic infections of the CNS, skeletal muscles, and the gastrointestinal system. Enterovirus infections occur also in children with X-linked agammaglobulinemia, with severe immunodeficiency syndrome (Fischmeister et al. 2000; Chakrabarti et al. 2004). When these persons are exposed to oral polio vaccine viruses, the virus multiplication for a long time in the bowel is followed by a high risk for the emergence of neurovirulent poliovirus strains. The persistent nonpolio enterovirus infections in CNS have been caused especially by echoviruses, and isolate by CVA4, CVA11, CVA15, and CVB2 and CVB3. The chronic progressive meningoencephalitis associated with a dermatomyositis-like syndrome and chronic hepatitis is characteristic for infection. The disease is progressive and the disorder is usually fatal because of the gliosis of gray and white matter and focal loss of neurons.

6.2.5 NONNEUROLOGICAL ASPECTS

6.2.5.1 Cardiovascular Diseases

Cardiac involvement of enterovirus infection occurs in the form of myopericarditis. The most frequent pathogens identified in myopericarditis include CVB and echoviruses (Kuhl et al. 2005). Inside the myocyte, the viral protease 2A of CVB cleaves a cytoskeletal protein dystrophin, leading to disruption of the dystrophin-glycoprotein complex that is essential for normal cardiac function (Badorff et al. 1999; Xiong et al. 2007). In neonates, enterovirus myocarditis is a rare and severe disease, and often results in chronic cardiac sequelae or leads to death (Freund et al. 2010).

6.2.5.2 Pleurodynia

Pleurodynia (Bornholm disease, devil's grippe) is an acute illness caused by CVB viruses (mainly CVB3 and CVB5), which are responsible for severe muscular pain in the chest and abdomen, sometimes mimicking serious surgical conditions. Symptoms as fever, headache, anorexia, nausea, and emesis are associated.

6.2.5.3 Autoimmune Diseases

Coxsackieviruses have been linked to the induction of autoimmune diseases such as chronic autoimmune myocarditis and type 1 diabetes. While myocarditis is considered to be a clinical precursor to dilated cardiomyopathy (DCM) (Richer and Horwitz 2009), type 1 diabetes is a disease characterized by a defect in insulin production caused by selective destruction of islet β cells (80%–90%) of the pancreas. A recent systematic review showed a clinically significant association between enterovirus infection and type 1 diabetes (T1D), with a more than nine times the risk of infection in cases of diabetes and three times the risk in children with autoimmunity (Yeung et al. 2011). CVB viruses (mainly CVB4) can play a role in the early phase of the disease through the infection of β cells and the activation of innate immunity and inflammation (Hober and Sauter 2010).

6.2.5.4 Epidemiology

Enterovirus infections are quite prevalent worldwide as sporadic infections or epidemic outbreaks. More than 50% of nonpolio enterovirus infections and more than 90% of poliovirus infections are asymptomatic. Only a minority of infections are associated with specific clinical syndromes. These infections occur throughout the year in the tropics, but in temperate climates, the rates of infection are highest in the summer and fall. The viruses spread mainly by the fecal-oral route, but can also be transmitted by respiratory droplets or indirectly via contaminated water or fomites. The transmission is higher in poor sanitation conditions and in crowded living conditions. Most of the infections occur in young children that are shedders of enteroviruses and are usually the index cases in family outbreaks. Host factors such as immunodeficiency, especially a deficient humoral immunity, and age, can predispose to severe infections.

Depending on environmental conditions, HEVs can remain viable at room temperature for several days and in contaminated soil and water for weeks or even months (Cohen 2006). Sewage contamination of water supplies or swimming in natural waters in areas where there is limited sewage treatment can result in enterovirus outbreaks (Begier et al. 2008). The information concerning circulations of HEV serotypes during any given year are important because changes in the predominant serotype can be accompanied by disease outbreaks (Leveque and Laurent 2008). The environmental surveillance takes place when there is the risk of reintroduction of wild poliovirus or the risk of the circulation of vaccine-derived poliovirus strains in population.

Enteroviral meningitis outbreaks with echovirus types 4, 9, 11, 30 involved many communities throughout Europe and also other continents (CDC 2000; Dalwai et al. 2010; Leveque et al. 2010; Wang et al. 2002; Yamashita et al. 1994). In the United States, between 1970 and 2005 was reported that echovirus 9 was the most commonly isolated enterovirus from cases with aseptic meningitis (Khetsuriani et al. 2006), whereas in 2007 CVB1 was implicated in an outbreak of severe neonatal infections (CDC 2008). Before 2000, sporadic cases of aseptic meningitis with echovirus type 13 were recorded worldwide. Since 2000, a number of countries, including Germany (Diedrich et al. 2001), the United States (CDC 2001), Spain (Avellon et al. 2003), France (Archimbaud et al. 2003), Belgium (Thoelen et al. 2003), Israel (Somekh et al. 2003), and Japan (Iwai et al. 2010) reported aseptic meningitis outbreaks associated with this serotype.

Since the first report about HEV71 isolation in 1969 in California from the stool sample of an infant with encephalitis (Schmidt et al. 1974), outbreaks of HEV71 disease have been reported worldwide (Alexander et al. 1994; Chan et al. 2003; Gilbert et al. 1998; Ho et al. 1999; Podin et al. 2006; Tu et al. 2007; Zhang et al. 2009). HEV71 circulation appears to be increasing in the United States (Perez-Velez et al. 2007). A 2–3 year cyclical pattern of these outbreaks was recorded in Malaysia (Podin et al. 2006), Japan (Ang et al. 2009), and the United Kingdom.

The earliest descriptions of epidemic poliomyelitis by using basic epidemiological methods were recorded in the United States between 1893 and 1894 (Caverly 1894; Putnam and Taylor 1893) and in Sweden in 1905 by Wickman. At the beginning of the 20th century, the polio outbreaks began to be more frequent, and widespread throughout Europe and the United States. The disease was controlled by using two vaccines: the formalin-inactivated vaccine (IPV) accomplished by Jonas Salk (1953), and live-attenuated vaccines (OPV) accomplished by Albert Sabin (1956) (Sabin 1985; Salk 1955). Both vaccines contain three components, one for each serotype of poliovirus. IPV, obtained by formaldehyde inactivation of tissue culture-propagated selected wild poliovirus strains, namely Mahoney (Salk type 1), MEF-1 (Salk type 2), and Saukett (Salk type 3), induces less mucosal immunity, in the intestin than OPV, requires a booster to achieve lifelong immunity, and poses no risk of vaccine-related disease. The OPV strains of Sabin consists of three live attenuated Sabin poliovirus strains obtained by sequential *in vitro* and *in vivo* passages of the wild strains, and it has now become the main instrument for the wild-type-poliovirus eradication program in the developing countries. The risks of OPV vaccination is the potential reversion to neurovirulence of the attenuated strains during their replication in the human intestine, with the emergence of virulent vaccine-derived poliovirus strains

(VDPVs) and vaccine-associated paralytic poliomyelitis (VAPP) (Ward et al. 1988). Vaccine-associated paralytic poliomyelitis may occur in recipients of OPV at a frequency of 1 case per 750,000 primary vaccinations and 1 per 1.2 million recipients of two vaccine doses (Nkowane et al. 1987; Prevots et al. 1994). VAPP occurs in both OPV recipients and their unimmunized contacts. The paralysis is most frequently associated with type 3 in vaccine recipients, and with type 2 among contacts of cases. The VDPV isolates have more than 1% nucleotide divergence in VP1 coding region as opposed to the original vaccine Sabin strains. These isolates can spread in populations with gaps in immunization (circulant cVDPV), and could be responsible for outbreaks. Such cVDPV outbreaks have occurred in countries such as Nigeria, Ethiopia, Congo, Myanmar, Niger, Indonesia, Madagascar, China, the Philippines, Dominican Republic, and Haiti since 2000 (WHO 2009). In most situations, these cVDPV strains were recombinants between OPV and HEV-C strains in the nonstructural coding region, excepting those from China (CDC 2006; Jiang et al. 2006). In developing countries, poliovirus infection in children at an early age has less often been associated with paralysis. In developed countries, poliovirus infection in older children and adults unprotected by vaccination could be followed by paralysis.

Genetic recombination appears to be an integral part of poliovirus evolution. Recombinant genomes are detected among OPV strains excreted by healthy vaccinated individuals, their contacts in the community (Blomqvist et al. 2003), and in patients with VAPP (Georgescu et al. 1997).

6.3   PATHOGENESIS

Transmission of enteroviruses occurs especially by ingestion of fecally contaminated material. The clinical manifestations of the diseases are due by the differences in tissue tropism and the cytolytic capacity of the viruses. According to the clinical syndrome, the incubation period varies between 3 and 5 days. From the port of entry (the mouth), viral multiplication takes place in the lymphoid organs of the oropharynx and in the small intestine. A transient minor viremia occurs, and the virus spreads to the reticuloendothelial system. Many of the enterovirus infections are asymptomatic and are limited at this stage. Further replication of the virus in the reticuloendothelial system is associated with minor illness. The virus spreads hematogenously to lymphoid tissue throughout the body. The virus replication at these sites, particularly the liver and spleen, produces a major viremia, which coincides with the onset of symptoms. In patients with persistent viremia, the virus spreads to target organs such as the CNS. Genomic differences among enterovirus serotypes might explain the tendency of some strains to cause aseptic meningitis and encephalitis. Poliomyelitis is characterized by a biphasic pattern with a nonspecific febrile illness occurring three to five days after exposure, followed by a period of relative well being, and then a recurrence of fever with CNS manifestations 9 to 12 days after exposure. In patients with persistent viremia, the poliovirus enters the nervous system by crossing the blood–brain barrier or by axonal transportation from a peripheral nerve (Ohka et al. 1992; Ren and Racaniello 1992). The poliovirus multiplies in the motor neurons of the anterior horn of the spinal cord, followed by denervation of the associated skeletal musculature (spinal poliomyelitis) or it multiplies in the neurons from the brain stem (bulbar poliomyelitis) (Modlin 2005; Muller 2005). After viral replication in the oropharynx and intestine, poliovirus is eliminated in oropharyngeal secretions for 1–3 weeks and in the stool for 1 or 2 months, until the virus is completely out of the body. During reinfection, the virus is eliminated in the stool within 3 weeks (Heymann 2004). The period of maximum communicability is probably the first two weeks after enterovirus infection. The potential for prolonged replication is higher in patients with immunodeficiency syndromes.

6.4 DIAGNOSIS

The diagnostic in suspected enterovirus infections is based on medical history and examination of a patient, followed by CSF analysis, and identification of the serotype by polymerase chain reaction amplification and serology. The history of a patient with suspected viral meningitis includes the presence of classic symptoms. Important aspects of the clinical examination include signs of meningeal inflammation (nuchal rigidity, Kernig and Brudzinski's signs), assessment of mental status (Glasgow coma scale), and findings associated with specific viruses (e.g., conjunctivitis, rash, herpangina, hand, foot, and mouth disease). The important distinguishing feature between encephalitis and meningitis is the brain function. Electroencephalography (EEG) is an indicator of cerebral involvement during the early stage of the disease. The presence of focal neurological signs is suggestive for encephalitis. In patients with signs or symptoms of increased intracranial pressure, computed tomography (CT) is recommended as a screening examination. Magnetic resonance imaging is more sensitive and specific than computed tomography (CT) for evaluation of the brain inflammation, and is useful before lumbar puncture (Fleischer 2006; Logan and MacMahon 2008; Steiner et al. 2010).

6.4.1 LABORATORY DIAGNOSIS

In aseptic meningitis and encephalitis with enteroviruses, the diagnosis requires identification of a viral pathogen from cerebrospinal fluid specimen (CSF) or other patient samples (e.g., throat swab, stool). The virus can be identified in a CSF sample only in the acute phase of infection. In infections with poliovirus or HEV71, weakness or paralysis may occur. The protocol for laboratory investigation of suspected cases of paralytic poliomyelitis includes two stool specimens and two throat swabs collected every 24 h at least, within 14 days since onset, a blood specimen for complete blood count, a cerebrospinal fluid specimen (CSF) for chemical and cytologic analysis, and acute and convalescent serum specimens, collected at an interval of at least 2–4 weeks for detection and titration of the neutralizing antibodies to the three poliovirus serotypes. The collection of CSF and throat swabs is not recommended by the WHO for the surveillance because the polioviruses are rarely detected in CSF and the titer of the virus in throat swabs is 10 fold lower than in stool specimens.

The laboratory tests show a peripheral leukocytosis and a pleocytosis in CSF [increase of white blood cell (WBC) count, but less than 250/mm^3 with predominance of neutrophils in early stage of infection, and shift from neutrophils to lymphocytes 8 h later in aseptic meningitis and few days later in poliomyelitis], an elevated protein concentration (usually less than 150 mg/dL in aseptic meningitis that may increase to 300 mg/dL for several weeks in poliomyelitis), and a normal level of glucose (Melnick 1996). In children, the enteroviral meningitis frequently occurs in the absence of either CSF pleocytosis or elevated protein levels. In this situation, the CSF profile alone cannot distinguish between enteroviral and bacterial meningitis, and the enteroviral polymerase chain reaction (PCR) must be performed as an additional diagnostic test (Graham and Murdoch 2005). The phenotypic and molecular laboratory techniques are important to rule out or confirm the diagnosis of infection with enteroviruses. The correct virological diagnosis depends on the timely collection, transportation, and storage of the specimens.

6.4.2 CONVENTIONAL TECHNIQUES

Traditionally, cell culture has been employed for the isolation of enteroviruses from clinical samples. Primary cells (primary monkey kidney cells) and suckling mice are unavailable for routine diagnosis of HEVs as a result of the international standards related to the care and management of experimental animals. The main cell cultures used today for HEV isolation are RD (a human rhabdomyosarcoma derived cell line recommended by the WHO), BGMK (Buffalo green monkey kidney cells), A549 (a human lung adenocarcinoma epithelial cell line), MRC-5 cells (derived from normal lung tissue of a 14-week-old male fetus), and HEp-2c cells (derived from a human larynx epidermoid carcinoma). A genetically engineered mouse cell line expressing the human poliovirus receptor PVR, L20B, recommended by the WHO is susceptible only to poliovirus infection (Pipkin et al. 1993). Enterovirus isolation needs inoculation of each specimen (directly or after pretreatment) onto continuous cell lines that are available for use in different laboratories. For poliovirus isolation, RD, HEp-2c, and L20B cell lines are recommended by the WHO. The cell lines must be examined daily, and once the complete cytopathic effect (CPE) occurs, the infected cells must be kept frozen (at −20°C) until viral identification. The time interval for enterovirus isolation and characterization must be at least 10 days (minimum of 5 days postinoculation and minimum of 5 days postpassage) before a reported negative test (WHO 2007). Rapid degeneration of the cell culture or cell death could appear in the nonspecific toxicity of the specimen or in microbial contamination of the culture maintenance medium (2% fetal calf serum), respectively. Characteristic CPE progresses from rounding, refractory individual cells within the monolayer to the detachment of the infected cell from the tissue culture tube.

The HEV identification and typing are carried out by seroneutralization with pools of antisera or by indirect immunofluorescence assay. The Lim Benyesh-Melnick (LBM) pools and the WHO enteroviral antisera pools are available for HEVs typing. The A-H and J-P pools from the LBM schedule identifies 42 serotypes including PV1–3 (Melnick et al. 1973) and 19 CVA strains, most of which can only be isolate in suckling mice (Melnick et al. 1997). The pools of polyclonal antisera against CVA9 and 20 echoviruses, CVB1–6, and PV1–3 have been developed by the National Institute of Public Health and the Environment (RIVM), Bilthoven, the Netherlands, and are supplied free of charge to WHO Polio Laboratory Network laboratories by WHO. The typing by seroneutralization with these pools has limitations because the newly discovered and circulating HEV strains are not recognized and these pools may not even recognize the progeny of previously identified HEV strains due to the antigenic drift that occurred over the years. Monospecific antisera have been used for confirmation of the serotype. The methods recommended by WHO for intratypic differentiation of poliovirus isolates are currently in use (van der Avoort et al. 1995). An enzyme-linked immunosorbent assay (ELISA) method developed by RIVM detects antigenic differences between wild and vaccine-related strains. The utilization of type-specific neutralizing monoclonal antibodies developed by the Pasteur Institute, Paris, and the National Institute for Biological Standards and Control, Potters Bar, was accepted, but it is not currently supported by the WHO Global Polio Laboratory Network.

The commercial Light Diagnostics™ Pan Enterovirus reagent (Millipore, Chemicon, Temecula, CA) is used for the preliminary identification of enteroviruses from cell culture by indirect immunofluorescence assay (IFA). The reagent contains a mixtures that recognize specific groups of HEV: the PV mixture for PV types 1, 2, and 3 detection, the enterovirus mixture for HEV70, 71, CVA16 detection, the Echo mixture for echovirus types 4, 6, 9, 11, 30 detection, and the CVB mixture for CVB types 1–6. The monovalent antibodies are available for each serotype included in the mixtures and for CVA9 and CVA24. By using of the Super E-Mix™ cell line combined with the D3 IFA enterovirus test (Diagnostic Hybrids, USA), the time for isolation and identification of the enteroviruses decrease as low as 16 h. Super E-Mix™ is a mixed cell monolayer in shell vials which contains human lung carcinoma (A-549) cells together with buffalo green monkey kidney (BGMK) cells, which have been genetically modified to produce large amounts of human decay-accelerating factor (DAF) on the cell surface. The D3 IFA enterovirus reagent uses a blend of Enterovirus VP1 antigen-specific murine monoclonal antibodies (MAbs) conjugated with a fluorescein isothiocyanate labelled antimouse antibody. Lin et al. (2008) described the development of an in-house indirect immunofluorescence assay (IFA) for rapid detection of CVA types 2, 4, 5, 6, and 10.

Antibodies to nontyped enteroviruses are measured from serum and CSF by enzyme immunoassay (EIA) tests. The presence of specific IgM in the CSF indicates CNS disease. The microneutralization test has limited utility in the routine diagnosis of nonpolio enterovirus infections because it is serotype specific, but it may be helpful in the diagnosis of paralytic poliomyelitis according to the vaccine history of the patient (the number of doses received, the time after the last vaccine dose received) and to the type of virus isolated. A 4-fold rise in serum antibody titer between the acute and convalescent serum is significant for diagnosis.

6.4.3 Molecular Techniques

For CNS infections, rapid identification of a viral pathogen by molecular diagnostic tests and prompt initiation of the therapy are potentially lifesaving, reduce hospitalization, and avoid the antibiotic use (King et al. 2007). The evidence of a microorganism in CSF, spinal, and brain tissue, which are normally sterile body sites, is probably an infection (usually monomicrobial). The CSF has no inhibitors of polymerase chain reaction (PCR) assays such as heme, endonucleases, and exonucleases. Nucleic acid amplification methods are often more sensitive than conventional culture-based or antigen detection methods. The molecular typing methods for HEVs are amplification (PCR) and sequencing targeting to specific coding regions for VP1 or VP2. The noncapsid encoding sequences are not highly conserved and may recombine with other enteroviruses (Lukashev et al. 2003). A small volume of sample of about 150–250 μl is enough for nucleic acid extraction. PCR allows exponential amplification of short DNA sequences within a longer double stranded DNA molecule by using a pair of primers (about 20 nucleotides in length, complementary to a sequence on each of the two strands of the DNA) and a DNA polymerase. The enterovirus RNA genome is converted initially into complementary DNA (cDNA), reverse transcription (RT) using the enzyme reverse transcriptase, followed by amplification of the correct amplicon using specific sets of primers and Taq polymerase, a thermostable DNA polymerase. The performance of the RT-PCR assays depends on optimization and standardization of the viral genome extraction, amplification, and detection. The manual extraction method using the Qiagen QIAamp viral RNA kit based on silica membrane columns (Qiagen GmbH, Hilden, Germany) is rapid and does not require the utilization of hazardous materials as phenol or chloroform. There were a few studies that compared the manual with the automated nucleic acid extraction (Knepp et al. 2003; Dundas et al. 2008). Amplification efficiency of nucleic acids extracted by automated methods was similar to that by the manual methods. The molecular techniques for amplification and detection of specific regions from HEV genome evolved from the RT-PCR (Chapman et al. 1990; Rotbart 1990) to the real-time RT-PCR assays (r-RT-PCR) (Archimbaud et al. 2009; Sofer et al. 2011; Baicus 2011). The primers targeting different genomic regions of nonpolio enteroviruses and polioviruses are reported by Balanant et al. (1991), Caro et al. (2001), Guillot et al. (2000), Kilpatrick et al. (1998, 2004, 2009), Oberste et al. (1999, 2002), and Yang et al. (1991), respectively. The relationships between isolates and enterovirus transmission could be detected by VP1 sequence analysis (Sambrook et al. 1989). The amplicons could be sequenced by the dideoxynucleotide method with the Big Dye Terminator Cycle Sequencing Ready Reaction kit (the procedure recommended by Applied Biosystems, Perkin-Elmer) and an ABI Prism automated sequencer (Applied Biosystems) using primers used for the PCR reaction. The alignment and comparison of the sequences can be done with a software (e.g., Clustal X version 2.0 or CLC Main Workbench software version 6.0.1). The MARSH assay (Microarrays for resequencing and sequence heterogeneity) can be applied to detect the point mutations present at a low level in heterogeneous populations and mixtures of different virus strains (Liu et al. 2007), and it has been used for studying the VDPV strains (Cherkasova et al. 2003).

6.5 PROGNOSIS, PREVENTION, AND TREATMENT

Most enterovirus infections are self-limited and do not require specific therapy. The prevention of the spreading of infection with enteroviruses is through measures of hygiene, such as hand washing. There are no vaccines available for protection against infections with nonpolio enteroviruses. For patients with enteroviral meningitis, acute encephalitis supportive therapy is required. The therapy with intravenous immune globulins has been useful in patients with agammaglobulinemia, chronic meningitis, or meningoencephalitis because the clearance of HEV by the host is primarily antibody mediated. Although there is no approved therapy, a variety of antiviral agents have shown activity against enteroviruses *in vitro*, and in early clinical trials. The capsid inhibiting class of drugs act by preventing the HEV uncoating or viral binding to a cellular receptor. Pleconaril is one of these drugs, an orally administered drug with a favorable pharmacokinetic and toxicity profile reaching higher concentrations within the CNS than in serum. In limited clinical studies on patients with enterovirus meningitis, pleconaril did not demonstrate overall clinical benefit (Abzug et al. 2003; Rotbart et al. 2001; Tormey et al. 2003), and the drug is not currently available for clinical use (Desmond et al. 2006). Aged and immunodeficient patients with aseptic meningitis may be considered for empiric therapy for 48 h until the diagnosis of viral meningitis is sure.

Treatment of poliomyelitis is supportive. Mechanical ventilation and close monitoring of cardiovascular status are necessary in patients with respiratory failure and bulbar poliomyelitis. The poliomyelitis has been virtually eliminated in most countries by the widespread immunization with the formalin-inactivated polio vaccine (IPV) or/and oral live-attenuated polio vaccine (OPV). After 22 years since the decision of the World Health Organization to globally eradicate poliomyelitis, circulation of wild poliovirus types 1 and 3 continues in 4 countries, India, Nigeria, Pakistan, and Afghanistan, because of underutilization of vaccine, vaccine failure, and the epidemiologic context (el-Sayed et al. 2008; Grassly et al. 2006; Jenkins et al. 2008). The indigenous wild type 2 poliovirus was eradicated in 1999 but a type 2 circulating vaccine-derived poliovirus (cVDPV) has persisted in northern Nigeria since 2006 (Adu et al. 2007). The supplementary immunization with monovalent strains of OPV (mOPV) type 1 (Grassly et al. 2007) or type 3 has been introduced (CDC 2009) in those regions where the virus has been difficult to control. A new bivalent oral poliovaccine bOPV (containing types 1 and 3 poliovirus) has been introduced into all 4 persistently endemic countries, beginning in 2009 with Afghanistan (WHO 2010). Low vaccination coverage, and the extent of immunization gaps increase the potential risk of emergence and circulation of VDPV strains (Nathanson and Kew 2010).

The WHO assists countries with decision-making on polio vaccination schedules and vaccines, given their risk of poliovirus importations and the probable transmission potential for polioviruses in their country. In a given country, once wild poliovirus was eliminated through the use of OPV, the public health authorities could decide continuation of OPV immunization or transition from OPV to IPV (Chumakov et al. 2007; Ehrenfeld et al. 2008; Fine and Ritchie 2006). Global vaccination with IPV is not yet possible because there are still financial, logistic, and scientific problems. The IPV was introduced to prevent VAPP, to close existing immunity gaps, or to optimize the administration of other antigens. A Poliovirus Antiviral Initiative (PAI) was proposed in 2006 by the Advisory Committee on Poliomyelitis Eradication (ACPE) and by the Task Force for Childhood Survival and Development (Task Force). The development of polio specific antiviral drugs, used with either IPV or OPV, will improve the control of outbreaks in the future (De Palma et al. 2008; Collett et al. 2008; Thys et al. 2008). Pleconaril was shown to be safe and effective in treating diseases caused by nonpolio enteroviruses (Bauer et al. 2002; Hayden et al. 2002; Utzig et al. 2003) but has shown little or no activity against polioviruses. V-073 was found to have potent, broad-spectrum antipoliovirus activity in cell culture (Thibaut et al. 2011).

6.6 CONCLUSIONS AND FUTURE PERSPECTIVES

The early clinical recognition and the rapid diagnosis by molecular techniques of the neurological infections are among the most important problems in medicine. Rapid detection of nonpolio enteroviruses in CSF within the first 24 h of hospitalization is followed by cessation of antibiotic administration and shortening of hospitalization time. The surveillance of the cocirculation and evolution of polioviruses and nonpolio enteroviruses must be increased by the fast detection of the emergence of new epidemic strains. The evaluation made in different scenarios concerning the risk and costs of the polio eradication was changed because the ability of VDPV strains to produce outbreaks. In April 2010, the first importation of wild PV type 1 from India was detected in Tajikistan, in the WHO European Region, since it was certified polio-free in 2002 (WHO 2010). In a polio-free region, the risk of importation and subsequent transmission of the poliovirus remains until polio is completely eradicated. In countries with otherwise adequate levels of vaccine coverage, the groups that are at high risk are the subpopulations that refuse immunization or with gaps in immunity (Alexander et al. 2009; Combiescu et al. 2007). Many countries have switched the schedule of vaccination against polio by using IPV instead of OPV to eliminate the risk of vaccine-associated paralytic poliomyelitis (VAPP). The barriers for the global introduction of IPV are its cost, the need for intramuscular injection, its inability to produce optimal intestinal immunity, and the biocontainment required for its production. A planning for the cessation of routine OPV immunization against type 2 polioviruses is taken into account (WHO 2011). A research program for obtaining an affordable IPV for developing countries was initiated and financed by GPEI/WHO (WHO 2009). A number of strategies are followed including a schedule reduction, a reduction of the antigen dose by intradermal administration (Mohammed et al. 2010; Resik et al. 2010), by using adjuvants (Baldwin et al. 2011), optimization of production processes, and development of an inactivated poliovirus vaccine produced from Sabin strains (Kreeftenberg et al. 2006; Simizu et al. 2006). Global Polio Eradication Initiative (GPEI) developed new tools for maintaining the comprehensive AFP surveillance, for achieving certification and containment of wild poliovirus, for preparing for VAPP and VDPV elimination and for the post-OPV era (GPEI 2009). A target of 90% routine vaccine coverage in low-income countries by 2010 has been an objective of the GPEI and the Global Alliance for Vaccines and Immunization (GAVI) (Fine and Griffiths 2007). After global cessation of OPV administration, the immunization by using IPV through the first 5 to 10 years is necessary (Aylward and Yamada 2011).

REFERENCES

Abzug, M. J., Cloud, G., Bradley, J., Sánchez, P. J., Romero, J., Powell, D., Lepow, M., Mani, C., Capparelli, E. V., Blount, S., Lakeman, F., Whitley, R. J., Kimberlin, D. W., and National Institute of Allergy and Infectious Diseases Collaborative Antiviral Study Group. 2003. Double blind placebo-controlled trial of pleconaril in infants with enterovirus meningitis. *Pediatr. Infect. Dis. J.* 22, 335–341.

Adu, F., Iber, J., Bukbuk, D., Gumede, N., Yang, S. J., Jorba, J., Campagnoli, R., Sule, W. F., Yang, C. F., Burns, C., Pallansch, M., Harry, T., and Kew, O. 2007. Isolation of recombinant type 2 vaccine-derived poliovirus (VDPV) from a Nigerian child. *Virus Res.* 127, 17–25.

Alexander, J. P., Baden, L., Pallansch, M., and Anderson, L. 1994. Enterovirus 71 infections and neurologic disease—United States, 1977–1991. *J. Infect. Dis.* 169, 905–908.

Alexander, J. P., Ehresmann, K., Seward, J., Wax, G., Harriman, K., Fuller, S., Cebelinski, E. A., Chen, Q., Jorba, J., Kew, O. M., Pallansch, M. A., Oberste, M. S., Schleiss, M., Davis, J. P., Warshawsky, B., Squires, S., Hull, H. F., and Vaccine-Derived Poliovirus Investigations Group. 2009. Transmission of imported vaccine-derived poliovirus in an undervaccinated community in Minnesota. *J. Infect. Dis.* 199, 391–397.

Amstey, M. S., Miller, R. K., Menegus, M. A., and di Sant'Agnese, P. A. 1988. Enterovirus in pregnant women and the perfused placenta. *Am. J. Obstet. Gynecol.* 158, 775–782.

Ang, L. W., Koh, B. K., Chan, K. P., Chua, L. T., James, L., and Goh, K. T. 2009. Epidemiology and control of hand, foot and mouth disease in Singapore, 2001–2007. *Ann. Acad. Med. Singapore.* 38, 106–112.

Archimbaud, C., Bailly, J. L., Chambon, M., Tournilhac, O., Travade, P., and Peigue-Lafeuille, H. 2003. Molecular evidence of persistent echovirus 13 meningoencephalitis in a patient with relapsed lymphoma after an outbreak of meningitis in 2000. *J. Clin. Microbiol.* 41, 4605–4610.

Archimbaud, C., Chambon, M., Bailly, J. L., Petit, I., Henquell, C., Mirand, A., Aublet-Cuvelier, B., Ughetto, S., Beytout, J., Clavelou, P., Labbé, A., Philippe, P., Schmidt, J., Regagnon, C., Traore, O., and Peigue-Lafeuille, H. 2009. Impact of rapid enterovirus molecular diagnosis on the management of infants, children, and adults with aseptic meningitis. *J. Med. Virol.* 81, 42–48.

Avellon, A., Casas, I., Trallero, G., Perez, C., Tenorio, A., and Palacios, G. 2003. Molecular analysis of echovirus 13 isolates and aseptic meningitis, Spain. *Emerg. Infect. Dis.* 9, 934–941.

Aylward, B., and Yamada, T. 2011. The Polio Endgame. *N. Engl. J. Med.* 364, 2273–2275.

Badorff, C., Lee, G. H., Lamphear, B. J., Martone, M. E., Campbell, K. P., Rhoads, R. E., and Knowlton, K. U. 1999. Enteroviral protease 2A cleaves dystrophin: evidence of cytoskeletal disruption in an acquired cardiomyopathy. *Nat. Med.* 5, 320–326.

Baicus, A. 2011. Poliovirus. In: Liu, D. (Ed.). *Molecular Detection of Human Viral Pathogens.* CRC Press, Taylor and Francis Group, Boca Raton, FL, USA, pp. 75–86.

Balanant, J., Guillot, S., Candrea, A., Delpeyroux, F., and Crainic, R. 1991. The natural genomic variability of poliovirus analyzed by a restriction fragment length polymorphism assay. *Virology.* 184, 645–654.

Baldwin, S. L., Fox, C. B., Pallansch, M. A., Coler, R. N., Reed, S. G., and Friede, M. 2011. Increased potency of an inactivated trivalent polio vaccine with oil-in-water emulsions. *Vaccine.* 29, 644–649.

Bauer, S., Gottesman, G., Sirota, L., Litmanovitz, I., Ashkenazi, S., and Levi, I. 2002. Severe Coxsackie virus B infection in preterm newborns treated with pleconaril. *Eur. J. Pediatr.* 161, 491–493.

Begier, E. M., Oberste, M. S., Landry, M. L., Brennan, T., Mlynarski, D., Mshar, P. A., Frenette, K., Rabatsky-Her, T., Purviance, K., Nepaul, A., Nix, W. A., Pallansch, M. A., Ferguson, D., Cartter, M. L., and Hadler, J. L. 2008. An outbreak of concurrent echovirus 30 and coxsackievirus A1 infections associated with sea swimming among a group of travelers to Mexico. *Clin. Infect. Dis.* 47, 616–623.

Blomqvist, S., Bruu, A. L., Stenvik, M., and Hovi, T. 2003. Characterization of a recombinant type 3/type 2 poliovirus isolated from a healthy vaccine and containing a chimeric capsid proteinVP1. *J Gen. Virol.* 84, 573–580.

Brown, B., Oberste, M. S., Maher, K., and Pallansch, M. A. 2003. Complete genomic sequencing shows that polioviruses and members of human enterovirus species C are closely related in the noncapsid coding region. *J. Virol.* 77, 8973–8984.

Burchett, S. K., and Dalgic, N. 2008. Viral infections. In: Cloherty, J. P., Eichenwald, E. C., and Stark, A. R. (Eds.). *Manual of Neonatal Care*, 6th ed., Lippincott, Williams & Wilkins, Philadelphia, p. 269.

Caro,V., Guillot, S., Delpeyroux, F., and Crainic, R. 2001. Molecular strategy for 'serotyping' of human enteroviruses. *J. Gen. Virol.* 82, 79–91.

Carstens, E. B., and Ball, L. A. 2009. Ratification vote on taxonomic proposals to the International Committee on Taxonomy of Viruses (2008). *Arch. Virol.* 154, 1181–1188.

Caverly, C. S., 1894. Preliminary report of an epidemic of paralytic disease, occurring in Vermont, in the summer of 1894. *Yale Med. J.* 1, 1–5.

Centers for Disease Control and Prevention (CDC). 2000. Outbreak of aseptic meningitis associated with multiple enterovirus serotypes—Romania, 1999. *M.M.W.R.* 49, 669–671.

Centers for Disease Control and Prevention (CDC). 2001. Echovirus type 13—United States 2001. *M.M.W.R.* 50, 777–780.

Centers for Disease Control and Prevention (CDC). 2006. Update on vaccine-derived polioviruses. *M.M.W.R.* 55, 1093.

Centers for Disease Control and Prevention (CDC). 2008. Increased detections and severe neonatal disease associated with coxsackievirus B1 infection—United States, 2007. *M.M.W.R.* 57, 553–556.

Centers for Disease Control and Prevention (CDC). 2009. Progress toward interruption of wild poliovirus transmission-worldwide, 2008. *M.M.W.R.* 58, 308–312.

Chakrabarti, S., Osman, H., Collingham, K. E., Fegan, C. D., and Milligan, D. W. 2004. Enterovirus infections following T-cell depleted allogeneic transplants in adults. *Bone Marrow Transplant.* 33, 425–430.

Chan, K. P., Goh, K. T., Chong, C. Y., Teo, E. S., Lau, G., and Ling, A. E. 2003. Epidemic hand, foot, and mouth disease caused by human enterovirus 71, Singapore. *Emerg. Infect. Dis.* 9, 78–85.

Chang, L. Y., Lin, T. Y., Hsu, K. H., Huang, Y. C., Lin, K. L., Hsueh, C., Shih, S. R., Ning, H. C., Hwang, M. S., Wang, H. S., and Lee, C. Y. 1999. Clinical features and risk factors of pulmonary oedema after enterovirus-71-related hand, foot, and mouth disease. *Lancet.* 354, 1862–1866.

Chapman, N. M., Tracy, S., Gauntt, C. J., and Fortmueller, U. 1990. Molecular detection and identification of enteroviruses using enzymatic amplification and nucleic acid hybridization. *J. Clin. Microbiol.* 28, 843–850.

Cherkasova, E., Laassri, M., Chizhikov, V., Korotkova, E., Dragunsky, E., Agol, V. I., and Chumakov, K. 2003. Microarray analysis of evolution of RNA viruses: evidence of circulation of virulent highly divergent vaccine-derived polioviruses. *Proc. Natl. Acad. Sci. U S A.* 100, 9398–9403.

Chumakov, K., Ehrenfeld, E., Wimmer, E, and Agol, V. I. 2007. Vaccination against polio should not be stopped. *Nat. Rev. Microbiol.* 5, 952–958.

Cohen, J. I. 2006. Enteroviruses and Reoviruses. In: Fauci, A. S., Braunwald, E., Kasper, D. L., Hauser, D. L., Longo, D. L., Jameson, J. L., and Loscalzo, J. (Eds). *Harrison's Principles of Internal Medicine*, 17th ed., McGrawHill, New York. pp.1208–1213.

Collett, M. S., Neyts, J., and Modlin, J. F. 2008. A case for developing antiviral drugs against polio. *Antiviral Res.* 79, 179–187.

Combiescu, M., Guillot, S., Persu, A., Baicus, A., Pitigoi, D., Balanant, J., Oprisan, G., Crainic, R., Delpeyroux, F., and Aubert-Combiescu, A. 2007. Circulation of a type 1 recombinant vaccine-derived poliovirus strain in a limited area in Romania. *Arch. Virol.* 152, 727–738.

Coyne, C. B., and Bergelson, J. M. 2006.Virus-induced Abl and Fyn kinase signals permit coxsackievirus entry through epithelial tight junctions. *Cell.* 124, 119–131.

Dalwai, A., Ahmad, S., and Al-Nakib, W. 2010. Echoviruses are a major cause of aseptic meningitis in infants and young children in Kuwait. *Virol. J.* 7, 236–241.

De Palma, A. M., Pürstinger, G., Wimmer, E., Patick, A. K., Andries, K., Rombaut, B., De Clercq, E., and Neyts, J. 2008. Potential use of antiviral agents in polio eradication. *Emerg. Infect. Dis.* 14, 545–551.

Desmond, R. A., Accortt, N. A., Talley, L., Villano, S. A., Soong, S. J., and Whitley, R. J. 2006. Enteroviral meningitis: natural history and outcome of pleconaril therapy. *Antimicrob. Agents Chemother.* 50, 2409–2414.

Diedrich, S., and Schreier, E. 2001. Aseptic meningitis in Germany associated with echovirus type 13. *BMC Infect. Dis.* 1, 14.

Dundas, N., Leos, N. K., Mitui, M., Revell, P., and Rogers, B. B. 2008. Comparison of automated nucleic acid extraction methods with manual extraction. *J. Mol. Diagn.* 10, 311–316.

Ehrenfeld, E., Glass, R. I., Agol, V. I., Chumakov, K., Dowdle, W., John, T. J., Katz, S. L., Miller, M., Breman, J. G., Modlin, J., and Wright, P. 2008. Immunisation against poliomyelitis: moving forward. *Lancet.* 371, 1385–1387.

el-Sayed, N., el-Gamal, Y., Abbassy, A. A., Seoud, I., Salama, M., Kandeel, A., Hossny, E., Shawky, A., Hussein, H. A., Pallansch, M. A., van der Avoort, H. G., Burton, A. H., Sreevatsava, M., Malankar, P., Wahdan, M. H., and Sutter, R. W. 2008. Monovalent type 1 oral poliovirus vaccine in newborns. *N. Engl. J. Med.* 359, 1655–1665.

Enders, J. F., Weller, T. H., and Robbins, F. C. 1949. Cultivation of the Lansing strain of poliovirus in cultures of various human embryonic tissue. *Science.* 109, 85–87.

Farbu, E., Gilhus, N. E., Barnes, M. P., Borg, K., de Visser, M., Driessen, A., Howard, R., Nollet, F., Opara, J., and Stalberg, E. 2006. EFNS guideline on diagnosis and management of post-polio syndrome. Report of an EFNS task force. *Eur. J. Neurol.* 13, 795–801.

Fine, P. E., and Griffiths, U. K. 2007. Global poliomyelitis eradication: status and implications. *Lancet.* 369, 1321–1322.

Fine, P. E., and Ritchie, S. 2006. Perspective: determinants of the severity of poliovirus outbreaks in the post eradication era. *Risk Anal.* 26, 1533–1540.

Fischmeister, G., Wiesbauer, P., Holzmann, H. M., Peters, C., Eibl, M., and Gadner, H. 2000. Enteroviral meningoencephalitis in immunocompromised children after matched unrelated donor-bone marrow transplantation. *Pediatr. Hematol. Oncol.* 17, 393–399.

Fleisher, G. R. 2006. Infectious disease emergencies. In: Fleisher, G. R., Ludwig, S., and Henretig, F. M. (Eds.) *Textbook of Pediatric Emergency Medicine*, 5th ed, Lippincott, Williams & Wilkins, Philadelphia, p. 783.

Flexner, S., and Lewis, P. A. 1910. Experimental poliomyelitis in monkeys; active immunization and passive serum protection. *J. Am. Med. Assoc.* 54, 1780–1782.

Fowlkes, A. L., Honarmand, S., Glaser, C., Yagi, S., Schnurr, D., Oberste, M. S., Anderson, L., Pallansch, M. A., and Khetsuriani, N. 2008. Enterovirus-associated encephalitis in the California encephalitis project, 1998–2005. *J. Infect. Dis.* 198, 1685–1691.

Freund, M. W., Kleinveld, G., Krediet, T. G., van Loon, A. M., and Verboon-Maciolek, M. A. 2010. Prognosis for neonates with enterovirus myocarditis. *Arch. Dis. Child. Fetal. Neonatal. Ed.* 95, F206–F212.

Georgescu, M. M., Balanant, J., Macadam, A., Otelea, D., Combiescu, M., Combiescu, A. A., Crainic, R., and Delpeyroux, F. 1997. Evolution of the Sabin type 1 poliovirus in humans: characterization of strains isolated from patients with vaccine-associated paralytic poliomyelitis. *J. Virol.* 71, 7758–7768.

Gilbert, G., Dickson, K., Waters, M., Kennett, M., Land, S., and Sneddon, M. 1988. Outbreak of enterovirus 71 infection in Victoria, Australia, with a high incidence of neurologic involvement. *Pediatr. Infect. Dis. J.* 7, 484–488.

Global Polio Eradication Initiative, 2009. Monthly Situation Report (online), Geneva: WHO. http://www.who.int/wer/2009/wer8443/en/index.html, last accessed on 17th of June 2011.

Godman, G. C., Bunting, H., and Melnick, J. L. 1952. The histopathology of coxsackie virus infection in mice. I. Morphologic observations with four different viral types. *Am. J. Pathol.* 28, 223–257.

Graham, A. K., and Murdoch, D. R. 2005. Association between cerebrospinal fluid pleocytosis and enteroviral meningitis. *J. Clin. Microbiol.* 43, 1491.

Grassly, N. C., Fraser, C., Wenger, J., Deshpande, J. M., Sutter, R. W., Heymann, D. L., and Aylward, R. B. 2006. New strategies for the elimination of polio from India. *Science.* 314, 1150–1153.

Grassly, N. C., Wenger, J., Durrani, S., Bahl, S., Deshpande, J. M., Sutter, R. W., Heymann, D. L., and Aylward, R. B. 2007. Protective efficacy of a monovalent oral type 1 poliovirus vaccine: a case-control study. *Lancet.* 369, 1356–1362.

Grimby, G., Stalberg, E., Sandberg, A., and Sunnerhagen, K. S. 1998. An 8-year longitudinal study of muscle strength, muscle fiber size, and dynamic electromyogram in individuals with late polio. *Muscle Nerve.* 21, 1428–1437.

Guillot, S., Caro, V., Cuervo, N., Korotkova, E., Combiescu, M., Persu, A., Aubert-Combiescu, A., Delpeyroux, F., and Crainic, R. 2000. Natural genetic exchanges between vaccine and wild poliovirus strains in humans. *J. Virol.* 74, 8434–8443.

Hamaguchi, T., Fujisawa, H., Sakai, K., Okino, S., Kurosaki, N., Nishimura, Y., Shimizu, H., and Yamada, M. 2008. Acute encephalitis caused by intrafamilial transmission of enterovirus 71 in adult. *Emerg. Infect. Dis.* 14, 828–830.

Hayden, F. G., Herrington, D. T., Coats, T. L., Kim, K., Cooper, E. C., Villano, S. A., Liu, S., Hudson, S., Pevear, D. C., Collett, M., McKinlay, M, and Pleconaril Respiratory Infection Study Group. 2003. Efficacy and safety of oral pleconaril for treatment of colds due to picornaviruses in adults: results of 2 double-blind, randomized, placebo controlled trials. *Clin. Infect. Dis.* 36, 1523–1532.

He, Y., Bowman, V. D., Mueller, S., Bator, C. M., Bella, J., Peng, X., Baker, T. S., Wimmer, E., Kuhn, R. J., and Rossmann, M. G. 2000. Interaction of the poliovirus receptor with poliovirus. *Proc. Natl. Acad. Sci. U S A.* 97, 79–84.

Hellen, C. U. T., and Wimmer, E. 1995. Enterovirus Structure and assembly, In: Rotbart, H. A. (Ed.). *Human Enterovirus Infections,* American Society for Microbiology, Washington, pp. 155–175.

Hendry, E., Hatanaka, H., Fry, E., Smyth, M., Tate, J., Stanway, G., Santti, J., Maaronen, M., Hyypiä, T., and Stuart, D. 1999. The crystal structure of coxsackievirus A9: new insights into the uncoating mechanisms of enteroviruses. *Structure.* 7, 1527–1538.

Heymann, D. L. 2004. Poliomyelitis acute. In: *Control of Communicable Diseases Manual*, 18th ed., American Public Health Association, Washington, pp. 425–431.

Ho, M., Chen, E. R., Hsu, K. H., Twu, S. J., Chen, K. T., Tsai, S. F., Wang, J. R., and Shih, S. R. 1999. An epidemic of enterovirus 71 infection in Taiwan. *New. Engl. J. Med.* 341, 929–35.

Hober, D., and Sauter, P. 2010. Pathogenesis of type 1 diabetes mellitus: interplay between enterovirus and host. *Nat. Rev. Endocrinol.* 6, 279–289.

Hogle, J. M., and Filman, D. J. 1989. Poliovirus: three-dimensional structure of a viral antigen. *Adv. Vet. Sci. Comp. Med.* 33, 65–91.

Hogle, J. M., Chow, M., and Filman, D. J. 1985. The three-dimensional structure of poliovirus at 2.9 Å resolution. *Science.* 229, 1358–1365.

Iwai, M., Yoshida, H., Obara, M., Horimoto, E., Nakamura, K., Takizawa, T., Kurata, T., Mizuguchi, M., Daikoku, T., and Shiraki, K. 2010. Widespread circulation of echovirus type 13 demonstrated by increased seroprevalence in Toyama, Japan, between 2000 and 2003. *Clin. Vaccine. Immunol.* 17, 764–770.

Jacques, J., Moret, H., Minette, D., Lévêque, N., Jovenin, N., Deslée, G., Lebargy, F., Motte, J., and Andréoletti, L. 2008. Epidemiological, molecular, and clinical features of enterovirus respiratory infections in french children between 1999 and 2005. *J. Clin. Microb.* 46, 206–213.

Jenkins, H. E., Aylward, R. B., Gasasira, A., Donnelly, C. A., Abanida, E. A., Koleosho-Adelekan, T., and Grassly, N. C. 2008. Effectiveness of immunization against paralytic poliomyelitis in Nigeria. *N. Engl. J. Med.* 359, 1666–1674.

Jiang, P., Faase, J. A., Toyoda, H., Paul, A., Wimmer, E., and Gorbalenya, A. E. 2007. Evidence for emergence of diverse polioviruses from C-cluster coxsackie A viruses: implications for global poliovirus eradication. *Proc. Natl. Acad. Sci. U S A.* 104, 9457–9462.

Johansson, M. E., Holmström, S., Abebe, A., Jacobsson, B., Ekman, G., Samuelson, A., and Wirgart, B. Z. 1992. Intrauterine fetal death due to echovirus 11. Scand. *J. Infect. Dis.* 24, 381–385.

Keels, M. A. 2012. Soft tissue lesions of the oral cavity in children. In: *UpToDate 20.3*, Waltham, MA, U S A.

Khetsuriani, N., Lamonte-Fowlkes, A., Oberst, S., and Pallansch, M. A. 2006. Enterovirus surveillance—United States, 1970–2005. *M.M.W.R.* 55, 1–20.

Kilpatrick, D. R., Ching, K., Iber, J., Campagnoli, R., Freeman, C. J., Mishrik, N., Liu, H. M., Pallansch, M. A., and Kew, O. M. 2004. Multiplex PCR method for identifying recombinant vaccine related polioviruses. *J. Clin Microbiol.* 42, 4313–4315.

Kilpatrick, D. R., Nottay, B., Yang, C. F., Yang, S. J., Mulders, M. N., Holloway, B. P., Pallansch, M. A., and Kew, O. M. 1998. Serotype-specific identification of polioviruses by PCR using primers containing mixed-base or deoxyinosine residues at positions of codon degeneracy. *J. Clin. Microbiol.* 36, 352–357.

Kilpatrick, D. R., Yang, C. F., Ching, K., Vincent, A., Iber, J., Campagnoli, R., Mandelbaum, M., De, L., Yang, S. J., Nix, A., and Kew, O. M. 2009. Rapid group-, serotype-, and vaccine strain-specific identification of poliovirus isolates by real-time reverse transcription-PCR using degenerate primers and probes containing deoxyinosine residues. *J. Clin. Microbiol.* 47, 1939–1941.

King, R. L., Lorch, S. A., Cohen, D. M., Hodinka, R. L., Cohn, K. A., and Shah, S. S. 2007. Routine cerebrospinal fluid enterovirus polymerase chain reaction testing reduces hospitalization and antibiotic use for infants 90 days of age or younger. *Pediatrics.* 120, 489–496.

Knepp, J. H., Geahr, M. A., Forman, M. S., and Valsamakis, A. 2003. Comparison of automated and manual nucleic acid extraction methods for detection of enterovirus RNA. *J. Clin. Microbiol.* 41, 3532–3536.

Kreeftenberg, H., van der Velden, T., Kersten, G., van der Heuvel, N., and de Bruijn, M. 2006. Technology transfer of Sabin-IPV to new developing country markets. *Biologicals.* 34, 155–158.

Kühl, U., Pauschinger, M., Seeberg, B., Lassner, D., Noutsias, M., Poller, W., and Schultheiss, H. P. 2005. Viral persistence in the myocardium is associated with progressive cardiac dysfunction. *Circulation.* 112, 1965–1970.

Landsteiner, K., and Popper, E. 1908. Mikroscopische Preparate von einen menschlichen und zwei Affenmeuckenmarken. *Wien. Klin. Wscgr.* 21, 1830.

Larkin, M. A., Blackshields, G., Brown, N. P., Chenna, R., McGettigan, P. A., McWilliam, H., Valentin, F., Wallace, I. M., Wilm, A., Lopez, R., Thompson, J. D., Gibson, T. J., and Higgins, D. G. 2007. Clustal W and Clustal X version 2.0. *Bioinformatics.* 23, 2947–2948.

Lee, B. E., and Davies, H. D. 2007. Aseptic meningitis. *Curr. Opin. Infect. Dis.* 20, 272–277.

Leveque, N., and Laurent, A. 2008. A novel mode of transmission for human enterovirus infection is swimming in contaminated seawater: implications in public health and epidemiological surveillance. *Clin. Infect. Dis.* 47, 624–626.

Leveque, N., Huguet, P., Norder, H., and Chomel, J. J. 2010. Enteroviruses responsible for acute hemorrhagic conjunctivitis. *Med. Mal. Infect.* 40, 212–218.

Leveque, N., Jacques, J., Renois, F., Antona, D., Abely, M., Chomel, J. J., and Andreoletti, L. 2010. Phylogenetic analysis of Echovirus 30 isolated during the 2005 outbreak in France reveals existence of multiple lineages and suggests frequent recombination events. *J. Clin. Virol.* 48, 137–141.

Lin, K. H., and Lim, Y. W. 2005. Post-poliomyelitis syndrome: case report and review of the literature. *Ann. Acad. Med. Singapore.* 34, 447–449.

Lin, T. L., Li, Y. S., Huang, C. W., Hsu, C. C., Wu, H. S., Tseng, T. C., and Yang, C. F. 2008. Rapid and highly sensitive coxsackievirus A indirect immunofluorescence assay typing kit for enterovirus serotyping. *J. Clin. Microbiol.* 46, 785–788.

Lin, T. Y., Kao, H. T., Hsieh, S. H., Huang, Y. C., Chiu, C. H., Chou, Y. H., Yang, P. H., Lin, R. I., Tsao, K. C., Hsu, K. H., and Chang, L. Y. 2003. Neonatal enterovirus infections: emphasis on risk factors of severe and fatal infections. *Pediatr. Infect. Dis. J.* 22, 889–894.

Liu, Q., Bai, Y., Ge, Q., Zhou, S., Wen, T., and Lu, Z. 2007. Microarray-in-a-tube for detection of multiple viruses. *Clin. Chem.* 53, 188–194.

Logan, S. A., and MacMahon, E. 2008. Viral meningitis. *BMJ.* 336, 36–40.

Lu, J. C., Koay, K. W., Ramers, C. B., and Milazzo, A. S. 2005. Neonate with coxsackie B1 infection, cardiomyopathy and arrhythmias. *J. Natl. Med. Assoc.* 97, 1028–1030.

Lukashev, A. N., Lashkevich, V. A., Ivanova, O. E., Koroleva, G. A., Hinkkanen, A. E., and Ilonen, J. 2003. Recombination in circulating enteroviruses. *J. Virol.* 77, 1423–1431.

Melnick, J. L. 1996. Current status of poliovirus infections. *Clin. Microbiol. Rev.* 9, 293–300.

Melnick, J. L., Rennick, V., Hampil, B., Schmidt, N. J., and Ho, H. H. 1973. Lyophilized combination pools of enterovirus equine antisera: preparation and test procedures for the identification of field strains of 42 enteroviruses. *Bull. World. Health. Organ.* 48, 263–268.

Melnick, J. L., Schmidt, N. J.,Hampil, B., and Ho, H. H. 1977. Lyophilized combination pools of enterovirus equine antisera: preparation and test procedures for the identification of field strains of 19 group A coxsackievirus serotypes. *Intervirology.* 8, 172–181.

Modlin, J. F. 2005. Poliovirus. In: Mandell, G. L., Bennett, J. E., and Dolin, R. (Eds). *Mandell, Douglas, and Bennett's Principles and Practice of Infectious Diseases*, 6th ed, Elsevier, Philadelphia, PA, pp. 2141–2148.

Mohammed, A. J., AlAwaidy, S., Bawikar, S., Kurup, P. J., Elamir, E., Shaban, M. M., Sharif, S. M., van der Avoort, H. G., Pallansch, M. A., Malankar, P., Burton, A., Sreevatsava, M., and Sutter, R. W. 2010. Fractional doses of inactivated poliovirus vaccine in Oman. *N. Engl. J. Med.* 362, 2351–2359.

Muckelbauer, J. K., Kremer, M., Minor, I., Diana, G., Dutko, F. J., Groarke, J., Pevear, D. C., and Rossmann, M. G. 1995. The structure of coxsackievirus B3 at 3.5 a resolution. *Structure.* 3, 653–667.

Mueller, S., Wimmer, E., and Cello, J. 2005. Poliovirus and poliomyelitis: a tale of guts, brains, and an accidental event. *Virus Res.* 111, 175–193.

Nathanson, N., and Kew, O. M. 2010. From emergence to eradication: the epidemiology of poliomyelitis deconstructed. *Am. J. Epidemiol.* 172, 1213–1229.

Nkowane, B. M., Wassilak, S. G., Orenstein, W. A., Bart, K. J., Schonberger, L. B., Hinman, A. R., and Kew, O. M. 1987. Vaccine-associated paralytic poliomyelitis: United States, 1973 through 1984. *JAMA.* 257, 1335–1340.

Oberste, M. S., Maher, K., and Pallansch, M. A. 2002. Molecular phylogeny and classification of the simian picornaviruses. *J. Virol.* 76, 1244–1251.

Oberste, M. S., Maher, K., Kilpatrick, D. R., Flemister, M. R, Brown, B. A., and Pallansch, M. A. 1999.Typing of human enteroviruses by partial sequencing of VP1. *J. Clin. Microbiol.* 37, 1288–1293.

Oberste, M. S., Maher, K., Schnurr, D., Flemister, M. R., Lovchik, J. C., Peters, H., Sessions, W., Kirk, C., Chatterjee, N., Fuller, S., Hanauer, J. M., and Pallansch, M. A. 2004. Enterovirus 68 is associated with respiratory illness and shares biological features with both the enteroviruses and the rhinoviruses. *J. Gen. Virol.* 85, 2577–2584.

Ohka, S., Yang, W. X., Terada, E., Iwasaki, K., and Nomoto, A. 1998. Retrograde transport of intact poliovirus through the axon via the fast transport system. *Virology.* 250, 67–75.

Ooi, M. H.,Wong, S. C., Lewthwaite, P., Cardosa, M. J., and Solomon, T. 2010. Clinical features, diagnosis, and management of enterovirus 71. *Lancet Neurol.* 9, 1097–1105.

Pallansch, M. A., and Ross, R. P. 2001. Enteroviruses: polioviruses, coxsackieviruses, echoviruses, and newer enteroviruses. In: Knipe, D. M., Howley, P. M., and Griffin, D. E., (Eds.). *Fields Virology*, 4th ed. Lippincott, Williams & Wilkins, Philadelphia, pp. 723–775.

Pérez-Vélez, C. M., Anderson, M. S., Robinson, C. C., McFarland, E. J., Nix, W. A., Pallansch, M. A., Oberste, M. S., and Glodé, M. P. 2007. Outbreak of neurologic enterovirus type 71 disease: a diagnostic challenge. *Clin. Infect. Dis.* 45, 950–957.

Pipkin, P. A., Wood, D. J., Racaniello, V. R., and Minor, P. D. 1993. Characterisation of L cells expressing the human poliovirus receptor for the specific detection of polioviruses *in vitro. J. Virol. Methods*. 41, 333–340.

Podin, Y., Gias, E. L., Ong, F., Leong, Y. W., Yee, S. F., Yusof, M. A., Perera, D., Teo, B., Wee, T. Y., Yao, S. C., Yao, S. K., Kiyu, A., Arif, M. T., and Cardosa, M. J. 2006. Sentinel surveillance for human enterovirus 71 in Sarawak, Malaysia: lessons from the first 7 years. *BMC Public Health*. 6, 180.

Prevots, D. R., Sutter, R. W., Strebel, P. M., Weibel, R. E., and Cochi, S. L. 1994. Completeness of reporting for paralytic poliomyelitis, United States, 1980 through 1991. Implications for estimating the risk of vaccine associated disease. *Arch. Pediatr. Adolesc. Med.* 148, 479–485.

Putnam, J. J., and Taylor, E. W. 1893. Is acute poliomyelitis unusually prevalent this season? *Boston Med. Surg. J.* 129, 502.

Racaniello, V. R. 2006. Picornaviridae: the viruses and their replication, In: Knipe, D. M., Howley, P. M., Griffin, D. E., Lamb, R. A., Martin, M. A., Roizman, B., and Straus, S. E. (Eds.). *Fields Virology*, 5th ed., Lippincott, Williams & Wilkins, Philadelphia, pp. 795–838.

Ren, R., and Racaniello, V. R. 1992. Poliovirus spreads from muscle to the central nervous system by neural pathways. *J. Infect. Dis.* 166, 747–752.

Resik, S., Tejeda, A., Lago, P. M., Diaz, M., Carmenates, A., Sarmiento, L., Alemañi, N., Galindo, B., Burton, A., Friede, M., Landaverde, M., and Sutter, R. W. 2010. Randomized controlled clinical trial of fractional doses of inactivated poliovirus vaccine administered intradermally by needle-free device in Cuba. *J. Infect. Dis.* 201, 1344–1352.

Richer, M. J., and Horwitz, M. S. 2009. The innate immune response: an important partner in shaping Coxsackievirus-mediated autoimmunity. *J. Innate. Immun.* 1, 421–434.

Rossmann, M. G., He, Y., and Kuhn, R. J. 2002. Picornavirus-receptor interactions. *Trends Microbiol.* 10, 324–31.

Rotbart, H. A. 1990. Enzymatic RNA amplification of the enteroviruses. *J. Clin. Microbiol.* 28, 438–442.

Rotbart, H. A., Brennan, P. J., Fife, K. H., Romero, J. R., Griffin, J. A., McKinlay, M. A., and Hayden, F. G. 1998. Enterovirus meningitis in adults. *Clin. Infect. Dis.* 27, 896–898.

Rotbart, H. A., Webster, A. D., and Pleconaril Treatment Registry Group, 2001. Treatment of potentially life-threatening enterovirus infections with pleconaril. *Clin. Infect. Dis.* 32, 228–235.

Sabin, A. B. 1985. Oral poliovirus vaccine: history of its development and use and current challenge to eliminate poliomyelitis from the world. *J. Infect. Dis.* 151, 420–436.

Salk, J. E. 1955. Consideration in the preparation and use of poliomyelitis virus vaccine. *J. Am. Med. Assoc.* 158, 1239–1248.

Sambrook, J., Fritsch, E. F., and Maniatis, T. 1989. *Molecular Cloning: A Laboratory Manual*, 2nd ed., vol 1. CSHL Press, Cold Spring Harbor, NY.

Sane, F., Sauter, P., Fronval, S., Goffard, A., Dewilde, A., and Hober, D. 2008. Fruit of the emergence of an enterovirus: acute haemorrhagic conjunctivitis. *Ann. Biol. Clin.* 66, 485–492.

Schmidt, N., Lennette, E., and Ho, H. 1974. An apparently new enterovirus isolated from patients with disease of the central nervous system. *J. Infect. Dis.* 129, 304–309.

Shafren, D. R., Dorahy, D. J., Ingham, R. A., Burns, G. F., and Barry, R. D. 1997. Coxsackievirus A21 binds to decay-accelerating factor but requires intercellular adhesion molecule 1 for cell entry. *J. Virol.* 71, 4736–4743.

Simizu, B., Abe, S., Yamamoto, H., Tano, Y., Ota, Y., Miyazawa, M., Horie, H., Satoh, K., and Wakabayashi, K. 2006. Development of inactivated poliovirus vaccine derived from Sabin strains. *Biologicals.* 34, 151–154.

Simmons, Z. 2012. Polio and infectious diseases of the anterior horn. In: *UpToDate 20.3*, Waltham, MA, U S A.

Sofer, D., Weil, M., Hindiyeh, M., Ram, D., Shulman, L. M., and Mendelson, E. 2011. Human Nonpolio Enteroviruses. In: Liu, D. (Ed.). *Molecular Detection of Human Viral Pathogens*, CRC Press, Taylor and Francis Group, Boca Raton, FL, USA, pp. 37–51.

Somekh, E., Cesar, K., Handsher, R., Hanukoglu, A., Dalal, I., Ballin, A., and Shohat, T. 2003. An outbreak of echovirus 13 meningitis in central Israel. *Epidemiol. Infect.* 130, 257–262.

Steiner, I., Budka, H., Chaudhuri, A., Koskiniemi, M., Sainio, K., Salonen, O., and Kennedy, P. G. 2010. Viral meningoencephalitis: a review of diagnostic methods and guidelines for management. *Eur. J. Neurol.* 17, e999–e57.

Thibaut, H. J., Leyssen, P., Puerstinger, G., Muigg, A., Neyts, J., and De Palma, A. M. 2011. Towards the design of combination therapy for the treatment of enterovirus infections. *Antiviral Res.* 90, 213–217.

Thoelen, I., Lemey, P., Van der Donck, I., Beuselink, K., Lindberg, A. M., and Van Ranst, M. 2003. Molecular typing and epidemiology of enteroviruses identified from an outbreak of aseptic meningitis in Belgium during the summer of 2000. *J. Med. Virol.* 70, 420–429.

Thorley, J. A., McKeating, J. A., and Rappoport, J. Z. 2010. Mechanisms of viral entry: sneaking in the front door. *Protoplasma.* 244, 15–24.

Thys, B., De Palma, A. M., Neyts, J., Andries, K., Vrijsen, R., and Rombaut, B. 2008. R75761, a lead compound for the development of antiviral drugs in late stage poliomyelitis eradication strategies and beyond. *Antiviral Res.* 78, 278–281.

Tormey, V. J., Buscombe, J. R., Johnson, M. A., Thomson, A. P., and Webster, A. D. 2003. SPECT scans for monitoring response to pleconaril therapy in chronic enteroviral meningoencephalitis. *J. Infect.* 46, 138–140.

Tu, P. V., Thao, N. T., Perera, D., Huu, T. K., Tien, N. T., Thuong, T. C., How, O. M., Cardosa, M. J., and McMinn, P. C. 2007. Epidemiologic and virologic investigation of hand, foot, and mouth disease, southern Vietnam, 2005. *Emerg. Infect. Dis.* 13, 1733–1741.

Utzig, N., Friedrich, B., Burtzlaff, C., and Lauffer, H. 2003. Polio-like myelitis due to Coxsackie-Virus B3: course under treatment with pleconaril. *Klin. Pediatr.* 215, 286–287.

van der Avoort, H. G., Hull, B. P., Hovi, T., Pallansch, M. A., Kew, O. M., Crainic, R., Wood, D. J., Mulders, M. N., and van Loon, A. M. 1995. Comparative study of five methods for intratypic differentiation of polioviruses. *J. Clin. Microbiol.* 33, 2562–2566.

Wang, J. R., Tsai, H. P., Huang, S. W., Kuo, P. H., Kiang, D., and Liu, C. C. 2002. Laboratory diagnosis and genetic analysis of an echovirus 30-associated outbreak of aseptic meningitis in Taiwan in 2001. *J. Clin. Microbiol.* 40, 4439–4444.

Ward, C. D., Stokes, M. A., and Flanegan, J. B. 1988. Direct measurement of the poliovirus RNA polymerase error frequency *in vitro. J. Virol.* 62, 558–562.

Wong, K. T., Munisamy, B., Ong, K. C., Kojima, H., Noriyo, N., Chua, K. B., Ong, B. B., and Nagashima, K. 2008. The distribution of inflammation and virus in human enterovirus 71 encephalomyelitis suggests possible viral spread by neural pathways. *J. Neuropathol. Exp. Neurol.* 67, 162–169.

World Health Organization (WHO), Regional Office for Europe, European Centre for Disease Prevention and Control, and World Health Organization Country Office Tajikistan. 2010. Outbreak of poliomyelitis in Tajikistan in 2010: risk of importation and impact on polio surveillance in Europe? *Euro Surveill.* 29, 15–17.

World Health Organization (WHO). 1997/2004. Polio laboratory manual WHO/IVB/04.10, WHO, Geneva, Switzerland.

World Health Organization (WHO). 2007. Summary of discussions and recommendations of the 13th informal consultation of the WHO Global Polio Laboratory Network. *Wkly. Epidemiol. Rec.* 82, 297.

World Health Organization (WHO). 2009. Circulating Vaccine Derived Poliovirus (cVDPV) 2000–2009. WHO/HQ. www.polioeradication.org/content/general/cvdpv_count.pdf.

World Health Organization (WHO). 2009. Polio Research Committee outcomes. PolioPipeline 3, 1.

World Health Organization (WHO). 2010. Polio vaccines and polio immunization in the pre-eradication era: WHO position paper. *Wkly. Epidemiol. Rec.* 85, 213–228.

World Health Organization (WHO). 2011. An update of ongoing research in the Global Polio Eradication Initiative. *PolioPipeline* 8.

Xiong, D., Yajima, T., Lim, B. K., Stenbit, A., Dublin, A., Dalton, N. D., Summers-Torres, D., Molkentin, J. D., Duplain, H., Wessely, R., Chen, J., and Knowlton, K. U. 2007. Inducible cardiac-restricted expression of enteroviral protease 2A is sufficient to induce dilated cardiomyopathy. *Circulation.* 115, 94–102.

Yamashita, K., Miyamura, K., Yamadera, S., Kato, N., Akatsuka, M., Hashido, M., Inouye, S., and Yamazaki, S. 1994. Epidemics of aseptic meningitis due to ECHO virus 30 in Japan. *Jpn. J. Med. Sci. Biol.* 47, 221–239.

Yang, C. F., De, L., Holloway, B. P., Pallansch, M. A., and Kew, O. M. 1991. Detection and identification of vaccine-related polioviruses by the polymerase chain reaction. *Virus. Res.* 20, 159–179.

Yeung, W. C., Rawlinson, W. D., and Craig, M. E. 2011. Enterovirus infection and type 1 diabetes mellitus:systematic review and meta-analysis of observational molecular studies. *BMJ.* 342, d35.

Zhang, Y., Tan, X. J., Wang, H. Y., Yan, D. M., Zhu, S. L., Wang, D. Y., Ji, F., Wang, X. J., Gao, Y. J., Chen, L., An, H. Q., Li, D. X., Wang, S. W., Xu, A. Q., Wang, Z. J., and Xu, W. B. 2009. An outbreak of hand, foot, and mouth disease associated with subgenotype C4 of human enterovirus 71 in Shandong. *China. J. Clin. Virol.* 44, 262–267.

7 Neurovirulence of the West Nile Virus

Kim-Long Yeo and Mah-Lee Ng

CONTENTS

7.1 INTRODUCTION

The West Nile virus (WNV) is an arbovirus that can cause significant and devastating neurological-related disease in infected persons. It was introduced into the Western hemisphere in 1999 and has remained endemic ever since. Although our understanding of the virus has expanded greatly in the past decade, treatment and prevention of WNV infection are still in progress. This chapter provides an introduction to the biology of the virus, its history and transmission, clinical symptoms and pathology of infection, and recent developments in treatment strategies.

7.1.1 MOLECULAR BIOLOGY OF WEST NILE VIRUS

The West Nile virus is an arthropod-borne virus that is closely related to approximately 70 other members of the family Flaviviridae. Specifically, it belongs to the

Japanese encephalitis serocomplex of the genus Flavivirus (Brinton 2002). The virus' small positive-sense, single-stranded genome of about 10.8 kilobases is contained within a capsid made of the viral capsid (C) protein. A 4-nm-thick host-derived lipid membrane further surrounds the capsid. Inserted into this lipid membrane are 180 copies of the virus-encoded envelope (E) and premembrane (prM) glycoproteins. Homodimers of the E protein lie in a herringbone-like arrangement that covers the lipid bilayer, whereas the prM protein forms homotrimers that cap the external tip of the E protein. Mature WNV particles have a distinctly smooth spikeless outer surface, are about 50 nm in diameter, and have isocahedral symmetry (Mukhopadhyay et al. 2003).

The infectious genome serves as a messenger RNA (mRNA) with a single long open reading frame (ORF) that encodes for a 3443-amino acid polyprotein. Both host and viral proteases cleave this polyprotein to form the C, prM, E, and 7 other nonstructural (NS) proteins (Brinton 2002). The NS proteins are named in the order that they are found in the genome NS1, NS2a, NS2b, NS3, NS4a, NS4b, and NS5. Whereas NS1 and N4 possess virus-antihost immunological-related functions, NS2, together with NS3, act as viral protease to cleave the viral polyprotein into its individual functional units. The largest NS protein, NS5, is the virus' RNA-dependent RNA polymerase. It synthesizes new copies of the viral genome from a negative-stranded viral RNA in an asymmetrical manner (Brinton 2002).

7.2 HISTORY

The virus was first isolated from a febrile female patient in the West Nile region of Uganda in 1937 (Smithburn et al. 1940), and is associated with periodic epidemics of febrile illness throughout Africa, Southwest Asia, and Eastern Europe (Murgue et al. 2002). Historically, WNV was found to cycle between *Culicine* mosquitoes and native birds. Birds served as the natural amplifying host, and humans were accidental secondary hosts. Symptoms of infection included dengue-like illness such as fever, malaise, lymphadenopathy, and rash. Most infections were self-limiting and resolved without much sequelae (Goldblum et al. 1954). In the 1990s however, fatal cases of encephalitis became a significant feature of WNV epidemics in Romania, Russia, and Israel. Approximately 60% of hospitalized patients had West Nile neuroinvasive disease (WNND) with a 4% to 7% mortality rate (Klein et al. 2005).

In 1999, WNV appeared for the first time in North America. This was marked by the simultaneous occurrence of an unusual number of deaths of exotic birds and crows in the New York City Metropolitan Area (Nash et al. 2001). Introduction of the virus has been largely attributed to infected migratory birds (Rappole et al. 2000) or possibly illegally imported exotic birds. A human source was ruled out since humans are dead-end hosts (Brinton 2002); this is with the exception of blood transfusion, an organ transplantation, or transplacental infection. There is also a small possibility that the virus was introduced via infected mosquitoes unintentionally carried by airplanes or other carriers (Davis et al. 2006). The notion that migratory birds were the origin of the virus in New York was supported by the fact that comparison of the nucleotide sequence of the envelope gene of the New York City virus (WNV-NY99) showed more than 99% homology in amino acid sequence to a virus isolated from a goose in Israel in 1998 (Lanciotti et al. 1999; Brinton 2002). This also suggested that WNV-NY99 originated from the Middle East or Eastern Europe, where a similar virus is circulating.

More recent genome sequencing of the E protein of the virus has revealed 2 distinct lineages of the virus (Lanciotti et al. 1999; Brinton 2002). Lineage 1 includes pathogenic strains from North America, Europe, Australia, Africa, and Asia, whereas lineage 2 includes strains from Africa and Madagascar. Lineage 1 viruses are further subdivided into four clades. In general, lineage 1 viruses are widespread and have caused recent epidemics of human encephalitis throughout western Africa, the Middle East, Eastern Europe, and more recently, North America. All North American isolates have so far been classified as lineage 1, clade B, and are closely related to strains from Israel (Lanciotti et al. 1999). Lineage 2 viruses, on the other hand, are associated with sporadic and endemic human cases of a less severe febrile illness without involvement of the central nervous system.

The initial outbreak in New York resulted in 62 cases of encephalitis in humans. Seven deaths occurred as a result of encephalitis (Nash et al. 2001). Over the past decade, WNV has shown to have an increased tendency to cause WNND. From 1999 to 2005, 19,506 cases of human WNV diseases were reported in the US. This included 8362 cases that were characterized as WNND, 782 of which resulted in death (Hayes et al. 2005; CDC). The geographic range and burden of disease has also greatly expanded to the 48 adjoining states of the US, as well as seven Canadian provinces, Mexico, the Carribean islands, and Colombia (Granwehr et al. 2004; Tyler 2004; Davis et al. 2005; Hayes et al. 2005; Public Health Agency of Canada). As such, it has become the most common cause of epidemic meningoencephalitis in the region.

7.3   TRANSMISSION

West Nile virus is maintained in nature by cycling between more than 200 species of birds and many species of mosquitoes (van der Meulen et al. 2005). The virus enters the mosquito via infected blood, penetrates the gut, and replicates in tissues including the nervous system and salivary glands. Infection of the mosquito is noncytopathic and persists for the life of the insect (Girard et al. 2005). Infected mosquitoes then infect susceptible birds by injecting about 10^4 plaque-forming units (PFU) of virus while feeding (Vanlandingham et al. 2004). Birds are the major amplifying host for WNV and can have viremia lasting for more than 100 days (Komar et al. 2003). This allows for repeated cycles of mosquito infection. The highest titer viremia of more than 10^{10} PFU has been reported (Komar et al. 2003). Viremia of this magnitude leads to subsequent transmission to more than 80% of biting mosquitoes (Turell et al. 2000). This is since the capacity to transmit infection increases dramatically as the level of viremia increases in the host.

In the United States, transmission of WNV to humans often results from an infected mosquito of the *Culex* species feeding on a human host (Campbell et al. 2002; Turell et al. 2002). This results in a dead end infection. Other modes of WNV transmission in humans have also been reported. Twenty-three blood transfusion recipients were infected with WNV in 2002 after given blood products obtained from viremic donors (Pealer et al. 2003; Centers for Disease Control and Prevention [CDC] 2004). This led to widespread screening of blood products using WNV-specific nucleic acid amplification tests. However, very low levels of viremia escape detection and contribute to transfusion-associated transmission. Human to human transmission has also occurred through transplantation of an organ harvested from a viremic donor (Iwamoto et al. 2003). Lastly, transplacental infection was confirmed in 2002 when an infant was found to have WNV-specific IgM antibody in the blood, and WNV nucleic acid was found in placental and umbilical cord tissue. The expecting mother had developed WNND in her 27th week of pregnancy, and gave birth to an infant with chorioretinitis and cystic cerebral lesion (CDC 2002; Alpert et al. 2003). Surveillance for WNV in pregnant women has thus been stepped up in light of these findings.

However, during the typical mode of infection, the biting mosquito injects saliva-containing WNV intradermally. The virus initially replicates in Langerhans dendritic cells (DC) (Chambers and Diamond 2003) before the infected DC migrates to draining lymph nodes (LNs). Viral replication then occurs within the lymphoid tissue (Johnston et al. 2000). Viremia peaks between 2 to 4 days after infection, and prior to illness onset in healthy persons (Southam and Moore 1952, 1954; Hayes and O'Leary 2004). Persistence of virus in immunocompromised persons may be more prolonged (Southam and Moore 1952; Iwamoto et al. 2003). The virus can be detected in blood within 1 to 2 days of a mosquito bite, and termination of viremia coincides with production of neutralizing IgM antibodies. The antibody response is the primary method by which WNV is cleared from the infected person. Interestingly, onset of illness coincides with IgM antibody production and a reduction in viremia. Delayed onset of illness in infected persons may thus be indicative that the immunological response of the individual plays a more important role in development of symptoms.

7.4   CLINICAL PRESENTATIONS

It has been estimated that more than 80% of infected persons remain asymptomatic, and 80%–90% of symptomatic patients develop a self-limiting febrile illness known as West Nile fever (WNF). Remaining persons can develop severe WNND-like aseptic meningitis (WNM), encephalitis (WNE), or an acute poliomyelitis-like syndrome (WNP) (Campbell et al. 2002). However, it should be noted that clinical classification of West Nile infection is often not clear-cut, as it can be hard to clinically distinguish among WNF, WNM, WNE, and WNP. For instance, a patient presenting fever, headache, and "neck stiffness" may not be subjected to lumbar puncture to demonstrate pleocytosis. As a result, a diagnosis of WNM may not be reported. Regardless, description of clinical syndrome in WNV-infected persons is reliable based on clinical grounds.

7.4.1   WEST NILE FEVER

The predominant clinical syndrome seen in most infected persons is WNF. Although WNF can develop in all ages, its incidence decreases with age (Brown 2004). After an incubation of about 2–14 days, the infected person can experience a sudden onset of fever, headache, fatigue, myalgia, and development of a transient maculopapular rash (Campbell et al. 2002; Anderson et al. 2004; Watson et al. 2004; Del Giudice et al. 2005; Ferguson et al. 2005; Gorsche and Tilley 2005). Rash development usually begins about 5 days after onset of illness and can last for about a week (Watson et al. 2004). Rash is more frequently observed in younger persons than in older persons (Ferguson et al. 2005). Although most patients experience complete and unremarkable recovery from WNF, some may experience fatigue lasting up to 36 days (Watson et al. 2004). Profound fatigue in particular can interfere with work or school activities (Gottfried et al. 2005).

7.4.2 WEST NILE NEUROINVASIVE DISEASE

In contrast to WNF, the incidence of WNND increases with age. It is significantly higher in the elderly and immunocompromised patients (Pepperell et al. 2003; O'Leary et al. 2004; Hayes and Gubler 2006). Although WNND is rarely reported in children or individuals younger than 30 years, 317 cases of WNV infection in children were categorized as WNND from 2002 to 2004 (Yim et al. 2004). However, this is not indicative of an increased incidence of WNND in younger individuals.

7.4.3 WEST NILE MENINGITIS

Development of WNM is similar to other viral meningitides. There is a sudden onset of fever, headache, and meningeal signs such as nuchal rigidity, photophobia, and phonophobia. Examination of the cerebral spinal fluid (CSF) often presents modest pleocytosis of less than 500/mm^3. Although pleocytosis is frequently lymphocytic in nature, CSF obtained during early onset of illness is predominantly neutrophilic (Crichlow et al. 2004; Sejvar et al. 2005). Other neurological features are usually absent and WNM is often associated with a good prognosis. However, some patients can experience persistent headache, fatigue, and myalgia (Sejvar et al. 2003a).

7.4.4 WEST NILE ENCEPHALITIS

West Nile encephalitis is more common in the elderly over the age of 55 (Nash et al. 2001; Weiss et al. 2001; O'Leary et al. 2004; Bode et al. 2006). During the 1999 outbreak, 88% of those affected were older than 50 years old, and 51% were older than 70 years of age (Nash et al. 2001). Immunocompromised individuals, for instance, organ transplant recipients taking immunosuppresive drugs, may be at high risk for WNE as well (Agamanolis et al. 2003; Armali et al. 2003; Ravindra et al. 2004).

The severity of WNE can range from a mild, self-limited confusional state to that of severe encephalopathy, coma, and death. Almost 100% of patients with WNE were reported to have fever, 42%–85% with fatigue, 47%–90% with headache, and 46%–74% with altered mental status (Davis et al. 2006). Patients also often develop a coarse postural tremor in the upper extremities during kinetic or rest (Sejvar et al. 2003a; Burton et al. 2004). Myoclonus was reported to occur in one-third of cases in a series and can be indicative of WNND since it is distinctly unusual in nonflaviviral encephalitis (Sejvar et al. 2003a). Parkinsonian-like features such as rigidity, bradykinesia, and postural instability have also been reported in up to two-thirds of WNND cases (Sejvar et al. 2003a).

Abnormalities noted above usually resolve over time, but persistence of tremor and parkinsonism have been observed in some patients recovering from severe encephalitis. More than 65% of encephalitic patients who underwent neuropsychological testing after being admitted to an acute rehabilitation center still present persisting cognitive deficits at discharge (Arciniegas and Anderson 2004). These included language/social communication deficits, memory impairment, executive dysfunction, and defects in attention and concentration. Approximately 25% of the patients had slowed processing speed. Emotional dysregulation such as depression, anxiety and irritability, and psychomotor abnormalities such as apathy and agitation, were found in more than 75% of these patients (Arciniegas and Anderson 2004).

Besides cognitive impairment, patients with WNE have been reported to develop a wide range of additional clinical signs and symptoms. These reflect the ability of WNV to affect areas as diverse as the cerebral cortex, basal ganglia, brainstem, and spinal cord. Patients with WNE who develop visual problems have also been increasingly recognized. They often describe blurry vision, trouble seeing, and photophobia (Anninger and Lubow 2004; Khairallah et al. 2004).

Fatality following an episode of WNE has ranged between 10% and 20% among patients with severe WNE. Although mortality is higher among the elderly and immunocompromised, independent risk factors for fatal outcome remain to be known (Kleinschmidt-DeMasters et al. 2004). Evidently, outcome after WNE is heterogeneous.

7.4.5 WEST NILE POLIOMYELITIS

Since WNV can infect neurons in the spinal cord, it can result in true poliomyelitis (Doron et al. 2003; Leis et al. 2003; Sejvar et al. 2003b, 2006). Recent data have suggested that WNP results from viral infection of the lower motor neurons in the anterior horn cells of the spinal cord (Glass et al. 2002; Leis et al. 2002; Jeha et al. 2003; Li et al. 2003; Sejvar et al. 2003b, 2006). Patients who develop WNP are usually younger than those who develop WNE (Sejvar et al. 2003b; Sayao et al. 2004; Sejvar et al. 2006).

Development of WNP can be abrupt and progress rapidly to weakness in one or more limbs, especially the legs (Jeha et al. 2003; Leis et al. 2003; Sejvar et al. 2003a,b, 2006). Weakness may develop concomitantly with signs of meningitis or encephalitis or several days after their onset (Leis et al. 2003; Sejvar et al. 2003a). It should be noted that clinical features of WNP are characteristic and dramatic in comparison to general muscle weakness experienced by many persons with WNV infection. Thus, WNP should be easily differentiated from general extreme fatigue.

Weakness tends to be asymmetric and may often result in monoplegia. Some patients with severe involvement may develop a more symmetric dense quadriplegia (Jeha et al. 2003; Leis et al. 2003; Sejvar et al. 2003a,b, 2006). Frequently, bilateral central facial weakness may also be seen (Li et al. 2003; Sejvar et al. 2006). Although numbness or sensory loss is usually absent, some patients experience intense pain in the affected limbs prior to or during the onset of weakness. The limb pain may become persistent in some affected patients (Sejvar et al. 2006).

Respiratory muscle innervation, leading to diaphragmatic and intercostal muscle paralysis, may also lead to respiratory failure in some persons (Fan et al. 2004; Sejvar et al. 2006). Affected persons would require emergent endotracheal intubation (Fan et al. 2004). Development of respiratory failure may be due to involvement of the lower brain stem, including the motor nuclei of the vagus and glossopharyngeal nerves (Agamanolis et al. 2003; Doron et al. 2003). Respiratory involvement in WNP is often associated with high morbidity and mortality. For survivors, prolonged ventilatory support may be required (Sejvar et al. 2006).

In addition to WNP, other forms of acute flaccid paralysis similar to Guillain-Barré syndrome have also been associated with WNV infection (Ahmed et al. 2000; Park et al. 2003). However, these appear to be less common than WNP and can be differentiated based on clinical and electrophysiological features.

Recovery of limb strength from WNP is variable. Generally, less profound initial weakness is associated with more rapid and complete strength recovery (Cao et al. 2005; Sejvar et al. 2006). In the short term, however, affected patients experience persistent weakness and associated functional disability. Prolonged physical and occupational therapy may be required to ensure complete recovery (Sejvar et al. 2006).

7.5 DIAGNOSIS

As with most viral infections, isolation of WNV from biological specimens such as blood, serum, CSF, or histology tissues is the gold standard for diagnosis of infection. However, this is rarely done due to the need for proper bio-safety containment facilities and bio-safety concerns. In addition, the virus is usually absent at the onset of illness (Lanciotti et al. 2000). Although nucleic acid based platforms are available for the detection of WNV nucleic acid in clinical samples, the technique has limited usefulness due to limited sensitivity and the absence of virus during onset of illness (Lanciotti et al. 2000). Thus, diagnosis is often done by demonstrating the presence of WNV-specific IgM antibodies in CSF or paired serum samples. Detection of WNV-specific IgM in the CSF of a patient, together with clinically compatible illness as mentioned above, is considered confirmatory.

However, confirmation of an acute infection requires demonstration of a four-fold increase in antibody titers using functional assays such as neutralization and hemagglutination inhibition. This is since WNV-specific IgM antibodies can persist in the serum for over a year (Kapoor et al. 2004). Diagnosis can also be complicated by serologic cross-reactivity between WNV and other closely related flaviviruses. This is especially so in areas where several flaviviruses such as WNV and St. Louis encephalitis coexist (Martin et al. 2002). In light of such complications, the plaque-reduction neutralization assay test is most widely utilized to circumvent the problem.

7.6 RISK FACTORS

Undoubtedly, the most important risk factor for acquiring WNV infection is exposure to infected mosquitoes (Hayes et al. 2005). People older than 50 years, especially

those between 60 and 89 years, have a 20-fold increase for developing WNM
(Petersen et al. 2002; O'Leary et al. 2004; Hayes et al. 2005). Recipients of organ
transplant who are under immunosuppressive therapy have up to a 40-fold increased
risk for developing WNND (DeSalvo et al. 2004; Kumar et al. 2004). Disease development is also often more severe in these patients as compared with immunocompetent individuals (Kleinschmidt-DeMasters et al. 2004). Although both children and
adults are equally susceptible to WNV infection, WNND is less common in children
(Yim et al. 2004).

A genetic determinant of WNV resistance, the 1B isoform of 2′–5′ oligoadenylate
synthetase (OAS) gene, has been found in mice (Mashimo et al. 2002; Perelygin et
al. 2002). The 2′–5′ OAS family of enzymes is activated in the presence of interferon
(IFN) and viral double stranded RNA (dsRNA). Activated 2′–5′ OAS synthesizes
oligoadenylates, which, in turn, bind to and activate RNase L. Activated RNase L
degrades viral RNA (Justesen et al. 2000; Mashimo et al. 2002; Perelygin et al.
2002; Lucas et al. 2003; Kajaste-Rudnitski et al. 2006). Mice resistant to WNV
infection have normal OAS genes while susceptible mouse strains have a truncated
form of the gene (Kajaste-Rudnitski et al. 2006).

However, the role of the OAS system in human susceptibility to WNV is still
unclear. A recent study demonstrated that there were differences in the frequency
distribution of at least one polymorphism in OAS genes in hospitalized patients with
WNV infection, as compared with controls (Yakub et al. 2005). This raised the possibility that the OAS system may play a role in human susceptibility to WNV infection. More work would need to be done to confirm this finding.

7.7 NEUROINVASIVENESS OF WEST NILE VIRUS

The frequency of invasion of the central nervous system (CNS) by WNV
increases with age and in immunocompromised individuals (Iwamoto et al. 2003;
Kleinschmidt-DeMasters et al. 2004; Hayes and Gubler 2006). This suggests that a
delayed production of neutralizing antibodies and a high viral load may be contribu-
tory factors to CNS infection (Iwamoto et al. 2003). However, the exact mechanism
by which WNV enters the CNS in humans remains unknown.

Murine models of infection have suggested that arrival of WNV in the LN triggers a series of events that determine either asymptomatic or neuroinvasive and fatal
infection. While WNV-infected DCs secrete type I IFN to inhibit viral infection in
the peripheral tissues (Scholle and Mason 2005; Liu et al. 2006), and also to aid in
inducing adaptive immune response by presenting viral antigen to B lymphocytes,
they can produce cytokines that affect the permeability of the blood–brain barrier
(BBB). Cytokines such as tumor necrosis factor (TNF)-α (Diamond et al. 2003) and
macrophage migration inhibitory factor (MIF) (Arjona et al. 2007) have been shown
to contribute to WNV neuroinvasion. Similarly, WNV infection of toll-like receptor
(TLR) 3 knockout mice (TLR-3$^{-/-}$) that have decreased levels of circulating inflammatory cytokines, show reduced permeability of their BBB (Wang et al. 2004).

In addition, neurotropic flaviviruses can enter the CNS after direct infection of
endothelial cells in the cerebral mircrovasculature or after viremic dissemination to
the olfactory bulb. The virus then spreads via the neurons to the CNS (Chambers

and Diamond 2003). Although passive transfer of WNV-specific antibodies to mice lacking functional B cells prevented viremia, the procedure could not completely block viral spread to the CNS. This suggested that other nonhematogenous pathways such as retrograde axonal transport from infected peripheral neurons might contribute to CNS entry (Engle and Diamond 2003).

In the CNS, WNV has a propensity to infect neurons. Glial cells in the cerebral cortex, basal ganglia, brain stem, and spinal cord are less often infected (Guarner et al. 2004). *In vitro* experiments show that both cultured neurons and astrocytes support WNV infection with differing kinetics (Cheeran et al. 2005). Although microglia do not support WNV growth, its infection leads to release of pro-inflammatory cytokines such as interleukin 6 (IL-6) and TNF-α. Chemokines such as CXCL-10, CCL-2, and CCL-5 are also produced. Both infected astrocytes and neurons also produce CXCL-10 and CCL-5. Production of these chemokines is essential for recruiting virus-specific T cells to clear the virus from the CNS (Cheeran et al. 2005; Glass et al. 2005).

7.8   VIRAL CLEARANCE

Although clearance of WNV from the brain and other organs is primarily antibody-mediated, WNV-specific CD8[+] cytotoxic T lymphocytes (CTL) have been shown to be crucial to prevent mortality in mice (Wang et al. 2003; Shrestha and Diamond 2004). Mice lacking CTL or the major histocompatibility (MHC) class 1a antigen have a 1000-fold increase in viral titer in the CNS. They also exhibit increased mortality after footpad viral challenge (Wang et al. 2003; Shrestha and Diamond 2004). Production of CXCL-10 by infected neurons facilitates recruitment of CXCR-3 receptor-bearing CTL to the CNS (Klein et al. 2005). Mice that lack CXCR-3 exhibit enhanced viral titer in the CNS and mortality after infection with WNV (Klein et al. 2005). This phenotype was similar in both CD8- (Klein et al. 2005) and CCR-5-deficient mice (Glass et al. 2005) that show defective T-cell recruitment into the CNS. Altogether, this demonstrates the underlying importance of CTL in clearing WNV from the CNS. However, studies have also suggested that CTL may be responsible for pathological outcome by injuring WNV-infected neurons (Wang et al. 2003).

Although the adaptive immune response plays a major role in viral clearance, the innate immune response is crucial in mounting an initial anti-viral response. Infected cells recognize and respond to WNV via endosomal dsRNA sensors such as TLR-3 (Wathelet et al. 1998; Alexopoulou et al. 2001; Iwamura et al. 2001; Wang and Fikrig 2004; Daffis et al. 2008; Wilson et al. 2008) and cytoplasmic dsRNA sensors such as retinoic-acid-inducible gene (RIG) 1 and melanoma-differentiation-associated gene (MDA) 5 (Andrejeva et al. 2004; Yoneyama et al. 2004; Rothenfusser et al. 2005; Yoneyama et al. 2005; Cárdenas et al. 2006; Chang et al. 2006; Fredericksen and Gale 2006). Binding of viral dsRNA to these pathogen-associated recognition receptors (PRR) induces phosphorylation and activation of downstream transcription factors such as interferon regulatory factor (IRF) 3 (Lin et al. 1998; Sato et al. 1998a; Weaver et al. 1998; Yoneyama et al. 1998; Suhara et al. 2000) and IRF-7 (Marié et al. 1998; Sato et al. 1998b). Phosphorylated forms of IRF-3 and IRF-7 homodimerize and heterodimerize to translocate to the nucleus to up-regulate production of type I IFN (Marié et al. 1998; Lin et al. 2000). Binding of secreted type I IFN to surface IFN-α/β receptor (IFN-α/βR) up-regulates production of various IFN-stimulated genes (ISG) such as 2′ 5′ OAS-2 and protein kinase R (PKR) to inhibit virus replication. While 2′ 5′ OAS-2 activates latent RNAses to degrade viral RNA (Justesen et al. 2000; Mashimo et al. 2002; Perelygin et al. 2002; Lucas et al. 2003; Kajaste-Rudnitski et al. 2006), viral dsRNA-induced dimerization and autophosphorylation of PKR activates it to phosphorylate eukaryotic initiation factor 2 (eIF-2α) and inhibit viral protein translation (Samuel et al. 2006).

Besides up-regulating various ISG with antiviral properties, type I IFN produced strongly augments its own production by establishing a positive feedback loop. Binding of type I IFN to IFN-α/βR up-regulates both IRF-1 and IRF-7 to further enhance the production of type I IFN (Marié et al. 1998; Sato et al. 1998b; Lin et al. 2000; Zhou et al. 2000). This establishes a strongly antiviral state to further inhibit viral progression. The importance of type I IFN in limiting viral infection was demonstrated in mice lacking the IFN-α/βR. Besides enhanced viremia and elevated viral titers in both the brain and peripheral organs, these mice had increased mortality after WNV infection (Samuel and Diamond 2005). Treatment of cells with type I IFN has been shown to reduce viral titer and inhibit cytopathicity (Anderson and Rahal 2002; Samuel and Diamond 2005).

7.9   TREATMENT

Despite extensive investigations studying essential antiviral immune responses to WNV in murine models, an efficacious treatment for WNV infection in humans remains elusive. The fact that viremia is usually short and precedes illness further compounds the problem. Thus, therapeutic agent(s) would have to be effective at reducing both intracellular concentration of virus and the inflammatory response to infection. Several agents have been tested recently to assess their potential as a therapeutic. These include antivirals, nucleic acid-based agents, and immunomodulating compounds.

The antiviral agent, ribavarin, is a guanosine analogue that can inhibit WNV replication and cytopathic effect *in vitro* (Jordan et al. 2000; Anderson and Rahal 2002). Although it demonstrated efficacy against WNV infection *in vitro*, its effectiveness *in vivo* was found wanting. Hepatitis C patients under a ribavarin treatment regime developed WNV infection despite presence of the agent (Hrnicek and Mailliard 2004). During an outbreak in Israel in 2000, patients treated with ribavarin fared worse than untreated patients. However, the unfavorable results could be biased by the fact that more seriously ill patients were selected for treatment (Chowers et al. 2001).

A proprietary antisense oligomer construct made by AVI BioPharma, AVI-4020, inhibited viral replication, and was found to be safe in a small pilot phase I human clinical trial (Deas et al. 2005). However, trials have since been terminated due to a limited pool of eligible WNV patients. Other RNA interference (RNAi)-based constructs have been studied *in vitro* but have yet to show efficacy as a therapeutic.

Use of immunomodulating compounds such as IFN have also showed limited efficacy. Although IFN treatment before WNV infection reduced mortality in murine models of infection, no such protection was observed when IFN was given 2 days after infection (Morrey et al. 2004). Efficacy of IFN treatment in humans is unclear due to the absence of data from randomized, placebo-controlled clinical trial. However, the use of an intravenous immunoglobulin containing high titers of anti-WNV IgG (Omr-IgG-am) has shown promising results (Shimoni et al. 2001; Agrawal and Petersen 2003; Diamond et al. 2003). Phase II trials have just been completed in March 2011, and Phase III trials are ongoing.

7.10 PREVENTION

In the absence of an effective therapeutic, prevention remains the key viable option against WNV infection. Effective prevention involves both the individual and the community. Reducing outdoor exposure during peak mosquito biting periods at dusk and dawn can mitigate risk of exposure to infected mosquitoes. Covering exposed skin and using mosquito repellent when outdoors for more than 30 minutes has been found to reduce the risk of WNV infection by 50% during an epidemic (Loeb et al. 2005). Community-wide mosquito eradication programs can also reduce the availability of transmitting vectors.

Currently, vaccines for WNV are being developed. Such vaccines include inactivated subunit vaccines, attenuated WNV vaccines, DNA-based vaccines, and chimeric vaccines. A phase II clinical trial in 200 subjects with a chimeric vaccine containing the WNV prM and E genes using the vaccine strain of Yellow Fever virus as a backbone has just been completed in February 2011. Results from the trial are pending (NIH Clinical Trials).

7.11 CONCLUSION

Arrival of WNV in the Western hemisphere has raised considerable awareness against this emerging pathogen. Despite extensive studies, an effective therapeutic antiviral agent is yet to become available. Recent vaccine developments hold great promise for future use to prevent WNV infection. In the meantime, it would be most prudent for persons most at risk for developing symptomatic WNV infection to take adequate personal precaution.

REFERENCES

Agamanolis, D. P., Leslie, M. J., Caveny, E. A., Guarner, J., Shieh, W.-J., and Zaki, S. R. 2003. Neuropathological findings in West Nile virus encephalitis: a case report. *Ann. Neurol.* 54, 547–551.

Agrawal, A. G., and Petersen, L. R. 2003. Human immunoglobulin as a treatment for West Nile virus infection. *J. Infect. Dis.* 188, 1–4.

Ahmed, S., Libman, R., Wesson, K., Ahmed, F., and Einberg, K. 2000. Guillain-Barré syndrome: an unusual presentation of West Nile virus infection. *Neurology* 55, 144–146.

Alexopoulou, L., Holt, A. C., Medzhitov, R., and Flavell, R. A. 2001. Recognition of double-stranded RNA and activation of NF-kappaB by Toll-like receptor 3. *Nature* 413, 732–738.

Alpert, S. G., Fergerson, J., and Noël, L. P. 2003. Intrauterine West Nile virus: ocular and systemic findings. *Am. J. Ophthalmol.* 136, 733–735.

Anderson, J. F., and Rahal, J. J. 2002. Efficacy of interferon alpha-2b and ribavirin against West Nile virus *in vitro. Emerg. Infect. Dis.* 8, 107–108.

Anderson, R. C., Horn, K. B., Hoang, M. P., Gottlieb, E., and Bennin, B. 2004. Punctate exanthem of West Nile virus infection: report of 3 cases. *J. Am. Acad. Dermatol.* 51, 820–823.

Andrejeva, J., Childs, K. S., Young, D. F., Carlos, T. S., Stock, N., Goodbourn, S., and Randall, R. E. 2004. The V proteins of paramyxoviruses bind the IFN-inducible RNA helicase, mda-5, and inhibit its activation of the IFN-beta promoter. *Proc. Natl. Acad. Sci. U S A.* 101, 17264–17269.

Anninger, W., and Lubow, M. 2004. Visual loss with West Nile virus infection: a wider spectrum of a "new" disease. *Clin. Infect. Dis.* 38, e55–e56.

Arciniegas, D. B., and Anderson, C. A. 2004. Viral encephalitis: neuropsychiatric and neurobehavioral aspects. *Curr. Psychiatry Rep.* 6, 372–379.

Arjona, A., Foellmer, H. G., Town, T., Leng, L., McDonald, C., Wang, T., Wong, S. J., Montgomery, R. R., Fikrig, E., and Bucala, R. 2007. Abrogation of macrophage migration inhibitory factor decreases West Nile virus lethality by limiting viral neuroinvasion. *J. Clin. Investig.* 117, 3059–3066.

Armali, Z., Ramadan, R., Chlebowski, A., and Azzam, Z. S. 2003. West Nile meningo-encephalitis infection in a kidney transplant recipient. *Transpl. Proc.* 35, 2935–2936.

Bode, A. V., Sejvar, J. J., Pape, W. J., Campbell, G. L., and Marfin, A. A. 2006. West Nile virus disease: a descriptive study of 228 patients hospitalized in a 4-county region of Colorado in 2003. *Clin. Infect. Dis.* 42, 1234–1240.

Brinton, M. A. 2002. The molecular biology of West Nile virus: a new invader of the western hemisphere. *Annu. Rev. Microbiol.* 56, 371–402.

Brown, J. D. 2004. West Nile virus in blood donors: Colorado cohort study, 2003. In *Fifth National Conference on West Nile virus in the United States*.

Burton, J. M., Kern, R. Z., Halliday, W., Mikulis, D., Brunton, J., Fearon, M., Pepperell, C., and Jaigobin, C. 2004. Neurological manifestations of West Nile virus infection. *Can. J. Neurol. Sci.* 31, 185–193.

Campbell, G. L., Marfin, A. A., Lanciotti, R. S., and Gubler, D. J. 2002. West Nile virus. *Lancet Infect. Dis.* 2, 519–529.

Cao, N. J., Ranganathan, C., Kupsky, W. J., and Li, J. 2005. Recovery and prognosticators of paralysis in West Nile virus infection. *J. Neurol. Sci.* 236, 73–80.

Cárdenas, W. B., Loo, Y.-M., Gale, M., Hartman, A. L., Kimberlin, C. R., Martínez-Sobrido, L., Saphire, E. O., and Basler, C. F. 2006. Ebola virus VP35 protein binds doublestranded RNA and inhibits alpha/beta interferon production induced by RIG-I signaling. *J. Virol.* 80, 5168–5178.

Centers for Disease Control and Prevention [http://www.cdc.gov] (Accessed September 2011).

Centers for Disease Control and Prevention CDC. 2002. Intrauterine West Nile virus infection—New York, 2002. *MMWR Morb. Mortal Wkly. Rep.* 51, 1135–1136.

Centers for Disease Control and Prevention CDC. 2004. Update: West Nile virus screening of blood donations and transfusion-associated transmission—United States, 2003. *MMWR Morb. Mortal Wkly. Rep.* 53, 281–284.

Chambers, T. J., and Diamond, M. S. 2003. Pathogenesis of flavivirus encephalitis. *Adv. Virus Res.* 60, 273–342.

Chang, T.-H., Liao, C.-L., and Lin, Y.-L. 2006. Flavivirus induces interferon-beta gene expression through a pathway involving RIG-I-dependent IRF-3 and PI3K-dependent NF-kappaB activation. *Microbes Infect.* 8, 157–171.

Cheeran, M. C.-J., Hu, S., Sheng, W. S., Rashid, A., Peterson, P. K., and Lokensgard, J. R. 2005. Differential responses of human brain cells to West Nile virus infection. *J. Neurovirol.* 11, 512–524.

Chowers, M. Y., Lang, R., Nassar, F., Ben-David, D., Giladi, M., Rubinshtein, E., Itzhaki, A., Mishal, J., Siegman-Igra, Y., Kitzes, R., Pick, N., Landau, Z., Wolf, D., Bin, H., Mendelson, E., Pitlik, S. D., and Weinberger, M. 2001. Clinical characteristics of the West Nile fever outbreak, Israel, 2000. *Emerg. Infect. Dis.* 7, 675–678.

Crichlow, R., Bailey, J., and Gardner, C. 2004. Cerebrospinal fluid neutrophilic pleocytosis in hospitalized West Nile virus patients. *J. Am. Board Fam. Pract.* 17, 470–472.

Daffis, S., Samuel, M. A., Suthar, M. S., Keller, B. C., Gale, M., and Diamond, M. S. 2008. Interferon regulatory factor IRF-7 induces the antiviral alpha interferon response and protects against lethal West Nile virus infection. *J. Virol.* 82, 8465–8475.

Davis, C. T., Ebel, G. D., Lanciotti, R. S., Brault, A. C., Guzman, H., Siirin, M., Lambert, A., Parsons, R. E., Beasley, D. W. C., Novak, R. J., Elizondo-Quiroga, D., Green, E. N., Young, D. S., Stark, L. M., Drebot, M. A., Artsob, H., Tesh, R. B., Kramer, L. D., and Barrett, A. D. T. 2005. Phylogenetic analysis of North American West Nile virus isolates, 2001–2004: evidence for the emergence of a dominant genotype. *Virology* 342, 252–265.

Davis, L. E., Debiasi, R., Goade, D. E., Haaland, K. Y., Harrington, J. A., Harnar, J. B., Pergam, S. A., King, M. K., DeMasters, B. K., and Tyler, K. L. 2006. West Nile virus neuroinvasive disease. *Ann. Neurol.* 60, 286–300.

Deas, T. S., Binduga-Gajewska, I., Tilgner, M., Ren, P., Stein, D. A., Moulton, H. M., Iversen, P. L., Kauffman, E. B., Kramer, L. D., and Shi, P.-Y. 2005. Inhibition of flavivirus infections by antisense oligomers specifically suppressing viral translation and RNA replication. *J. Virol.* 79, 4599–4609.

Del Giudice, P., Schuffenecker, I., Zeller, H., Grelier, M., Vandenbos, F., Dellamonica, P., and Counillon, E. 2005. Skin manifestations of West Nile virus infection. *Dermatology (Basel)* 211, 348–350.

DeSalvo, D., Roy-Chaudhury, P., Peddi, R., Merchen, T., Konijetti, K., Gupta, M., Boardman, R., Rogers, C., Buell, J., Hanaway, M., Broderick, J., Smith, R., and Woodle, E. S. 2004. West Nile virus encephalitis in organ transplant recipients: another high-risk group for meningoencephalitis and death. *Transplantation* 77, 466–469.

Diamond, M. S., Shrestha, B., Marri, A., Mahan, D., and Engle, M. 2003. B cells and antibody play critical roles in the immediate defense of disseminated infection by West Nile encephalitis virus. *J. Virol.* 77, 2578–2586.

Diamond, M. S., Sitati, E. M., Friend, L. D., Higgs, S., Shrestha, B., and Engle, M. 2003. A critical role for induced IgM in the protection against West Nile virus infection. *J. Exp. Med.* 198, 1853–1862.

Doron, S. I., Dashe, J. F., Adelman, L. S., Brown, W. F., Werner, B. G., and Hadley, S. 2003. Histopathologically proven poliomyelitis with quadriplegia and loss of brainstem function due to West Nile virus infection. *Clin. Infect. Dis.* 37, e74–e77.

Engle, M. J., and Diamond, M. S. 2003. Antibody prophylaxis and therapy against West Nile virus infection in wild-type and immunodeficient mice. *J. Virol.* 77, 12941–12949.

Fan, E., Needham, D. M., Brunton, J., Kern, R. Z., and Stewart, T. E. 2004. West Nile virus infection in the intensive care unit: a case series and literature review. *Can. Respir. J.* 11, 354–358.

Ferguson, D. D., Gershman, K., LeBailly, A., and Petersen, L. R. 2005. Characteristics of the rash associated with West Nile virus fever. *Clin. Infect. Dis.* 41, 1204–1207.

Fredericksen, B. L., and Gale, M. 2006. West Nile virus evades activation of interferon regulatory factor 3 through RIG-I-dependent and -independent pathways without antagonizing host defense signaling. *J. Virol.* 80, 2913–2923.

Girard, Y. A., Popov, V., Wen, J., Han, V., and Higgs, S. 2005. Ultrastructural study of West Nile virus pathogenesis in Culex pipiens quinquefasciatus (Diptera: Culicidae). *J. Med. Entomol.* 42, 429–444.

Glass, J. D., Samuels, O., and Rich, M. M. 2002. Poliomyelitis due to West Nile virus. *N. Engl. J. Med.* 347, 1280–1281.

Glass, W. G., Lim, J. K., Cholera, R., Pletnev, A. G., Gao, J.-L., and Murphy, P. M. 2005. Chemokine receptor CCR5 promotes leukocyte trafficking to the brain and survival in West Nile virus infection. *J. Exp. Med.* 202, 1087–1098.

Goldblum, N., Sterk, V. V., and Paderski, B. 1954. West Nile fever; the clinical features of the disease and the isolation of West Nile virus from the blood of nine human cases. *Am. J. Hyg.* 59, 89–103.

Gorsche, R., and Tilley, P. 2005. The rash of West Nile virus infection. *CMAJ* 172, 1440.

Gottfried, K., Quinn, R., and Jones, T. 2005. Clinical description and follow-up investigation of human West Nile virus cases. *South. Med. J.* 98, 603–606.

Granwehr, B. P., Lillibridge, K. M., Higgs, S., Mason, P. W., Aronson, J. F., Campbell, G. A., and Barrett, A. D. T. 2004. West Nile virus: where are we now? *Lancet Infect. Dis.* 4, 547–556.

Guarner, J., Shieh, W.-J., Hunter, S., Paddock, C. D., Morken, T., Campbell, G. L., Marfin, A. A., and Zaki, S. R. 2004. Clinicopathologic study and laboratory diagnosis of 23 cases with West Nile virus encephalomyelitis. *Human Pathol.* 35, 983–990.

Hayes, E. B., and Gubler, D. J. 2006. West Nile virus: epidemiology and clinical features of an emerging epidemic in the United States. *Annu. Rev. Med.* 57, 181–194.

Hayes, E. B., Komar, N., Nasci, R. S., Montgomery, S. P., O'Leary, D. R., and Campbell, G. L. 2005. Epidemiology and transmission dynamics of West Nile virus disease. *Emerg. Infect. Dis.* 11, 1167–1173.

Hayes, E. B., and O'Leary, D. R. 2004. West Nile virus infection: a pediatric perspective. *Pediatrics* 113, 1375–1381.

Hayes, E. B., Sejvar, J. J., Zaki, S. R., Lanciotti, R. S., Bode, A. V., and Campbell, G. L. 2005. Virology, pathology, and clinical manifestations of West Nile virus disease. *Emerg. Infect. Dis.* 11, 1174–1179.

Hrnicek, M. J., and Mailliard, M. E. 2004. Acute west nile virus in two patients receiving interferon and ribavirin for chronic hepatitis C. *Am. J. Gastroenterol.* 99, 957.

Iwamoto, M., Jernigan, D. B., Guasch, A., Trepka, M. J., Blackmore, C. G., Hellinger, W. C., Pham, S. M., Zaki, S., Lanciotti, R. S., Lance-Parker, S. E., DiazGranados, C. A., Winquist, A. G., Perlino, C. A., Wiersma, S., Hillyer, K. L., Goodman, J. L., Marfin, A. A., Chamberland, M. E., Petersen, L. R., and West Nile Virus in Transplant Recipients Investigation Team, 2003. Transmission of West Nile virus from an organ donor to four transplant recipients. *N. Engl. J. Med.* 348, 2196–2203.

Iwamura, T., Yoneyama, M., Yamaguchi, K., Suhara, W., Mori, W., Shiota, K., Okabe, Y., Namiki, H., and Fujita, T. 2001. Induction of IRF-3/-7 kinase and NF-kappaB in response to double-stranded RNA and virus infection: common and unique pathways. *Genes Cells* 6, 375–388.

Jeha, L. E., Sila, C. A., Lederman, R. J., Prayson, R. A., Isada, C. M., and Gordon, S. M. 2003. West Nile virus infection: a new acute paralytic illness. *Neurology* 61, 55–59.

Johnston, L. J., Halliday, G. M., and King, N. J. 2000. Langerhans cells migrate to local lymph nodes following cutaneous infection with an arbovirus. *J. Invest. Dermatol.* 114, 560–568.

Jordan, I., Briese, T., Fischer, N., Lau, J. Y., and Lipkin, W. I. 2000. Ribavirin inhibits West Nile virus replication and cytopathic effect in neural cells. *J. Infect. Dis.* 182, 1214–1217.

Justesen, J., Hartmann, R., and Kjeldgaard, N. O. 2000. Gene structure and function of the 2"-5-"oligoadenylate synthetase family. Cellular and molecular life sciences. *CMLS.* 57, 1593–1612.

Kajaste-Rudnitski, A., Mashimo, T., Frenkiel, M.-P., Guénet, J.-L., Lucas, M., and Desprès, P. 2006. The 2",5-"oligoadenylate synthetase 1b is a potent inhibitor of West Nile virus replication inside infected cells. *J. Biol. Chem.* 281, 4624–4637.

Kapoor, H., Signs, K., Somsel, P., Downes, F. P., Clark, P. A., and Massey, J. P. 2004. Persistence of West Nile virus (WNV) IgM antibodies in cerebrospinal fluid from patients with CNS disease. *J. Clin. Virol.* 31, 289–291.

Khairallah, M., Ben Yahia, S., Ladjimi, A., Zeghidi, H., Ben Romdhane, F., Besbes, L., Zaouali, S., and Messaoud, R. 2004. Chorioretinal involvement in patients with West Nile virus infection. *Ophthalmology* 111, 2065–2070.

Klein, R. S., Lin, E., Zhang, B., Luster, A. D., Tollett, J., Samuel, M. A., Engle, M., and Diamond, M. S. 2005. Neuronal CXCL10 directs CD8+ T-cell recruitment and control of West Nile virus encephalitis. *J. Virol.* 79, 11457–11466.

Kleinschmidt-DeMasters, B. K., Marder, B. A., Levi, M. E., Laird, S. P., McNutt, J. T., Escott, E. J., Everson, G. T., and Tyler, K. L. 2004. Naturally acquired West Nile virus encephalomyelitis in transplant recipients: clinical, laboratory, diagnostic, and neuropathological features. *Arch. Neurol.* 61, 1210–1220.

Komar, N., Langevin, S., Hinten, S., Nemeth, N., Edwards, E., Hettler, D., Davis, B., Bowen, R., and Bunning, M. 2003. Experimental infection of North American birds with the New York 1999 strain of West Nile virus. *Emerg. Infect. Dis.* 9, 311–322.

Kumar, D., Drebot, M. A., Wong, S. J., Lim, G., Artsob, H., Buck, P., and Humar, A. 2004. A seroprevalence study of west nile virus infection in solid organ transplant recipients. *Am. J. Transplant.* 4, 1883–1888.

Lanciotti, R. S., Kerst, A. J., Nasci, R. S., Godsey, M. S., Mitchell, C. J., Savage, H. M., Komar, N., Panella, N. A., Allen, B. C., Volpe, K. E., Davis, B. S., and Roehrig, J. T. 2000. Rapid detection of west nile virus from human clinical specimens, field-collected mosquitoes, and avian samples by a TaqMan reverse transcriptase-PCR assay. *J. Clin. Microbiol.* 38, 4066–4071.

Lanciotti, R. S., Roehrig, J. T., Deubel, V., Smith, J., Parker, M., Steele, K., Crise, B., Volpe, K. E., Crabtree, M. B., Scherret, J. H., Hall, R. A., Mackenzie, J. S., Cropp, C. B., Panigrahy, B., Ostlund, E., Schmitt, B., Malkinson, M., Banet, C., Weissman, J., Komar, N., Savage, H. M., Stone, W., McNamara, T., and Gubler, D. J. 1999. Origin of the West Nile virus responsible for an outbreak of encephalitis in the northeastern United States. *Science* 286, 2333–2337.

Leis, A. A., Stokic, D. S., Polk, J. L., Dostrow, V., and Winkelmann, M. 2002. A poliomyelitis-like syndrome from West Nile virus infection. *N. Engl. J. Med.* 347, 1279–1280.

Leis, A. A., Stokic, D. S., Webb, R. M., Slavinski, S. A., and Fratkin, J. 2003. Clinical spectrum of muscle weakness in human West Nile virus infection. *Muscle Nerve* 28, 302–308.

Li, J., Loeb, J. A., Shy, M. E., Shah, A. K., Tselis, A. C., Kupski, W. J., and Lewis, R. A. 2003. Asymmetric flaccid paralysis: a neuromuscular presentation of West Nile virus infection. *Ann. Neurol.* 53, 703–710.

Lin, R., Heylbroeck, C., Pitha, P. M., and Hiscott, J. 1998. Virus-dependent phosphorylation of the IRF-3 transcription factor regulates nuclear translocation, transactivation potential, and proteasome-mediated degradation. *Mol. Cell. Biol.* 18, 2986–2996.

Lin, R., Mamane, Y., and Hiscott, J. 2000. Multiple regulatory domains control IRF-7 activity in response to virus infection. *J. Biol. Chem.* 275, 34320–34327.

Liu, W. J., Wang, X. J., Clark, D. C., Lobigs, M., Hall, R. A., and Khromykh, A. A. 2006. A single amino acid substitution in the West Nile virus nonstructural protein NS2A disables its ability to inhibit alpha/beta interferon induction and attenuates virus virulence in mice. *J. Virol.* 80, 2396–2404.

Loeb, M., Elliott, S. J., Gibson, B., Fearon, M., Nosal, R., Drebot, M., D'Cuhna, C., Harrington, D., Smith, S., George, P., and Eyles, J. 2005. Protective behavior and West Nile virus risk. *Emerg. Infect. Dis.* 11, 1433–1436.

Lucas, M., Mashimo, T., Frenkiel, M.-P., Simon-Chazottes, D., Montagutelli, X., Ceccaldi, P.-E., Guénet, J.-L., and Desprès, P. 2003. Infection of mouse neurones by West Nile virus is modulated by the interferon-inducible 2"–5" oligoadenylate synthetase 1b protein. *Immunol. Cell Biol.* 81, 230–236.

Marié, I., Durbin, J. E., and Levy, D. E. 1998. Differential viral induction of distinct interferon-alpha genes by positive feedback through interferon regulatory factor-7. *EMBO J.* 17, 6660–6669.

Martin, D. A., Biggerstaff, B. J., Allen, B., Johnson, A. J., Lanciotti, R. S., and Roehrig, J. T. 2002. Use of immunoglobulin m cross-reactions in differential diagnosis of human flaviviral encephalitis infections in the United States. *Clin Diagn Lab Immunol* 9, 544–549.

Mashimo, T., Lucas, M., Simon-Chazottes, D., Frenkiel, M.-P., Montagutelli, X., Ceccaldi, P.-E., Deubel, V., Guénet, J.-L., and Desprès, P. 2002. A nonsense mutation in the gene encoding 2"-5-"oligoadenylate synthetase/L1 isoform is associated with West Nile virus susceptibility in laboratory mice. *Proc. Natl. Acad. Sci. U S A.* 99, 11311–11316.

Morrey, J. D., Day, C. W., Julander, J. G., Blatt, L. M., Smee, D. F., and Sidwell, R. W. 2004. Effect of interferon-alpha and interferon-inducers on West Nile virus in mouse and hamster animal models. *Antivir. Chem. Chemother.* 15, 101–109.

Mukhopadhyay, S., Kim, B.-S., Chipman, P. R., Rossmann, M. G., and Kuhn, R. J. 2003. Structure of West Nile virus. *Science* 302, 248.

Murgue, B., Zeller, H., and Deubel, V. 2002. The ecology and epidemiology of West Nile virus in Africa, Europe and Asia. *Curr. Top. Microbiol. Immunol.* 267, 195–221.

Nash, D., Mostashari, F., Fine, A., Miller, J., O'Leary, D., Murray, K., Huang, A., Rosenberg, A., Greenberg, A., Sherman, M., Wong, S., Layton, M., 1999 and West Nile Outbreak Response Working Group, 2001. The outbreak of West Nile virus infection in the New York City area in 1999. *N. Engl. J. Med.* 344, 1807–1814.

NIH Clinical Trials. Sanofi-Aventis. Safety and Immunogenicity Study of ChimeriVax West Nile Vaccine in Healthy Adults (WinVax004) http://clinicaltrials.gov/ct2/show/ NCT00746798 (Accessed September 2011).

O'Leary, D. R., Marfin, A. A., Montgomery, S. P., Kipp, A. M., Lehman, J. A., Biggerstaff, B. J., Elko, V. L., Collins, P. D., Jones, J. E., and Campbell, G. L. 2004. The epidemic of West Nile virus in the United States, 2002. *Vector Borne Zoonotic Dis.* 4, 61–70.

Park, M., Hui, J. S., and Bartt, R. E. 2003. Acute anterior radiculitis associated with West Nile virus infection. *J. Neurol. Neurosurg. Psychiatr.* 74, 823–825.

Pealer, L. N., Marfin, A. A., Petersen, L. R., Lanciotti, R. S., Page, P. L., Stramer, S. L., Stobierski, M. G., Signs, K., Newman, B., Kapoor, H., Goodman, J. L., Chamberland, M. E., and West Nile Virus Transmission Investigation Team. 2003. Transmission of West Nile virus through blood transfusion in the United States in 2002. *N. Engl. J. Med.* 349, 1236–1245.

Pepperell, C., Rau, N., Krajden, S., Kern, R., Humar, A., Mederski, B., Simor, A., Low, D. E., McGeer, A., Mazzulli, T., Burton, J., Jaigobin, C., Fearon, M., Artsob, H., Drebot, M. A., Halliday, W., and Brunton, J. 2003. West Nile virus infection in 2002: morbidity and mortality among patients admitted to hospital in southcentral Ontario. *CMAJ* 168, 1399–1405.

Perelygin, A. A., Scherbik, S. V., Zhulin, I. B., Stockman, B. M., Li, Y., and Brinton, M. A. 2002. Positional cloning of the murine flavivirus resistance gene. *Proc. Natl. Acad. Sci. U S A.* 99, 9322–9327.

Petersen, L. R., Roehrig, J. T., and Hughes, J. M. 2002. West Nile virus encephalitis. *N. Engl. J. Med.* 347, 1225–1226.

Public Health Agency of Canada: West Nile Virus Surveillance Information [http://www.phac aspc.gc.ca/wnv-vwn] (Accessed September 2011).

Rappole, J. H., Derrickson, S. R., and Hubálek, Z. 2000. Migratory birds and spread of West Nile virus in the Western Hemisphere. *Emerg. Infect. Dis.* 6, 319–328.

Ravindra, K. V., Freifeld, A. G., Kalil, A. C., Mercer, D. F., Grant, W. J., Botha, J. F., Wrenshall, L. E., and Stevens, R. B. 2004. West Nile virus-associated encephalitis in recipients of renal and pancreas transplants: case series and literature review. *Clin. Infect. Dis.* 38, 1257–1260.

Rothenfusser, S., Goutagny, N., DiPerna, G., Gong, M., Monks, B. G., Schoenemeyer, A., Yamamoto, M., Akira, S., and Fitzgerald, K. A. 2005. The RNA helicase Lgp2 inhibits TLR-independent sensing of viral replication by retinoic acid-inducible gene-I. *J. Immunol.* 175, 5260–5268.

Samuel, M. A., and Diamond, M. S. 2005. Alpha/beta interferon protects against lethal West Nile virus infection by restricting cellular tropism and enhancing neuronal survival. *J. Virol.* 79, 13350–13361.

Samuel, M. A., Whitby, K., Keller, B. C., Marri, A., Barchet, W., Williams, B. R. G., Silverman, R. H., Gale, M., and Diamond, M. S. 2006. PKR and RNase L contribute to protection against lethal West Nile virus infection by controlling early viral spread in the periphery and replication in neurons. *J. Virol.* 80, 7009–7019.

Sato, M., Tanaka, N., Hata, N., Oda, E., and Taniguchi, T. 1998a. Involvement of the IRF family transcription factor IRF-3 in virus-induced activation of the IFN-beta gene. *FEBS Lett.* 425, 112–116.

Sato, M., Hata, N., Asagiri, M., Nakaya, T., Taniguchi, T., and Tanaka, N. 1998b. Positive feedback regulation of type I IFN genes by the IFN-inducible transcription factor IRF-7. *FEBS Lett.* 441, 106–110.

Sayao, A.-L., Suchowersky, O., Al-Khathaami, A., Klassen, B., Katz, N. R., Sevick, R., Tilley, P., Fox, J., and Patry, D. 2004. Calgary experience with West Nile virus neurological syndrome during the late summer of 2003. *Can. J. Neurol. Sci.* 31, 194–203.

Scholle, F., and Mason, P. W. 2005. West Nile virus replication interferes with both poly(I:C)-induced interferon gene transcription and response to interferon treatment. *Virology.* 342, 77–87.

Sejvar, J. J., Bode, A. V., Marfin, A. A., Campbell, G. L., Pape, J., Biggerstaff, B. J., and Petersen, L. R. 2006. West Nile virus-associated flaccid paralysis outcome. *Emerg. Infect. Dis.* 12, 514–516.

Sejvar, J. J., Labutta, R. J., Chapman, L. E., Grabenstein, J. D., Iskander, J., and Lane, J. M. 2005. Neurologic adverse events associated with smallpox vaccination in the United States, 2002–2004. *JAMA* 294, 2744–2750.

Sejvar, J. J., Haddad, M. B., Tierney, B. C., Campbell, G. L., Marfin, A. A., Van Gerpen, J. A., Fleischauer, A., Leis, A. A., Stokic, D. S., and Petersen, L. R. 2003a. Neurologic manifestations and outcome of West Nile virus infection. *JAMA* 290, 511–515.

Sejvar, J. J., Leis, A. A., Stokic, D. S., Van Gerpen, J. A., Marfin, A. A., Webb, R., Haddad, M. B., Tierney, B. C., Slavinski, S. A., Polk, J. L., Dostrow, V., Winkelmann, M., and Petersen, L. R. 2003b. Acute flaccid paralysis and West Nile virus infection. *Emerg. Infect. Dis.* 9, 788–793.

Shimoni, Z., Niven, M. J., Pitlick, S., and Bulvik, S. 2001. Treatment of West Nile virus encephalitis with intravenous immunoglobulin. *Emerg. Infect. Dis.* 7, 759.

Shrestha, B., and Diamond, M. S. 2004. Role of CD8+ T cells in control of West Nile virus infection. *J. Virol.* 78, 8312–8321.

Smithburn, K., Hughes, T., Burke, A., and Paul, J. 1940. A neurotropic virus isolated from the blood of a native of Uganda. *Am. J. Trop. Med. Hyg.* 1, 471–492.

Southam, C. M., and Moore, A. E. 1952. Clinical studies of viruses as antineoplastic agents with particular reference to Egypt 101 virus. *Cancer* 5, 1025–1034.

Southam, C. M., and Moore, A. E. 1954. Induced virus infections in man by the Egypt isolates of West Nile virus. *Am. J. Trop. Med. Hyg.* 3, 19–50.

Suhara, W., Yoneyama, M., Iwamura, T., Yoshimura, S., Tamura, K., Namiki, H., Aimoto, S., and Fujita, T. 2000. Analyses of virus-induced homomeric and heteromeric protein associations between IRF-3 and coactivator CBP/p300. *J. Biochem.* 128, 301–307.

Turell, M. J., O'Guinn, M., and Oliver, J. 2000. Potential for New York mosquitoes to transmit West Nile virus. *Am. J. Trop. Med. Hyg.* 62, 413–414.

Turell, M. J., O'Guinn, M. L., Dohm, D. J., Webb, J. P., and Sardelis, M. R. 2002. Vector competence of Culex tarsalis from Orange County, California, for West Nile virus. *Vector Borne Zoonotic Dis.* 2, 193–196.

Tyler, K. L. 2004. West Nile virus infection in the United States. *Arch. Neurol.* 61, 1190–1195.

van der Meulen, K. M., Pensaert, M. B., and Nauwynck, H. J. 2005. West Nile virus in the vertebrate world. *Arch. Virol.* 150, 637–657.

Vanlandingham, D. L., Schneider, B. S., Klingler, K., Fair, J., Beasley, D., Huang, J., Hamilton, P., and Higgs, S. 2004. Real-time reverse transcriptase-polymerase chain reaction quantification of West Nile virus transmitted by Culex pipiens quinquefasciatus. *Am. J. Trop. Med. Hyg.* 71, 120–123.

Wang, T., and Fikrig, E. 2004. Immunity to West Nile virus. *Curr. Opin. Immunol.* 16, 519–523.

Wang, T., Town, T., Alexopoulou, L., Anderson, J. F., Fikrig, E., and Flavell, R. A. 2004. Toll-like receptor 3 mediates West Nile virus entry into the brain causing lethal encephalitis. *Nat. Med.* 10, 1366–1373.

Wang, Y., Lobigs, M., Lee, E., and Müllbacher, A. 2003. CD8+ T cells mediate recovery and immunopathology in West Nile virus encephalitis. *J. Virol.* 77, 13323–13334.

Wathelet, M. G., Lin, C. H., Parekh, B. S., Ronco, L. V., Howley, P. M., and Maniatis, T. 1998. Virus infection induces the assembly of coordinately activated transcription factors on the IFN-beta enhancer *in vivo*. *Mol. Cell.* 1, 507–518.

Watson, J. T., Pertel, P. E., Jones, R. C., Siston, A. M., Paul, W. S., Austin, C. C., and Gerber, S. I. 2004. Clinical characteristics and functional outcomes of West Nile Fever. *Ann. Intern. Med.* 141, 360–365.

Weaver, B. K., Kumar, K. P., and Reich, N. C. 1998. Interferon regulatory factor 3 and CREB-binding protein/p300 are subunits of double-stranded RNA-activated transcription factor DRAF1. *Mol. Cell. Biol.* 18, 1359–1368.

Weiss, D., Carr, D., Kellachan, J., Tan, C., Phillips, M., Bresnitz, E., and Layton, M., West Nile Virus Outbreak Response Working Group, 2001. Clinical findings of West Nile virus infection in hospitalized patients, New York and New Jersey, 2000. *Emerg. Infect. Dis.* 7, 654–658.

Wilson, J. R., de Sessions, P. F., Leon, M. A., and Scholle, F. 2008. West Nile virus nonstructural protein 1 inhibits TLR3 signal transduction. *J. Virol.* 82, 8262–8271.

Yakub, I., Lillibridge, K. M., Moran, A., Gonzalez, O. Y., Belmont, J., Gibbs, R. A., and Tweardy, D. J. 2005. Single nucleotide polymorphisms in genes for 2"–5-"oligoadenylate synthetase and RNase L inpatients hospitalized with West Nile virus infection. *J. Infect. Dis.* 192, 1741–1748.

Yim, R., Posfay-Barbe, K. M., Nolt, D., Fatula, G., and Wald, E. R. 2004. Spectrum of clinical manifestations of West Nile virus infection in children. *Pediatrics* 114, 1673–1675.

Yoneyama, M., Kikuchi, M., Matsumoto, K., Imaizumi, T., Miyagishi, M., Taira, K., Foy, E., Loo, Y.-M., Gale, M., Akira, S., Yonehara, S., Kato, A., and Fujita, T. 2005. Shared and unique functions of the DExD/H-box helicases RIG-I, MDA5, and LGP2 in antiviral innate immunity. *J. Immunol.* 175, 2851–2858.

Yoneyama, M., Kikuchi, M., Natsukawa, T., Shinobu, N., Imaizumi, T., Miyagishi, M., Taira, K., Akira, S., and Fujita, T. 2004. The RNA helicase RIG-I has an essential function in double-stranded RNA-induced innate antiviral responses. *Nat. Immunol.* 5, 730–737.

Yoneyama, M., Suhara, W., Fukuhara, Y., Fukuda, M., Nishida, E., and Fujita, T. 1998. Direct triggering of the type I interferon system by virus infection: activation of a transcription factor complex containing IRF-3 and CBP/p300. *EMBO J.* 17, 1087–1095.

Zhou, Y., Wang, S., Gobl, A., and Oberg, K. 2000. The interferon-alpha regulation of interferon regulatory factor 1 (IRF-1) and IRF-2 has therapeutic implications in carcinoid tumors. *Ann. Oncol.* 11, 707–714.

8 Murray Valley Encephalitis Virus

Natalie A. Prow, Roy A. Hall, and Mario Lobigs

CONTENTS

8.1 INTRODUCTION

Murray Valley encephalitis (MVE) is an important mosquito-borne viral disease of Australia that causes annual, sporadic cases and occasional epidemics of potentially fatal encephalitis in man. Although human cases of the disease are most commonly reported in the tropical areas of Northern Australia, ecological factors and climatic conditions occasionally result in cases appearing in more southerly areas of the country, sometimes involving large-scale outbreaks of the disease. As there are no virus-specific vaccines or treatment options currently available, this vector-borne viral disease continues to represent a major public health threat in Australia. In this chapter we discuss properties of the virus, cellular infection, clinical disease and the host immune response to infection. We also describe recent advances in diagnosis of the disease and strategies for disease prevention.

8.2   STRUCTURE AND REPLICATION

MVE virus (MVEV) is a spherical, enveloped particle with a positive strand, nonsegmented RNA genome of about 11,000 nucleotides. The virus is a member of the flaviviruses, family Flaviviridae. The replication and molecular biology of the flaviviruses have been reviewed in detail by others (Chambers et al. 1990; Fernandez-Garcia et al. 2009; Lindenbach and Rice 2003; Mukhopadhyay et al. 2005). Briefly, the viral RNA is translated into a polyprotein precursor, which is cleaved into at least 10 viral proteins. These include three structural (capsid [C], envelope [E], and premembrane/membrane [prM]), and seven nonstructural proteins (NS1, NS2A, NS2B, NS3, NS4A, NS4B, and NS5). The structural proteins together with the viral genomic RNA assemble into the virion particle by a process that involves budding across the membranes of the endoplasmic reticulum. The virion surface consists of 180 copies of the envelope (E) protein, which are arranged in icosahedral organization consisting of 30 rafts, each of which is composed of 3 E protein dimers oriented in parallel and lying flat on the virus surface. Structural studies show that the flavivirus E protein is organized into 3 domains: the central structural domain (domain I) is flanked on one side by an elongated dimerization domain (domain II) and on the other by an immunoglobulin-like domain (domain III), which makes the highest protrusion from the otherwise smooth particle. The fusion peptide is located at the distal end of domain II, and the receptor-binding sites are thought to be located on domain III. The MVEV E protein is modified by a single glycan linked to residue 154 on domain I (Dalgarno et al. 1986), which facilitates virus morphogenesis and is a virulence determinant (see Section 8.10). Most flavivirus-neutralizing antibodies recognize epitopes on the E protein: in murine infections, serotype-specific neutralizing antibodies are mostly elicited by epitopes on domain III and are thought to inhibit virus infectivity by preventing virus binding to cell surface receptors; antibodies that recognize epitopes in domain II are often cross-reactive with other flaviviruses, and can have neutralizing activity due to inhibition of membrane fusion, while antibodies against epitopes in domain I are generally nonneutralizing (Nybakken et al. 2005; Oliphant et al. 2007; Oliphant et al. 2006). Studies in humans suggest that the antibody response against West Nile virus (WNV) is biased to epitopes on domain II, especially the fusion loop, rather than against domain III (Throsby et al. 2006).

Virus particles are transported from the intracellular site of assembly via the secretory pathway to the cell surface to be released into the extracellular milieu. During this process, virus maturation occurs, which requires the furin-catalyzed cleavage of the small, virion surface prM to M protein. This triggers a conformational rearrangement in E protein required for activation of the fusion function (reviewed by Harrison 2008). A specific host receptor for MVEV has not been identified; given the wide host and vector tropism of the virus, it is likely that it can employ multiple cell surface receptors for establishment of productive infection. Heparan sulfate proteoglycans are sulphated polysaccharides ubiquitous found on cellular surfaces and extracellular matrices, and have been shown to facilitate attachment/ entry of MVEV in cell culture (Lee and Lobigs 2000). However, in mice variants of MVEV and other flaviviruses selected for high binding-affinity to these cell surface molecules display a complete loss of neuroinvasiveness due to a mechanism involving rapid virus clearance from the blood stream, thereby preventing virus dissemination (see Section 8.10). This suggests that heparan sulfate proteoglycans do not function as uptake receptors in the transmission cycle of the virus, but may still play a role in initial low-affinity attachment to cellular surfaces. MVEV enters the cell via receptor-mediated endocytosis. Fusion of the viral membrane with the endosomal membrane occurs after exposure to low pH in the endosomal compartment, allowing viral RNA release into the cytoplasm of the newly infected cell.

8.3 EPIDEMIOLOGY

MVEV is the main cause of arboviral encephalitis in Australia (reviewed by Doherty 1974; French 1973; Mackenzie and Broom 1995; Marshall 1988) and was first isolated from fatal human cases of encephalitis during an epidemic in 1951 in the Murray Valley in the south-east of the continent (French 1952; Miles et al. 1951). The virus is a member of the Japanese encephalitis virus (JEV) serological complex within the genus Flavivirus, family Flaviviridae (Thiel et al. 2005). MVEV circulates in Australia, Papua New Guinea (PNG), and probably on islands in the eastern part of the Indonesian archipelago (Mackenzie et al. 1994). The virus is thought to be enzootic in tropical northern Australia, mainly the Kimberley region of Western Australia and the "Top End" of the Northern Territory, and to a lesser extent in northern Queensland (Mackenzie et al. 1994; Mackenzie and Williams 2009). Intermittent virus activity occurs in the Pilbara region of Western Australia, as indicated by sentinel chicken seroconversion, virus isolations from mosquitoes, and cases of MVE (Broom et al. 1989). MVEV is sporadically found in central, south-eastern and south-western regions of Australia, where epidemics of viral encephalitis can occur (Figure 8.1). It has been proposed that during extended periods of above average rainfall MVEV may be transmitted from enzootic northern regions to temperate zones by the southward movement of viremic birds (Johansen et al. 2007; Lobigs et al. 1986, 1988). Such climatic conditions also result in the surge in abundance of vertebrate hosts (water birds) and mosquito vectors necessary for the appearance of clinical disease in humans and horses.

Several large epidemics of encephalitis were observed in eastern Australia during 1917, 1918, 1922, and 1925 and were designated Australian X disease (Anderson 1954). In 1951, 45 cases of encephalitis were attributed to MVEV, where all but two cases from the epidemic originated from the Murray Valley. The next major epidemic occurring in 1974 resulted in MVE spreading to all mainland states with 54 cases, including the first recorded West Australian case. From 1975 to 1999, all cases of MVE (48 cases) were acquired in northern Australia with the majority from the Kimberley region (Burrow et al. 1998; Mackenzie et al. 1993). An MVEV epidemic in 2000 resulted in 15 human cases of encephalitis, 9 in Western Australia, 3 in the

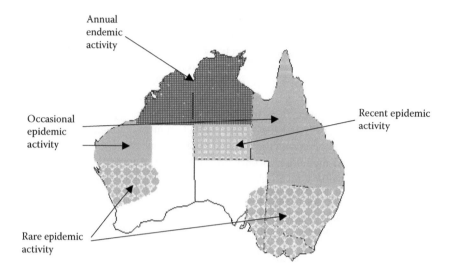

FIGURE 8.1 MVEV activity in Australia.

Northern Territories, and one in South Australia, the latter being the first recorded case of MVE in the dry inland region of central Australia in 26 years (Brown et al. 2002). Also remarkable in this epidemic was the acquisition of MVE as close as 315 km north of the Western Australian capital, Perth. During the 2000 outbreak, West Australian patients ranged in age from 10 months to 79 years, were predominately male, and were largely non-Aboriginal adult visitors or residents. Nine patients developed encephalitis and one died. From 2001 to 2008 there were 11 human cases of MVE recorded from Western Australia, the Northern Territories, Queensland, and New South Wales (Johansen et al. 2008). This marked the reappearance of MVE in New South Wales after an absence of 24 years, and although there was evidence that MVEV activity occurred in previous years, as indicated by seroconversions in sentinel chickens and mosquito isolates (Doggett et al. 2008), no cases of human disease were reported in the intervening years. In 2011, a significant outbreak of arboviral encephalitis occurred in humans and horses in south-eastern Australia. Although more than 1000 cases of equine disease were reported (Frost et al. 2012) only a handful of human cases occurred. Interesting, the vast majority of confirmed equine cases were caused by infections with a new strain of Kunjin virus (KUNV), a subtype of WNV, while all confirmed human cases were shown to be associated with MVEV infection. This was the first report of human cases in south-eastern Australia since 1974. During the first five months of 2011, there have been a total of 14 notifications of MVE (National Communicable Diseases surveillance report, Fortnight 09 2011; http://www.health.gov.au/internet/main/publishing.nsf/Content/cdnareport-fn9-11.htm.)

8.4   ECOLOGY

Culex annulirostris is the major mosquito species involved in MVEV transmission (Kay et al. 1989). It is a widely distributed, highly adaptable, freshwater mosquito that inhabits permanent and semipermanent water bodies, and has the ability to colonize rain water pools within a day of their formation (Doherty et al. 1963). In addition, the virus has also been isolated from numerous other mosquito species in Australia (Broom and Whelan 2005; Broom et al. 1989; Kay and Carley 1980; Russell 1998; van den Hurk et al. 2010). Ardeid water birds of the order *Ciconiiformes*, particularly the rufous night heron (*Nycticorax calendonicus*), and other herons and egrets are thought to be the major vertebrate hosts for MVEV (Anderson 1952; Boyle et al. 1983). Other avian and mammalian vertebrates have shown serological evidence of infection and may play a role in virus transmission, although this is yet to be confirmed (Kay et al. 1985a,b).

MVEV co-circulates with several other flaviviruses in Australia, including KUNV. In northwestern Australia, MVEV is more frequently isolated from mosquitoes than KUNV, while in Queensland and south-eastern Australia KUNV is isolated more frequently (Mackenzie et al. 1994). The vector competence of different regional populations of *Cx. annulirostris* may contribute to the varying prevalence of the viruses in the different locations (Kay et al. 1984, 1989), in addition to host biology. Carver et al. (2009) have reviewed mechanisms by which hosts influence MVEV and related virus transmission, and have identified five areas: host immunity, cross-protective immunity and antibody-dependent enhancement, host abundance, host diversity, and pathogen spill-over and dispersal.

Widespread transmission of JEV in the Torres Strait of northern Australia and subsequent virus isolation on the Australian mainland have raised the possibility that JEV would become enzootic in Australia, where suitable host and vector species are thought to be abundant (reviewed by van den Hurk et al. 2009). This scenario would greatly increase the complexity of the Australian flavivirus ecology with the likely concurrent circulation of MVEV with JEV, the most important human and veterinary pathogen of the JEV serocomplex. Both viruses coexist in PNG, which shows that the two closely related viruses can be maintained in the same ecosystem. However, it appears that JEV has, so far, not become established in natural transmission cycles on the Australian mainland. Possible reasons for this include cross-protective immunity to JEV in susceptible hosts, suboptimal vector competence of the lineages of *Cx. annulirostris* to JEV, and the propensity of *Cx. annulirostris* to feed on marsupials (which do not produce high levels of viremia) and not pigs (an important amplified host for JEV) (van den Hurk et al. 2009).

Global warming and associated climate change have been postulated to lead to increased activity of vector-borne diseases, such as MVEV (reviewed by Colwell et al. 1998; Mackenzie and Williams 2009). Warmer, wetter, and more humid conditions could lead to increases in both mosquito abundance and distribution. These conditions could also lengthen the seasonal activity of some mosquito vectors. Rising sea levels may lead to extensive flooding, leading to increases in mosquito numbers (Mellor and Leake 2000). However, Russell et al. (2009) have suggested that any evaluation of the potential effects of climate change will need a detailed examination of at least site-specific vector and host factors and other aspects likely to influence the outcomes of virus activity on human health. The authors suggest that climate change, as currently projected, is unlikely to significantly change the distribution and transmission of endemic arboviruses and is not likely to provide cause for public health concern regarding mosquito-borne diseases in Australia.

8.5   SEROPREVALENCE

Antibody levels within a population provide information about the frequency of infection in a community. Calculation of antibody seroprevalence rates of MVEV is problematic due to the sporadic nature of epidemics and cases of disease throughout Australia. Furthermore, the inability to serologically distinguish between MVEV and KUNV in early epidemics added further ambiguity to the determination of prevalence rates. Seroprevalence of MVEV and KUNV differ based on geographical location (Hawkes et al. 1985, 1993). Antibody prevalence rates were higher for KUNV than for MVEV in sera collected in New South Wales during 1981–1982 (Hawkes et al. 1985). In a second study of the same regions from 1981 to 1991, KUNV antibody was detected, whereas MVEV antibody was relatively uncommon (Hawkes et al. 1993). In Western Australia, MVEV and KUNV antibody prevalence tends to decrease geographically from the north of the State to the south. The highest MVEV seroprevalence (52.6%) was reported from the southeast Kimberley region, where MVEV and KUNV are considered to be enzootic (Broom et al. 2002). A serosurvey of human samples collected between 1999 and 2001 from the mid-west region of Western Australia, where MVEV activity is epizootic, showed that only 2.3% of samples contained antibodies against MVEV (Sturrock 2009). The seroprevalence of MVEV antibodies in humans tends to increase with increasing age in enzootic areas, as MVEV-specific antibodies are life-long (Broom et al. 2002); there is little or no difference between antibody seroprevalence in males and females (Broom et al. 2002; Hawkes et al. 1985).

8.6   CLINICAL PRESENTATION

MVEV commonly infects humans without producing apparent illness. It has been estimated that only about 1 in 1000 infections results in clinical disease (reviewed by Burrow et al. 1998; Mackenzie et al. 1993; Marshall 1988). Cases are reported mostly among resident Aboriginal children and interstate or international travellers to regions where the virus is endemic, indicating that natural exposure provides long-lived immunity. The clinical aspects of MVEV infection (previously called Australian encephalitis, which also included a rare disease caused by KUNV) have been described for the 1951 (Robertson and McLorinan 1952) and 1974 (Bennett 1976) epidemics in south-eastern Australia, and in studies of more recent cases in Western Australia (Mackenzie et al. 1993) and the Northern Territories (Burrow et al. 1998). MVEV infection involves a prodromal stage with fever in all patients, commonly with features such as severe frontal headache, nausea, vomiting, dizziness, increasing confusion, and convulsions frequent among children. Within a period of ~5 days of onset, this progresses to obvious neurological disease resulting in encephalitis of variable severity. Signs of brain dysfunction such as drowsiness, irritability, confusion, fitting, ataxia, neck stiffness, speech disturbance, cranial nerve palsies, and movement disorders, which include parkinsonism and other tremors, indicate onset of encephalitis. In severe cases, this will progress to respiratory failure, coma, and death. The case fatality rate is high (15%–32%), while significant neurological sequelae with physical and/or intellectual handicap are seen in ~50% of survivors (Burrow et al. 1998; Mackenzie et al. 1993). Burrows et al. observed four clinical patterns of disease: (i) relentless progression to death, (ii) prominent spinal cord involvement, ("poliomyelitis-like"), (iii) cranial nerve/brainstem involvement and tremor, and (iv) encephalitis with complete recovery (Burrow et al. 1998). Flaccid paralysis with rapid progression to respiratory failure is a predictor of poor neurological outcome and death, and electrophysiological studies in these cases indicate extensive anterior horn cell involvement (Burrow et al. 1998; Einsiedel et al. 2003). Magnetic resonance imaging (MRI) reveals extensive and bilateral thalamic injury, and may prove helpful in assessing the clinical long-term outcomes of patients infected with MVEV (Burrow et al. 1998; Douglas et al. 2007; Einsiedel et al. 2003; Kienzle and Boyes 2003): mild cases of MVE have no apparent MRI changes with an excellent outcome, while more severe cases have striking changes and poor outcome. In one case report, MRI findings showed typical temporal lobe changes, suggesting that MVE can mimic herpes simplex encephalitis clinically and radiologically (Wong et al. 2005). An accurate and detailed travel history of patients, where there is a risk of exposure to MVEV, combined with serological testing are therefore important for correct diagnosis and patient management. Notably, MVE is after herpes simplex encephalitis, the second most serious acute viral encephalitis to be encountered in Australia, and the most common cause of viral encephalitis in tropical Australia (Burrow et al. 1998).

8.7 LABORATORY DIAGNOSIS OF MVEV INFECTIONS

8.7.1 SEROLOGICAL TESTS

Diagnosis of clinical MVEV infections in humans is based on the signs and symptoms at presentation (see above), but must be supported by laboratory confirmation using serological and/or molecular tests. Standard assays used to diagnose arbovirus infections in previous decades (e.g., haemagglutination inhibition and virus neutralization) have largely been replaced by ELISA, immunofluorescence assays, and more recently microsphere immunoassays (MIA) (Johnson et al. 2005). A diagnostic requirement for detection of virus-specific IgM in patient serum and preferably a 4-fold rise in virus-specific IgG between presentation (acute sample) and follow-up testing (convalescent sample) has been recommended for conclusive diagnosis (Mackenzie et al. 1993). Detection of MVEV-specific IgM in CSF samples has also been used successfully for laboratory diagnosis. Similar symptoms can present with infections in related flaviviruses that occur in Australia (e.g., MVEV, JEV, KUNV) and the high level of serological cross-reactivity observed between these viruses. It is highly recommended that samples must be tested against a complete panel of antigens prepared from local flaviviruses and at least a four-fold differential in antibody titer be determined to identify the infecting virus (Taylor et al. 2005).

8.7.2 VIRAL PROTEINS TARGETED IN SEROLOGICAL ASSAYS

Currently, high throughput serological assays used for the routine diagnosis of infections with MVEV and other flaviviruses are based on virion antigens in direct binding assay formats such as ELISA and MIA. These antigens have been successfully produced in large quantities from infected cell culture fluid by chemical inactivation of the virion with binary ethyleneimine and partial purification and concentration by lateral flow filtration (Pyke et al. 2004). However, the relatively high level of antigenic conservation of the envelope (E) protein between members of the JEV serogroup often results in a cross-reactive primary response or original antigenic sin compounded by previous infections with heterologous flaviviruses (Crill and Chang 2004).

More recently, serum antibody to other viral proteins such as NS1 (Blitvich et al. 2003a,b; Hall et al. 1995), prM (Hobson-Peters 2010; Setoh et al. 2011) or subdomains and peptides of the E protein (Estrada-Franco et al. 2003; Hobson-Peters et al. 2008a,b; Hobson-Peters 2010) or NS5 have also been suggested as more specific markers of infection with JEV serogroup viruses. Recombinantly expressed peptides or domains of E (DI and DIII), NS1, prM, and NS5 are currently being assessed by our laboratory and our collaborators to differentiate between members of the JEV serogroup in multiplexed MIAs (Johnson et al. 2005).

Blocking ELISAs have been developed to specifically identify antibodies of MVEV and KUNV in sentinel birds based on monoclonal antibodies to immuno-genic epitopes on the E and NS1 proteins (Hall et al. 1995; Hawkes et al. 1990). To some extent these assay have also been useful for screening for infections in horses; however, their use for human diagnosis has been limited due to inability to differentiate IgM from IgG responses and confounding results from previous infections with heterologous flaviviruses (Hall et al. 1995; Spicer et al. 1999).

The development of high throughput RT-PCR technology has enabled the use of molecular testing for RNA in viral infections on a routine basis. McMinn et al. described the use of RT-PCR to detect MVEV RNA in the serum of a 4-year-old boy suffering viral encephalitis at days 4 and 7 postonset (McMinn et al. 2000). This was crucial in the diagnosis of the disease as virus-specific IgM was undetectable and cross-reactive IgG responses due to a prior KUNV infection rendered the serological diagnosis inconclusive. Consistent with previous reports, virus could not be isolated from the PCR positive samples. These findings suggested that RT-PCR analysis of acute phase specimens is a useful complement to serological testing. More recently, Pyke et al. (2004) have described sensitive qRT-PCR protocols to test for MVEV, JEV, and KUNV in clinical specimens.

8.8 MVEV INFECTION IN ANIMALS

8.8.1 MICE

Mice provide an excellent animal model for MVE in humans. MVEV is neurotropic in mice; when small virus doses are injected directly into the brain it grows to high titers and uniformly causes fatal encephalitis (Licon Luna et al. 2002; MacDonald 1952a). In contrast, and similar to human infections, MVEV does not grow to detectable virus titers in extraneural tissues of adult immunocompetent mice following peripheral inoculation of the virus (Licon Luna et al. 2002; Lobigs et al. 2009; MacDonald 1952b), and often fails to produce morbidity or mortality over a wide dose-range (up to 10^6 PFU) (Licon Luna et al. 2002). This dose-independence of mortality and average survival time in peripherally infected adult mice has been reported for other flaviviruses (Larena et al. 2011; Wang et al. 2003), and suggests that equalizing factors exist: one such factor could be interferon (IFN) and other innate immune responses, the magnitude of which may inversely correlate with the virus dose inoculated.

The disease outcome in mice infected with MVEV is strongly age-dependent, where the animals are highly susceptible to a low-dose peripheral virus inoculum until the age of ~3 weeks (Lobigs et al. 1988; MacDonald 1952a; McMinn et al. 1996). In the weanling mouse model, MVEV is first detected in the lymph node draining the inoculation site at 24 h after inoculation into the footpad. Further replication at these sites generates a viremia between 2 and 3 days postinfection (pi) prior to entry of the virus into the CNS at 4 days pi, where peak virus titers occur between 6 and 9 days pi; the virus appears to enter the CNS via the olfactory lobes and spreads throughout the brain in the following 3 to 4 days, producing neuronal necrosis in the presence of inflammatory infiltrates, particularly noticeable in regions of the hippocampus (Matthews et al. 2000; McMinn et al. 1996). While the olfactory neuroepithelium is not protected by the blood-brain-barrier and is richly supplied with capillaries having fenestrated endothelia, thereby providing a potential route for virus entry into the CNS, other mechanisms by which MVEV may breach the blood-brain-barrier have also been canvassed, such as (i) virus infection of vascular endothelial cells of capillaries in the brain and release of virus into the brain parenchyma (Dropulic and Masters 1990; Licon Luna et al. 2002) or (ii) by diffusion of virus between capillary endothelial cells in individuals displaying leakiness of the blood-brain-barrier due to factors unrelated or secondary to the virus infection (reviewed by Mullbacher et al. 2003). The magnitude of viral load in the circulation, while mostly below the detection limit in adult immunocompetent mice, is a factor that contributes to virus infection of the CNS, based on two observations: extraneural infection of adult mice with a high dose (10^8 PFU) of MVEV results in early appearance of signs of encephalitis and high mortality (Colombage et al. 1998; Licon Luna et al. 2002) and infection of type I IFN response-defective mice produces high viremia, which correlates with infection of the CNS in all infected animals (Lobigs et al. 2003b).

Genetic resistance of wild and some inbred strains of mice to disease induced by MVEV and other flaviviruses has been described (Brinton and Perelygin 2003; Sangster et al. 1993, 1998; Silvia et al. 2004). Resistance is flavivirus-specific and is controlled by a single dominant autosomal gene. Resistant animals are infected productively, but produce significantly lower virus titers in brain relative to susceptible mice. The resistance gene (*Flv*) has been identified as an IFN-inducible gene encoding 2′-5′-oligoadenylate synthetase (Mashimo et al. 2002; Perelygin et al. 2002).

8.8.2 VETERINARY SPECIES AND WILDLIFE

Among domestic animals, potentially lethal nervous system disease associated with MVEV infection of horses is of concern. The limited reports of naturally acquired or experimental infections have documented nervous system disease in horses following an outbreak of MVEV in 1974 in south-eastern Australia, and only trace amounts of virus in blood in the absence of clinical signs other than a transient rise in temperature, respectively (Gard et al. 1977; Kay et al. 1987). Thus, MVEV infection of horses resembles that of humans in terms of low apparent to non-apparent infection ratio, and low or undetectable viremia, but high morbidity and mortality in clinical cases. Although currently a low incidence disease, demand for a vaccine against MVEV for use in horses may arise with increased agricultural development and human activity in MVEV endemic regions in northern Australia or altered frequency/severity of epidemic outbreaks of MVEV in south-eastern and Western Australia as a possible consequence of climate change. Indeed, recent incidents of fatal equine encephalitis in 2008 and 2011 have been associated with MVEV infection, as determined by detection of viral RNA or isolation of virus from necroscopy brain samples, and represent the first laboratory confirmed cases of MVE in horses (Gordon et al. 2012; Holmes et al. 2012). No clinical signs have been observed in a range of domestic animals and wildlife infected with MVEV, although some species (rabbits, gray kangaroos, native birds, pigs, dogs, and chicken) show evidence of moderate to high viremia (Kay et al. 1985a,b; Sanderson 1968).

8.9 GENETIC HETEROGENEITY AMONG NATURAL ISOLATES

Molecular epidemiological investigations on MVEV show only limited genetic differentiation of the majority of virus isolates over time and geographic distance in Australia (Lobigs et al. 1986, 1988; Coelen et al. 1988; Johansen et al. 2007). This observation that most MVEV isolates belong to a single genetic lineage has provided the strongest evidence, so far, for the hypothesis that the virus moves from enzootic foci in northern Australia to areas further south under the influence of particular climatic conditions. A second lineage of MVEV detected only in the Kimberley region of Western Australia may have been introduced from outside Australia (Johansen et al. 2007). In contrast to the overall genetic homogeneity of MVEV in Australia, virus strains from PNG display marked genetic divergence both between isolates and from the Australian genotype (Johansen et al. 2007; Lobigs et al. 1986). A major question relating to MVEV infections of humans is the reason for the high ratio of subclinical to clinical infection. One possibility is that certain strains are inherently more virulent than others; however, this is most likely not the case, (i) given the absence of genetic differences between virus isolated from fatal human cases and from other sources (mosquitoes or birds) and (ii) in view of their identical virulence profile in a mouse model of encephalitis (Lobigs et al. 1988). A naturally-occurring subtype of MVEV, Alfuy virus, also circulates in Australia but has neither been associated with human disease nor is it neuroinvasive in weanling mice even at high doses (May et al. 2006; Thiel et al. 2005).

8.10 MOLECULAR DETERMINANTS OF VIRULENCE

Field isolates of MVEV do not show significant variation in virulence in mouse models of MVE (Lobigs et al. 1988). In contrast, virus propagation in the laboratory and reverse genetics with the use of full-length infectious cDNA clones of MVEV (Hurrelbrink et al. 1999; Lee and Lobigs 2000) has allowed the generation of variants with altered virulence phenotypes. Studies on these variants are instrumental in structure–function analyses of virus replication and *in vivo* pathogenesis, and have identified molecular determinants of virulence attenuation with potential application in live vaccine development. The latter should involve mutations in the viral genome, which are not deleterious for replication, per se, but prevent disease in the mammalian host. We have shown that host cell adaptation of MVEV by serial passage in mammalian cell culture (human adenocarcinoma [SW13] and baby hamster kidney [BHK] cells) rapidly selects for variants with single amino acid changes in E protein domain III, which give rise to a high level of virulence attenuation (Lobigs et al. 1990). The substitutions in E protein (at residue 390) involve the acquisition of an increase in net positive charge on the virion surface that accounts for augmented binding affinity to heparan sulfate proteoglycans (Lee and Lobigs 2000). While this change in receptor usage benefits growth of the host cell-adapted variants in cell culture, it dramatically reduces their capacity to spread into the CNS from an extraneural site of infection in the mouse (Lee et al. 2004; Lee and Lobigs 2002). This loss of neuroinvasiveness is due to rapid clearance of variant virus from the blood as a result of nonproductive binding to glycosaminoglycans in tissues such as liver and on extracellular matrices. This *in vivo* mechanism of virulence attenuation also accounts, at least in part, for the loss of viscerotropism of yellow fever 17D vaccine (Lee and Lobigs 2008) and the attenuation of a JEV live vaccine (SA-14-14-2 strain) widely used in China (Lee and Lobigs 2002).

The E protein glycan of MVEV is conserved among all natural isolates and is an important marker of virulence: removal of the glycosylation site in the protein results in a marked reduction in neurovirulence and is associated with a reduced level of virus in the blood (Prow et al. 2011). Our studies and those of others show that virulence attenuation is due to less efficient secretion of the nonglycosylated than glycosylated virus from infected cells (Beasley et al. 2005; Hanna et al. 2005; Lee et al. 2010; Shirato et al. 2004; Setoh et al. 2012). Interestingly, this defect does not reduce the efficiency of virus growth in mosquito cells, where loss of the glycan markedly enhances infectivity of MVEV and other flaviviruses, albeit at the expense of efficient virus release (Lee et al. 2010).

Studies by McMinn and colleagues (Hurrelbrink and McMinn 2001; McMinn et al. 1995) and in our laboratory (Prow et al. 2011) have identified residues in the flexible hinge region of the MVEV E protein (residues 273–277) that are critical for virulence in mice. Amino acid substitutions introduced in this region are thought to inhibit pH-dependant rearrangement of the E protein required for efficient fusion triggered by mildly acidic pH, thereby reducing virus infectivity. Nevertheless, wildtype and hinge region variants of MVEV grow equally well in both vertebrate and invertebrate cell cultures, indicating that the reduced neuroinvasiveness of the latter is not due to a major abnormality of replication (Prow et al. 2011).

In contrast to the virulence variants described above, we have also identified molecular determinants of virulence attenuation, which impact on efficient virus replication. A single amino acid substitution in NS1 (residue 250) eliminates dimerization of the protein, but allows virus replication to continue; however, growth in Vero cells of the variant is retarded and levels of viremia and virulence in mice are markedly lower than those for wild-type MVEV (Clark et al. 2007). Similarly, amino acid changes at the junction of the prM and E proteins of MVEV, which uncouple the cleavage coordination between the two proteins required for efficient virus assembly, reduce growth in mammalian cell culture by ~10-fold (Lobigs and Lee 2004), and markedly reduce neuroinvasiveness in weanling mice (Lobigs et al. 2010a). Interestingly, a compensatory mutation in the prM signal peptide, which restores virus growth in cell culture to wild-type levels, does not repair the growth and virulence phenotype of the mutant virus in mice (Lobigs et al. 2010a). This demonstrates the greater sensitivity of animal models to reflect the impact of mutations that reduce the efficiency of virus replication that is found in cell culture.

The ability of flaviviruses to replicate efficiently in the mammalian host is dependent on their ability to evade, at least in part, the innate immune responses, particularly the antiviral activity of type 1 IFNs (Section 8.11.1). Recent studies on WNV and JEV have identified critical motifs in the viral nonstructural proteins that are responsible for enhanced resistance to the effects of IFN (Audsley et al. 2011; Daffis et al. 2011; Laurent-Rolle et al. 2010; Lin et al. 2008). Although similar studies have, so far, not been performed with MVEV, it is assumed that this virus also encodes IFN-resistance markers, which are important determinants of virulence.

8.11 IMMUNOBIOLOGY

8.11.1 INNATE IMMUNITY

Among the innate immune responses, type I IFN is of critical importance in recovery from infection with MVEV (Lobigs et al. 2003b). In response to cytosolic viral infection, activation of RIG-1-like receptors triggers IFN production, while specialized immune cells (dendritic cells and macrophages) can also produce type I IFNs following extracellular stimuli of viral origin by toll-like receptor (TLR) engagement. Type I IFNs (IFN-α and -β) then induce immediate antiviral effects in infected and neighboring cells and thereby limit viral spread. Mice that are deficient in IFN-α/β responses show sustained viremia, fulminant disease, rapid virus entry into the brain, and 100% mortality following administration of a low dose of MVEV by the intravenous route (Lobigs et al. 2003b). Given their exquisite sensitivity to infection with MVEV, type I IFN response-defective mice serve as an excellent model for virulence testing of attenuated variants of the virus (Clark et al. 2007; Lee and Lobigs 2002; Lobigs et al. 2010a; May et al. 2006). The therapeutic potential of recombinant IFN in human cases of MVE has not been investigated, although in the case of the closely related JEV, IFN therapy did not improve the outcome of patients with encephalitis (Solomon et al. 2003).

IFN-γ is made exclusively by natural killer (NK) and T cells, and has important immunoregulatory functions as well as antiviral activity. The latter is mostly mediated by nitric oxide (NO) synthesized by monocytes, following induction of the enzyme NO synthase by the cytokine. IFN-γ knock-out mice show a marginal increase in susceptibility to MVEV relative to wild-type mice, which is reflected in a small increase in virus titers in spleen, more rapid virus spread into the CNS and increased mortality (Lobigs et al. 2003b). The marginally protective role of IFN-γ against MVEV appears to be, at least in part, mediated by NO, given that mice deficient in NO synthase 2 also display a slight increase susceptibility to infection with MVEV in comparison to congenic control mice (Lobigs et al. 2003b). In contrast to this investigation in adult mice, a pathological contribution of NO production in the CNS following neutrophil infiltration has been described in the weanling mouse model for MVE (Andrews et al. 1999). This discrepancy on the role of NO in recovery from MVEV infection probably reflects the increased level of immunopathology in infected weanling relative to adult mice as a consequence of not yet fully competent regulation of innate immune responses of the developing immune system in the former, in combination with the higher viral burden in the young relative to adult mice.

NK cells are part of the innate immune response and have been implicated in the early defense against numerous viral infections (reviewed by Biron 2010). They are activated by type I IFNs, are important producers of IFN-γ, and mediators of cytotoxicity by causing apoptotic lysis of virally infected cells. While the induction of classical NK cell cytolytic activity as a result of flavivirus infection has been reported in mice (Mullbacher et al. 2003), it is thought that flaviviruses employ a strategy to evade the NK cell-mediated host defense, which involves up-regulation of major histocompatibility class I (MHC-I) molecules at the surface of infected cells (Lobigs et al. 1996, 2003a; Momburg et al. 2001). MHC-I engages with NK cell inhibitory receptors and can thereby down-regulate the NK cell response. To assess whether NK cell cytotoxicity plays a role in recovery of MVEV infection, we infected adult *beige* mice, which are deficient in the cytolytic function of NK cells (Roder and Duwe 1979), with a low dose of MVEV (10^2 PFU), intravenously. No significant difference in susceptibility of mice to the virus infection relative to wild-type mice (60% and 46% mortality, respectively [n = 10]) was observed (Licon Luna and Lobigs, unpublished).

8.11.2   HUMORAL IMMUNITY

To investigate whether the adaptive immune responses are required in resistance against MVEV, we compared the susceptibility of mice genetically deficient of both B and T cells (RAG-1$^{-/-}$ mice) to that of wild-type mice (Table 8.1). A low dose (10^2 PFU) intravenous infection with MVEV resulted in almost complete mortality of RAG-1$^{-/-}$ mice, while ~50% of congenic wild-type mice did not develop signs of encephalitis and survived. Interestingly, the average time to death of RAG-1$^{-/-}$ mice was significantly delayed relative to that in groups of wild-type mice, demonstrating an immunopathological contribution of the adaptive cellular immune responses to mortality with MVEV, which is T-cell-mediated (Licon Luna et al. 2002) (and see below). In a second experiment we show that virus-immune B cells but not T cells are required for the control of infection with MVEV (Table 8.1). Thus, transfer of MVEV-immune B cells completely protected against challenge with a ~50% lethal

TABLE 8.1
Role of Adaptive Immune Responses in Recovery from Infection with MVEV

Mouse Strain and Treatment[a]	No[b]	% Mortality[c]	ATD ± SEM[d]
Experiment 1			
B/6 (wt)	17	47	11.5 ± 0.6
RAG-1[-/-]	23	91 ($P = 0.003$)	17.1 ± 2.2
Experiment 2			
B/6 (wt) mock-treated	13	46	10.5 ± 1.0
B/6 (wt) + MVEV-immune B cells	5	0	
B/6 (wt) + MVEV-immune T cells	6	67	13.0 ± 0.8

Source:　R. M. Licon Luna (2004). On the role of cell-mediated cytotoxicity in a mouse model of flavivirus encephalitis. PhD thesis. The Australian National University, Canberra.

[a]　Six-week-old C57Bl/6 (B/6) or congenic recombinant activating gene (RAG) 1 knock-out mice (Mombaerts et al. 1992) were used. RAG-1-/- mice fail to produce mature B or T cells. Mice were challenged with 10^2 PFU MVEV by the intravenous route. For isolation of MVEV-immune B or T cell-enriched splenocytes, donor B/6 mice were infected with 10^2 PFU MVEV, i.v., and spleens collected at 6 days pi. B and T cell-enriched fractions (78 and 73% pure, respectively) were isolated by nylon wool separation and transferred (4×10^7 cells) into recipient mice at 3 days after challenge with MVEV.

[b]　Number of infected mice/group.

[c]　Difference in survival ratio relative to control mice was assessed using Fisher's exact test.

[d]　Average time to death, calculated in days, ± standard error of the mean (SEM).

dose of MVEV; in contrast, transfer of immune T cells failed to provide a survival advantage in comparison to a group of mock-treated mice infected with MVEV. This highlights the critical importance of the humoral immune response in recovery from infection with MVEV.

Mechanistically, antibodies elicited against infection with flaviviruses exhibit their action directly by neutralization of virus infectivity or indirectly by antibody-mediated cytotoxicity, Fc-γ-receptor-mediated clearance of virus/antibody complexes or complement-mediated cytotoxicity (Pierson et al. 2008). Neutralizing antibodies predominantly target the E protein, and several groups have isolated neutralizing monoclonal antibodies against MVEV and mapped the corresponding epitopes on the E protein (Hall et al. 1990; Hawkes et al. 1988; McMinn et al. 1995). Passive transfer of neutralizing monoclonal antibody offers significant protection in mice from otherwise lethal intraperitoneal virus challenge (Hawkes et al. 1988). Monoclonal antibodies against the MVEV NS1 protein have also been described (Clark et al. 2007; Hall et al. 1990); these can control flavivirus infection by their complement-mediated cytolytic potential (Hall et al. 1996; Schlesinger et al. 1986; Schlesinger et al. 1985).

8.11.3　CD4+ T-Cell Immunity

There are two predominant lineages of peripheral T cells that can be differentiated on the basis of their co-receptor expression (CD4+ vs. CD8+). CD4+ T cells contribute to the control of infection by various mechanisms, including antiviral and immunoregulatory cytokine production, antibody class switching, direct cytotoxicity and maintenance of CD8+ T-cell activity (Zhu et al. 2010). They recognize MHC-II/peptide complexes on antigen presenting cells (dendritic cells, macrophages, and B cells), and following activation proliferate and mature into one of three T helper subsets, Th1, Th2, or Th17, depending on the cytokine milieu. Similar to most viruses, infection with MVEV induces a strong Th1 response, which is reflected in the mouse in antibody isotype switching toward the biased production of IgG2a and IgG2b antibodies, while antibodies of the IgG1 isotype are rare (Colombage et al. 1998). While production of early IgM antibodies in flavivirus infection is T cell-independent, the sustained antibody response essential for virus clearance and immunological memory requires CD4+ T-cell help (Larena et al. 2011). Two early studies have mapped the source of peptide determinants recognized in association with MHC-II by MVEV-immune CD4+ T cells to the E protein and show cross-reactivity of the responses with related flaviviruses (Mathews et al. 1991, 1992).

8.11.4 CD8+ T-CELL IMMUNITY

CD8+ T cells destroy cells that they recognize as virally infected via two distinct mechanisms: ligation of the death receptor, Fas, on the target cell by FasL on the T cell or via exocytosis of specialized granules that contain the pore-forming protein perforin and the pro-apoptotic granzymes (reviewed by Chowdhury and Lieberman 2008; Voskoboinik, Smyth, and Trapani 2006). In addition, CD8+ T cells secrete IFN-γ and tumour necrosis factor (TNF) α in response to cognate antigen. Infection of mice with MVEV elicits functional, virus-specific, CD8+ T-cell responses characterized by *in vitro* cytotoxicity and ex vivo IFN-γ production (Licon Luna et al. 2002; Lobigs et al. 1994; Lobigs et al. 1997; Regner et al. 2001a,b,c). However, the memory cytotoxic T-cell response against MVEV exhibits the unusual feature that restimulation of MVEV-primed splenocytes with virus, after lengthy periods following priming, triggers high lysis of uninfected target cells; in contrast, re-stimulation with MVEV peptide-pulsed target cells boosts a potent virus-specific response (Mullbacher et al. 2003; Regner et al. 2001c). Accordingly, memory MVEV-immune CD8+ T cells are clearly generated as a consequence of a primary infection or immunization with recombinant subunit vaccines; however, the protective value of CD8+ T cells against secondary MVEV infection is probably relatively poor, given the high self-reactive component among the memory cytotoxic T cells.

To investigate the contribution of CD8+ T cells to recovery from primary infection in a mouse model of MVE, Licon Luna et al. compared the pathogenesis and mortality of mice with genetic defects in either or both of the cytolytic pathways relative to that of congenic wild-type mice, using low-dose, extraneural infection with MVEV (Licon Luna et al. 2002). This study showed that the cytolytic effector functions of CD8+ T cells facilitate invasion of MVEV into the brain and that MVEV-immune CD8+ T cells are detrimental in disease progression: mice deficient in either the granule-exocytosis or Fas-mediated pathway of cytotoxicity show delayed and reduced mortality, while mice deficient in both pathways are resistant to infection. While the mechanism that allows MVEV to breach the blood-brain-barrier remains uncertain, the above finding suggests that CD8$^+$ T-cell cytotoxicity may induce local breakdown (by killing virus-infected vascular endothelial cells of capillaries in the brain) and thereby facilitate virus entry into the CNS. CD8$^+$ T cells also increase pathology due to the inflammatory response in the infected brain. This is reflected in prolonged survival of mice defective in both granule exocytosis- and Fas-mediated pathways of cytotoxicity relative to immunocompetent mice, following peripheral infection with a high dose (10^8 PFU) of MVEV, which results in uniform and rapid virus entry into the CNS in both mouse strains (Licon Luna et al. 2002).

Regions in the viral polyprotein encompassing epitopes recognized in association with MHC-I by mouse MVEV-immune CD8$^+$ T cell have been mapped. Similar to other flaviviruses, the determinants are almost exclusively derived from the nonstructural proteins and are clustered in the region from NS3 to NS4B (Lobigs et al. 1994; Lobigs et al. 1997; Regner et al. 2001c). Two immunodominant H-2K^k-restricted peptides (MVE$_{1785}$: REHSGNEI and MVE$_{1971}$: DEGEGRVI) have been described (Lobigs et al. 1994; Regner et al. 2001c). The response against these determinants is broadly flavivirus cross-reactive, and paradoxically recognizes disparate epitopes from corresponding regions in NS3 from other flaviviruses but ignores more similar peptides from "self" and other virus families (Regner et al. 2001a). This suggests that primary sequence homology is not always the crucial factor in peptide recognition in the cross-reactive cellular immune responses against flaviviruses.

8.12   VACCINATION

There are no vaccines or antiviral agents available against MVEV and, given the relatively small number of human cases of encephalitic disease, there is no commercial interest for development of an MVEV-specific vaccine. However, it should be anticipated that the incidence of MVE increases as a consequence of ongoing industrial and agricultural development in northern Australia and associated increase of the "at-risk" population in regions of seasonal MVEV activity. Furthermore, it is unclear whether climate change will impact on the frequency and/ or severity of epidemic outbreaks of MVEV in southeastern and western Australia. Consequently, a public health demand for vaccination against the virus may arise and justify production of an MVEV-specific vaccine, most likely in public-private partnership. Given the vast worldwide expertise in vaccine research and development against the closely related JEV (reviewed by Beasley et al. 2008; Monath 2002), it is almost certain that manufacture of an effective and safe MVEV vaccine is feasible within a relatively short period of time. The induction of potent and durable memory B cells that produce high-affinity, neutralizing antibody against the E protein should be considered as the prime criterion for efficacy of a putative MVEV vaccine, based on our understanding of the immunological correlates for protection against the virus (Section 8.11). Several studies in mice illustrate that experimental vaccines encoding the viral prM and E proteins, which are secreted in the form of highly immunogenic subviral particles (Lobigs 1993), induce protective humoral immunity; these include DNA-based, alphavirus-vectored and vaccinia virus-vectored delivery of the MVEV structural proteins (Colombage et al. 1998; Hall et al. 1996; Kroeger and McMinn 2002; Lobigs et al. 2003c).

An alternative approach to vaccination against MVEV is the use of available vaccines against JEV, which can protect against the former (reviewed in Lobigs and Diamond 2012). It has been known for many years that at least in animal models, live viral infection with one virus belonging to the JEV serocomplex will induce cross-protective immunity against other members of the serocomplex (Fang and Reisen 2006; Goverdhan et al. 1992; Hammon and Sather 1956; Tesh et al. 2002; Williams et al. 2001). Consistent with this observation, preclinical vaccine trials in mice and horses have shown potent cross-protective immunity against MVEV induced by live (ChimeriVax-JE) or inactivated (Advax-ccJE) candidate vaccines against JEV (Lobigs et al. 2009, 2010b). ChimeriVax-JE is constructed from yellow fever virus cDNA by replacement of the prM-E proteins with those of an attenuated JEV strain and has undergone phase 2 and phase 3 trials for safety and efficacy in humans (reviewed by Appaiahgari and Vrati 2010); Advax-ccJE is a cell-culture-grown JEV antigen formulated with a carbohydrate-based adjuvant that potently stimulates vaccine immunogenicity without the increased reactogenicity seen with other adjuvants (Petrovsky 2008).

Vaccine efficacy in terms of magnitude and/or quality of the vaccine-elicited immune response is most likely the critical property of the novel JEV vaccines for successful vaccination against MVEV. The first internationally licensed but recently discontinued JE vaccine (JE-VAX; Biken Institute) does not efficiently cross-protect, and the poor immunity induced with JE-VAX can result, under specific experimental conditions, in infection-enhancement in mice following challenge with MVEV (Broom et al. 2000; Lobigs et al. 2009, 2003c; Wallace et al. 2003). The phenomenon of antibody-mediated enhancement of infection was discovered in studies using MVEV and related flaviviruses (Hawkes 1964). The mechanism for this finding is thought to involve the enhanced uptake into Fc receptor-bearing cells of virus, when bound to an antibody that fails to neutralize, resulting in an increase in viral burden and disease severity. While the remote risk of immune enhancement was a consideration against recommendation of the emergency use of JE-VAX in the face of an epidemic of MVEV (Marshall 1988), the significantly enhanced immunogenicity of adjuvanted and live, recombinant candidate JEV vaccines (Lobigs et al. 2009, 2010b) strongly indicates that protection against multiple viruses belonging to the serocomplex can be achieved with the one vaccine. An additional public health consideration for the availability of JEV vaccines with cross-protective value against MVEV in Australia is the ongoing threat of emergence of JEV on the Australian mainland (Mackenzie et al. 2004). This scenario would necessitate extensive vaccination against JEV, where the choice of vaccine should be guided by its immunogenic potency to prevent the remote risk of immune-enhancement of infection with MVEV with the benefit of protection against the endemic pathogen.

REFERENCES

Anderson, S. G. (1952). Murray Valley encephalitis; epidemiological aspects. *Med J Aust* 1(4), 97–100.

Anderson, S. G. (1954). Murray Valley encephalitis and Australian X disease. *J Hyg (Lond)* 52(4), 447–68.

Andrews, D. M., Matthews, V. B., Sammels, L. M., Carrello, A. C., and McMinn, P. C. (1999). The severity of murray valley encephalitis in mice is linked to neutrophil infiltration and inducible nitric oxide synthase activity in the central nervous system. *J Virol* 73, 8781–8790.

Appaiahgari, M. B., and Vrati, S. (2010). IMOJEV((R)): a Yellow fever virus-based novel Japanese encephalitis vaccine. *Exp Rev Vaccines* 9, 1371–1384.

Audsley, M., Edmonds, J., Liu, W., Mokhonov, V., Mokhonova, E., Melian, E. B., Prow, N., Hall, R. A., and Khromykh, A. A. (2011). Virulence determinants between New York 99 and Kunjin strains of West Nile virus. *Virology* 414(1), 63–73.

Beasley, D. W., Lewthwaite, P., and Solomon, T. (2008). Current use and development of vaccines for Japanese encephalitis. *Exp Opin Biol Ther* 8, 95–106.

Beasley, D. W., Whiteman, M. C., Zhang, S., Huang, C. Y., Schneider, B. S., Smith, D. R., Gromowski, G. D., Higgs, S., Kinney, R. M., and Barrett, A. D. (2005). Envelope protein glycosylation status influences mouse neuroinvasion phenotype of genetic lineage 1 West Nile virus strains. *J Virol* 79, 8339–8347.

Bennett, N. M. (1976). Murray Valley encephalitis 1974: clinical features. *Med J Aust* (12), 446–450.

Biron, C. A. (2010). Expansion, maintenance, and memory in NK and T cells during viral infections: responding to pressures for defense and regulation. *PLoS Pathog* 6(3), e1000816.

Blitvich, B. J., Bowen, R. A., Marlenee, N. L., Hall, R. A., Bunning, M. L., and Beaty, B. J. (2003a). Epitope-blocking enzyme-linked immunosorbent assays for detection of west nile virus antibodies in domestic mammals. *J Clin Microbiol* 41(6), 2676–2679.

Blitvich, B. J., Marlenee, N. L., Hall, R. A., Calisher, C. H., Bowen, R. A., Roehrig, J. T., Komar, N., Langevin, S. A., and Beaty, B. J. (2003b). Epitope-blocking enzyme-linked immunosorbent assays for the detection of serum antibodies to west nile virus in multiple avian species. *J Clin Microbiol* 41(3), 1041–1047.

Boyle, D. B., Marshall, I. D., and Dickerman, R. W. (1983). Primary antibody responses of herons to experimental infection with Murray Valley encephalitis and Kunjin viruses. *Aust J Exp Biol Med Sci* 61 (Pt 6), 665–674.

Brinton, M. A., and Perelygin, A. A. (2003). Genetic resistance to flaviviruses. *Adv Virus Res* 60, 43–85.

Broom, A. K., Lindsay, M. D., Plant, A. J., Wright, A. E., Condon, R. J., and Mackenzie, J. S. (2002). Epizootic activity of Murray Valley encephalitis virus in an aboriginal community in the southeast Kimberley region of Western Australia: results of cross-sectional and longitudinal serologic studies. *Am J Trop Med Hyg* 67(3), 319–323.

Broom, A. K., Wallace, M. J., Mackenzie, J. S., Smith, D. W., and Hall, R. A. (2000). Immunization with gamma globulin of Murray Valley encephalitis virus and with an inactivated Japanese encephalitis virus vaccine as prophylaxis against Australian encephalitis: Evaluation in a mouse model. *J Med Virol* 61, 259–265.

Broom, A. K., and Whelan, P. I. (2005). Sentinel Chicken Surveillance Program in Australia, July 2003 to June 2004. *Commun Dis Intell* 29(1), 65–70.

Broom, A. K., Wright, A. E., MacKenzie, J. S., Lindsay, M. D., and Robinson, D. (1989). Isolation of Murray Valley encephalitis and Ross River viruses from Aedes normanensis (Diptera: Culicidae) in Western Australia. *J Med Entomol* 26(2), 100–103.

Brown, A., Bolisetty, S., Whelan, P., Smith, D., and Wheaton, G. (2002). Reappearance of human cases due to Murray Valley encephalitis virus and Kunjin virus in central Australia after an absence of 26 years. *Commun Dis Intell* 26(1), 39–44.

Burrow, J. N., Whelan, P. I., Kilburn, C. J., Fisher, D. A., Currie, B. J., and Smith, D. W. (1998). Australian encephalitis in the Northern Territory: clinical and epidemiological features 1987–1996. *Aust N Z J Med* 28, 590–596.

Carver, S., Bestall, A., Jardine, A., and Ostfeld, R. S. (2009). Influence of hosts on the ecology of arboviral transmission: potential mechanisms influencing dengue, murray valley encephalitis, and ross river virus in australia. *Vector Borne Zoonotic Dis* 9(1), 51–64.

Chambers, T. J., Hahn, C. S., Galler, R., and Rice, C. M. (1990). Flavivirus genome organization, expression, and replication. *Annu Rev Microbiol* 44, 649–88.

Chowdhury, D., and Lieberman, J. (2008). Death by a thousand cuts: granzyme pathways of programmed cell death. *Annu Rev Immunol* 26, 389–420.

Clark, D. C., Lobigs, M., Lee, E., Howard, M. J., Clark, K., Blitvich, B. J., and Hall, R. A. (2007). *In situ* reactions of monoclonal antibodies with a viable mutant of Murray Valley encephalitis virus reveal an absence of dimeric NS1 protein. *J Gen Virol* 88, 1175–1183.

Coelen, R. J., and Mackenzie, J. S. (1988). Genetic variation of Murray Valley encephalitis virus. *J Gen Virol* 69 (Pt 8), 1903–1912.

Colombage, G., Hall, R., Pavy, M., and Lobigs, M. (1998). DNA-based and alphavirus-vectored immunisation with prM and E proteins elicits long-lived and protective immunity against the flavivirus, Murray Valley encephalitis virus. *Virology* 250, 151–163.

Colwell, R. R., Epstein, P. R., Gubler, D., Maynard, N., McMichael, A. J., Patz, J. A., Sack, R. B., and Shope, R. (1998). Climate change and human health. *Science* 279(5353), 968–969.

Crill, W. D., and Chang, G. J. (2004). Localization and characterization of flavivirus envelope glycoprotein cross-reactive epitopes. *J Virol* 78(24), 13975–13986.

Daffis, S., Lazear, H. M., Liu, W. J., Audsley, M., Engle, M., Khromykh, A. A., and Diamond, M. S. (2011). The naturally attenuated Kunjin strain of West Nile virus shows enhanced sensitivity to the host type I interferon response. *J Virol* 85(11), 5664–5668.

Dalgarno, L., Trent, D. W., Strauss, J. H., and Rice, C. M. (1986). Partial nucleotide sequence of the Murray Valley encephalitis virus genome. Comparison of the encoded polypeptides with yellow fever virus structural and non-structural proteins. *J Mol Biol* 187(3), 309–323.

Doggett, S., Clancy, J., Haniotis, J., Webb, C., Russell, R. and Institute for Clinical Pathology & Medical Research (2008). The New South Wales Arbovirus Surveillance and mosquito monitoring program: Annual Report 2007–2008.

Doherty, R. L. (1974). Arthropod-borne viruses in Australia and their relation to infection and disease. *Prog Med Virol* 17(0), 136–192.

Doherty, R. L., Carley, J. G., Mackerras, M. J., and Marks, E. N. (1963). Studies of arthropod-borne virus infections in Queensland. III. Isolation and characterization of virus strains from wild-caught mosquitoes in North Queensland. *Aust J Exp Biol Med Sci* 41, 17–39.

Douglas, M. W., Stephens, D. P., Burrow, J. N., Anstey, N. M., Talbot, K., and Currie, B. J. (2007). Murray Valley encephalitis in an adult traveller complicated by long-term flaccid paralysis: case report and review of the literature. *Trans R Soc Trop Med Hyg* 101, 284–288.

Dropulic, B., and Masters, C. L. (1990). Entry of neurotropic arboviruses into the central nervous system: an *in vitro* study using mouse brain endothelium. *J Infect Dis* 161, 685–691.

Einsiedel, L., Kat, E., Ravindran, J., Slavotinek, J., and Gordon, D. L. (2003). MR findings in Murray Valley encephalitis. *AJNR Am J Neuroradiol* 24, 137913–137982.

Estrada-Franco, J. G., Navarro-Lopez, R., Beasley, D. W., Coffey, L., Carrara, A. S., Travassos da Rosa, A., Clements, T., Wang, E., Ludwig, G. V., Cortes, A. C., Ramirez, P. P., Tesh, R. B., Barrett, A. D., and Weaver, S. C. (2003). West Nile virus in Mexico: evidence of widespread circulation since July 2002. *Emerg Infect Dis* 9(12), 1604–1607.

Fang, Y., and Reisen, W. K. (2006). Previous infection with West Nile or St. Louis encephalitis viruses provides cross protection during reinfection in house finches. *Am J Trop Med Hyg* 75, 480–485.

Fernandez-Garcia, M. D., Mazzon, M., Jacobs, M., and Amara, A. (2009). Pathogenesis of flavivirus infections: using and abusing the host cell. *Cell Host Microbe* 5(4), 318–328.

French, E. L. (1952). Murray Valley encephalitis isolation and characterization of the aetiological agent. *Med J Aust* 1(4), 100–103.

French, E. L. (1973). A review of arthropod-borne virus infections affecting man and animals in Australia. *Aust J Exp Biol Med Sci* 51(2), 131–158.

Frost, M. J., Zhang, J., Edmonds, J. H., Prow, N. A., Gu, X., Davis, R., Hornitzky, C., Arzey, K. E., Finlaison, D., Hick, P., Read, A., Hobson-Peters, J., May, F. J., Doggett, S. L., Haniotis, J., Russell, R. C., Hall, R. A., Khromykh, A. A., and Kirkland, P. D. (2012). Characterization of virulent West Nile virus Kunjin strain, Australia, 2011. *Emerg Infect Dis* 18(5), 792–800.

Gard, G. P., Marshall, I. D., Walker, K. H., Acland, H. M., and Saren, W. G. (1977). Association of Australian arboviruses with nervous disease in horses. *Aust Vet J* 53, 61–66.

Gordon, A. N., Marbach, C. R., Oakey, J., Edmunds, G., Condon, K., Diviney, S. M., Williams, D. T., and Bingham, J. (2012). Confirmed case of encephalitis caused by Murray Valley encephalitis virus infection in a horse. *J Vet Diagn Invest* 24(2), 431–436.

Goverdhan, M. K., Kulkarni, A. B., Gupta, A. K., Tupe, C. D., and Rodrigues, J. J. (1992). Two-way cross-protection between West Nile and Japanese encephalitis viruses in bonnet macaques. *Acta Virol* 36, 277–283.

Hall, R. A., Brand, T. N. H., Lobigs, M., Sangster, M. Y., Howard, M. J., and Mackenzie, J. S. (1996). Protective immune responses to the E and NS1 proteins of Murray Valley encephalitis virus in hybrids of flavivirus-resistant mice. *J Gen Virol* 77, 1287–1294.

Hall, R. A., Broom, A. K., Hartnett, A. C., Howard, M. J., and Mackenzie, J. S. (1995). Immunodominant epitopes on the NS1 protein of MVE and KUN viruses serve as targets for a blocking ELISA to detect virus-specific antibodies in sentinel animal serum. *J Virol Methods* 51(2–3) 201–10.

Hall, R. A., Kay, B. H., Burgess, G. W., Clancy, P., and Fanning, I. D. (1990). Epitope analysis of the envelope and non-structural glycoproteins of Murray Valley encephalitis virus. *J Gen Virol* 71, 2923–2930.

Hammon, W. M., and Sather, G. E. (1956). Immunity of hamsters to West Nile and Murray Valley viruses following immunization with St. Louis and Japanese B. *Proc Soc Exp Biol Med* 91, 521–524.

Hanna, S. L., Pierson, T. C., Sanchez, M. D., Ahmed, A. A., Murtadha, M. M., and Doms, R. W. (2005). N-linked glycosylation of west nile virus envelope proteins influences particle assembly and infectivity. *J Virol* 79(21), 13262–13274.

Harrison, S. C. (2008). Viral membrane fusion. *Nat Struct Mol Biol* 15(7), 690–698.

Hawkes, R. A. (1964). Enhancement of the infectivity of arboviruses by specific antisera produced in domestic fowls. *Aust J Exp Biol Med Sci* 42, 465–482.

Hawkes, R. A., Boughton, C. R., Naim, H. M., Wild, J., and Chapman, B. (1985). Arbovirus infections of humans in New South Wales. Seroepidemiology of the flavivirus group of togaviruses. *Med J Aust* 143(12–13), 555–561.

Hawkes, R. A., Pamplin, J., Boughton, C. R., and Naim, H. M. (1993). Arbovirus infections of humans in high-risk areas of south-eastern Australia: a continuing study. *Med J Aust* 159(3), 159–162.

Hawkes, R. A., Roehrig, J. T., Boughton, C. R., Naim, H. M., Orwell, R., and Anderson-Stuart, P. (1990). Defined epitope blocking with Murray Valley encephalitis virus and monoclonal antibodies: laboratory and field studies. *J Med Virol* 32(1), 31–38.

Hawkes, R. A., Roehrig, J. T., Hunt, A. R., and Moore, G. A. (1988). Antigenic structure of the Murray Valley encephalitis virus E glycoprotein. *J Gen Virol* 69, 1105–1109.

Hobson-Peters, J. (2010). Characterisation and recombinant expression of antigens for the rapid diagnosis of West Nile virus infection. PhD thesis. The University of Queensland.

Hobson-Peters, J., Shan, J., Hall, R. A., and Toye, P. (2008a). Mammalian expression of functional autologous red cell agglutination reagents for use in diagnostic assays. *J Virol Methods* 168(1–2), 177–190.

Hobson-Peters, J., Toye, P., Sanchez, M. D., Bossart, K. N., Wang, L. F., Clark, D. C., Cheah, W. Y., and Hall, R. A. (2008b). A glycosylated peptide in the West Nile virus envelope protein is immunogenic during equine infection. *J Gen Virol* 89(Pt 12), 3063–3072.

Holmes, J. M., Gilkerson, J. R., El Hage, C. M., Slocombe, R. F., and Muurlink, M. A. (2012). Murray Valley encephalomyelitis in a horse. *Aust Vet J* 90(7), 252–254.

Hurrelbrink, R. J., and McMinn, P. C. (2001). Attenuation of Murray Valley encephalitis virus by site-directed mutagenesis of the hinge and putative receptor-binding regions of the envelope protein. *J Virol* 75(16), 7692–7702.

Hurrelbrink, R. J., Nestorowicz, A., and McMinn, P. C. (1999). Characterization of infectious Murray Valley encephalitis virus derived from a stably cloned genome-length cDNA. *J Gen Virol* 80 (Pt 12), 3115–3125.

Johansen, C., Avery, V., Power, S., Zammit, C., Masters, L., Frestel, S., Geerlings, K., Sturrock, K., Gordon, C., Smith, D., and Shellam, G. (2008). The University of Western Australia Arbovirus Surveillance and Research Laboratory Annual Report: 2007–2008. The University of Western Australia.

Johansen, C. A., Susai, V., Hall, R. A., Mackenzie, J. S., Clark, D. C., May, F. J., Hemmerter, S., Smith, D. W., and Broom, A. K. (2007). Genetic and phenotypic differences between isolates of Murray Valley encephalitis virus in Western Australia 1972–2003. *Virus Genes* 35(2), 147–154.

Johnson, A. J., Noga, A. J., Kosoy, O., Lanciotti, R. S., Johnson, A. A., and Biggerstaff, B. J. (2005). Duplex microsphere-based immunoassay for detection of anti-West Nile virus and anti-St. Louis encephalitis virus immunoglobulin m antibodies. *Clin Diagn Lab Immunol* 12(5), 566–574.

Kay, B. H., and Carley, J. G. (1980). Transovarial transmission of Murray Valley encephalitis virus by Aedes aegypti (L). *Aust J Exp Biol Med Sci* 58(5), 501–504.

Kay, B. H., Fanning, I. D., and Carley, J. G. (1984). The vector competence of Australian Culex annulirostris with Murray Valley encephalitis and Kunjin viruses. *Aust J Exp Biol Med Sci* 62 (Pt 5), 641–650.

Kay, B. H., Fanning, I. D., and Mottram, P. (1989). The vector competence of Culex annulirostris, Aedes sagax and Aedes alboannulatus for Murray Valley encephalitis virus at different temperatures. *Med Vet Entomol* 3(2), 107–112.

Kay, B. H., Hall, R. A., Fanning, I. D., and Young, P. L. (1985a). Experimental infection with Murray Valley encephalitis virus: galahs, sulphur-crested cockatoos, corellas, black ducks and wild mice. *Aust J Exp Biol Med Sci* 63 (Pt 5), 599–606.

Kay, B. H., Young, P. L., Hall, R. A., and Fanning, I. D. (1985b). Experimental infection with Murray Valley encephalitis virus. Pigs, cattle, sheep, dogs, rabbits, macropods and chickens. *Aust J Exp Biol Med Sci* 63(Pt 1), 109–126.

Kay, B. H., Pollitt, C. C., Fanning, I. D., and Hall, R. A. (1987). The experimental infection of horses with Murray Valley encephalitis and Ross River viruses. *Aust Vet J* 64, 52–55.

Kienzle, N., and Boyes, L. (2003). Murray Valley encephalitis: case report and review of neuroradiological features. *Australas Radiol* 47, 61–63.

Kroeger, M. A., and McMinn, P. C. (2002). Murray Valley encephalitis virus recombinant subviral particles protect mice from lethal challenge with virulent wild-type virus. *Arch Virol* 147, 1155–1172.

Larena, M., Regner, M., Lee, E., and Lobigs, M. (2011). Pivotal Role of Antibody and Subsidiary Contribution of CD8+ T Cells to Recovery from Infection in a Murine Model of Japanese Encephalitis. *J Virol* 85, 5446–5455.

Laurent-Rolle, M., Boer, E. F., Lubick, K. J., Wolfinbarger, J. B., Carmody, A. B., Rockx, B., Liu, W., Ashour, J., Shupert, W. L., Holbrook, M. R., Barrett, A. D., Mason, P. W., Bloom, M. E., Garcia-Sastre, A., Khromykh, A. A., and Best, S. M. (2010). The NS5 protein of the virulent West Nile virus NY99 strain is a potent antagonist of type I interferon-mediated JAK-STAT signaling. *J Virol* 84(7), 3503–3515.

Lee, E., Hall, R. A., and Lobigs, M. (2004). Common E protein determinants for attenuation of glycosaminoglycan-binding variants of Japanese encephalitis and West Nile viruses. *J Virol* 78, 8271–8280.

Lee, E., Leang, S. K., Davidson, A., and Lobigs, M. (2010). Both E protein glycans adversely affect dengue virus infectivity but are beneficial for virion release. *J Virol* 84(10), 5171–5180.

Lee, E., and Lobigs, M. (2000). Substitutions at the putative receptor-binding site of an encephalitic flavivirus alter virulence and host cell tropism and reveal a role for glycosaminoglycans in entry. *J Virol* 74(19), 8867–8875.

Lee, E., and Lobigs, M. (2002). Mechanism of virulence attenuation of GAG-binding variants of Japanese encephalitis and Murray Valley encephalitis viruses. *J Virol* 76, 4901–4911.

Lee, E., and Lobigs, M. (2008). E protein domain III determinants of yellow fever virus 17D vaccine strain enhance binding to glycosaminoglycans, impede virus spread, and attenuate virulence. *J Virol* 82(12), 6024–6033.

Licon Luna, R. M., Lee, E., Müllbacher, A., Blanden, R. V., Langman, R., and Lobigs, M. (2002). Lack of both Fas ligand and perforin protects from flavivirus-mediated encephalitis in mice. *J Virol* 76, 3202–3211.

Lin, C. W., Cheng, C. W., Yang, T. C., Li, S. W., Cheng, M. H., Wan, L., Lin, Y. J., Lai, C. H., Lin, W. Y., and Kao, M. C. (2008). Interferon antagonist function of Japanese encephalitis virus NS4A and its interaction with DEAD-box RNA helicase DDX42. *Virus Res* 137(1), 49–55.

Lindenbach, B. D., and Rice, C. M. (2003). Molecular biology of flaviviruses. *Adv Virus Res* 59, 23–61.

Lobigs, M. (1993). Flavivirus premembrane protein cleavage and spike heterodimer secretion require the function of the viral proteinase NS3. *Proc Natl Acad Sci U S A* 90, 6218–6222.

Lobigs, M., Arthur, C. E., Müllbacher, A., and Blanden, R. V. (1994). The flavivirus nonstructural protein, NS3, is a dominant source of cytotoxic T cell peptide determinants. *Virology* 202, 195–201.

Lobigs, M., Blanden, R. V., and Müllbacher, A. (1996). Flavivirus-induced up-regulation of MHC class I antigens; implications for the induction of CD8+ T-cell-mediated autoimmunity. *Immunol Rev* 152, 5–19.

Lobigs, M., and Diamond, M. S. (2012). Feasibility of cross-protective vaccination against flaviviruses of the Japanese encephalitis serocomplex. *Expert Rev Vaccines* 11(2), 177–187.

Lobigs, M., Larena, M., Alsharifi, M., Lee, E., and Pavy, M. (2009). Live chimeric and inactivated Japanese encephalitis virus vaccines differ in their cross-protective values against Murray Valley encephalitis virus. *J Virol* 83, 2436–2445.

Lobigs, M., and Lee, E. (2004). Inefficient signalase cleavage promotes efficient nucleocapsid incorporation into budding flavivirus membranes. *J Virol* 78, 178–186.

Lobigs, M., Lee, E., Ng, M. L., Pavy, M., and Lobigs, P. (2010a). A flavivirus signal peptide balances the catalytic activity of two proteases and thereby facilitates virus morphogenesis. *Virology* 401, 80–89.

Lobigs, M., Marshall, I. D., Weir, R. C., and Dalgarno, L. (1986). Genetic differentiation of Murray Valley encephalitis virus in Australia and Papua New Guinea. *Aust J Exp Biol Med Sci* 64 (Pt 6), 571–585.

Lobigs, M., Marshall, I. D., Weir, R. C., and Dalgarno, L. (1988). Murray Valley encephalitis virus field strains from Australia and Papua New Guinea: studies on the sequence of the major envelope protein gene and virulence for mice. *Virology* 165(1), 245–255.

Lobigs, M., Müllbacher, A., and Pavy, M. (1997). The CD8+ cytotoxic T cell response to flavivirus infection. *Arbovirus Res Aust* 7, 160–165.

Lobigs, M., Mullbacher, A., and Regner, M. (2003a). MHC class I up-regulation by flaviviruses: Immune interaction with unknown advantage to host or pathogen. *Immunol Cell Biol* 81, 217–223.

Lobigs, M., Mullbacher, A., Wang, Y., Pavy, M., and Lee, E. (2003b). Role of type I and type II interferon responses in recovery from infection with an encephalitic flavivirus. *J Gen Virol* 84, 567–572.

Lobigs, M., Pavy, M., and Hall, R. A. (2003c). Cross-protective and infection-enhancing immunity In mice vaccinated against flaviviruses belonging to the japanese encephalitis virusserocomplex. *Vaccine* 21(15), 1572–1579.

Lobigs, M., Pavy, M., Hall, R. A., Lobigs, P., Cooper, P., Komiya, T., Toriniwa, H., and Petrovsky, N. (2010b). An inactivated Vero cell-grown Japanese encephalitis vaccine formulated with Advax, a novel inulin-based adjuvant, induces protective neutralizing antibody against homologous and heterologous flaviviruses. *J Gen Virol* 91, 1407–1417.

Lobigs, M., Usha, R., Nestorowicz, A., Marshall, I. D., Weir, R. C., and Dalgarno, L. (1990). Host cell selection of Murray Valley encephalitis virus variants altered at an RDG sequence in the envelope protein and in mouse virulence. *Virology* 176, 587–595.

MacDonald, F. (1952a). Murray Valley encephalitis infection in the laboratory mouse. I. Influence of age on the susceptibility of infection. *Aust J Exp Biol Med Sci* 30, 319–324.

MacDonald, F. (1952b). Murray Valley encephalitis infection in the laboratory mouse. II. Multiplication of virus inoculated intramuscularly. *Aust J Exp Biol Med Sci* 30, 325–332.

Mackenzie, J. S., and Broom, A. K. (1995). Australian X disease, Murray Valley encephalitis and the French connection. *Vet Microbiol* 46(1–3), 79–90.

Mackenzie, J. S., Gubler, D. J., and Petersen, L. R. (2004). Emerging flaviviruses: the spread and resurgence of Japanese encephalitis, West Nile and dengue viruses. *Nat Med* 10(12 Suppl), S98–S109.

Mackenzie, J. S., Lindsay, M. D., Coelen, R. J., Broom, A. K., Hall, R. A., and Smith, D. W. (1994). Arboviruses causing human disease in the Australasian zoogeographic region. *Arch Virol* 136(3–4), 447–467.

Mackenzie, J. S., Smith, D. W., Broom, A. K., and Bucens, M. R. (1993). Australian encephalitis in Western Australia 1978–1991. *Med J Aust* 158, 591–595.

Mackenzie, J. S., and Williams, D. T. (2009). The zoonotic flaviviruses of southern, southeastern and eastern Asia, and Australasia: the potential for emergent viruses. *Zoonoses Publ Health* 56(6–7), 338–356.

Marshall, I. D. (1988). Murray Valley and Kunjin encephalitis. *In* "The Arboviruses: Epidemiology and Ecology" (T. P. Monath, Ed.), Vol. III, pp. 151–189. Boca Raton, FL, CRC Press.

Mashimo, T., Lucas, M., Simon-Chazottes, D., Frenkiel, M. P., Montagutelli, X., Ceccaldi, P. E., Deubel, V., Guenet, J. L., and Despres, P. (2002). A nonsense mutation in the gene encoding 2′–5′-oligoadenylate synthetase/L1 isoform is associated with West Nile virus susceptibility in laboratory mice. *Proc Natl Acad Sci U S A* 99, 11311–11316.

Mathews, J. H., Allan, J. E., Roehrig, J. T., Brubaker, J. R., Uren, M. F., and Hunt, A. R. (1991). T-helper cell and associated antibody response to synthetic peptides of the E glycoprotein of Murray Valley encephalitis virus. *J Virol* 65, 5141–5148.

Mathews, J. H., Roehrig, J. T., Brubaker, J. R., Hunt, A. R., and Allan, J. E. (1992). A synthetic peptide to the E glycoprotein of Murray Valley encephalitis virus defines multiple virus-reactive T- and B-cell epitopes. *J Virol* 66, 6555–6562.

Matthews, V., Robertson, T., Kendrick, T., Abdo, M., Papadimitriou, J., and McMinn, P. (2000). Morphological features of Murray Valley encephalitis virus infection in the central nervous system of Swiss mice. *Int J Exp Pathol* 81, 31–40.

May, F. J., Lobigs, M., Lee, E., Gendle, D. J., Mackenzie, J. S., Broom, A. K., Conlan, J. V., and Hall, R. A. (2006). Biological, antigenic and phylogenetic characterization of the flavivirus Alfuy. *J Gen Virol* 87, 329–337.

McMinn, P. C., Carman, P. G., and Smith, D. W. (2000). Early diagnosis of Murray Valley encephalitis by reverse transcriptase-polymerase chain reaction. *Pathology* 32(1), 49–51.

McMinn, P. C., Dalgarno, L., and Weir, R. C. (1996). A comparison of the spread of Murray Valley encephalitis viruses of high or low neuroinvasiveness in the tissues of Swiss mice after peripheral inoculation. *Virology* 220, 414–423.

McMinn, P. C., Lee, E., Hartley, S., Roehrig, J. T., Dalgarno, L., and Weir, R. C. (1995). Murray valley encephalitis virus envelope protein antigenic variants with altered hemagglutination properties and reduced neuroinvasiveness in mice. *Virology* 211, 10–20.

Mellor, P. S., and Leake, C. J. (2000). Climatic and geographic influences on arboviral infections and vectors. *Rev Sci Tech* 19(1), 41–54.

Miles, J. A., Chir, B., Fowler, M. C., and Howes, D. W. (1951). Isolation of a virus from encephalitis in South Australia: a preliminary report. *Med J Aust* 1(22), 799–800.

Mombaerts, P., Iacomini, J., Johnson, R. S., Herrup, K., Tonegawa, S., and Papaioannou, V. E. (1992). RAG–1-deficient mice have no mature B and T lymphocytes. *Cell* 68, 869–877.

Momburg, F., Mullbacher, A., and Lobigs, M. (2001). Modulation of transporter associated with antigen processing (TAP)-mediated peptide import into the endoplasmic reticulum by flavivirus infection. *J Virol* 75, 5663–5671.

Monath, T. P. (2002). Japanese encephalitis vaccines: current vaccines and future prospects. *Curr Top Microbiol Immunol* 267, 105–138.

Mukhopadhyay, S., Kuhn, R. J., and Rossmann, M. G. (2005). A structural perspective of the flavivirus life cycle. *Nat Rev Microbiol* 3(1), 13–22.

Mullbacher, A., Lobigs, M., and Lee, E. (2003). Immunobiology of mosquito-borne encephalitic flaviviruses. *Adv Virus Res* 60, 87–120.

Nybakken, G. E., Oliphant, T., Johnson, S., Burke, S., Diamond, M. S., and Fremont, D. H. (2005). Structural basis of West Nile virus neutralization by a therapeutic antibody. *Nature* 437(7059), 764–769.

Oliphant, T., Nybakken, G. E., Austin, S. K., Xu, Q., Bramson, J., Loeb, M., Throsby, M., Fremont, D. H., Pierson, T. C., and Diamond, M. S. (2007). Induction of epitope-specific neutralizing antibodies against West Nile virus. *J Virol* 81(21), 11828–11839.

Oliphant, T., Nybakken, G. E., Engle, M., Xu, Q., Nelson, C. A., Sukupolvi-Petty, S., Marri, A., Lachmi, B. E., Olshevsky, U., Fremont, D. H., Pierson, T. C., and Diamond, M. S. (2006). Antibody recognition and neutralization determinants on domains I and II of West Nile Virus envelope protein. *J Virol* 80(24), 12149–12159.

Perelygin, A. A., Scherbik, S. V., Zhulin, I. B., Stockman, B. M., Li, Y., and Brinton, M. A. (2002). Positional cloning of the murine flavivirus resistance gene. *Proc Natl Acad Sci U S A* 99, 9322–9327.

Petrovsky, N. (2008). Freeing vaccine adjuvants from dangerous immunological dogma. *Exp Rev Vaccines* 7, 7–10.

Pierson, T. C., Fremont, D. H., Kuhn, R. J., and Diamond, M. S. (2008). Structural insights into the mechanisms of antibody-mediated neutralization of flavivirus infection: implications for vaccine development. *Cell Host Microbe* 4, 229–238.

Prow, N. A., May, F., Westlake, D. J., Hurrelbrink, R. J., Biron, R. M., Leung, J. Y., McMinn, P. C., Clark, D. C., Mackenzie, J. S., Lobigs, M., Khromykh, A. A., and Hall, R. A. (2011). Determinants of attenuation in the envelope protein of the flavivirus Alfuy. *J Gen Virol* 92(10), 2286–2296.

Pyke, A. T., Smith, I. L., van den Hurk, A. F., Northill, J. A., Chuan, T. F., Westacott, A. J., and Smith, G. A. (2004). Detection of Australasian flavivirus encephalitic viruses using rapid fluorogenic TaqMan RT-PCR assays. *J Virol Methods* 117(2), 161–167.

Regner, M., Lobigs, M., Blanden, R. V., Milburn, P., and Mullbacher, A. (2001a). Antiviral cytotoxic T cells cross-reactively recognize disparate peptide determinants from related viruses but ignore more similar self- and foreign determinants. *J Immunol* 166(6), 3820–3828.

Regner, M., Lobigs, M., Blanden, R. V., and Mullbacher, A. (2001b). Effector cytolotic function but not IFN-gamma production in cytotoxic T cells triggered by virus-infected target cells *in vitro*. *Scand J Immunol* 54, 366–374.

Regner, M., Müllbacher, A., Blanden, R. V., and Lobigs, M. (2001c). Immunogenicity of two peptide determinants in the cytolytic T cell response to flavivirus infection: Inverse correlation between peptide affinity for MHC class I and T cell precursor frequency. *Viral Immunol* 14, 135–149.

Robertson, E. G., and McLorinan, H. (1952). Murray Valley encephalitis; clinical aspects. *Med J Aust* 1, 103–107.

Roder, J., and Duwe, A. (1979). The beige mutation in the mouse selectively impairs natural killer cell function. *Nature* 278(5703), 451–453.

Russell, R. C. (1998). Vectors vs. humans in Australia—who is on top down under? An update on vector-borne disease and research on vectors in Australia. *J Vector Ecol* 23(1), 1–46.

Russell, R. C., Currie, B. J., Lindsay, M. D., Mackenzie, J. S., Ritchie, S. A., and Whelan, P. I. (2009). Dengue and climate change in Australia: predictions for the future should incorporate knowledge from the past. *Med J Aust* 190(5), 265–268.

Sanderson, C. J. (1968). The immune response to viruses in calves. I. Response to Murray Valley encephalitis virus. *J Hygiene* 66, 451–460.

Sangster, M. Y., Heliams, D. B., MacKenzie, J. S., and Shellam, G. R. (1993). Genetic studies of flavivirus resistance in inbred strains derived from wild mice: evidence for a new resistance allele at the flavivirus resistance locus (Flv). *J Virol* 67(1), 340–347.

Sangster, M. Y., Mackenzie, J. S., and Shellam, G. R. (1998). Genetically determined resistance to flavivirus infection in wild Mus musculus domesticus and other taxonomic groups in the genus Mus. *Arch Virol* 143, 697–715.

Schlesinger, J. J., Brandriss, M. W., Cropp, C. B., and Monath, T. P. (1986). Protection against yellow fever in monkeys by immunization with yellow fever virus nonstructural protein NS1. *J Virol* 60, 1153–1155.

Schlesinger, J. J., Brandriss, M. W., and Walsh, E. E. (1985). Protection against 17D yellow fever encephalitis in mice by passive transfer of monoclonal antibodies to the nonstructural glycoprotein gp48 and by active immunization with gp48. *J Immunol* 135, 2805–2809.

Setoh, Y. X., Hobson-Peters, J., Prow, N. A., Young, P. R., and Hall, R. A. (2011). Expression of recombinant West Nile virus prM protein fused to an affinity tag for use as a diagnostic antigen. *J Virol Methods* 175(1) 20–27.

Setoh, Y. X., Prow, N. A., Hobson-Peters, J., Lobigs, M., Young, P. R., Khromykh, A. A., and Hall, R. A. (2012). Identification of residues in West Nile virus pre-membrane protein that influence viral particle secretion and virulence. *J Gen Virol* 93(Pt 9), 1965–1975.

Shirato, K., Miyoshi, H., Goto, A., Ako, Y., Ueki, T., Kariwa, H., and Takashima, I. (2004). Viral envelope protein glycosylation is a molecular determinant of the neuroinvasiveness of the New York strain of West Nile virus. *J Gen Virol* 85(Pt 12), 3637–3645.

Silvia, O. J., Pantelic, L., Mackenzie, J. S., Shellam, G. R., Papadimitriou, J., and Urosevic, N. (2004). Virus spread, tissue inflammation and antiviral response in brains of flavivirus susceptible and resistant mice acutely infected with Murray Valley encephalitis virus. *Arch Virol* 149, 447–464.

Solomon, T., Dung, N. M., Wills, B., Kneen, R., Gainsborough, M., Diet, T. V., Thuy, T. T., Loan, H. T., Khanh, V. C., Vaughn, D. W., White, N. J., and Farrar, J. J. (2003). Interferon alfa-2a in Japanese encephalitis: a randomised double-blind placebo-controlled trial. *Lancet* 361, 821–826.

Spicer, P. E., Phillips, D., Pike, A., Johansen, C., Melrose, W., and Hall, R. A. (1999). Antibodies to Japanese encephalitis virus in human sera collected from Irian Jaya. Follow-up of a previously reported case of Japanese encephalitis in that region. *Trans R Soc Trop Med Hyg* 93(5), 511–514.

Sturrock, K. (2009). The changing epidemiology of Murray Valley encephalitis virus and West Nile virus (Kunjin strain) in epizootic regions of Western Australia. PhD thesis. The University of Western Australia, Perth.

Taylor, C., Simmons, R., and Smith, I. (2005). Development of immunoglobulin M capture enzyme-linked immunosorbent assay to differentiate human flavivirus infections occurring in Australia. *Clin Diagn Lab Immunol* 12(3), 371–374.

Tesh, R. B., Travassos da Rosa, A. P., Guzman, H., Araujo, T. P., and Xiao, S. Y. (2002). Immunization with heterologous flaviviruses protective against fatal West Nile encephalitis. *Emerg Infect Dis* 8, 245–251.

Thiel, H. J., Collett, M. S., Gould, E. A., Heinz, F. X., Meyers, G., Purcell, R. H., Rice, C. M., and Houghton, M. (2005). Flaviviridae. *In* "Virus Taxonomy, Eighth Report of the International Committee for the taxonomy of Viruses" (C. M. Fauquet, M. A. Mayo, J. Maniloff, U. Desselberger, and L. A. Ball, Eds.), pp. 981–998. Academic Press, San Diego.

Throsby, M., Geuijen, C., Goudsmit, J., Bakker, A. Q., Korimbocus, J., Kramer, R. A., Clijsters-van der Horst, M., de Jong, M., Jongeneelen, M., Thijsse, S., Smit, R., Visser, T. J., Bijl, N., Marissen, W. E., Loeb, M., Kelvin, D. J., Preiser, W., ter Meulen, J., and de Kruif, J. (2006). Isolation and characterization of human monoclonal antibodies from individuals infected with West Nile Virus. *J Virol* 80(14), 6982–6992.

van den Hurk, A. F., Craig, S. B., Tulsiani, S. M., and Jansen, C. C. (2010). Emerging tropical diseases in Australia. Part 4. Mosquitoborne diseases. *Ann Trop Med Parasitol* 104(8), 623–640.

van den Hurk, A. F., Ritchie, S. A., and Mackenzie, J. S. (2009). Ecology and geographical expansion of Japanese encephalitis virus. *Annu Rev Entomol* 54, 17–35.

Voskoboinik, I., Smyth, M. J., and Trapani, J. A. (2006). Perforin-mediated target-cell death and immune homeostasis. *Nat Rev Immunol* 6(12), 940–952.

Wallace, M. J., Smith, D. W., Broom, A. K., Mackenzie, J. S., Hall, R. A., Shellam, G. R., and McMinn, P. C. (2003). Antibody-dependent enhancement of Murray Valley encephalitis virus virulence in mice. *J Gen Virol* 84, 1723–1728.

Wang, Y., Lobigs, M., Lee, E., and Mullbacher, A. (2003). CD8+ T cells mediate recovery and immunopathology in West Nile virus encephalitis. *J Virol* 77, 13323–13334.

Williams, D. T., Daniels, P. W., Lunt, R. A., Wang, L. F., Newberry, K. M., and Mackenzie, J. S. (2001). Experimental infections of pigs with Japanese encephalitis virus and closely related Australian flaviviruses. *Am J Trop Med Hyg* 65, 379–387.

Wong, S. H., Smith, D. W., Fallon, M. J., and Kermode, A. G. (2005). Murray valley encephalitis mimicking herpes simplex encephalitis. *J Clin Neurosci* 12, 822–824.

Zhu, J., Yamane, H., and Paul, W. E. (2010). Differentiation of effector CD4 T cell populations (*). *Annu Rev Immunol* 28, 445–489.

9 Japanese Encephalitis Virus and Human CNS Infection

Kallol Dutta, Arshed Nazmi, and Anirban Basu

CONTENTS

9.1 A BRIEF HISTORY OF JAPANESE ENCEPHALITIS

9.1.1 INTRODUCTION

The antecedents of Japanese encephalitis (JE) can be traced back to the days of the "Yoshiwara cold" (Miyake 1964) even though cases of summer-fall disease outbreaks bearing symptomatic similarity to JE was reported from Japan since 1871. The largest outbreak was reported in 1924 in which there were more than 6000 reported cases of which about 3600–4000 were fatal (Hiroyama 1962). The first clinical isolate of the Japanese encephalitis virus was prepared in 1933 from human brain tissue in rabbits (Hayashi 1934) and was initially referred to as Japanese "B" encephalitis virus to indicate its association with the "B" or summer type of epidemic encephalitis in Japan. Von Economo's encephalitis lethargica, prevalent throughout the world in the years immediately following World War I, was type "A," which had different clinical and epidemiologic characteristics (Rosen 1986).

9.1.2 DISEASE VECTORS IN JE

JE is maintained in nature by extra-human hosts. Human beings are incidental hosts and are known not to play any role in perpetuating the virus. The role of mosquitoes as vectors for this disease was suggested when the virus was isolated from *Culex tritaeniorhynchus* in 1938. Since then, this virus has been isolated from several other culicine mosquitoes such as *Culex fuscocephala*, *Culex vishnui*, *Culex sitiens*, *Culex annulirostris*, *Culex gelidus*, *Culex bitaeniorhynchus*, *Culex epidesmus*, *Culex pseudovishnui*, and *Culex whitmorei*, four species of anophelines *Anopheles annularis*, *Anopheles barbirostris*, *Anopheles hyrcanus*, and *Anopheles subpictus*, and five species of other mosquito genera *Armigeres subalbatus*, *Mansonia annulifera*, *Mansonia bonneal dives*, *Mansonia uniformis*, and *Aedes vigilax* (Muangman et al. 1972; Reid et al. 2006; Rosen 1986; Trosper et al. 1980; Vythilingam et al. 1994). Even though JEV has been reported to effectively replicate in other arthropod hosts when infected parentally (Hurlbut and Thomas 1969), isolation of the virus from arthropods other than mosquito in nature has been reported only twice; the first case was from midges, *Lasiohelea taiwana*, collected while biting humans in China (Wu and Wu 1957), and the second case was from ixodid ticks, *Haemaphysalis japonica*, in the erstwhile USSR (Lvov 1978).

9.1.3 ENZOOTIC LIFE CYCLE OF THE JE VIRUS

The virus is able to replicate within the salivary glands of mosquitoes. Mature JE virions remain entrapped in intracellular vacuoles and are later released into the apical cavity of salivary gland cells through the fusion of these vacuoles with the apical plasma membrane. This process is associated with primary re-synthesis of saliva in mosquitoes following blood feeding activity. Another type of shedding involves virus particles, either singly or in mass, being released directly through the apical plasma membrane (Takahashi and Suzuki 1979). Components of the mosquito saliva may also modulate infection by altering the local cytokine milieu. Feeding by mosquitoes of Culex sp or administration of sialokinin-I, a mosquito salivary protein, has been found to down-regulate IFN-γ production and up-regulate the TH_2 cytokines, IL-4 and IL-10 (Zeidner et al. 1999).

Large perennial lakes, swamps, and rice fields provide a wintering and staging ground for several migratory waterfowl; such areas also favor breeding and survival of mosquitoes. Human infections are mainly spread by *Culex tritaeniorrhynchus*, which breeds in pools of stagnant water such as rice paddy fields (Innis 1995). Because the rice paddy is unavoidable, the majority of the population in rural Asia has been infected with the virus by early adulthood (Solomon 2003). Wading ardeid water birds, particularly the black-crowned night heron (*Nycticorax nycticorax*) and the Asiatic cattle egret (*Bubulcus ibis coromandus*), and bats serve as virus reservoirs or maintenance hosts, but the virus regularly spills over into pigs, members of the family of equidae (e.g., horses, donkeys), and humans. Interestingly, the Asiatic cattle egret's range dramatically expanded across Asia in the 19th century following changing agricultural practices (Hancock and Kushlan 1984), which coincides with the evolution and spread of the more recent JEV genotypes. Pigs are considered as the main amplifications hosts as viremia results with a high titer. Due to the close proximity of pigs with human dwellings these animals are considered main components in the transmission cycle with respect to human infection (Ghosh and Basu 2009). JEV infection in other domestic animals does not result in high viremia and thus they are not expected to transmit the virus to humans.

9.1.4 ORIGIN, SPREAD, AND CURRENT GEOGRAPHIC REALM OF JE

Traditionally, Africa is considered to be the cradle of all emerging pathogens. However, a closer look at the various genotypes of JEV (I, II, III, IV, and V) showed that the virus could have evolved from the present day Indonesia-Malaysia region (also known as the Malay Archipelago). This tropical climate and great diversity of insect and vertebrate life may also facilitate the emergence and rapid evolution of viruses (Solomon et al. 2003). This is supported by the fact that all the five genotypes including the most divergent types IV and V, which are believed to represent the oldest lineages, are found in this region. From there, the virus has spread to the islands of Japan and subsequently spread over the entire eastern and south-east Asian region. Currently, the JE endemic region extends from the islands of Japan in the east to Pakistan, in the west (Igarashi et al. 1994) and parts of Russia (former USSR) in the north (Grascenkov 1964) to northern parts of Australia in the south (Hanna et al. 1996, 1999).

Analysis of the different strains of JEV isolated from different countries has suggested shifts in circulating genotypes (Fulmali et al. 2011; Nga et al. 2004). This may be possible due to several factors such as bird migration, new irrigation projects, and increasing animal husbandry (Innis 1995; Pfeffer and Dobler 2010; van den Hurk et al. 2009). Wind-blown mosquitoes caught in air currents during the typhoon season have been suggested to play a role in viral transmission from one country to another (Mackenzie et al. 2001; Ritchie and Rochester 2001). This has been found to be the case for the introduction of JEV to the Torres Strait region of Australia from Papua New Guinea (Hanna et al. 1996). Due to these reasons, it is possible that in the not so distant future, the geographic realm of JE may expand from its current state and may even cross the Pacific to enter the United States (Nett et al. 2009). A recent serosurvey from various bird species in Spain has confirmed the presence of viruses belonging to the JEV antigenic group (Garcia-Bocanegra et al. 2010). This shows that parts of the European continent can also come under the radar of this disease.

9.1.5 MOLECULAR ARCHITECTURE OF THE JE VIRUS

The JE virion consists of a single strand of positive-sense RNA of around 11 kb, inside a nucleocapsid, and is surrounded by a glycoprotein-containing envelope. The RNA comprises a short 5′ untranslated region (UTR), a longer 3′UTR, and with a single open reading frame between them. It codes for a single polyprotein, which is translationally and posttranslationally cleaved by viral and host proteases into three structural proteins (core-C, premembrane-PrM, and envelope-E), and seven nonstructural (NS) proteins (NS1, NS2A, NS2B, NS3, NS4A, NS4B, and NS5). The C protein (12–14 kDa) is highly basic and combines with the RNA to form

the nucleocapsid (Chang et al. 1999). The prM is closely associated with the E protein, forming a heterodimer, and is thought to act as a "chaperone" to it, impairing
its function until after virion release. Immediately prior to virion release, the prM
protein (18–19 kDa) is cleaved to its mature M protein (8–9 kDa) form (Figure 9.1).
This allows the formation of E protein homodimers, which are thus "activated." The
prM protein of JEV contains a single N-linked glycosylation site, which is highly
conserved among the JEV strains. Researchers indicated that this highly conserved
N glycosylation motif in prM is crucial for multiple stages of JEV biology; prM biogenesis, virus release, and pathogenesis (Kim et al. 2008). Depending on about 12%
genetic divergence in the C-prM region, the virus is classified into the four genotypes
(Chen et al. 1990). The E protein is the largest structural protein (53–55 kDa), with
up to two potential gylcosylation sites. It is the major target for the humoral immune
response, and is thought to be important for viral entry into host cells. It is worth
mentioning that low pH is extremely important for viral entry into the cell to trigger viral membrane fusion with host endosomal membrane, thereby releasing the
nucleoplasmid in the cytosol.

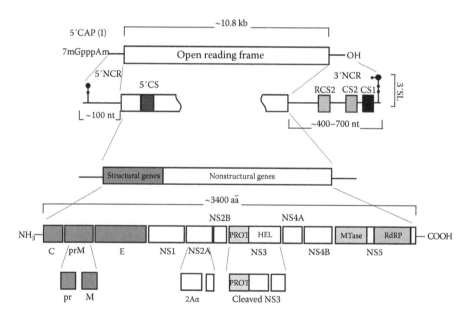

FIGURE 9.1 JEV genome structure and expression. The viral genome is depicted with the
structural and nonstructural protein coding regions, the 5′ cap, open reading frame and the
5′ and 3′ noncoding regions (NCR). Models of functionally important secondary and tertiary
structures within the 5′ and 3′ NCR and the coding region are shown with predicted hairpin
loops. Boxes below the genome indicate precursors and mature proteins generated by the
proteolytic processing cascade. Structural proteins are in grayscale, whereas nonstructural
(NS) proteins are white. The proposed topology of the flavivirus polyprotein cleavage products is also depicted. The proteins are arranged in order (left to right) of their appearance in
the polyprotein.

9.2   HUMAN INFECTIONS

Owing to the highly effective neuroinvasive nature of the JEV, it has been difficult to study the virus peripherally in clinical cases, as a result of which a lot remains unanswered. How the virus reaches the central nervous system (CNS) following peripheral inoculation or how it evades the hosts' immune system still remains enigmatic. Of the nearly 10,000 cases that are fatal out of 30,000–50,000 reported cases of JE per year, most are children belonging to age groups younger than 15 years. Adults living in the epidemic zones are not prone to be symptomatic for this disease; however, it is reported that they may become so in cases of spread to virgin territories. Although human beings are considered as incidental dead-end hosts of the JEV, mother to child transmission of the virus has been reported in the past (Chaturvedi et al. 1980; Mathur et al. 1981). However, the clinical impact of such could not be established. JEV persists in the human brain for 8 to 15 years after the onset of encephalitis (Shiraki 1970); however, whether it reactivates during immunosuppression or has any long-term neuropathological effect is unknown.

Neurovirulence of the JEV involves a combination of infection and dysfunction of neurons, caused by direct viral damage, and indirect damage mediated by the generation of an inflammatory milieu in the CNS, and other mechanisms such as apoptosis. In the following sections, we shall try to link available laboratory research reports along with clinical case studies so as to gain a better understanding of this disease.

9.2.1   Virus Transmission from the Periphery to the CNS

Human infections of Japanese encephalitis are common throughout the endemic region. Despite the enormity of the disease, not enough is known about the neuropathogenesis of this disease, including the exact mechanism of spread to the CNS (Myint et al. 2007). However studies regarding other flaviviral infections or *in vitro* studies have shown that following intracutaneous inoculation by mosquito bite, the virus enters the Langerhan's dendritic cells in the skin, which carry the virus into the nearest draining lymph nodes (Johnston et al. 2000). From there it is carried out into the general circulation via the thoracic duct, where the virus probably infects cells of myeloid lineage. From the general circulation, the JEV is hypothesized to enter the CNS, but the exact mechanism/s is yet to be elucidated. There are three possible mechanisms by which the virus is expected to enter the CNS by crossing the blood brain barrier (BBB)—passive transport across the endothelium, by active replication in endothelial cells or by a "Trojan horse" mechanism in which the virus is carried into the brain by infected peripheral inflammatory cells (Diamond 2003). Investigations in mice models (Dutta et al. 2010a) and study of human autopsy samples (Miyake 1964; Mukherji and Biswas 1976) have confirmed that the JEV infects and is able to replicate in peripheral organs such as lymph nodes, spleen, kidney, and lungs before crossing the BBB. Hematogenous spread of the virus from the periphery to the CNS is supported by the observation that in intranasally JEV inoculated monkeys, virus replication was widespread in the CNS, but not always identified in the olfactory bulb (Myint et al. 1999). The hematogenous route is also supported by observations that led to isolation of the virus from blood clots collected during the acute phase of infection (Sapkal et al. 2007).

Perivascular cuffing is a common occurrence in human infections of JEV. This leads to invasion of peripheral inflammatory cells into the CNS parenchyma. Inflammatory cells invading the parenchyma are shown to be predominantly macrophages with small numbers of T cells (Johnson et al. 1985), though the role of these cells in transporting the virus from periphery into the CNS remains ambiguous. Some *in vitro* studies have reported that JEV is capable of surviving within cells of monocyte/macrophage lineage for prolonged time periods (Aleyas et al. 2009; Dutta et al. 2010b). Although human data are lacking, studies in the mouse model of JE has shown that there is up-regulation of the cellular adhesion molecules ICAM and VCAM in the brain (Mishra et al. 2009a), which may be important in initiating adhesion and migration of neutrophils and macrophages. This was also associated with elevated levels of MMP-9 in the brain which could also contribute to increased BBB permeability. Taken together, these findings could indicate a "Trojan horse" role of these cells at a later stage of infection.

The disruptive role of cytokines on BBB has also been reported. In a mice model, macrophage-derived neutrophil chemotactic factor was shown to alter the BBB permeability in a dose dependent manner (Mathur et al. 1992). Tumor necrosis factor α (TNF-α) and interleukin 8, which is involved in polymorphonuclear cell recruitment, have also been reported to be elevated in cerebrospinal fluid (CSF) and serum of humans with JE and are higher in fatal than nonfatal cases (Ravi et al. 1997; Singh et al. 2000).

How the virus actually gains entry to infect the neurons is not well understood. JEV is believed to enter target cells through receptor-mediated endocytosis involving both clathrin-dependent and caveola-dependent pathways, low pH-triggered membrane fusion and then replicate in intracellular membrane structures (Nawa et al. 2003). The host membrane may play critical roles in various stages of the viral life cycle—from entry, replication, assembly, and egress of the virus particles. A recent study has claimed the involvement of host membrane lipid rafts in JEV entry and life cycle into neural stem/progenitor cells (Das et al. 2010).

9.2.2 NEUROPATHOLOGY ASSOCIATED WITH JEV INFECTIONS

JEV causes neuronal death. Time and again; various investigations involving human autopsy samples or animal models or even *in vitro* studies with neuronal cell lines, have shown conclusively that JEV infection leads to massive neuronal loss. Human autopsy studies as early as 1933 identified severe damage to nerve cells and the brain parenchyma including minute necroses, softening, and perivascular cuffing. The majority of the lesions were observed in the diencephalon and the mesencephalon. The overall inflammatory changes in the CNS were identified with marked increase in the number of glial cells. This led early investigators to believe that Japanese encephalitis was a "generalized toxic inflammation." However, it should be kept in perspective that this was before the isolation of the causative agent for the disease, i.e., the JEV. Later, histopathological studies on autopsy samples by Drs. M. Miyake and T. Ogota concluded that the disease was associated with "perivascular cell infiltration or cuffing, glial proliferation, glial nodules, chromolysis of Nissl's bodies, neuronophagia, haemorrhages, necrosis, softening and calcification" in the CNS (Miyake 1964). These observations were confirmed from investigations of several autopsy samples in the early 1960s. It was observed that these changes were scattered widely from the cerebrum, cerebellum, and brain stem to the spinal cord and most prominently in the cerebral cortex, thalamus, and substantia nigra.

JEV infection has been reported to initiate apoptotic death in neurons. The tumor necrosis factor receptor (TNFR)-associated death domain (TRADD) has been suggested to be the crucial signal adaptor that mediates all intracellular responses from TNFR-1. Using an *in vitro* approach it has been shown that the altered expression of TNFR-1 and TRADD following JEV infection regulates the downstream apoptotic cascades (Swarup et al. 2007, 2008). However, even though the infected neurons eventually die, recent evidences suggests that a possible intracellular innate immune response against the virus is mounted following viral recognition through the retinoic-acid-inducible gene I (RIG-I) (Nazmi et al. 2011).

Even in the early days of investigations it was known that this disease was accompanied with inflammation in the CNS. The CNS is a unique organ where the movement of cells or molecules is restricted by the BBB. Even though immune cells from periphery do infiltrate into the CNS at different stages of the disease, the initial inflammation is due to the activity of resident immune cells. The microglia and the astrocytes have been reported to play extensive roles following JEV infection. In animal models as well as *in vitro* models of JE, it has been reported that there is microglial activation characterized by distinct morphological changes along with heightened release of pro-inflammatory cyto/chemokines such as TNF-α, IL-6, MCP-1, IFN-γ, and IL-1β and other mediators. A region specific analysis showed that these releases were the highest from the hippocampus region (Ghoshal et al. 2007). This inflammatory milieu in the brain has a severe detrimental effect on neurons, leading to their death. Neuronal death also acts as a stimulator for further microglial activation, thereby creating a vicious cycle. Even though it is difficult to ascertain the extent of direct viral killing or the 'bystander' death, the net effect of JEV infection remains neuronal death. Astrocytes, on the other hand, also respond to the infection by increasing cytokine production, lactic acid release, and glucose mobilization (Chen et al. 2000) even though it does not confer significant neuroprotection (Mishra et al. 2007).

9.2.3 Clinical Features of JE

Infection with JE virus (JEV) may be asymptomatic or manifest as a mild febrile illness, aseptic meningitis, or classic severe meningomyeloencephalitis. The case fatality rate is approximately 25%, with 50% having neuropsychiatric sequelae and 25% recovering fully. Long term sequelae in survivors include weakness, ataxia, tremors, athetoid movements, paralysis, memory loss, and abnormal emotional behavior (Simpson and Meiklejohn 1947).

Based on the clinical observations of development and progression of this disease, it can be conveniently divided into three stages:

1. A prodromal stage preceding signs of involvement of the CNS.
2. An acute encephalitic stage marked by CNS signs and continuing fever.
3. Late stage marked by recovery or the persistence of cognitive dysfunction as a result of irreversible CNS damage.

The essential features of the prodromal stage are general malaise, headache, and fever. The onset of the illness is usually acute and is heralded with fever. Headache is often accompanied by vomiting. However, these symptoms are common to various other diseases that are not even related to flaviviral infections. Thus, a clinical diagnosis at this stage is absolutely impossible. A good example is the characterization of some U.S. military personnel serving during the Korean conflict, who were suffering from war neurosis when they were actually infected with JEV (Solomon and Vaughn 2002). The onset of this stage may be abrupt (1–6 h), acute (6–24 h), or subacute (2–5 days). In more than 75% of patients, the onset is subacute. Although spontaneous recovery (the so-called abortive encephalitis) is known following this stage, the disease usually progresses to the acute encephalitis phase (Gourie-Devi et al. 1995).

The acute encephalitis stage is marked by continuous fever, nuchal rigidity, convulsions, and altered sensorium, progressing in many cases to coma, focal CNS signs, polymorphonuclear leucocytosis in the peripheral blood, and CSF changes marked by pleocytosis with a normal or raised glucose or protein content. Seizures occur in approximately 85% of children and 10% of adults with JE (Kumar et al. 1990). Continuous unremitting seizure lasting longer than 30 minutes (status epilepticus) or multiple recurrent seizures are common in JE. Also, subtle motor status epilepticus, in which the only clinical manifestation might be the twitching of a finger or eyebrow, is important in JE (Solomon et al. 2002). Approximately 50% of the patients with JE suffer from high CSF opening pressure. Brain swelling is a common feature that is observed during autopsy, although herniation is not reported (Johnson et al. 1985). Multiple uncontrolled seizures may be associated with this raised intracranial pressure.

Movement disorders are common in JE, both in the acute encephalitis stages and also in survivors with neuropsychiatric sequelae. The characteristic features include mask-like faces, abulia, tremors, and cogwheel rigidity that bear similarity to Parkinson's disease. Other movement disorders include generalized rigidity, jaw dystonias, opisthotonus, choreoathetosis, orofacial dyskinesias (involuntary tongue protrusions), oromandibular dystonia, myoclonic jerks, and opsoclonus myoclonus (Kalita et al. 2011; Misra and Kalita 1997b). These clinical features grossly correlate with changes observed by MRI scans of patients. The role of basal ganglia, particularly the thalamus and the substantia nigra, have long been considered to be significant in eliciting such responses. MRI reveals prominent changes in thalamus, basal ganglia, substantia nigra, cerebellum, pons, cerebral cortex, and spinal cord. These MRI lesions are generally hypointense on T1 and hyperintense on T2 and fluid attenuation inversion recovery (FLAIR) sequence. The thalamic lesions may be of mixed intensity on T1 and T2 in the subacute stage and may suggest hemorrhagic changes (Figure 9.2). Follow-up MRI after several months reveals shrinkage of acute lesions which are hypointense on T1 and T2 sequences (Misra and Kalita 2010). In a comparative study of CT and MRI, the CT scan was abnormal in 55.3%; MRI was abnormal in all the patients and revealed thalamic lesions in 94%, basal ganglia in 35%, midbrain in 58%, pons in 26%, and cerebellum and cerebral cortex in 19% each (Kalita and Misra 2000a,b). In JE, involvement of the temporal lobe has also been reported in approximately 17% of the patients, but all of them had thalamic and substantia nigra involvement (Handique et al. 2006). Diffusion-weighted brain magnetic resonance imaging demonstrated abnormal high intensity lesions

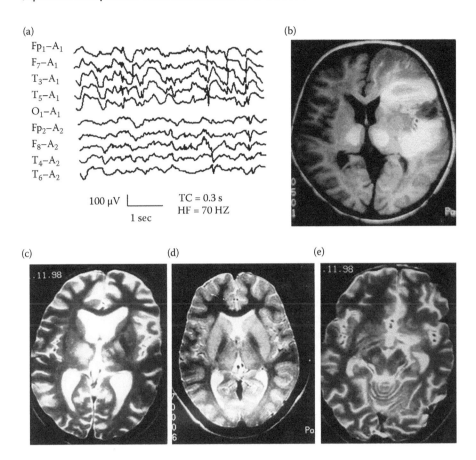

FIGURE 9.2 Representative EEG and MRI patterns observed in JE. Typical electroencephalographic (EEG) and MRI patterns observed from JE patients are shown here. EEG of a patient with secondary generalized seizure shows epileptiform (spike and wave) discharges mainly on the left side (a). T1 sequence of cranial MRI of the same patient shows hemorrhagic lesions on the left frontoparietal and bilateral thalami (b). Characteristic cranial MRI changes on T2 sequence showing bilateral thalamic lesion (c), thalamic and basal ganglia lesions (d), and substantial nigra (e) involvement on the right side are observed. Bilateral hyperintense thalamic lesion are seen in T1 sequence (f) which are also hyperintense in T2 sequence (g) suggesting subacute hemorrhage. (Reprinted from *Prog. Neurobiol.* 91(2), Misra, U. K. and Kalita, J., Overview: Japanese encephalitis, pp. 108–20. Copyright (2010), with permission from Elsevier.)

in the bilateral pulvinar and gray matter, with an abnormal appearance mimicking pulvinar sign (Toshio et al. 2011). Single photon emission computed tomography (SPECT) analysis of JE patients show thalamic hyperperfusion in the acute stage, which is replaced by hypoperfusion in the subacute or chronic stage (Kalita et al. 1999; Kimura et al. 1997). EEG recordings during the acute stage were found to be grossly abnormal. The outstanding features are diminution of electrical activity, dysrhythmia, and slowing with periodic lateralized epileptiform discharges (PLEDS).

(f)   (g)

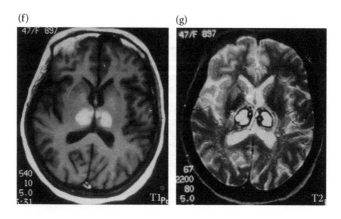

FIGURE 9.2   (Continued)

In some patients, intention tremors and ataxia that are indicative of the cerebellar involvement are observed. Other focal neurological signs include cranial nerve palsies, upper motor neuron weakness (in 30%–50% of patients), and flaccid limb weakness, with reduced or absent reflexes, which is often associated with respiratory or bulbar paralysis (Misra and Kalita 1997a). This disease is also referred to as encephalomyelitis. The combination of upper and lower motor neuron damage can lead to bizarre mixtures of clinical signs that can change hourly during the acute stage (Solomon et al. 2007). JEV can also cause a poliomyelitis-like acute flaccid paralysis in fully conscious patients. Acute retention of urine, due to an atonic bladder, may be an early clue that paralysis is due to a flavivirus (Solomon et al. 1998).

The late stage of the disease begins when active inflammation is at an end, i.e., when body temperature is normal and the neurological signs are stationary or tending to improve. When the encephalitic stage is short, recovery occurs rapidly and the patient becomes normal within 2–4 weeks of the onset of illness. However, a prolonged encephalitic stage corresponded to slower recovery or prolonged sequel to the disease. The neuropsychiatric problems in the survivors (in about 50% of cases) include learning and memory deficits, behavioral abnormalities, and speech disorders. The cellular or molecular basis of the persistence of these changes is not well understood. JEV predominantly infects children who are in a dynamic state of brain development, and so insult on the CNS may have consequences later in life. Since JEV infection leads to massive neuronal death, effective CNS repair processes which restore the neuronal loss are imperative for complete recovery from JE. In the postnatal/adult CNS, neuronal regeneration is primarily dependent on the pool of neural stem/progenitor cells (NSPCs) and their ability to generate cells of both neuronal and astrocyctic lineage. It is hypothesized that JEV infection and the associated inflammation disrupt the NSPC pool in the germinal niches and their efficacy of generating functional neurons, thereby stalling the neuronal repair. The lack of functional CNS repair/regeneration possibly culminates in long-term neurological consequences in JE survivors. In animal models and *in vitro* models of JE it has been shown that NSPCs are permissive to infection, which leads to their growth retardation. The pathophysiological relevance of these observations was supported by profound decrement in actively proliferating NSPCs in the subventricular zone (SVZ) of JEV-infected animals. Infection of the NSPCs and suppression of their proliferation might be primarily responsible for dysregulated neurogenesis and development of cognitive deficits in survivors of JE (Das and Basu 2008; Das et al. 2009).

Most of the symptoms associated with JE are also common to various other diseases. Due to the close genetic similarity of flaviviruses, some or most of these clinical characteristics are common to all human infections, thereby making differential diagnosis difficult. Other than flaviviral infections, encephalitis due to viral or nonviral reasons may also be characterized with some of these features. JE has also been associated with other diseases. Cysticercosis is a risk factor for JE that is attributed to the disruption of the BBB (Desai et al. 1997; Liu et al. 1957). JEV infection may also predispose patients to Guillain-Barré syndrome in endemic areas (Ravi et al. 1994).

9.2.4 Diagnosis, Prophylaxis, and Therapy

The diagnosis of the disease is currently based on immunological detection of the viral antigen or the detection of viral RNA or particles from patient samples. The low viremia in blood has always been a problem in rapid diagnosis of JEV. IgM capture ELISA had been the most widely used diagnostic method for JEV infection detection, but the kit is expensive and not suitable for low-cost, large-scale diagnosis in rural conditions for its short shelf life. A rapid IgM capture ELISA called JEV-Chex was developed having more stable reagents useful under rural conditions (Ravi et al. 2006). A comparative study carried out between IgM capture ELISA and nested reverse transcription-polymerase chain reaction (RT-PCR) for the diagnosis of Japanese encephalitis from the samples of CSF and blood revealed that RT-PCR is also useful for an early detection of JEV (Swami et al. 2008). At present, though many advancements and modifications have been done on the ELISA methods, such as introduction of the dipstick method (Shrivastva et al. 2008), but going by the principle of detection, IgM capture ELISA remains the very principle in clinical and laboratory confirmatory diagnosis of JEV, but of course a positive detection from a gene amplification analysis reinforces the confirmation.

A sensitive quantitative assay for JEV RNA has been reportedly developed using real-time RT-PCR. The assay was performed using LightCycler and RNA amplification kit SYBR Green I by selecting the JEV specific primer from the 3'UTR. On comparing results obtained by real-time RT-PCR assay for JEV and infectivity titrations, it was suggested that the real-time RT-PCR assay could have an additive effect on the interpretation and evaluation of virus clearance, especially during the virus removal process (Jeong et al. 2003). Again, a one step TaqMan RT-PCR using a TaqMan probe has also been developed for detection of JEV, where it was shown to be 10-fold more sensitive than the conventional two-step RT-PCR method (Yang et al. 2004).

Therapy for JE is entirely supportive and currently there are no specific drugs to target the virus. Over the years, various drugs—natural or synthetic—have been tried out either singly or in combination with other compounds with limited or no success. Even compounds that had shown promising results *in vitro* or in animal models have failed in human trials. Interferon alpha and ribavirin are two such compounds. Details about these drugs and their mode of action can be found in a review by these authors (Dutta et al. 2011). The latest and most promising candidate for therapy in JE is minocycline, a second generation tetracycline. Minocycline has been found to be highly effective in preventing animal mortality following acute challenge with the virus (Mishra and Basu 2008; Mishra et al. 2009a,b) and is slated for a randomized double blind phase II clinical trial.

Due to lack of definitive therapeutic countermeasures to combat JE, vaccination in humans remains, to date, the most effective measure to prevent JE. Multiple vaccines exist to control JE, but all have limitations. The formalin-inactivated vaccine against JEV was produced from infected mouse brain-derived tissue soon after the virus was discovered. This type of vaccine, manufactured by the Research Foundation for Microbial Diseases of Osaka University, Japan, became commercially available in Japan (as the Japanese Biken vaccine JE-VAX) and was produced in Korea by the Green Cross Vaccine company. These were later licensed to be produced also in the United States (Solomon 2008). This is the only JE vaccine recommended by the World Health Organization (WHO), but there have been several concerns with its side effects (Shlim and Solomon 2002). These vaccines are expensive and require multiple doses to maintain efficacy and immunity. An inexpensive, live attenuated vaccine (SA14-14-2) 48 was licensed by China in 1988, but WHO does not approve it for human use because it is produced in primary hamster kidney cells. Although the vaccine was adjudged to be safe and efficacious by the WHO's Global Advisory Committee on Vaccine Safety, several parameters such as safety in immunocompromised individuals and pregnant women, viral shedding in vaccines and implications of the shedding, and efficacy in infants younger than 1 year old, remains to be ascertained (Dutta et al. 2011). The recently developed Vero cell-derived inactivated JE vaccine containing the purified, inactivated JEV strain SA14-14-2 with aluminum hydroxide as adjuvant seems to be a promising candidate and has passed the phase III randomized controlled trial (Tauber et al. 2007). Several efforts have been and are still being made to develop recombinant vaccines for JE, with some of them in preclinical or various phases of clinical trial.

Even though vaccination is effective and has considerably lowered the incidence of JE in many endemic regions, reports are available of their ineffectiveness in some cases. A young adult man, who received four doses of JEV (Nakayama strain) vaccination in childhood, reportedly developed acute JEV infection that was characterized with acute flaccid paralysis. His deep tendon reflexes were decreased except for the Achilles reflex. Following supportive care, one month after his discharge, his muscle power level and deep tendon reflexes recovered partially (Chung et al. 2007).

REFERENCES

Aleyas, A. G., George, J. A., Han, Y. W., Rahman, M. M., Kim, S. J., Han, S. B., Kim, B. S., Kim, K., and Eo, S. K. (2009). Functional modulation of dendritic cells and macrophages by Japanese encephalitis virus through MyD88 adaptor molecule-dependent and -independent pathways. *J. Immunol.* 183(4), 2462–74.

Chang, Y. S., Liao, C. L., Tsao, C. H., Chen, M. C., Liu, C. I., Chen, L. K., and Lin, Y. L. (1999). Membrane permeabilization by small hydrophobic nonstructural proteins of Japanese encephalitis virus. *J. Virol.* 73(8), 6257–64.

Chaturvedi, U. C., Mathur, A., Chandra, A., Das, S. K., Tandon, H. O., and Singh, U. K. (1980). Transplacental infection with Japanese encephalitis virus. *J. Infect Dis.* 141(6), 712–5.

Chen, C. J., Liao, S. L., Kuo, M. D., and Wang, Y. M. (2000). Astrocytic alteration induced by Japanese encephalitis virus infection. *Neuroreport.* 11(9), 1933–7.

Chen, W. R., Tesh, R. B., and Rico-Hesse, R. (1990). Genetic variation of Japanese encephalitis virus in nature. *J. Gen. Virol.* 71(Pt 12), 2915–22.

Chung, C. C., Lee, S. S., Chen, Y. S., Tsai, H. C., Wann, S. R., Kao, C. H., and Liu, Y. C. (2007). Acute flaccid paralysis as an unusual presenting symptom of Japanese encephalitis: a case report and review of the literature. *Infection* 35(1), 30–2.

Das, S., and Basu, A. (2008). Japanese encephalitis virus infects neural progenitor cells and decreases their proliferation. *J. Neurochem.* 106(4), 1624–36.

Das, S., Chakraborty, S., and Basu, A. (2010). Critical role of lipid rafts in virus entry and activation of phosphoinositide 3′ kinase/Akt signaling during early stages of Japanese encephalitis virus infection in neural stem/progenitor cells. *J. Neurochem.* 115(2), 537–49.

Das, S., Ghosh, D., and Basu, A. (2009). Japanese encephalitis virus induce immuno-competency in neural stem/progenitor cells. *PLoS One* 4(12), e8134.

Desai, A., Shankar, S. K., Jayakumar, P. N., Chandramuki, A., Gourie-Devi, M., Ravikumar, B. V., and Ravi, V. (1997). Co-existence of cerebral cysticercosis with Japanese encephalitis: a prognostic modulator. *Epidemiol. Infect.* 118(2), 165–71.

Diamond, M. S. (2003). Evasion of innate and adaptive immunity by flaviviruses. *Immunol. Cell Biol.* 81(3), 196–206.

Dutta, K., Kumawat, K. L., Nazmi, A., Mishra, M. K., and Basu, A. (2010a). Minocycline differentially modulates viral infection and persistence in an experimental model of Japanese encephalitis. *J. Neuroimmune Pharmacol.* 5(4), 553–65.

Dutta, K., Mishra, M. K., Nazmi, A., Kumawat, K. L., and Basu, A. (2010b). Minocycline differentially modulates macrophage mediated peripheral immune response following Japanese encephalitis virus infection. *Immunobiology* 215(11), 884–93.

Dutta, K., Nazmi, A., and Basu, A. (2011). Chemotherapy in Japanese encephalitis: are we there yet? *Infect. Disord. Drug Targets* 11(3), 300–14.

Fulmali, P. V., Sapkal, G. N., Athawale, S., Gore, M. M., Mishra, A. C., and Bondre, V. P. (2011). Introduction of Japanese encephalitis virus genotype I, India. *Emerg. Infect. Dis.* 17(2), 319–21.

Garcia-Bocanegra, I., Busquets, N., Napp, S., Alba, A., Zorrilla, I., Villalba, R., and Arenas, A. (2010). Serosurvey of West Nile Virus and other flaviviruses of the Japanese encephalitis antigenic complex in birds from Andalusia, Southern Spain. *Vector Borne Zoonotic Dis.* 11(8), 1107–13.

Ghosh, D., and Basu, A. (2009). Japanese encephalitis—a pathological and clinical perspective. *PLoS Negl. Trop. Dis.* 3(9), e437.

Ghoshal, A., Das, S., Ghosh, S., Mishra, M. K., Sharma, V., Koli, P., Sen, E., and Basu, A. (2007). Proinflammatory mediators released by activated microglia induces neuronal death in Japanese encephalitis. *Glia* 55(5), 483–96.

Gourie-Devi, M., Ravi, V., and Shankar, S. K. (1995). Japanese encephalitis: An overview. In. *Recent Advances in Tropical Neurology*, ed. F. C. Rose. Elsevier Sciences B.V. Amsterdam, 217–35.

Grascenkov, N. I. (1964). Japanese encephalitis in the USSR. *Bull. World Health Organ* 30, 161–72.

Hancock, J., and Kushlan, J. (1984). *The Herons Handbook.* Harper and Row, New York.

Handique, S. K., Das, R. R., Barman, K., Medhi, N., Saharia, B., Saikia, P., and Ahmed, S. A. (2006). Temporal lobe involvement in Japanese encephalitis: problems in differential diagnosis. *AJNR Am. J. Neuroradiol.* 27(5), 1027–31.

Hanna, J. N., Ritchie, S. A., Phillips, D. A., Lee, J. M., Hills, S. L., van den Hurk, A. F., Pyke, A. T., Johansen, C. A., and Mackenzie, J. S. (1999). Japanese encephalitis in north Queensland, Australia, 1998. *Med. J. Aust.* 170(11), 533–6.

Hanna, J. N., Ritchie, S. A., Phillips, D. A., Shield, J., Bailey, M. C., Mackenzie, J. S., Poidinger, M., McCall, B. J., and Mills, P. J. (1996). An outbreak of Japanese encephalitis in the Torres Strait, Australia, 1995. *Med. J. Aust.* 165(5), 256–60.

Hayashi, M. (1934). Ubertragung des virus von encephalitis epidemica auf Affen. *Proc. Imp. Acad. Tokyo.* 10, 41–4.

Hiroyama, T. (1962). Epidemiology of Japanese encephalitis (in Japanese). *Saishin-Igaku.* 17, 1272–80.

Hurlbut, H. S., and Thomas, J. I. (1969). Further studies on the arthropod host range of arboviruses. *J. Med. Entomol.* 6(4), 423–7.

Igarashi, A., Tanaka, M., Morita, K., Takasu, T., Ahmed, A., Akram, D. S., and Waqar, M. A. (1994). Detection of west Nile and Japanese encephalitis viral genome sequences in cerebrospinal fluid from acute encephalitis cases in Karachi, Pakistan. *Microbiol. Immunol.* 38(10), 827–30.

Innis, B. L. (1995). Japanese encephalitis. In. *Kass Handbook of Infectious Diseases: Exotic Viral infections*, ed. J. S. Porterfield. Chapman and Hall Medical, London, 147–74.

Jeong, H. S., Shin, J. H., Park, Y. N., Choi, J. Y., Kim, Y. L., Kim, B. G., Ryu, S. R., Baek, S. Y., Lee, S. H., and Park, S. N. (2003). Development of real-time RT-PCR for evaluation of JEV clearance during purification of HPV type 16 L1 virus-like particles. *Biologicals* 31(3), 223–9.

Johnson, R. T., Burke, D. S., Elwell, M., Leake, C. J., Nisalak, A., Hoke, C. H., and Lorsomrudee, W. (1985). Japanese encephalitis: immunocytochemical studies of viral antigen and inflammatory cells in fatal cases. *Ann. Neurol.* 18(5), 567–73.

Johnston, L. J., Halliday, G. M., and King, N. J. (2000). Langerhans cells migrate to local lymph nodes following cutaneous infection with an arbovirus. *J. Invest. Dermatol.* 114(3), 560–8.

Kalita, J., and Misra, U. K. (2000a). Comparison of CT scan and MRI findings in the diagnosis of Japanese encephalitis. *J. Neurol. Sci.* 174(1), 3–8.

Kalita, J., and Misra, U. K. (2000b). Markedly severe dystonia in Japanese encephalitis. *Mov. Disord.* 15(6), 1168–72.

Kalita, J., Das, B. K., and Misra, U. K. (1999). SPECT studies of regional cerebral blood flow in 8 patients with Japanese encephalitis in subacute and chronic stage. *Acta Neurol. Scand.* 99(4), 213–8.

Kalita, J., Misra, U. K., and Pradhan, P. K. (2011). Oromandibular dystonia in encephalitis. *J. Neurol. Sci.* 304(1–2), 107–10.

Kim, J. M., Yun, S. I., Song, B. H., Hahn, Y. S., Lee, C. H., Oh, H. W., and Lee, Y. M. (2008). A single N-linked glycosylation site in the Japanese encephalitis virus prM protein is critical for cell type-specific prM protein biogenesis, virus particle release, and pathogenicity in mice. *J. Virol.* 82(16), 7846–62.

Kimura, K., Dosaka, A., Hashimoto, Y., Yasunaga, T., Uchino, M., and Ando, M. (1997). Single-photon emission CT findings in acute Japanese encephalitis. *AJNR Am. J. Neuroradiol.* 18(3), 465–9.

Kumar, R., Mathur, A., Kumar, A., Sharma, S., Chakraborty, S., and Chaturvedi, U. C. (1990). Clinical features & prognostic indicators of Japanese encephalitis in children in Lucknow (India). *Indian J. Med. Res.* 91, 321–7.

Liu, Y. F., Teng, C. L., and Liu, K. (1957). Cerebral cysticercosis as a factor aggravating Japanese B encephalitis. *Chin. Med. J.* 75(12), 1010–7.

Lvov, D. K. (1978). The role of ixodid ticks in the reservation and transmission of arboviruses in the USSR. In. *Tick-Borne Diseases and Their Vectors*, ed. T. K. H. Wilde. Lewis Reprints, Tonbridge, UK, 482–6.

Mackenzie, J. S., Chua, K. B., Daniels, P. W., Eaton, B. T., Field, H. E., Hall, R. A., Halpin, K., Johansen, C. A., Kirkland, P. D., Lam, S. K., McMinn, P., Nisbet, D. J., Paru, R., Pyke, A. T., Ritchie, S. A., Siba, P., Smith, D. W., Smith, G. A., van den Hurk, A. F., Wang, L. F., and Williams, D. T. (2001). Emerging viral diseases of Southeast Asia and the Western Pacific. *Emerg. Infect. Dis.* 7(3 Suppl), 497–504.

Mathur, A., Arora, K. L., and Chaturvedi, U. C. (1981). Congenital infection of mice with Japanese encephalitis virus. *Infect. Immun.* 34(1), 26–9.

Mathur, A., Khanna, N., and Chaturvedi, U. C. (1992). Breakdown of blood-brain barrier by virus-induced cytokine during Japanese encephalitis virus infection. *Int. J. Exp. Pathol.* 73(5), 603–11.

Mishra, M. K., and Basu, A. (2008). Minocycline neuroprotects, reduces microglial activation, inhibits caspase 3 induction, and viral replication following Japanese encephalitis. *J. Neurochem.* 105(5), 1582–95.

Mishra, M. K., Dutta, K., Saheb, S. K., and Basu, A. (2009a). Understanding the molecular mechanism of blood-brain barrier damage in an experimental model of Japanese encephalitis: correlation with minocycline administration as a therapeutic agent. *Neurochem. Int.* 55(8), 717–23.

Mishra, M. K., Ghosh, D., Duseja, R., and Basu, A. (2009b). Antioxidant potential of Minocycline in Japanese Encephalitis Virus infection in murine neuroblastoma cells: correlation with membrane fluidity and cell death. *Neurochem. Int.* 54(7), 464–70.

Mishra, M. K., Koli, P., Bhowmick, S., and Basu, A. (2007). Neuroprotection conferred by astrocytes is insufficient to protect animals from succumbing to Japanese encephalitis. *Neurochem. Int.* 50(5), 764–73.

Misra, U. K., and Kalita, J. (1997a). Anterior horn cells are also involved in Japanese encephalitis. *Acta Neurol. Scand.* 96(2), 114–7.

Misra, U. K., and Kalita, J. (1997b). Movement disorders in Japanese encephalitis. *J. Neurol.* 244(5), 299–303.

Misra, U. K., and Kalita, J. (2010). Overview: Japanese encephalitis. *Prog. Neurobiol.* 91(2), 108–20.

Miyake, M. (1964). The pathology of Japanese encephalitis. A review. *Bull. World Health Organ.* 30, 153–60.

Muangman, D., Edelman, R., Sullivan, M. J., and Gould, D. J. (1972). Experimental transmission of Japanese encephalitis virus by Culex fuscocephala. *Am. J. Trop. Med. Hyg.* 21(4), 482–6.

Mukherji, A. K., and Biswas, S. K. (1976). Histopathological studies of brains (and other viscera) from cases of JE virus encephalitis during 1973 epidemic at Bankura. *Indian J. Med. Res.* 64(8), 1143–9.

Myint, K. S., Gibbons, R. V., Perng, G. C., and Solomon, T. (2007). Unravelling the neuropathogenesis of Japanese encephalitis. *Trans. R. Soc. Trop. Med. Hyg.* 101(10), 955–6.

Myint, K. S., Raengsakulrach, B., Young, G. D., Gettayacamin, M., Ferguson, L. M., Innis, B. L., Hoke, C. H., Jr., and Vaughn, D. W. (1999). Production of lethal infection that resembles fatal human disease by intranasal inoculation of macaques with Japanese encephalitis virus. *Am. J. Trop. Med. Hyg.* 60(3), 338–42.

Nawa, M., Takasaki, T., Yamada, K., Kurane, I., and Akatsuka, T. (2003). Interference in Japanese encephalitis virus infection of Vero cells by a cationic amphiphilic drug, chlorpromazine. *J. Gen. Virol.* 84(Pt 7), 1737–41.

Nazmi, A., Dutta, K., and Basu, A. (2011). RIG-I mediates innate immune response in mouse neurons following Japanese encephalitis virus infection. *PLoS One* 6(6), e21761.

Nett, R. J., Campbell, G. L., and Reisen, W. K. (2009). Potential for the emergence of Japanese encephalitis virus in California. *Vector Borne Zoonotic Dis.* 9(5), 511–7.

Nga, P. T., del Carmen Parquet, M., Cuong, V. D., Ma, S. P., Hasebe, F., Inoue, S., Makino, Y., Takagi, M., Nam, V. S., and Morita, K. (2004). Shift in Japanese encephalitis virus (JEV) genotype circulating in northern Vietnam: implications for frequent introductions of JEV from Southeast Asia to East Asia. *J. Gen. Virol.* 85(Pt 6), 1625–31.

Pfeffer, M., and Dobler, G. (2010). Emergence of zoonotic arboviruses by animal trade and migration. *Parasit. Vectors* 3(1), 35.

Ravi, V., Desai, A., Balaji, M., Apte, M. P., Lakshman, L., Subbakrishna, D. K., Sridharan, G., Dhole, T. N., and Ravikumar, B. V. (2006). Development and evaluation of a rapid IgM capture ELISA (JEV-Chex) for the diagnosis of Japanese encephalitis. *J. Clin. Virol.* 35(4), 429–34.

Ravi, V., Parida, S., Desai, A., Chandramuki, A., Gourie-Devi, M., and Grau, G. E. (1997). Correlation of tumor necrosis factor levels in the serum and cerebrospinal fluid with clinical outcome in Japanese encephalitis patients. *J. Med. Virol.* 51(2), 132–6.

Ravi, V., Taly, A. B., Shankar, S. K., Shenoy, P. K., Desai, A., Nagaraja, D., Gourie-Devi, M., and Chandramuki, A. (1994). Association of Japanese encephalitis virus infection with Guillain-Barre syndrome in endemic areas of south India. *Acta Neurol. Scand.* 90(1), 67–72.

Reid, M., Mackenzie, D., Baron, A., Lehmann, N., Lowry, K., Aaskov, J., Guirakhoo, F., and Monath, T. P. (2006). Experimental infection of Culex annulirostris, Culex gelidus, and Aedes vigilax with a yellow fever/Japanese encephalitis virus vaccine chimera (ChimeriVax-JE). *Am. J. Trop. Med. Hyg.* 75(4), 659–63.

Ritchie, S. A., and Rochester, W. (2001). Wind-blown mosquitoes and introduction of Japanese encephalitis into Australia. *Emerg. Infect. Dis.* 7(5), 900–3.

Rosen, L. (1986). The natural history of Japanese encephalitis virus. *Annu. Rev. Microbiol.* 40, 395–414.

Sapkal, G. N., Wairagkar, N. S., Ayachit, V. M., Bondre, V. P., and Gore, M. M. (2007). Detection and isolation of Japanese encephalitis virus from blood clots collected during the acute phase of infection. *Am. J. Trop. Med. Hyg.* 77(6), 1139–45.

Shiraki, H. (1970). Japanese encephalitis. In. *Clinical Virology*, ed. R. Debre, and J. Celers. W. B. Saunders, Philadelphia, 155–75.

Shlim, D. R., and Solomon, T. (2002). Japanese encephalitis vaccine for travelers: exploring the limits of risk. *Clin. Infect. Dis.* 35(2), 183–8.

Shrivastva, A., Tripathi, N. K., Parida, M., Dash, P. K., Jana, A. M., and Lakshmana Rao, P. V. (2008). Comparison of a dipstick enzyme-linked immunosorbent assay with commercial assays for detection of Japanese encephalitis virus-specific IgM antibodies. *J. Postgrad. Med.* 54(3), 181–5.

Simpson, T. W., and Meiklejohn, G. (1947). Sequelae of Japanese B encephalitis. *Am. J. Trop. Med. Hyg.* 27(6), 727–31.

Singh, A., Kulshreshtha, R., and Mathur, A. (2000). Secretion of the chemokine interleukin-8 during Japanese encephalitis virus infection. *J. Med. Microbiol.* 49(7), 607–12.

Solomon, T. (2003). Recent advances in Japanese encephalitis. *J. Neurovirol.* 9(2), 274–83.

Solomon, T. (2008). New vaccines for Japanese encephalitis. *Lancet Neurol.* 7(2), 116–8.

Solomon, T., and Vaughn, D. W. (2002). Pathogenesis and clinical features of Japanese encephalitis and West Nile virus infections. *Curr. Top. Microbiol. Immunol.* 267, 171–94.

Solomon, T., Dung, N. M., Kneen, R., Thao le, T. T., Gainsborough, M., Nisalak, A., Day, N. P., Kirkham, F. J., Vaughn, D. W., Smith, S., and White, N. J. (2002). Seizures and raised intracranial pressure in Vietnamese patients with Japanese encephalitis. *Brain* 125(Pt 5), 1084–93.

Solomon, T., Kneen, R., Dung, N. M., Khanh, V. C., Thuy, T. T., Ha, D. Q., Day, N. P., Nisalak, A., Vaughn, D. W., and White, N. J. (1998). Poliomyelitis-like illness due to Japanese encephalitis virus. *Lancet* 351(9109), 1094–7.

Solomon, T., Ni, H., Beasley, D. W., Ekkelenkamp, M., Cardosa, M. J., and Barrett, A. D. (2003). Origin and evolution of Japanese encephalitis virus in southeast Asia. *J. Virol.* 77(5), 3091–8.

Solomon, T., Ooi, M. H., and Mallewa, M. (2007). Chapter 10 Viral infections of lower motor neurons. *Handb. Clin. Neurol.* 82, 179–206.

Swami, R., Ratho, R. K., Mishra, B., and Singh, M. P. (2008). Usefulness of RT-PCR for the diagnosis of Japanese encephalitis in clinical samples. Scand. *J. Infect Dis.* 40(10), 815–20.

Swarup, V., Das, S., Ghosh, S., and Basu, A. (2007). Tumor necrosis factor receptor-1-induced neuronal death by TRADD contributes to the pathogenesis of Japanese encephalitis. *J. Neurochem.* 103(2), 771–83.

Swarup, V., Ghosh, J., Das, S., and Basu, A. (2008). Tumor necrosis factor receptor-associated death domain mediated neuronal death contributes to the glial activation and subsequent neuroinflammation in Japanese encephalitis. *Neurochem. Int.* 52(7), 1310–21.

Takahashi, M., and Suzuki, K. (1979). Japanese encephalitis virus in mosquito salivary glands. *Am. J. Trop. Med. Hyg.* 28(1), 122–35.

Tauber, E., Kollaritsch, H., Korinek, M., Rendi-Wagner, P., Jilma, B., Firbas, C., Schranz, S., Jong, E., Klingler, A., Dewasthaly, S., and Klade, C. S. (2007). Safety and immunogenicity of a Vero-cell-derived, inactivated Japanese encephalitis vaccine: a non-inferiority, phase III, randomised controlled trial. *Lancet* 370(9602), 1847–53.

Toshio, S., Saito, T., Takahashi, Y., Kokunai, Y., and Fujimura, H. (2011). [Encephalitis associated with positive anti-GluR antibodies showing abnormal appearance in basal ganglia, pulvinar and gray matter on MRI—case report]. *Rinsho Shinkeigaku* 51(3), 192–6.

Trosper, J. H., Ksiazek, T. G., and Cross, J. H. (1980). Isolation of Japanese encephalitis virus from the Republic of the Philippines. *Trans. R. Soc. Trop. Med. Hyg.* 74(3), 292–5.

van den Hurk, A. F., Ritchie, S. A., and Mackenzie, J. S. (2009). Ecology and geographical expansion of Japanese encephalitis virus. *Annu. Rev. Entomol.* 54, 17–35.

Vythilingam, I., Oda, K., Tsuchie, H., Mahadevan, S., and Vijayamalar, B. (1994). Isolation of Japanese encephalitis virus from Culex sitiens mosquitoes in Selangor, Malaysia. *J. Am. Mosq. Control Assoc.* 10(2 Pt 1), 228–9.

Wu, C. J., and Wu, S. Y. (1957). Isolation of virus of B type encephalitis from Lasiohelea taiwana Shiraki-a blood sucking midge. *Acta Microbial. Sin.* 5, 22–6.

Yang, D. K., Kweon, C. H., Kim, B. H., Lim, S. I., Kim, S. H., Kwon, J. H., and Han, H. R. (2004). TaqMan reverse transcription polymerase chain reaction for the detection of Japanese encephalitis virus. *J. Vet. Sci.* 5(4), 345–51.

Zeidner, N. S., Higgs, S., Happ, C. M., Beaty, B. J., and Miller, B. R. (1999). Mosquito feeding modulates Th1 and Th2 cytokines in flavivirus susceptible mice: an effect mimicked by injection of sialokinins, but not demonstrated in flavivirus resistant mice. *Parasite Immunol.* 21(1), 35–44.

10 Tick-Borne Encephalitis

Daniel Růžek, Bartosz Bilski, and Göran Günther

CONTENTS

10.1 INTRODUCTION

Tick-borne encephalitis is recognized from 18th-century parish records in Åland Islands in Finland. A virus, as the causative agent, was first isolated in 1937 by Zilber and collaborators in the Far Eastern Soviet Union (Zilber 1939). In 1937–1939, the Russian Ministry of Health organized three successive expeditions to the Far East, with the purpose to reveal the origin of severe outbreaks of meningoencephalitis, called "Taiga encephalitis" or "biphasic minogoencehalitis," a disease that had been observed in the Far East since 1914, but more frequently had occurred since 1933. The expeditions revealed the viral origin of the disease and the tick *Ixodes persulcatus* as the main vector of the disease (Zilber 1939; Chumakov and Zeitlenok 1940).

In the European part of Russia (in Ural), the disease seems to have been known since 1898. However, the well-documented history of TBE on the European continent starts with an outbreak in the Volkhov Front's armies in 1942–1943. During that time, the TBE virus of the Siberian subtype was isolated from *Ixodes ricinus* ticks (Petrishcheva and Levkovich 1945). In 1943, the TBE virus of the western type was isolated for the first time from human patients and *I. ricinus* ticks by Zilber and collaborators in Belarus (Pogodina et al. 2004).

Tick-borne encephalitis in Central Europe was first described by Austrian physician Schneider, who had studied clinical cases of TBE in the area of Neunkirchen (Lower Austria) since 1927, but without knowing its etiology (Schneider 1931). In 1957, Moritsch and Krausler isolated the TBE virus in Neunkirchen and proved that the so-called Schneider's disease represented in fact TBE (Moritsch and Krausler 1957). However, the first successful isolation of the TBE virus in the central and western part of Europe was performed in Czechoslovakia in 1948 by Gallia and coworkers (Rampas and Gallia 1949), when local outbreaks of meningoencephalitis occurred in several regions in Bohemia and Moravia (Hloucal 1949, 1960; Hloucal and Gallia 1949; Hloucal and Rampas 1953; Krejčí 1949a). Virus isolated from patient samples was pathogenic for white mice and was filterable through Seitz and Chamberland filters. In the same year, Krejčí, with assistance from Gallia and Blaškovič, isolated the virus during an outbreak of meningoencephalitis in South Moravia (Krejčí 1949b). Gallia, Edward, and others demonstrated a close similarity of the new virus with Russian spring–summer encephalitis virus and louping-ill virus. Approximately 80% of the TBE patients recorded a tick bite before the illness, suggesting the role of ticks as vectors of the virus. This was confirmed in 1949 by Rampas and Gallia and subsequently by Krejčí, when the virus was successfully isolated from different stages of ticks *Ixodes ricinus* collected in the endemic areas.

Shortly after the isolation of the TBE virus in Czechoslovakia, the virus was isolated in Hungary, Poland, Bulgaria, Yugoslavia (Slovenia) (Bedjanič et al. 1955; Vesenjak-Zmijanac et al. 1955), Austria, Romania, and Germany, but also in Finland, Sweden, Northern China, and Japan.

There are several synonyms known for TBE, based on historical descriptions of TBE in different countries. These include "Taiga encephalitis," "Kumlinge disease," "Central European encephalitis," "Czechoslovak encephalitis," "Russian spring–summer encephalitis," "Far East Russian encephalitis," "Biphasic milk fever," "Biundulating meningoencephalitis," etc.

TBE after drinking raw goat milk was first reported in the Leningrad region in Russia in 1948 (Smorodintsev et al. 1953). This so-called biphasic miningoencephalitis was characterized with a milder clinical course and, unlike the classical form of TBE, a family character of the disease. Initially, this illness was considered to be a different disease from TBE. The same disease occurring after drinking raw milk was observed in the Moscow region in 1951, and was called milk fever (Drozdov 1959). In the same year, a large outbreak of milk-borne TBE was reported in Slovakia, when at least 660 people become infected, and 271 of those were hospitalized. During this outbreak, extensive scientific investigation under supervision by Raška, Bárdoš, and Blaškovič was performed, and the etiology and mode of transmission (i.e., by goat milk) was successfully revealed (Blaškovič 1954). Transmission of TBE by milk of infected dairy animals or by milk products (yogurt, cheese) was experimentally confirmed by Grešíková (Grešíková 1957, 1958). Historically, most of the pioneer research work on TBE has been done in Russia and the Czech Republic (Czechoslovakia).

10.2 BIOLOGICAL PROPERTIES

TBEV is the most medically important member of the tick-borne serocomplex group of the genus *Flavivirus*, family Flaviviridae. The TBE serocomplex includes Langat virus, louping-ill virus, Negishi virus, Kyasanur Forest disease virus, Omsk hemorrhagic fever virus, Powassan virus, and others. TBE virus is subdivided into three antigenic subtypes corresponding to three genotypes: European (previously Central European encephalitis; with Neudoerfl strain as prototype), Far Eastern (previously Russian spring–summer encephalitis; prototype strain Sofjin), and Siberian (previously Western Siberian encephalitis; prototype strains Zausaev and Vasilchenko)

(Ecker et al. 1999). However, based on antigenic properties, the European TBEV strains are more closely related rather to Louping ill virus than to the Far Eastern and Siberian strains (Hubálek et al. 1995).

Recently, a new taxonomic scheme based on the comparison of the complete coding sequences of all recognized tick-borne flavivirus species has been proposed. This suggests the assignment of TBEV and Louping ill virus to a unique species (TBEV) including four viral types (i.e., Western Tick-borne encephalitis virus, Eastern Tick-borne encephalitis virus, Turkish sheep Tick-borne encephalitis virus, and Louping ill Tick-borne encephalitis virus) (Grard et al. 2007). However, this classification has not been approved by the International Committee for Taxomony of Viruses yet, and it is not widely accepted since it combines viruses with different biological characteristics into one species.

More recently, a comparison of higher number of TBEV isolates from Siberia resulted in identification of two separate groups of TBEV strains, which meet the criteria to be classified as new genotypes. These new genotypes are phylogenetically different from the three previously established TBEV genotypes. One of the new possible genotypes is represented by only one isolate, 178–79, originated from the Irkutsk region, Russia. The second new genotype is tentatively named as "group 866" and is represented by 10 isolates (Zlobin et al. 2001; Tkachev et al. 2011). In summary, the most up-to-date taxonomical study indicates TBEV species divided into six subtypes/genotypes. The differences of biological properties of the members of the newly described genotypes in comparison with strains from the previously established genotypes are currently under investigation.

The TBEV virions are spherical, lipid-enveloped particles, approximately 50–60 nm in diameter (Slávik et al. 1967). The genome consists of a linear positive single-stranded RNA molecule, which is deposited in a capsid formed by C (capsid) protein. Two virus proteins are integrated in the viral envelope, namely E (envelope; M_r 55,000) and M (membrane; M_r 8000) proteins. Viral RNA consists of one open reading frame (ORF), which is flanked by untranslated (noncoding) regions (UTRs). The 5′UTR contains a type 1 cap (m7GpppAmG), followed by a conserved stem-loop structure. The 3′UTR is not polyadenylated and is characterized by extensive length and sequential heterogeneity (Wallner et al. 1995). This part of the viral genome can be divided into two parts: a proximal (localized behind the "stop" codon of the open reading frame) and a distal ("core," the 3′ terminus itself). The distal part of this region (approximately 340 nt) is highly conserved, while the proximal part is a noticeably variable segment with common deletions and insertions (Proutski et al. 1997; Gritsun et al. 1997). The untranslated regions form secondary stem-loop structures that probably serve as *cis*-acting elements for genome replication, translation and/or packaging (Gritsun et al. 1997; Proutski et al. 1997a,b). The ORF encodes one large polyprotein, which is co- and post-translationally cleaved by viral and cellular proteases into three structural proteins (C, prM, and E) and seven nonstructural proteins (NS1, NS2A, NS2B, NS3, NS4A, NS4B, and NS5).

C protein is a relatively small basic protein with lower sequence homology between different flaviviruses (Lindenbach and Rice 2003). The carboxyl terminus of C protein serves as an internal signal sequence leading the structural protein prM into the membrane of endoplasmic reticulum (ER). The viral protease NS2B-NS3 cleaves this signal sequence, releasing the N-terminus of prM protein (Kofler et al. 2002). prM protein is a glycosylated precursor of the membrane protein M. The prM protein shows a chaperon-like activity during the envelope protein E folding (Lorenz 2002; Lorenz et al. 2002).

The E protein is the site of the major viral antigens and the main target for neutralizing antibodies (although antibodies directed by prM/M and NS1 also provide some protection). Moreover, it is responsible for specific binding to a cellular receptor and penetration of the virus into the host cell. It is supposed to be a main determinant of the virulence (Gritsun et al. 1995). Three-dimensional structure of the protein E was studied at the resolution of 2.0 Å by x-ray crystallography (Rey et al. 1995).

The protein forms two monomers anchored in the membrane by their distal parts at physiological pH. After virus uptake by receptor-mediated endocytosis into the host cell, acidic pH in endosomes triggers irreversible changes in the E protein structure including its re-arrangement to trimeric forms and this leads to the initiation of the fusion process between the viral and endosomal membrane (Holzmann et al. 1995). Conserved histidines in the E protein function as molecular switches and, by their protonation at acidic pH, control the fusion process (Fritz et al. 2008).

Each E protein monomer is composed of three domains (I–III). Domain I is located in the central part of the protein. It is formed by eight antiparallel beta sheets, contains the N-terminus of the protein, two disulfide bridges, and an N-glycosylation site.

Domain II is formed by two long loops that extend out of domain I and form a finger-like structure. The domain contains a number of beta sheets and three disulfide bridges (Rey et al. 1995; Heinz 2003). Part of the domain responsible for the fusion of the viral envelope with the membrane of the endosome is called fusion peptide (Heinz and Allison 2003).

The domain III has a typical fold of an IgC molecule (Heinz 2003). It contains a beta barrel composed of seven antiparallel beta sheets. It is supposed that the lateral part of the domain III is responsible for binding to a specific cellular receptor (Rey et al. 1995).

Among the most conserved parts of the E protein, there are 12 cysteine residues forming six disulfide bridges with conserved localization in comparison with all known flaviviruses (Nowak and Wengler 1987).

NS1 is a glycoprotein containing two or three potential glycosylation sites (Lee et al. 1989) with not exactly defined functions. It exists in dimeric forms localized freely in the cytoplasm or associated with membranes. This protein is also secreted into the extracellular space particularly as a pentamer or hexamer and occasionally as a decamer or dodecamer (Crooks et al. 1994). This so-called soluble antigen induces protective immune response in the host (Gould et al. 1986).

NS2A is a small, hydrophobic protein with undefined function. It is supposed that it plays a role in the forming of a replication complex (Lindenbach and Rice 2003). A small membrane-associated protein NS2B serves as a crucial cofactor for protease activity of the NS3 protein (Yamschikov and Compans 1995). The central hydrophilic domain of the NS2B protein possibly interacts with the NS3 protein and it is flanked by hydrophobic regions probably anchored in the membrane (Chambers et al. 1993).

NS3 is the second largest viral protein. It contains conserved regions important for the function of the NS3 as a serine protease, helicase, and RNA triphosphatase (reviewed by Lindenbach and Rice 2003).

NS4A and NS4B are small, hydrophobic proteins. NS4A is probably part of the replication complex (Uchil and Satchidanandam 2003), while the function of NS4B is not known.

NS5 is the largest and highly conserved viral protein serving as a viral RNA-dependent RNA polymerase (Steffens et al. 1999). Its C-terminus shares a sequence homology with RNA-dependent RNA polymerases of other (+)RNA viruses (Lindenbach and Rice 2003). Apart from their main function as RNA dependent RNA polymerase the TBEV NS5 protein is able to interfere with type I IFN JAK-STAT signaling (Werme et al. 2008).

The infection of the host cell with TBEV (Figure 10.1) begins with the binding of the virus to a cell receptor, which has not been sufficiently identified until now. Kopecký et al. (1999) identified two polypeptides of 35 and 18 kD as putative vertebrate receptors for TBEV using viroblot technique with anti-idiotypic monoclonal antibodies directed against antibodies that neutralize the infectivity of TBEV. However, the anti-idiotypic monoclonal antibodies did not bind effectively to tick cells indicating that different receptors are used by vertebrate and invertebrate cells for the binding of TBE virus (Kopecký et al. 1999). It remains unclear whether TBEV uses single or multiple receptors on susceptible cells. Apparently, just the ability to use multiple receptors can be responsible for the very wide host range of flaviviruses, which replicate in arthropods and in a broad range of vertebrates. After binding to the receptor, virus is internalized by the process of endocytosis. As already mentioned above, the acidification within the endosomal vesicle triggers conformational changes of the E proteins leading to rearrangement of the dimers to trimeric forms

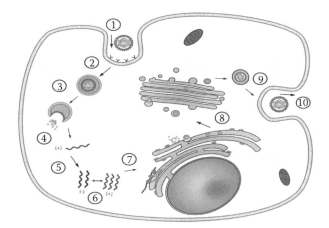

FIGURE 10.1   Replication machinery of TBEV in mammalian host cell. (1) Interaction of TBEV with host cell receptor. (2) Receptor mediated endocytosis of TBEV. (3) Fusion of viral and host cell membrane. (4) Release of the viral genome into the cytoplasm. (5, 6) Replication of the viral genome. (7) Transcription. (8) Viral particles assembly occurs in the endoplasmic reticulum. (9) Maturation of viral particles in the Golgi complex. (10) Release of mature virus.

and subsequent fusion of the viral envelope with the membrane of the vesicle. The viral nucleocapsid is then released into the cytoplasm and viral RNA is uncoated. The positive-stranded RNA is used for translation, and negative-stranded RNA that serves as a template for the RNA is synthesized. The polyprotein is cleaved by viral and cellular proteases into individual viral proteins. The surface structural proteins prM and E are translocated into lumen of the ER and their amino termini are liberated through proteolytic cleavage by the host signalase. The newly synthesized RNA is packaged by protein C into nucleocapsids on the cytoplasmic site of ER. Viral envelope is acquired by budding of the nucleocapsid into ER. The immature non-infectious virions containing proteins prM and E in heterodimeric association are transported into Golgi complex, where prM is cleaved, and the E protein is reorganized to the form of fusion-competent homodimers. These mature virions are finally released from the host cell by fusion of the transport vesicle membrane with plasma membrane (Mandl 2005).

TBEV infection is associated with dramatic morphological changes occurring in the infected cells. These include formation of smooth membrane structures, proliferation of endoplasmic reticulum, and accumulation and convolution of membranes. The infected cells often die by apoptosis or necrosis (Růžek et al. 2009).

The TBEV maturation process in tick cells seems, however, to be very different from the cells of vertebrates. In cell lines derived from the tick *Rhipicephalus appendiculatus* infected with TBEV, nucleocapsids occur in cytoplasm and the envelope is acquired by budding onto the cytoplasmic membrane or into cell vacuoles (Šenigl et al. 2006).

10.3 MICROEVOLUTION OF TBEV

It has been recognized since the 1960s that TBEV isolated from field-collected ticks contains a heterogeneous population of variants that produce a range of plaque sizes, express different levels of temperature-sensitivity, and neuroinvasiveness (Mayer and Kožuch 1969). Tick-adapted variants of TBEV were shown to exhibit small-plaque phenotype and slower replication in mammal cells and decreased neuroinvasiveness in laboratory mice (Bakhvalova et al. 2011). In nature, such low-virulent virus variants could emerge after several generations spent in ticks after transovarial and transstadial transmission and direct transfer from one tick to another during co-feeding on the same host.

The relatively rapid phenotype change of TBEV was first mentioned when the TBEV passaged in ticks *Hyalomma plumbeum* noticeably decreased the virulence for laboratory mouse and subsequent passaging through mouse brains led to restoring of the former phenotype (Dzhivanyan et al. 1988). Similarly, passaging of TBEV through salivary glands of ticks *Ixodes ricinus* led to reduction of neuroinvasiveness (Labuda et al. 1994). Analogously, the attenuated phenotype of the passaged virus was not stable; when the attenuated virus was passaged through mouse brains, the virulent phenotype was restored and after additional passages, the virus was more virulent than the parental strain (Kaluzová et al. 1994).

A Siberian strain isolated from *I. persulcatus* and passaged in mouse brain was subsequently passaged in *H. marginatum* by artificial inoculation and then again through mice. The tick-adapted virus exhibited small-plaque phenotype and slower replication in pig embryo kidney cells, higher yield in ticks, and decreased neuroinvasiveness in mice. A total of six amino acid substitutions distinguishing genomes of the variants were identified and two of them located in the E protein are supposed to be responsible for the phenotypic differences (Romanova et al. 2007).

In another study, an attenuated temperature-sensitive TBEV strain (263), isolated from field ticks *I. ricinus*, was either serially subcultured 5 times in mice or at 40°C in PS cells, producing two independent strains, 263-m5 and 263-TR with identical genomes; both strains exhibited increased plaque size, neuroinvasiveness, and temperature-resistance. Sequencing revealed two unique amino acid substitutions, one mapping close to the catalytic site of the viral protease NS2B-NS3 (Růžek et al. 2008b).

The selection, during serial passage, of preexisting quasi-species was postulated to be the explanation for the rapid shift of virus phenotypic characteristics. All the results lead to the suggestion that TBE virus exists as a heterogeneous population that contains virus variants most adapted to reproduction in either ticks or mammals. Host switch results in a change in the ratio of these variants in the population (Romanova et al. 2007). In other words, virulent and attenuated viruses may coexist as quasi-species in the same TBEV population and rapid conversion of neuro-virulence during virus tick/mammal adaptation is mediated by selection from the quasi-species population rather than random mutagenesis during virus passage in the laboratory (Růžek et al. 2008b).

10.4   ECOLOGY AND EPIDEMIOLOGY

In Europe, the main vector as well as reservoir of TBEV is the tick *Ixodes ricinus* (Ixodidae) (Rampas and Gallia 1949), a dominant hard tick across the European continent (Figure 10.2). *I. trianguliceps*, *I. hexagonus*, and *I. arboricola* are considered as amplifying vector ticks of TBEV (Grešíková 1972; Křivanec et al. 1988).

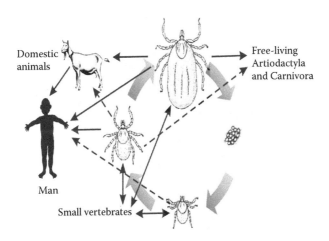

FIGURE 10.2   Life cycle of ixodid tick and transmission cycle of TBEV.

Infected secondary vector ticks, such as *Haemaphysalis inermis* and *Dermacentor reticulatus* exhibit lower transmission rates (Grešíková and Kaluzová 1997). The virus was also isolated from *H. inermis* in the Czech Republic (Grešíková and Nosek 1966), and *H. spinigera* and *H. turturis* were shown to be able to transmit TBEV under laboratory conditions (Nosek et al. 1967). Kožuch and Nosek (1971) confirmed *D. marginatus* and *D. reticulatus* as possible TBEV vectors, though the infection and transmission rates were lower than in vector species of the genera *Ixodes* and *Haemaphysalis* (Nosek et al. 1967).

Far Eastern and Siberian subtypes are transmitted predominantly by *I. persulcatus*. This tick comprises 80%–97% of all tick species in the Urals, Siberia, and the Far East region of Russia. *Dermacentor pictus*, *Dermacentor silvarum*, and *Hyalomma concinna* have also been associated with local TBE outbreaks in some areas of Siberia and the Far East, where *I. persulcatus* is not the predominant species (Zlobin and Gorin 1996). However, TBEV has been isolated from 15 other tick species in Russia and also sporadically from other parasitic invertebrates (e.g., fly, flea, lice; reviewed by Gritsun et al. 2003b).

The life cycle of *I. ricinus* consists of three stages: six-legged larva molds to eight-legged nymph, which develops to similar but larger imago (adult). Each stage takes approximately 1 year to develop to the next stage. However, the life cycle can take from 2 to 6 years, depending on various factors, including climatic conditions, availability of suitable hosts, etc. Each developmental stage prefers different vertebrate hosts for feeding. Larvae feed on small rodents, but also insectivores or birds. Nymphs prefer larger animals such as squirrels, hedgehogs, hares, and birds. Adults feed on deer, foxes, goats, sheep, cows, dogs, etc. The fertilized engorged female lays 500–5000 eggs and dies. The virus infects ticks chronically for the duration of their life. It is transmitted from transstadially from one developmental stage to the next and transovarially from infected female to eggs. The frequency of transovarial transmission seems to be very low, but under certain conditions it can be sufficient to ensure the continuity of virus populations. Sexual transmission from infected male to uninfected female has been also suggested and verified experimentally (Chunikhin et al. 1983). TBE virus can be transmitted to man or other hosts by all the tick stages, i.e., larvae, nymphs, as well as adult ticks. The seasonal activity of *I. ricinus* has two peaks: April–May and September–October. Comparison of the tick population curves and the morbidity rate in humans shows that there is a difference of approximately 14 days between the peaks of the two curves. The gap between the peak of tick activity and the highest morbidity rate in humans corresponds to the incubation period of the disease, which is between 4 and 14 days. The activity of *I. persulcatus* has only one peak and lasts from the end of April to the beginning of June. During July only some sporadic cases can be seen (Süss 2003).

A tick can be infected with TBEV following feeding on viremic animal hosts or following co-feeding of infected and uninfected ticks on the same host (nonviremic transmission) (Labuda et al. 1993, 1997). Virus crossing from tick esophagus to subesophageal ganglion represents the main route of tick infection. Epidermal cells are the primary site of virus replication in the tick body. Immunofluorescence detection of TBEV antigen in sections of virophoric female ticks feeding for 36 hours shows clear infection of epidermal cells and salivary glands (Nosek et al. 1972). In the period that precedes molting, the virus multiplies in the tick and invades almost all the tick's organs (Benda 1958).

Virus transmission from the infected tick to the host is quite fast. Theoretically, the virus can be transmitted by saliva during the first minutes of feeding. Experimentally, it was demonstrated that TBEV was transmitted from infected *Haemaphysalis inermis* ticks to lab mice within the first 3 hours of feeding (Grešíková and Nosek 1966). A number of pharmacologically active compounds is secreted in tick saliva. These modify the microenvironment in the site of feeding and control the hemostatic, inflammatory, and immune responses in the vertebrate host in order to facilitate blood feeding. Such bioactive saliva molecules include immunoglobulin-binding proteins, histamine-binding proteins, interferon regulators, and inhibitors of natural killer cells and complement. The action of the bioactive saliva molecules can facilitate TBEV transmission to the vertebrate host (Nuttall and Labuda 2004).

Hosts of TBEV include various rodents (*Clethrionomys*, *Apodemus*, *Mus*, *Microtus*, *Micromys*, *Pitymys*, *Arvicola*, *Glis*, *Sciurus*, and *Citellus*) and insectivores (*Sorex*, *Talpa*, *Erinaceus*), but also reptiles, birds, bats, carnivores (*Meles*, *Vulpes*, *Mustela*), and large vertebrates. Rodents, insectivores, bats, and probably some birds and carnivores serve as reservoirs of TBEV in nature, i.e., these animals develop viremia for a long period without becoming clinically ill and thus can serve as a source of TBEV for the virus transmission to uninfected ticks. Small rodents and insectivores exhibit unapparent infection after experimental TBEV inoculation with long-lasting viremia (Kožuch et al. 1967; Achazi et al. 2011). The virus can be detected in various organs for long time periods (Achazi et al. 2011; Knap et al. 2012). Experimentally, the transmission of TBEV from ticks to rodents and insectivores, as well as from these hosts to ticks, was demonstrated. The virus has been successfully isolated from various rodents and insectivores captured in the field (e.g., *Apodemus flavicollis*, *Clethrionomys glareolus*, *Erinaceus roumanicus*, etc.; Kožuch et al. 1967; Weidmann et al. 2006). This all clearly demonstrates the crucial role of rodents as well as insectivores in TBEV circulation in nature. Moreover, these animals serve as a bridge for TBEV transmission by co-feeding of infected and uninfected ticks. The same has been verified experimentally even on immune individuals (Labuda et al. 1997). The importance of co-feeding in the virus maintenance in nature is not clearly determined, since it requires common feeding of larvae and nymphs on the same host, which is not, however, a frequent event.

Lizards are frequently infested with ticks in the field. Experimentally inoculated lizards *Lacerta viridis* with TBEV develop viremia lasting up to 7 days and antibody response (Grešíková and Albrecht 1959; Sekeyová et al. 1970).

The role of birds in the circulation of TBEV is not fully clear (Ernek et al. 1968), but the virus was isolated from several species, especially from water birds (Grešíková 1972). Experimentally infected wild ducks (*Anas platyrhynchos*) develop chronic infection with viremia detectable from 4 to 36 weeks postinoculation (Ernek et al. 1969). On the other hand, viremia was not detected in the inoculated great tit (*Parus major*), blackbird (*Turdus merula*), common buzzard (*Buteo buteo*), common kestrel (*Falco tinnunculus*), common pheasant (*Phasianus colchichus*) (Grešíková 1972).

High and long-lasting viremia (7–23 days p.i.) was observed in bats (*Myotis myotis*, *Barbastella barbastella*, *Plecotus auritus*) inoculated with TBEV (Kolman et al. 1960; Nosek et al. 1961). TBEV persisted in bats during their hibernation and posthibernation viremia was observed (Nosek et al. 1961).

Indicator hosts have only brief viremia with low virus production and are not able to transmit the virus to vectors. Dogs or roe deer represent examples of indicator hosts. Dogs develop low and short viremia (Grešíková et al. 1972) and seroconvert upon infection but they are not capable to further spread the virus (Pfeffer and Dobler 2011). Low and short viremia and seroconversion was also observed in roe deer (*Capreolus capreolus*) after experimental inoculation with TBEV or after experimental transmission of TBEV from infected ticks (Nosek et al. 1967). Dairy animals (goats, sheep, cows) develop viremia after the infection, the virus can pass from the blood of the livestock into the mammary gland and is present in milk (Grešíková 1957, 1958; Grešíková and Řeháček 1959), but their role in TBEV circulation in nature is not known.

Humans are accidental and dead-end hosts of TBEV, i.e., they can develop a disease with viremia, but they do not participate in TBEV circulation in nature. In most cases, people are infected by a bite of an infected tick. Less frequent cases of TBE occur after drinking infected unboiled milk or eating unpasteurized milk products. In the Czech Republic, retrospective analysis revealed that, between 1997 and 2008, 64 cases of TBE were recorded in patients who reported consumption of unpasteurized goats' and dairy milk or unpasteurized sheep's milk cheese (0.9% of the total 7288 number of TBE cases). The majority of cases involved goats' milk (36 patients, i.e., 56.3%) and sheep's milk cheese (21 patients, i.e., 32.8%). Dairy milk-borne infection was responsible for 7 TBE cases (10.9%). Thirty-three cases (51.6%) occurred in family outbreaks following purchase of cheese or milk from animal breeders (Kříž et al. 2009). In Slovakia, 33 TBE cases after drinking raw milk were reported during 5 years (about 9% all cases) (Labuda et al. 2002). In Poland, 119 unpasteurized milk samples from 63 cows, 29 goats, 27 sheep from 8 farms in eastern Poland were analyzed (Cisak et al. 2010). The most common TBEV occurrence was in the milk of sheep (22.2%), milk of goats (20.7%), and cows (11.1%) (as determined by the RT-PCR method). By the ELISA method, the highest prevalence of anti-TBEV antibodies was found in the milk of sheep (14.8%), milk of cows in 3.2%, and none in milk of goats.

Sporadic laboratory-based infections caused by inhaling infected aerosol or by accidental needle-stick injury were reported before the availability of effective TBEV vaccine (Gallia et al. 1949; Molnár and Fornosi 1952; Bodemann et al. 1977; Avšič-Županc et al. 1995).

Based on the biology of ticks as the vectors of TBEV, TBE has two main epidemiological characteristics: seasonal character of the disease and territorial distribution. The case distribution according to age, sex, and occupation is determined by contact with the source of infection, particularly in forested areas. TBEV is endemic in areas extending from Central and Eastern Europe to Siberia and parts of Asia. More and more TBEV endemic areas are being detected, especially in Asia (Lu et al. 2008). In Russia, the highest TBE incidence is reported in Western Siberia and Ural. In the European part of Russia, especially the northern part and Crimea exhibit high TBE incidence. The countries and regions in Central and Eastern Europe with a high risk of exposure to TBEV in 2011 are the following: Latvia, Lithuania, Estonia, Belarus, Sweden (eastern coast, Gotland, Oland, and endemic foci in northern part),

Finland (Åland Islands, and west coast), Poland (Mazury, Podlasie, Opole, Lublin, Warsaw, and Gdańsk Regions, single endemic areas in central part of Poland), Czech Republic (whole country but especially South Bohemia, Plzen Region, Moravia), Slovakia (especially between Bratislava and Banska Bystrica), Germany (south part and endemic areas in Sachsen and in the northern Germany), Austria (area between Vienna and Klagenfurt and between Vienna and Linz), Hungary (west part and scattered endemic areas in eastern part of this country), Slovenia, Croatia (northern part), Albania (southern part), and Norway (southern coast). Small, single endemic areas occur in Switzerland, France, and Italy. No TBE cases were reported, e.g., in Great Britain, Ireland, Iceland, the Netherlands, Luxemburg, Spain, and Portugal. TBEV represents a potential risk for people traveling to endemic countries for leisure activities in nature (Rendi-Wagner 2004; Reusken et al. 2011; Chaudhuri and Růžek 2012). During the past decades, an increase in TBE incidence has been reported in most European countries as well as in Russia. This might be caused by several factors, which include ecological (climatic changes), agricultural, but also social factors (changes in leisure activities) (Korenberg 2009). In relation to the climatic changes, a shift of the upper limit of the geographical habitats of ticks to higher altitudes has been observed. Previously, a limit of occurrence of ticks was at 700–750 m above sea level and ticks were not able to finish their life cycle at higher altitudes. It was revealed recently that ticks shifted to the altitudes up to 1000 m above sea level (Danielová et al. 2008). Because these mountain zones are often used for leisure and outdoor activities, the risk of TBEV infection in these areas increased considerably (Daniel et al. 2003). Socioeconomic factors may exert a powerful effect on the frequency of population contact with TBEV, which leads to an explosive increase in general morbidity. But attributing the increasing incidence of TBE cases to "the collapse of communism" in Eastern Europe as repeatedly published by some authors (Randolph 2004, 2008) is too simplistic and has a poor epidemiological basis (Korenberg 2009).

The most exposed groups to TBEV are forestry workers and farmers. For example, in serological studies in Poland, seropositivity was found in about 20%–30% of farmers and forestry workers (Cisak et al. 1998). Children and youth include 25% of sick persons in Poland.

10.5   CLINICAL FEATURES

It is assumed that the majority of TBEV infections are asymptomatic. Although the proportion of these cases is difficult to determine, serological surveys suggest 70%–95% of the infections occurring asymptomatically (Kaiser 2008; Shapoval 1976, 1977; Pogodina et al. 1979).

In case of symptomatic infection, the incubation period is usually 7–14 days, but it may vary from 2 to 28 days. Two-thirds of patients with TBE caused by European TBEV strains have a characteristic biphasic course (Kaiser 1999; Günther et al. 1997a; Holzmann 2003). The first, viremic phase is generally sudden and is characterized with nonspecific influenza-like symptoms lasting 2–4 days, with moderate fever (sometimes with chills), fatigue, malaise, headache, myalgia, gastrointestinal symptoms, leukocytopenia, thrombocytopenia (Lotrič-Furlan 1995), and sometimes with elevated liver enzymes. This is followed by a symptom-free interval of about 1 week (range 1–33 days) before the second phase develops. The second phase presents as meningitis (50% of all adult patients), meningoencephalitis (40%), or as meningoencephalomyelitis (10%) (Bogovič et al. 2010). During the second phase, an elevated white blood cell count can be seen, but rarely exceeds $15 \times 10^9/L$. The C-reactive protein concentration and erythrocyte sedimentation is usually normal but may be elevated in some cases. In CSF, moderately raised protein levels and lymphocytic pleocytosis is seen (only during the early phases of the disease polymorphonuclear cells may predominate in CSF) (Bogovič et al. 2010).

The meningeal form is usually manifested by high fever, headache, nausea, vomiting, and vertigo. Encephalitis is characterized by restlessness, tremor of extremities, fasciculations of the tongue, concentration disturbances, and cognitive function disturbances. Other symptoms include global latent paresis of the limbs, hyperesthesia, impaired micturition, and increased physiology reflexes. Disturbance of consciousness ranges from somnolence to stupor or very rarely to coma (Fališevac and Balus 1981; Bogovič et al. 2010). Seizures are rare.

The meningoencephalomyelitis and meningoencephalomyeloradiculitis represent the most severe form of TBE. In these forms, flaccid paralyses of the limbs are present, but also the paralyses of pharyngeal or respiratory muscles can develop. The upper extremities are affected more frequently than the lower ones (Bogovič et al. 2010).

Far Eastern TBEV strains cause more frequently a disease with a monophasic course; the biphasic form occurs in only 3%–8% of the patients (Votiakov et al. 2002). Focal encephalitic symptoms appear in 31%–64% of the patients, meningeal form is seen in about 26%, febrile form in 14%–16% (Votiakov et al. 2002). In about 0.5% of cases, the infection progresses into a chronic form.

The Siberian subtype is associated with focal encephalitis in 5%, meningeal in about 47%, and febrile form in 40% of the cases. Biphasic course is seen in about 20% of patients (Votiakov et al. 2002). About 1.7% of patients with acute illness develop a chronic progressive form of TBE (Popponikova 2008). The chronic form of TBE is not seen in Europe; only two cases have been reported with some controversy (Mickiene et al. 2002). However, in Russia, several cases are well documented, although they vary in the clinical presentation, and the time of onset of the individual neurological symptoms (Bogovič et al. 2010). Clinical manifestations include Kozhevnikov's epilepsy (epilepsia partialis continua), progresive neuritis, lateral sclerosis, progressive muscle atrophy, and a Parkinson's-like disease (Bogovič et al. 2010).

The fatality rate in adult patients in Europe is less than 1%. Far Eastern TBEV subtype is associated with more severe disease with case fatality rate up to 40%. The disease caused by Siberian TBEV strains has a case fatality rate of 2%–3% (Lindquist and Valapathi 2008; Bogovič et al. 2011; Mickiene et al. 2002). Severe courses of TBE infection with higher mortality and long-lasting sequelae often affecting the quality of life are in correlation with increased age (>60 years of age) (Haglund and Günther 2003).

A postencephalitic syndrome has been identified in 35%–58% of patients after acute TBE. The patients have permanent sequelae; the most commonly reported problems include cognitive or neuropsychiatric complaints, balance disorders, headache, dysphasia, hearing defects, and spinal paralysis (Růžek et al. 2011).

TBE in children is generally milder, although severe illness may occur and even lead to permanent impairment of the quality of life due to neuropsychological sequelae (Kunze et al. 2004). Encephalomyelitic manifestation of TBE is very rare in children. The paralytic form usually heals without sequelae. The prognosis of TBE in children is usually favorable (Falk and Lazarini 1981; Messner 1981).

TBE following alimentary infection is about 50% monophasic. In this form, the symptoms include fever, intracranial hypertension, sharp headache, nausea, vomiting, weakness, loss of appetite, dizziness, drowsiness, gastrointestinal problems, epistaxis, pharyngitis, laryngitis, and photophobia. After 2–7 days, these symptoms disappear and the patients recover (Kubánka and Pór 1954). The biphasic form of alimentary TBE is more severe, but benign. The first phase takes about 7 days and is characterized with the same symptoms as the monophasic form, but in addition with very high fever, blurred vision, and diplopia. The second phase appears after approximately 8 days of remission and is characterized with meningeal irritation and/or encephalitis. Hypersomnia and diplopia are typical signs. In mild cases, the second phase lasts 3–4 days; in more serious cases, 14–21 days (Henner 1954; Hympán 1954; Dudáš et al. 1954; Černáček et al. 1954).

Treatment is symptomatic only, with strict bed rest. Maintenance of water and electrolyte balance is important. Analgesics, vitamins, and antipyretics are administered. Corticoids have a favorable effect during the acute stage of TBE (intravenously 5–10 mg/kg/day) (Dunyewicz et al. 1981), but the use of corticosteroids may be questioned, as it has not been shown to be useful in prospective studies (Mickiene et al. 2002). Administration of hyperimmunoglobulin is not recommended due to concerns about antibody-dependent enhancement of the infection (Kaiser 1999; Waldvogel et al. 1996; Jones et al. 2007).

Besides preventive measures, such as wearing appropriate clothing or checking the skin for attached ticks after returning from activities in nature, TBE can be successfully prevented by active immunization (Kunz 2003). In Russia, several inactivated vaccines are available (vaccine produced by the Institute of Poliomyelitis and Viral Encephalitis [IPVE] in Moscow and EnceVir produced by Virion, Tomsk). The IPVE vaccine is applied for adults and children of three years and more. The basic vaccination scheme consists of two doses within 5–7 months with revaccination after 1 year and a booster every 3 years. The EnceVir vaccine is administered to adults (>18 years of age) with the same vaccination scheme. In case of rapid immunization, the first two doses are administered within 1–2 months (Donoso Mantke et al. 2011). In Europe, two inactivated vaccines are available (FSME-Immun by Baxter Bioscience, Austria; Encepur by Novartis Vaccines and Diagnostics, Germany). The vaccination scheme is analogous for both vaccines with three doses given on 0, 1–3 months, 5–12 months after the second (FSME-Immun), or 9–12 months (Encepur). First booster vaccination should be after 3 years, and the next booster vaccinations every 5 years (or every 3 years for people older than 50 years [Encepur] or 60 years [FSME-Immun]) (Rendi-Wagner et al. 2004; Hainz et al. 2005). Both vaccines are comparable in terms of efficacy and tolerability. FSME-Immun has shown a protective effect of >95% after three doses (Heinz 2007). TBE cases are observed despite immunization with both available vaccines (Anderson et al. 2010; Stiasny 2009). Persons older than 50 years show a significantly lower antibody response (Weinberger et al. 2010), with a higher frequency of low responders and vaccine failures. Therefore, people older than 50–60 years of age may be recommended three doses as basic immunization, day 0, 1 month, and 3 months. The next booster dose should be administrated as early as possible before the next season. Rapid schedules with an interval shortened to 2 weeks between the first and second dose should be avoided in people older than 60 years.

Vaccination is especially recommended for forestry workers, farmers, hunters, people who are in contact with forests (collectors of mushrooms, etc.), and tourists and children staying in those places. Most common adverse reactions after immunization are itching, local swelling, pain, rash, fever, or moderate elevated body temperature (especially in children), nausea, malaise, pain of the skeletal system and muscles, headache, and vomiting. Contraindications for immunization include hypersensitivity (allergy) to chicken protein, formalin, neomycin, gentamicin, and/or acute reaction to previous immunization. There are no data available concerning the influence of TBEV vaccines on pregnancy. Immunization of pregnant women and children <12 months of age is not recommended. Other contraindications include acute infections.

10.6 PATHOLOGY AND PATHOGENESIS

After the tick bite, the virus replicates in subcutaneous tissues. Various cell types in the skin including keratinocytes become infected by the virus. Langerhans cells (LCs) are probably the first distinct dendritic cells subset that present antigens of TBEV to T cells and activate their differentiation to T helper type 1 (Th1), Th2, and cytotoxic T lymphocyte (CTL) effector cells. However, LCs are likely to serve also as a vehicle for the transport of the virus to draining lymph nodes (Chambers and Diamond 2003). The lymph nodes play an important part in the pathogenesis of TBE, although virus replication is not accompanied by virus-specific histological changes and no marked destruction of infected lymph node cells is observed (Málková and Filip 1968). Within the lymph nodes, macrophages represent the target cells for TBEV infection. The interaction between TBEV and macrophages is crucial, and the inability of the virus to multiply in macrophages is in association with the inability to induce an infection of the individual (Ahantarig et al. 2009; Plekhova et al. 2011). Massive viral multiplication in the nodes leads to the spread of the virus into the bloodstream and induction of viremia (Málková and Fraňková 1959; Málková and Kolman 1964). Temporary leukopenia in the white blood picture is observed. A significant decrease is recorded in all cellular elements. In regional lymph nodes, a significant decrease in lymphocytes appears (Málková et al. 1961). TBEV can be isolated from blood leukocytes during the first days of infection, which indicates virus replication in immunocompetent blood cells (Leonova et al. 1996). The virus is probably cleared when protecting antibodies appear in serum and the encephalitic symptoms are probably due to an intense inflammatory reaction in the brain.

During the primary viremic phase, several extraneural tissues are infected (especially spleen, liver, and bone marrow cells). The release of the virus from these cells induces secondary viremia, which continues for a couple of days. During the secondary viremia, the virus crosses the blood–brain barrier and reaches the CNS. The mode of virus crossing the blood–brain barrier remains unknown. Four potential routes were postulated: (i) by neuronal route after infection of peripheral nerves or by olfactory neurons, (ii) by so-called Trojan horse mechanism when TBEV-infected immune cells migrate into the CNS, (iii) by infection of vascular endothelial cells of brain capillaries, and (iv) by diffusion of virus between the capillary endothelial cells under the conditions of increased blood–brain barrier permeability (Růžek et al. 2010) (Figure 10.3). Experiments with mice infected with TBEV showed that the breakdown of the blood–brain barrier occurs at later stages of the neuroinfection when a high virus load is present in the brain; therefore, the breakdown of the

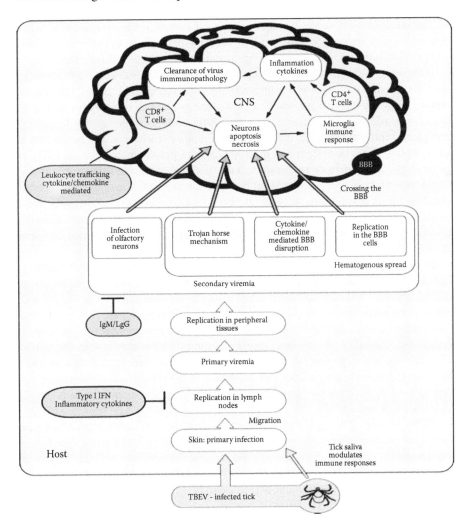

FIGURE 10.3 Schematic drawing of the steps during TBEV infection in the mammalian host. BBB, blood–brain barrier; CNS, central nervous system.

blood–brain barrier is not necessary for TBEV entry into the brain and more likely is in association with dramatic up-regulation of proinflammatory cytokine/chemokine expression in the infected brain (Růžek et al. 2011).

In most cases, the morphological picture of TBE in the CNS has the characteristics of nodular polioencephalomyelitis with meningeal involvement. The histopathological picture involves (i) damage to the nervous parenchyma with cell necrosis and neuronophagy, (ii) perivascular inflammatory reaction with serous exudation, (iii) spongiform focal necrosis in the form of facultative lesions and secondary damage or anoxic vassal lesions (Jellinger 1981).

Viral antigens can be demonstrated in perikarya and processes of Purkinje cells and large neurons of dentate nucleus, inferior olives, anterior horns, neurons of other brainstem nuclei, isocortex, and basal ganglia (Gelpi et al. 2005).

The infected neurons are damaged—there is necrosis and neurolysis. The degradation products are phagocyted by microglia cells (neurophagy). Astroglial swelling and proliferation and increase of glycogen content take place (Jelliger 1981).

Interestingly, there is a poor topographical correlation between inflammatory changes and distribution of viral antigen in the brain (Gelpi et al. 2005). The inflammatory response has two phases. The first phase is characterized by an unspecific resorptive inflammatory reaction of granulocytes and macrophages, while the second phase represents specific, defensive inflammatory reaction in which elements of the lymphomonocytic system and macrophages are predominant (Jelliger 1981). In general, the inflammatory response includes nodular and flaky tissue infiltrates of histiocytes and rod-shaped microglia, perivascular cell cuffs, meningeal infiltrates, and less frequent infiltrates in cerebral nerve roots, spinal nerve roots, and spinal ganglia. The perivascular cuffs consist predominantly of T-lymphocytes, histiocytes, plasma cells, and macrophages (Jelliger 1981). B-cells are only rarely found (Gelpi et al. 2005).

In most cases, the spinal gray matter is infected with preference for the anterior horns and the cervical region. There is a disseminated infection in the brainstem. The cerebellum is mostly affected; massive infection is seen in the dentate nucleus, cortex, and white matter. In the diencephalon, thalamus nuclei are highly infected. The putamen and caudate nucleus are severely affected, whereas the pallidum is only slightly affected. Widespread dissemination of the nodules is seen throughout the cortex of telencephalon, with frontal accumulation, in insula of Reil, claustrum, basal rhinencephalic gray matter and amygdala, in the subcortical white matter, and less in the deep cerebral white matter and fiber systems. The hippocampus is usually uninfected (Jelliger 1981).

TBEV induces a strong intrathecal immune activation, as demonstrated by a massive up-regulation of proinflammatory cytokines and other inflammatory mediators. Patients with TBE react with stronger immune activation than patients with other forms of encephalitis (enterovirus, HSV2) as indicated by CSF neopterin response (Günther et al. 1996). The immune activation in brain involves production of various inflammatory cytokines including IFN-γ, IL-2, IL5, IL-6, and IL-10. The importance of IL-10 during TBE has been demonstrated; low levels of IL-10 in CSF aggravate the course of TBE (Günther et al. 2011) (Figure 10.4). Although IL-6 production is generally associated with a protective immune response, it may also contribute to

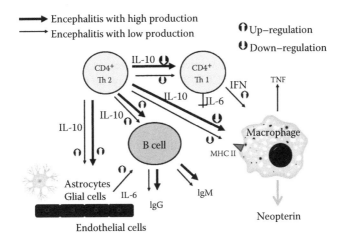

FIGURE 10.4 Interaction of intrathecal inflammatory mediatos in TBE with different clinical course. Proposed pathogenesis resulting in severe encephalitic or mild disease. (From Günther, G. 1997. *Tick-borne encephalitis—on pathogenesis and prognosis.* Dissertation Thesis, Karolinska Institutet, Stockholm. With permission.)

disease progression. Interestingly, an inverse correlation between raised IL-6 levels and IgG titers was observed in TBE patients.

It has been hypothesized that the immunological mechanisms activated in the brain can contribute to the nerve destruction during TBE, i.e., the host immune response can act as a double-edged sword during TBE. Experiments with mice demonstrated that mice immunosuppressed by cyclophosphamide or sublethal X-irradiation exhibited prolonged survival after TBEV inoculation when compared with untreated individuals (Semenov et al. 1981; Vince and Grčević 1981). Adoptive transfer of sensitized splenocytes to immunosuppressed mice significantly decreased the mean survival time of the infected animals (Semenov et al. 1981). The important role of CD8+ T-cells in immunopathology during TBE has been revealed (Růžek et al. 2009). Based on these results, it seems that the outcome of TBE represents a result of certain "immunological conflict" between the infection control mediated by immunity and damage to the host mediated by immunopathology (Růžek et al. 2010; Rouse and Sehrawat 2010).

IgM and IgG antibodies against TBEV antigens are found in serum as well as in the CSF. TBEV-IgM antibodies are detectable at an early stage of the infection when the first symptoms appear. The level of IgM in CSF starts to increase between day 0 and day 6 after onset of encephalitic symptoms and reaches its peak approximately 2 weeks later, but variations were found in individual patients. Although in most cases IgM antibodies are not detectable after 6–7 weeks, they may persist for several months. In contrast, the IgG level increases only moderately at the beginning and during the whole encephalitic phase. These TBEV-specific IgG antibodies confer a long-term or even life-long immunity (Růžek et al. 2011). In CSF, IgG antibodies are detectable as long as 11–13 months (Günther et al. 1996).

The course and outcome of TBE can be influenced by several factors. These include virulence of the particular TBEV strain, and dose of the virus, but also age, sex, immune status, and genetic background of the host. Interestingly, a functional toll-like receptor 3 gene may be a risk factor for TBEV infection (Kindberg et al. 2011). A deletion within the chemokine receptor CCR5 (CCR5Δ32), which plays an important role in leukocyte transmigration across the blood–brain barrier, is significantly more frequent in patients with TBE than in TBE-naive patients with aseptic meningitis (Kindberg et al. 2008). Moreover, the severity and outcome of TBE is associated with variability in the 2′–5′-oligoadenylate synthetase gene cluster (family members are interferon-induced antiviral proteins) (Barkhash et al. 2010), and the rs2287886 single nucleotide polymorphism located in the promoter region of the human CD209 gene (Barkhash et al. 2012). This gene encodes dendritic cell-specific ICAM3-grabbing nonintegrin (DC-SIGN), a C-type lectin pathogen-recognition receptor expressed on the surface of dendritic cells and some types of macrophages (Barkhash et al. 2012). Taken together, polymorphism in various genes may largely influence the sensitivity of the host to the infection and determine the severity of the disease.

10.7 DIAGNOSIS

In the later stage of the infection, specific antibodies are formed. They cut off viremia and at the beginning of the second phase, no infective virus can be found in the blood. Therefore, the most important laboratory techniques for the diagnosis of TBE are not those of virus isolation but serological ones. Antibodies occur as early as the beginning of the second phase, which represents the actual disease. If specific antibodies are found, it is necessary to exclude that these are old antibodies caused by a previous TBE infection or by TBEV vaccination (Hofmann 1981). This is ruled out by intrathecally detecting the produced antibodies that indicate actual TBEV infection. IgM activity can be demonstrated in 96% of patients, a median of 3 days, after onset of encephalitis, later, serum from all patients are positive (Günther et al. 1997b). Maximum IgG activity can be detected in serum after 6 weeks and decreases thereafter, but persists for many years (>30 years). IgG should be analyzed in paired sera. Intrathecal antibodies are seen in 97% of patients after a median of 9 days (Günther et al. 1997b) and the analysis may be of value in certain cases.

It is recommended to test paired sera with 1 or 2 weeks' interval using ELISA or by classical methods, which include virus neutralization, inhibition of hemagglutination, and complement fixation tests. Diagnosis is established when at least a fourfold rise of antibodies is demonstrated. However, if the patient is hospitalized at the peak of the second phase or even later, further increase of the already high antibody titer cannot be often observed. In this case, the analysis of IgM antibodies is crucial; the presence of specific IgM antibodies indicates recent infection (Hofmann 1981). Generally, ELISA is the method of choice due to its simple performance. New diagnostic ELISA kits are available, which have very high specificity and sensitivity (Holzmann 2003). Isolation of TBEV or detection of viral RNA by RT-PCR in serum or CSF have large limitations and is rarely used in clinical practice (Saksida et al. 2005; Bogovič et al. 2011).

Antibodies against TBEV can be also assayed directly from CSF. Most patients suffering from acute TBE have IgG antibodies in CSF, but IgM antibodies are present only in about 80% of the cases. Sometimes, it is not clear if these antibodies are actually produced in the brain or if they penetrate to the CSF though the broken blood–brain barrier (Hofmann 1981).

In the postmortem material, the virus can be demonstrated in brain tissue by immunofluorescence, RT-PCR, or by cultivation techniques (Hofmann 1981).

Tissue destruction in the CNS is rare. Abnormalities on MRI are seen in up to 18% in TBE-Eu with lesions confined to the thalamus, cerebellum, brainstem, and nucleus caudatus (Lorenzl et al. 1996; Marjelund et al. 2004). Electroencephalogram is abnormal in 77% (Kaiser 1999). Both MRI and EEG abnormalities are unspecific, not diagnostic, and no direct correlation to the prognosis has been shown.

ACKNOWLEDGEMENTS

The authors acknowledge financial support by the Czech Science Foundation project P302/10/P438 and P502/11/2116 and grant Z60220518 from the Ministry of Education, Youth, and Sports of the Czech Republic. We thank Patrik Kilian for the preparation of the figures.

REFERENCES

Achazi, K., Růžek, D., Donoso-Mantke, O., Schlegel, M., Ali, H. S., Wenk, M., Schmidt-Chanasit, J., Ohlmeyer, L., Rühe, F., Vor, T., Kiffner, C., Kallies, R., Ulrich, R. G., and Niedrig, M. 2011. Rodents as sentinels for the prevalence of tick-borne encephalitis virus. *Vector Borne Zoonotic Dis.* 11(6), 641–7.

Ahantarig, A., Růžek, D., Vancová, M., Janowitz, A., Šťastná, H., Tesařová, M., and Grubhoffer, L. 2009. Tick-borne encephalitis virus infection of cultured mouse macrophages. *Intervirology.* 52(5), 283–90.

Andersson, C. R., Vene, S., Insulander, M., Lindquist, L., Lundkvist, A., and Günther, G. 2010 Vaccine failures after active immunisation against tick-borne encephalitis. *Vaccine.* 28(16), 2827–31.

Avšič-Županc, T., Poljak, M., Maticic, M., Radsel-Medvescek, A., LeDuc, J. W., Stiasny, K., Kunz, C., and Heinz, F. X. 1995. Laboratory acquired tick-borne meningoencephalitis: characterisation of virus strains. *Clin. Diagn. Virol.* 4(1), 51–9.

Bakhvalova, V. N., Panov, V. V., and Morozova, O. V. 2011. Tick-borne encephalitis virus quasispecies rearrangements in ticks and mammals. In: Růžek, D. (ed.) *Flavivirus Encephalitis.* InTech, Rijeka, 213–34.

Barkhash, A. V., Perelygin, A. A., Babenko, V. N., Brinton, M. A., and Voevoda, M. I. 2012. Single nucleotide polymorphism in the promoter region of the CD209 gene is associated with human predisposition to severe forms of tick-borne encephalitis. *Antiviral. Res.* 93(1), 64–8.

Barkhash, A. V., Perelygin, A. A., Babenko, V. N., Myasnikova, N. G., Pilipenko, P. I., Romaschenko, A. G., Voevoda, M. I., and Brinton, M. A. 2010. Variability in the 2′–5′-oligoadenylate synthetase gene cluster is associated with human predisposition to tick-borne encephalitis virus-induced disease. *J. Infect. Dis.* 202(12), 1813–8.

Bedjanič, M. 1959. Tick-borne meningoencephalitis. *Minerva Med.* 50(33), 1220–4.

Benda, R. 1958. The common tick "Ixodes ricinus" as a reservoir and vector of tick-borne encephalitis. I. Survival of the virus (strain B3) during the development of ticks under laboratory condition. *J. Hyg. Epidemiol. (Prague)* 2, 314.

Blaškovič, D. (ed.) 1954. *The Epidemic of Encephalitis in Rožňava Natural Focus of Infection.* Slovak Academy of Sciences, Bratislava. (in Slovak).

Bodemann, H. H., Pausch, J., Schmitz, H., Hoppe-Seyler, G. 1977. Tick-borne encephalitis (ESME) as laboratory infection. *Med. Welt.* 28(44), 1779–81.

Bogovič, P., Lotrič-Furlan, S., and Strle, F. 2010. What tick-borne encephalitis may look like: clinical signs and symptoms. *Travel Med. Infect. Dis.* 8(4), 246–50.

Černáček, J., Hanzal, F., Henner, K., and Hympán, J. 1954. Clinical features of the Rožňava epidemic. In: Blaškovič, D. (ed.) *An Epidemic of Encephalitis in the Natural Focus of Infection in Rožňava*. Slovak Academy of Sciences, Bratislava, 56–63.

Chambers, T. J., and Diamond, M. S. 2003. Pathogenesis of flavivirus encephalitis. *Adv. Virus Res.* 60, 273–342.

Chambers, T. J., Nestorowicz, A., Amberg, S. M., and Rice, C. M. 1993. Mutagenesis of the yellow fever virus NS2B protein: effects on proteolytic processing, NS2B-NS3 complex formation, and viral replication. *J. Virol.* 67(11), 6797–807.

Chaudhuri, A., and Růžek, D. 2012. First documented case of imported tick-borne encephalitis in Australia. *Int. Med. J.*, in press.

Chumakov, M. P., and Zeitlenok, N. A. 1940. Tick-borne spring–summer encephalitis in the Ural region. In: Neuroinfections in the Ural. *Sverdlovsk* 23–30. (in Russian).

Chunikhin, S. P., Stefuktina, L. F., Korolev, M. B., Reshetnikov, I. A., and Khozinskaia, G. A. 1983. Sexual transmission of the tick-borne encephalitis virus in ixodid ticks (Ixodidae). *Parazitologiia* 17(3), 214–7.

Cisak, E., Sroka, J., Zwoliński, J., and Umiński, J. 1998. Seroepidemiologic study on tick-borne encephalitis among forestry workers and farmers from the Lublin region (eastern Poland). *Ann. Agric. Environ. Med.* 5(2), 177–81.

Cisak, E., Wójcik-Fatla, A., Zając, V., Sroka, J., Buczek, A., and Dutkiewicz, J. 2010. Prevalence of tick-borne encephalitis virus (TBEV) in samples of raw milk taken randomly from cows, goats and sheep in eastern Poland. *Ann. Agric. Environ. Med.* 17(2), 283–6.

Crooks, A. J., Lee, J. M., Easterbrook, L. M., Timofeev, A. V., and Stephenson, J. R. 1994. The NS1 protein of tick-borne encephalitis virus forms multimeric species upon secretion from the host cell. *J. Gen. Virol.* 75(Pt 12), 3453–60.

Daniel, M., Danielová, V., Kříž, B., Jirsa, A., and Nožička, J. 2003. Shift of the tick Ixodes ricinus and tick-borne encephalitis to higher altitudes in central Europe. *Eur. J. Clin. Microbiol. Infect. Dis.* 22(5), 327–8.

Danielová, V., Kliegrová, S., Daniel, M., and Beneš, C. 2008. Influence of climate warming on tickborne encephalitis expansion to higher altitudes over the last decade (1997–2006) in the Highland Region (Czech Republic). *Cent. Eur. J. Public. Health.* 16(1), 4–11.

Donoso-Mantke, O., Karan, L. S., and Růžek, D. 2011. Tick-borne encephalitis virus: a general overview. In: Růžek, D. (ed.) *Flavivirus Encephalitis*. Intech, Rijeka, 133–156.

Drozdov, S. G. 1959. The role of domestic animals in the epidemiology of biphasic milk fever. *J. Microbiol. Epidemiol. Immunol.* 30(4), 103.

Dudáš, D., Havlík, M., Hympán, J., Magdo, J., and Trebula, J. 1954. Symptomatology of the disease and evaluation of 50 control examinations at a time 5 months after onset of the disease. In: Blaškovič, D. (ed.) *An Epidemic of Encephalitis in the Natural Focus of Infection in Rožňava*. Slovak Academy of Sciences, Bratislava, 43–49.

Duniewicz, M., Mertenová, J., Moravcová, E., and Kulková, H. 1981. Corticoids in the therapy of TBE and other viral encephalitides. In: Kunz, C. H. (ed.) *Tick-Borne Encpehalitis*. International Symposium Baden/Vienna 19–20 October 1979. 36–44.

Dzhivanian, T. I., Korolev, M. B., Karganova, G. G., Lisak, V. M., and Kashtanova, G. M. 1988. Changes in the host-dependent characteristics of the tick-borne encephalitis virus during its adaptation to ticks and its readaptation to white mice. *Vopr. Virusol.* 33(5), 589–95.

Ecker, M., Allison, S. L., Meixner, T., and Heinz, F. X. 1999. Sequence analysis and genetic classification of tick-borne encephalitis viruses from Europe and Asia. *J. Gen. Virol.* 80(Pt 1), 179–85.

Ernek, E., Kožuch, O., and Nosek, J. 1969. The relation between tick-borne encephalitis virus and the wild duck (Anas platyrhynchos). II. Chronic latent infection. *Acta Virol.* 13, 303–8.

Ernek, E., Kožuch, O., Lichard, M., and Nosek, J. 1968. The role of birds in the circulation of tick-borne encephalitis virus in the Tribec region. *Acta Virol.* 12(5), 468–70.

Ernek, E., Kožuch, O., Nosek, J., and Hudec, K. 1969. The relation between tick-borne encephalitis virus and the wild duck (Anas platyrhynchos). I. Acute infection. *Acta Virol.* 13, 296–302.

Fališevac, J., and Beus, I. 1981. Clinical manifestation of TBE in Croatia. In: Kunz, C. H. (ed.) *Tick-Borne Encephalitis.* International Symposium Baden/Vienna 19–20 October 1979. 13–19.

Falk, W., and Lazarini, W. 1981. TBE in childhood. In: Kunz, C. H. (ed.) *Tick-Borne Encpehalitis.* International Symposium Baden/Vienna 19–20 October 1979. 20–24.

Fritz, R., Stiasny, K., and Heinz, F. X. 2008. Identification of specific histidines as pH sensors in flavivirus membrane fusion. *J. Cell Biol.* 183(2), 353–61.

Gallia, F., Rampas, J., and Hollender, L. 1949. Laboratory infection caused by tick-borne encephalitis virus. *Čas. Lék. Čes.* 88, 224–9.

Gelpi, E., Preusser, M., Garzuly, F., Holzmann, H., Heinz, F. X., and Budka, H. 2005. Visualization of Central European tick-borne encephalitis infection in fatal human cases. *J. Neuropathol. Exp. Neurol.* 64(6), 506–12.

Gould, E. A., Buckley, A., Barrett, A. D., and Cammack, N. 1986. Neutralizing (54K) and non-neutralizing (54K and 48K) monoclonal antibodies against structural and non-structural yellow fever virus proteins confer immunity in mice. *J. Gen. Virol.* 67(Pt 3), 591–5.

Grard, G., Moureau, G., Charrel, R. N., Lemasson, J. J., Gonzalez, J. P., Gallian, P., Gritsun, T. S., Holmes, E. C., Gould, E. A., and de Lamballerie, X. 2007. Genetic characterization of tick-borne flaviviruses: new insights into evolution, pathogenetic determinants and taxonomy. *Virology.* 361(1), 80–92.

Grešíková, M. 1957. Secretion of tick-borne encephalitis virus in goat milk. *Veter. Čas.* 5, 177–82.

Grešíková, M. 1958. Excretion of the tickborne encephalitis virus in the milk of subcutaneously infected cows. *Acta Virol.* 2(3), 188–92.

Grešíková, M. 1972. Studies on tick-borne arvobiruses isolated in Central Europe. *Biological Works* XVIII(2), 1–111.

Grešíková, M., and Albrecht, P. 1959. Experimental pathogenicity of the tick-borne encephalitis virus for the green lizard, Lacerta viridis (Laurenti 1768). *J. Hyg. Epidemiol. Microbiol. Immunol.* 3, 258–63.

Grešíková, M., and Kaluzová, M. 1997. Biology of tick-borne encephalitis virus. *Acta Virol.* 41(2), 115–24.

Grešíková, M., and Nosek, J. 1966. Isolation of tick-borne encephalitis virus from Haemaphysalis inermis ticks. *Acta Virol.* 10, 359–361.

Grešíková, M., and Řeháček, J. 1959. Isolation of the tick encephalitis virus from the blood and milk of domestic animals (sheep and cow) after infection by ticks of the family Ixodes ricinus L. *Arch. Gesamte Virusforsch.* 9, 360–4.

Grešíková, M., Sekeyová, M., Weidnerová, K., Blaškovič, D., Steck, F., and Wandeler, A. 1972. Isolation of tick-borne encephalitis virus from the brain of a sick dog in Switzerland. *Acta Virol.* 16(1), 88.

Grešíková, M., Weidnerová, K., Nosek, J., and Rajčáni, J. 1972. Experimental pathogenicity of tick-borne encephalitis virus for dogs. *Acta Virol.* 16(4), 336–40.

Gritsun, T. S., Holmes, E. C., and Gould, E. A. 1995. Analysis of flavivirus envelope proteins reveals variable domains that reflect their antigenicity and may determine their pathogenesis. *Virus Res.* 35(3), 307–21.

Gritsun, T. S., Lashkevich, V. A., and Gould, E. A. 2003. Tick-borne encephalitis. *Antiviral. Res.* 57(1–2), 129–46.

Gritsun, T. S., Venugopal, K., Zanotto, P. M., Mikhailov, M. V., Sall, A. A., Holmes, E. C., Polkinghorne, I., Frolova, T. V., Pogodina, V. V., Lashkevich, V. A., and Gould, E. A. 1997. Complete sequence of two tick-borne flaviviruses isolated from Siberia and the UK: analysis and significance of the 5′ and 3′-UTRs. *Virus Res.* 49(1), 27–39.

Günther, G. 1997. Tick-borne encephalitis—on pathogenesis and prognosis. Dissertation Thesis, Karolinska Instituted, Stockholm.

Günther, G., Haglund, M., Lindquist, L., Forsgren, M., and Sköldenberg, B. 1997a. Tick-borne encephalitis in Sweden in relation to aseptic meningo-encephalitis of other etiology: a prospective study of clinical course and outcome. *J. Neurol.* 244(4), 230–8.

Günther, G., Haglund, M., Lindquist, L., Forsgren, M., Andersson, J., Andersson, B., and Sköldenberg, B. 2011. Tick-borne encephalitis is associated with low levels of interleukin-10 in cerebrospinal fluid. *Infect. Ecol. Epid.* 1, 6029. DOI: 10.3402/iee.v1i0.6029.

Günther, G., Haglund, M., Lindquist, L., Sköldenberg, B., and Forsgren, M. 1997b. Intrathecal IgM, IgA and IgG antibody response in tick-borne encephalitis. Long-term follow-up related to clinical course and outcome. *Clin. Diagn. Virol.* 8(1), 17–29.

Günther, G., Haglund, M., Lindquist, L., Sköldenberg, B., and Forsgren, M. 1996. Intrathecal production of neopterin and beta 2 microglobulin in tick-borne encephalitis (TBE) compared to meningoencephalitis of other etiology. *Scand. J. Infect. Dis.* 28(2), 131–8.

Haglund, M., and Günther, G. 2003. Tick-borne encephalitis—pathogenesis, clinical course and long-term follow-up. *Vaccine* 21(Suppl 1), S11–8.

Hainz, U., Jenewein, B., Asch, E., Pfeiffer, K. P., Berger, P., and Grubeck-Loebenstein, B. 2005. Insufficient protection for healthy elderly adults by tetanus and TBE vaccines. *Vaccine* 23(25), 3232–5.

Heinz, F. X. 2003. Molecular aspects of TBE virus research. *Vaccine* 21(Suppl 1), S3–S10.

Heinz, F. X., and Allison, S. L. 2001. The machinery for flavivirus fusion with host cell membranes. *Curr. Opin. Microbiol.* 4(4), 450–5.

Henner, K. 1954. Comments to the clinical features of the Rožňava epidemic. In: Blaškovič, D. (ed.) *An Epidemic of Encephalitis in the Natural Focus of Infection in Rožňava.* Slovak Academy of Sciences, Bratislava, 24–27.

Hloucal, L. 1949. Abortive viral meningoencephalitis. *Čas. Lék. Čes.* 88, 1390.

Hloucal, L. 1960. Tick-borne encephalitis as observed in Czechoslovakia. *J. Trop. Med. Hyg.* 63, 293–6.

Hloucal, L., and Gallia, F. 1949. An epidemic of neutropic virus disease in the district of Strakonice 1948. *Sborn. lék.* 51, 374.

Hloucal, L., and Rampas, J. 1953. Czechoslovak tick-borne encephalitis. *Thomayerova sbírka.* 311/1, 1–22.

Hofmann, H. 1981. Diagnosis of TBE in the virological routine laboratory. In: Kunz, C. H. (ed.) *Tick-Borne Encephalitis.* International Symposium Baden/Vienna 19–20 October 1979. 129–32.

Holzmann, H. 2003. Diagnosis of tick-borne encephalitis. *Vaccine* 21(Suppl 1), S36–S40.

Holzmann, H., Stiasny, K., York, H., Dorner, F., Kunz, C., and Heinz, F. X. 1995. Tick-borne encephalitis virus envelope protein E-specific monoclonal antibodies for the study of low pH-induced conformational changes and immature virions. *Arch. Virol.* 140(2), 213–21.

Hubálek, Z., Pow, I., Reid, H. W., and Hussain, M. H. 1995. Antigenic similarity of central European encephalitis and louping-ill viruses. *Acta Virol.* 39(5–6), 251–6.

Jellinger, K. 1981. The histopathology of TBE. In: Kunz, C. H. (ed.) *Tick-Borne Encephalitis.* International Symposium Baden/Vienna 19–20 October 1979. 59–75.

Jones, N., Sperl, W., Koch, J., Holzmann, H., and Radauer, W. 2007. Tick-borne encephalitis in a 17-day-old newborn resulting in severe neurologic impairment. *Pediatr. Infect. Dis. J.* 26(2), 185–6.

Kaiser, R. 1999. The clinical and epidemiological profile of tick-borne encephalitis in southern Germany 1994–98: a prospective study of 656 patients. *Brain*. 122 (Pt 11). 2067–78.

Kaiser, R. 2008. Tick-borne encephalitis. *Infect. Dis. Clin. North. Am.* 22(3), 561–75.

Kaluzová, M., Elečková, E., Žuffová, E., Pastorek, J., Kaluz, S., Kožuch, O., and Labuda, M. 1994. Reverted virulence of attenuated tick-borne encephalitis virus mutant is not accompanied with the changes in deduced viral envelope protein amino acid sequence. *Acta Virol.* 38(3), 133–40.

Kindberg, E., Mickiene, A., Ax, C., Akerlind, B., Vene, S., Lindquist, L., Lundkvist, A., and Svensson, L. 2008. A deletion in the chemokine receptor 5 (CCR5) gene is associated with tickborne encephalitis. *J. Infect. Dis.* 197(2), 266–9.

Kindberg, E., Vene, S., Mickiene, A., Lundkvist, Å., Lindquist, L., and Svensson, L. 2011. A functional Toll-like receptor 3 gene (TLR3) may be a risk factor for tick-borne encephalitis virus (TBEV) infection. *J. Infect. Dis.* 203(4), 523–8.

Knap, N., Korva, M., Dolinšek, V., Sekirnik, M., Trilar, T., and Avšič-Županc, T. 2012. Patterns of tick-borne encephalitis virus infection in rodents in Slovenia. *Vector Borne Zoonotic Dis.* 12(3), 236–42.

Kofler, R. M., Heinz, F. X., and Mandl, C. W. 2002. Capsid protein C of tick-borne encephalitis virus tolerates large internal deletions and is a favorable target for attenuation of virulence. *J. Virol.* 76(7), 3534–43.

Kolman, J. M., Fischer, J., and Havlík, O. 1960. Experimental infection of bats species Myotis myotis Borkhausen with the Czechoslovak tick-borne encephalitis virus. *Acta Univ. Carol. Med. (Praha)* 6, 147–80.

Kopecký, J., Grubhoffer, L., Kovář, V., Jindrák, L., and Vokurková, D. 1999. A putative host cell receptor for tick-borne encephalitis virus identified by anti-idiotypic antibodies and virus affinoblotting. *Intervirology* 42(1), 9–16.

Korenberg, E. I. 2009. Recent epidemiology of tick-borne encephalitis an effect of climate change? *Adv. Virus. Res.* 74, 123–44.

Kožuch, O., and Nosek, J. 1971. Transmission of tick-borne encephalitis (TBE) virus by Dermacentor marginatus and D. reticulatus ticks. *Acta Virol.* 15(4), 334.

Kožuch, O., Grešíková, M., Nosek, J., Lichard, M., and Sekeyová, M. 1967. The role of small rodents and hedgehogs in a natural focus of tick-borne encephalitis. *Bull. World Health Organ.* 36(Suppl), 61–6.

Krejčí, J. 1949. Isolement d'un virus noveau en course d'un epidémie de meningoencephalite dans la region de Vyškov (Moraviae). *Presse Méd. (Paris).* 74, 1084, 1949.

Krejčí, J. 1949. Outbreak of encephalitis virus in the region of Vyškov. *Lék. Listy (Brno).* 4, 73–75, 112–116, 132–134.

Křivanec, K., Kopecký, J., Tomková, E., and Grubhoffer, L. 1988. Isolation of TBE virus from the tick Ixodes hexagonus. *Folia Parasitol.* 35(3), 273–6.

Kříž, B., Beneš, C., and Daniel, M. 2009. Alimentary transmission of tick-borne encephalitis in the Czech Republic (1997–2008). *Epidemiol. Mikrobiol. Imunol.* 58(2), 98–103.

Kubánka, Š., and Pór, F. 1954. Comments of internists to the epidemic of encephalitis. In: Blaškovič, D. (ed.) *An epidemic of Encephalitis in the Natural Focus of Infection in Rožňava.* Slovak Academy of Sciences, Bratislava, 28–30.

Kunz, C. 2003. TBE vaccination and the Austrian experience. *Vaccine* 21(Suppl 1), S50–5.

Kunze, U., Asokliene, L., Bektimirov, T., Busse, A., Chmelik, V., Heinz, F. X., Hingst, V., Kadar, F., Kaiser, R., Kimmig, P., Kraigher, A., Krech, T., Linquist, L., Lucenko, I., Rosenfeldt, V., Ruscio, M., Sandell, B., Salzer, H., Strle, F., Süss, J., Zilmer, K., and Mutz, I. 2004. Tick-borne encephalitis in childhood-consensus 2004. *Wien. Med. Wochenschr.* 154(9–10), 242–5.

Labuda, M., Danielová, V., Jones, L. D., and Nuttall, P. A. 1993. Amplification of tick-borne encephalitis virus infection during co-feeding of ticks. *Med. Vet. Entomol.* 7(4), 339–42.

Labuda, M., Elečková, E., Licková, M., and Sabó, A. 2002. Tick-borne encephalitis virus foci in Slovakia. *Int. J. Med. Microbiol.* 291(Suppl 33), 43–7.

Labuda, M., Jiang, W. R., Kaluzová, M., Kožuch, O., Nuttall, P. A., Weismann, P., Elečková, E., Žuffová, E., and Gould, E. A. 1994. Change in phenotype of tick-borne encephalitis virus following passage in Ixodes ricinus ticks and associated amino acid substitution in the envelope protein. *Virus Res.* 31(3), 305–15.

Labuda, M., Kozuch, O., Žuffová, E., Elečková, E., Hails, R. S., and Nuttall, P. A. 1997. Tick-borne encephalitis virus transmission between ticks cofeeding on specific immune natural rodent hosts. *Virology* 235(1), 138–43.

Lee, J. M., Crooks, A. J., and Stephenson, J. R. 1989. The synthesis and maturation of a non-structural extracellular antigen from tick-borne encephalitis virus and its relationship to the intracellular NS1 protein. *J. Gen. Virol.* 70 (Pt 2), 335–43.

Leonova, G. N., and Maĭstrovskaia, O. S. 1996. Viremia in patients with tick-borne encephalitis and in persons with attached ixodes ticks. *Vopr. Virusol.* 41(5), 224–8.

Lindenbach, B. D., and Rice, C. M. 2003. Molecular biology of flaviviruses. *Adv. Virus Res.* 59, 23–61.

Lindquist, L., and Vapalahti, O. 2008. Tick-borne encephalitis. *Lancet.* 371(9627), 1861–71.

Lorenz, I. C., Allison, S. L., Heinz, F. X., and Helenius, A. 2002. Folding and dimerization of tick-borne encephalitis virus envelope proteins prM and E in the endoplasmic reticulum. *J. Virol.* 76(11), 5480–91.

Lorenzl, S., Pfister, H. W., Padovan, C., and Yousry, T. 1996. MRI abnormalities in tick-borne encephalitis. *Lancet* 347(9002), 698–9.

Lotrič-Furlan, S., and Strle, F. 1995. Thrombocytopenia—a common finding in the initial phase of tick-borne encephalitis. *Infection* 23(4), 203–6.

Lu, Z., Bröker, M., and Liang, G. 2008. Tick-borne encephalitis in mainland China. *Vector Borne Zoonotic Dis.* 8(5), 713–20.

Málková, D., and Filip, O. 1968. Histological picture in the place of inoculation and in lymph nodes of mice after subcutaneous infection with tick-borne encephalitis virus. *Acta Virol.* 12(4), 355–60.

Málková, D., and Fraňková, V. 1959. The lymphatic system in the development of experimental tick-borne encephalitis in mice. *Acta Virol.* 3, 210–4.

Málková, D., and Kolman, J. M. 1964. Role of the regional lymphatic system of the immunized mouse in penetration of the tick-borne encephalitis virus into the bloodstream. *Acta Virol.* 8, 10–3.

Málková, D., Pala, F., and Šidák, Z. 1961. Cellular changes in the white cell count, regional lymph node and spleen during infection with tick-borne encephalitis virus in mice. *Acta Virol.* 5, 101–111.

Mandl, C. W. 2005. Steps of the tick-borne encephalitis virus replication cycle that affect neuropathogenesis. *Virus Res.* 111(2), 161–74.

Marjelund, S., Tikkakoski, T., Tuisku, S., and Raisanen, S. 2004. Magnetic resonance imaging findings and outcome in severe tick-borne encephalitis. Report of four cases and review of the literature. *Acta Radiol.* 45(1), 88–94.

Mayer, V., and Kožuch, O. 1969. Study of the virulence of tick-borne encephalitis virus. XI. Genetic heterogeneity of the virus from naturally infectious Ixodes ricinus ticks. *Acta Virol.* 13(6), 469–82.

Messner, H. 1981. Pediatric problems of TBE. In: Kunz Ch. (ed.) *Tick-Borne Encephalitis.* International Symposium Baden/Vienna 19–20 October 1979. 25–27.

Mickiene, A., Laiskonis, A., Günther, G., Vene, S., Lundkvist, A., and Lindquist, L. 2002. Tickborne encephalitis in an area of high endemicity in Lithuania: disease severity and long-term prognosis. *Clin. Infect. Dis.* 35(6), 650–8.

Molnár, E., and Fornosi, F. 1952. Accidental laboratory infection with the Czechoslovakian strain of tick encephalitis. *Orv. Hetil.* 93(36), 1032–3.

Moritsch, H., and Krausler, J. 1957. Die endemische Frühsommer-Meningo-Encephalitis im Wiener Becken (Schneidersche Krankheit). *Wien. Klin. Wochenschrift.* 69, 921–6.

Moritsch, H., and Krausler, J. 1957. Endemic early summer meningoencephalomyelitis in the Vienna area (Schneider's disease). *Wien. Klin. Wochenschr.* 69(49), 921–6, 69(50), 952–6, 69(51), 965–70.

Nosek, J., Čiampor, F., Kožuch, O., and Rajčáni, J. 1972. Localization of tick-borne encephalitis virus in alveolar cells of salivary glands of Dermacentor marginatus and Haemaphysalis inermis ticks. *Acta Virol.* 16(6), 493–7.

Nosek, J., Grešíková, M., and Řeháček, J. 1961. Persistence of TBE virus in hibernating bats. *Acta Virol.* 5, 112–116.

Nosek, J., Kožuch, O., and Lichard, M. 1967. Persistence of tick-borne encephalitis virus in, and its transmission by Haemaphysalis spinigera and H. turturis ticks. *Acta Virol.* 11(5), 479.

Nosek, J., Kožuch, O., Ernek, E., and Lichard, M. 1967. Übertragung des Zeckenenzephalitis-Virus (TBE) durch die Weibchen von Ixodes ricinus und Nymphen von Haemophysalis inermis auf den Rehkitzen (Capreolus capreolus). *Zbl. Bakt. I Orig.* 203, 162–6.

Nowak, T., and Wengler, G. 1987. Analysis of disulfides present in the membrane proteins of the West Nile flavivirus. *Virology* 156(1), 127–37.

Nuttall, P. A., and Labuda, M. 2004. Tick-host interactions: saliva-activated transmission. *Parasitology* 129(Suppl), S177–89.

Petrishcheva, P. A., and Levkovich, E. N. 1945. Spring-summer encephalitis in Leningrad region. *Papers of Medical Officers of the Volkhov Front.* Leningrad, Russia.

Pfeffer, M., and Dobler, G. 2011. Tick-borne encephalitis virus in dogs—is this an issue? *Parasit. Vectors.* 4, 59.

Plekhova, N. G., Somova, L. M., Lyapun, I. N., Kondrashova, N. N., Krylova, N. V., Leonova, G. N., and Pustovalov, E. V. 2011. The cells of innate systems in tick-borne encephalitis. In Růžek, D. (ed.) *Flavivirus Encephalitis.* InTech, Rijeka, 167–94.

Pogodina, V. V., Bochkova, N. G., Karan, L. S., Frolova, M. P., Trukhina, A. G., Malenko, G. V., Levina, L. S., and Platonov, A. E. 2004. Comparative analysis of virulence of the Siberian and Far-East subtypes of the tick-born encephalitis virus. *Vopr. Virusol.* 49(6), 24–30.

Pogodina, V. V., Frolova, M. P., and Erman, B. A. 1979. *Chronic Tick-Borne Encephalitis.* Nauka, Moscow.

Popponikova, T. V. 2006. Specific clinical and epidemiological features of tick-borne encephalitis in Western Siberia. *Int. J. Med. Microbiol.* 296(Supp. 40), 59–62.

Proutski, V., Gould, E. A., and Holmes, E. C. 1997. Secondary structure of the 3′ untranslated region of flaviviruses: similarities and differences. *Nucl. Acids Res.* 25(6), 1194–202.

Proutski, V., Gritsun, T. S., Gould, E. A., and Holmes, E. C. 1997. Biological consequences of deletions within the 3′-untranslated region of flaviviruses may be due to rearrangements of RNA secondary structure. *Virus Res.* 64(2), 107–23.

Rampas, J., and Gallia, F. 1949. Isolation of tick-borne encephalitis virus from ticks Ixodes ricinus. *Čas. Lék. Čes.* 88, 1179–80.

Randolph, S. E. 2004. Evidence that climate change has caused 'emergence' of tick-borne diseases in Europe? *Int. J. Med. Microbiol.* 293(Suppl 37), 5–15.

Randolph, S. E. 2008. Dynamics of tick-borne disease systems: minor role of recent climate change. *Rev. Sci. Tech.* 27(2), 367–81.

Rendi-Wagner, P. 2004. Risk and prevention of tick-borne encephalitis in travelers. *J. Travel Med.* 11(5), 307–12.

Rendi-Wagner, P., Kundi, M., Zent, O., Banzhoff, A., Jaehnig, P., Stemberger, R., Dvorak, G., Grumbeck, E., Laaber, B., and Kollaritsch, H. 2004. Immunogenicity and safety of a booster vaccination against tick-borne encephalitis more than 3 years following the last immunisation. *Vaccine* 23(4), 427–34.

Reusken, C., Reimerink, J., Verduin, C., Sabbe, L., Cleton, N., and Koopmans, M. 2011. *Case Report: Tick-Borne Encephalitis in Two Dutch Travellers Returning From Austria, Netherlands,* July and August 2011. *Euro Surveill.* 16(44). pii: 20003.

Rey, F. A., Heinz, F. X., Mandl, C., Kunz, C., and Harrison, S. C. 1995. The envelope glycoprotein from tick-borne encephalitis virus at 2 A resolution. *Nature* 375(6529), 291–8.

Romanova, L.Iu., Gmyl, A. P., Dzhivanian, T. I., Bakhmutov, D. V., Lukashev, A. N., Gmyl, L. V., Rumyantsev, A. A., Burenkova, L. A., Lashkevich, V. A., and Karganova, G. G. 2007. Microevolution of tick-borne encephalitis virus in course of host alternation. *Virology* 362(1), 75–84.

Rouse, B. T., and Sehrawat, S. 2010. Immunity and immunopathology to viruses: what decides the outcome? *Nat. Rev. Immunol.* 10(7), 514–26.

Růžek, D., Dobler, G., and Donoso Mantke, O. 2011. Tick-borne encephalitis: pathogenesis and clinical implications. *Travel Med. Infect. Dis.* 8(4), 223–32.

Růžek, D., Gritsun, T. S., Forrester, N. L., Gould, E. A., Kopecký, J., Golovchenko, M., Rudenko, N., and Grubhoffer, L. 2008. Mutations in the NS2B and NS3 genes affect mouse neuroinvasiveness of a Western European field strain of tick-borne encephalitis virus. *Virology* 374(2), 249–55.

Růžek, D., Salát, J., Palus, M., Gritsun, T. S., Gould, E. A., Dyková, I., Skallová, A., Jelínek, J., Kopecký, J., and Grubhoffer, L. 2009. CD8+ T-cells mediate immunopathology in tick-borne encephalitis. *Virology* 384(1), 1–6.

Růžek, D., Salát, J., Singh, S. K., and Kopecký, J. 2011. Breakdown of the blood–brain barrier during tick-borne encephalitis in mice is not dependent on CD8+ T-cells. *PLoS One* 6(5), e20472.

Růžek, D., Vancová, M., Tesařová, M., Ahantarig, A., Kopecký, J., and Grubhoffer, L. 2009. Morphological changes in human neural cells following tick-borne encephalitis virus infection. *J. Gen. Virol.* 90(Pt 7), 1649–58.

Saksida, A., Duh, D., Lotrič-Furlan, S., Strle, F., Petrovec, M., and Avšič-Županc, T. 2005. The importance of tick-borne encephalitis virus RNA detection for early differential diagnosis of tick-borne encephalitis. *J. Clin. Virol.* 33(4), 331–5.

Schneider, H. 1939. Über Epidemische akute Meningitis Serosa. *Wien. Klin. Woch.* 44, 350–2.

Sekeyová, M., Grešíková, M., and Lesko, J. 1970. Formation of antibody to tick-borne encephalitis virus in Lacerta viridis and L. agilis lizards. *Acta Virol.* 14(1), 87.

Semenov, B. F., Khozinsky, V. V., and Vargin, V. V. 1981. Immunopathology and immunotherapy of tick-borne encephalitis. In: Kunz, C. H. (ed.) *Tick-Borne Encephalitis.* International Symposium Baden/Vienna 19–20 October 1979. 45–58.

Šenigl, F., Grubhoffer, L., and Kopecky, J. 2006. Differences in maturation of tick-borne encephalitis virus in mammalian and tick cell line. *Intervirology* 49(4), 239–48.

Shapoval, A. N. 1976. Chronic forms of tick-borne encephalitis. *Med. Leningrad.*

Shapoval, A. N. 1977. Inapparent forms of tick-borne encephalitis. *Zh. Mikrobiol. Epidemiol. Immunobiol.* 5, 11–7.

Slávik, I., Mayer, V., and Mrena, E. 1967. Morphology of purified tick-borne encephalitis virus. *Acta Virol.* 11, 66.

Smorodintsev, A. A., Alekseyev, B. P., Gulamova, V. P., Drobyshevskaya, A. I., Ilyenko, V. I., Klenov, K. N., and Churilova, A. A. 1953. The epidemiologic characteristics of biphasic virus meningoencephalitis. *Z. Mikrobiol. (Mosk.)* (5), 54 (in Russian).

Steffens, S., Thiel, H. J., and Behrens, S. E. 1999. The RNA-dependent RNA polymerases of different members of the family Flaviviridae exhibit similar properties *in vitro. J. Gen. Virol.* 80(Pt 10), 2583–90.

Stiasny, K. Holzmann, H., and Heinz, F. X. 2009. Characteristics of antibody responses in tick-borne encephalitis vaccination breakthroughs. *Vaccine* 27, 7021–26.

Süss, J. 2003. Epidemiology and ecology of TBE relevant to the production of effective vaccines. *Vaccine* 21(Suppl 1), S19–35.

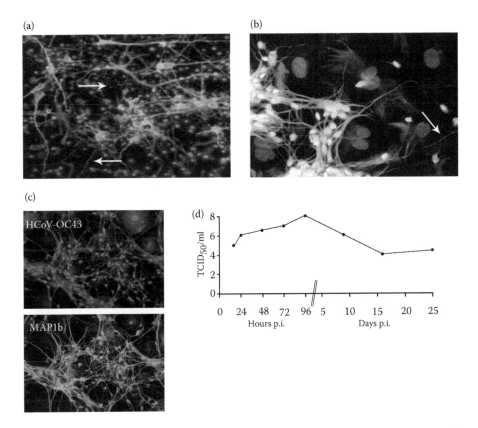

FIGURE 5.4 The main target of HCoV-OC43 infection is the neuron in mouse and human cell cultures. (a) Mixed primary cultures from the murine CNS. (b) Cocultures of human neurons and astrocytes obtained from differentiated human NT2 cell line using a protocol, which gives rise to a mixture of neurons and astrocytes. In both type of cultures, HCoV-OC43 primarily targets the neuron for infection leading to axonal beading (white arrows in a and b). The +viral S protein is in green in infected neurons and red represents the glial fibrillary acidic protein (GFAP) in activated astrocytes. The blue signal is the nucleus detected by the DNA-specific dye DAPI. (c) NT2-N cells (95% pure human neuronal culture) infected by HCoV-OC43. The viral S protein is in red in infected neurons and green represents the microtubule associated protein 1b (MAP1b) expression in differentiated neurons. (d) HCoV-OC43 can establish a long term infection of the NT2-N cells for up to 25 days postinfection even though cell death occurred in a portion of the NT2-N cells after acute infection.

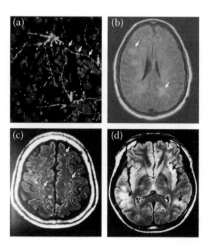

FIGURE 15.1 (a) Detection of the N protein of MV in a 7-μm section obtained from an SSPE case by indirect immunofluorescence (green). Nuclei from uninfected neurons are counterstained with propidium iodide (red). Interconnecting neuronal processes (arrows) and cell bodies (asterisk) are indicated. (b) T2-weighted MRI sequence of a patient with MuV encephalitis. T2-signal hyperintensities are indicated (arrows). (Copyright © MedReviews®, LLC. Adapted and reprinted with permission of MedReviews, LLC. Cooper A.D. et al. Mumps encephalitis: return with a vengeance. *Rev Neurol Dis.* 2007; 4:100–102. *Reviews in Neurological Diseases* is a copyrighted publication of MedReviews, LLC. All rights reserved.) (c) T2-weighted MRI sequence of a patient with acute NiV encephalitis. Selected punctate T2-signal hyperintensities are indicated (arrows). (d) T2-weighted MRI sequence of a patient with relapsed NiV encephalitis. Selected confluent T2-signal hyperintensities are indicated (arrows). (Adapted and reprinted from Goh, K. J. et al., 2000, *N. Engl. J. Med.* 342, 1229–1235.)

FIGURE 17.4 Macular–papular rash in postnatally acquired rubella infection. (Reproduced from Dr. D. Wallach and Editions De Boeck/Estem. With permission.)

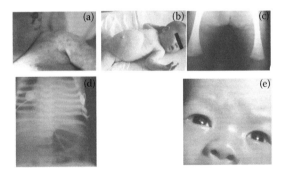

FIGURE 17.5 Congenital anomalies in congenital rubella syndrome (CRS). (a) Case of CRS with maculo-papular rash and purpura; (b) case of CRS with hepatosplenomegaly; (c) case of CRS with radiolucencies of long bones; (d) case of CRS with cardiac dilatation; (e) cataracts (opacity of the lens). (Kindly provided by Dr. C. A. Bouhanna and Dr. J. C. Janaud, Hôpital intercommunal, Créteil, France, with permission from Dr. D. Wallach and Editions De Boeck/Estem.)

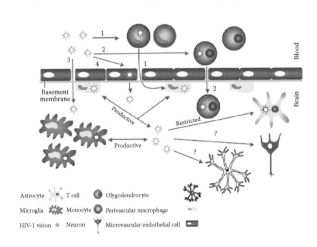

FIGURE 19.1 HIV-1 neuroinvasion. (1) According to the "Trojan horse" hypothesis, the entry of HIV-1 into the brain takes place by the migration of infected monocytes, which differentiate into perivascular macrophage. (2) The passage of infected CD4+ T cells can be another source of infection in the brain. Other probable causes of CNS infection might be (3) the direct entrance of the virus or (4) entrance of HIV-1 by transcytosis of brain microvascular endothelial cells. Once the virus is in the brain, it productively infects macrophages and microglia. Astrocyte infection is known to be restricted. The infection of oligodendrocytes, especially neurons, is questionable. (Reproduced from Ghafouri, M. et al., 2006, *Retrovirology* 3, 28. With permission.)

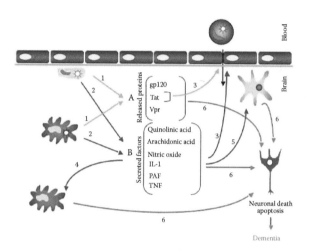

FIGURE 19.2 Mechanism of neuropathogenesis. Two components of this mechanism are (A) the direct effect of the HIV-1 infection, including HIV-1 proteins, and (B) the indirect consequence of infection comprising the secretion of cytokines and neurotoxins. The infected macrophages and microglia participate actively in the neurodegeneration by (1) shedding viral proteins and (2) releasing a significant amount of cytokines and neurotoxins into the CNS. (3) Tat and TNF-α contribute to the disruption of the BBB, which in turn become more permeable to infected monocytes and cytokines present in the periphery. The secreted proinflammatory cytokines activates (4) microglia and (5) astrocytes, which in turn secrete neurotoxins; moreover, the alteration of astrocytes function results in an increase in the level of neurotoxicity in the brain. (6) Multifactorial neuronal injury: neurotoxins released from several sources, as the direct and indirect consequences of HIV-1 infection lead to neuronal injury. (Reproduced from Ghafouri, M. et al., 2006, *Retrovirology* 3, 28. With permission.)

Tkachev, S. E., Demina, T. V., Dzhioev, Yu. P., Kozlova, I. V., Verkohozina, M. M., Doroshchenko, E. K., Lisak, O. V., Bakhvalova, V. N., Paramonov, A. I., and Zlobin, V. I. 2011. Genetic studies of tick-borne encephalitis virus strains from Western and Easter Siberia. In: Růžek, D. (ed.) *Flavivirus Encephalitis*. InTech, Rijeka, 235–54.

Uchil, P. D., and Satchidanandam, V. 2003. Architecture of the flaviviral replication complex. Protease, nuclease, and detergents reveal encasement within double-layered membrane compartments. *J. Biol. Chem.* 278(27), 24388–98.

Vesenjak-Zmijanac, J., Bedjanič, M., Rus, S., and Kmet, J. 1955. Virus meningo-encephalitis in Slovenia. *Bull. World Health Organ.* 12(4), 513–20.

Vince, V., and Grčević, N. 1981. Pathogenetic problems arising from experiences in series of experiments with TBE in mice. In: Kunz Ch. (ed.) *Tick-Borne Encephalitis*. International Symposium Baden/Vienna 19–20 October 1979. 76–92.

Votiakov, V. I., Zlobin, V. I., and Mishayeava, N. P. 2002. Tick-borne encephalitis of Eurasia. Ecology, molecular epidemiology, nosology, evolution. *Nauka, Novosibirsk*.

Waldvogel, K., Bossart, W., Huisman, T., Boltshauser, E., and Nadal, D. 1996. Severe tick-borne encephalitis following passive immunization. *Eur. J. Pediatr.* 155(9), 775–9.

Wallner, G., Mandl, C. W., Kunz, C., and Heinz, F. X. 1995. The flavivirus 3′-noncoding region: extensive size heterogeneity independent of evolutionary relationships among strains of tick-borne encephalitis virus. *Virology* 213(1), 169–78.

Weidmann, M., Schmidt, P., Hufert, F. T., Krivanec, K., and Meyer, H. 2006. Tick-borne encephalitis virus in Clethrionomys glareolus in the Czech Republic. *Vector Borne Zoonotic Dis.* 6(4), 379–81.

Weinberger, B., Keller, M., Fischer, K. H., Stiasny, K., Neuner, C., Heinz, F. X., and Grubeck-Loebenstein, B. 2010. Decreased antibody titers and booster responses in tick-borne encephalitis vaccinees aged 50–90 years. *Vaccine* 28(20), 3511–5.

Werme, K., Wigerius, M., and Johansson, M. 2008. Tick-borne encephalitis virus NS5 associates with membrane protein scribble and impairs interferon-stimulated JAK-STAT signalling. *Cell. Microbiol.* 10(3), 696–712.

Yamshchikov, V. F., and Compans, R. W. 1995. Formation of the flavivirus envelope: role of the viral NS2B-NS3 protease. *J. Virol.* 69(4), 1995–2003.

Zilber, L. A. 1939. Spring- and spring–summer-endemic tick-borne encephalitis. *Arch. Boil. Nauk.* 56, 9–37 (in Russian).

Zlobin, V. I., and Gorin, O. Z. 1996. *Tick-borne Encephalitis: Etiology, Epidemiology and Prophylactics in Siberia*, Nauka, Novosibirsk, p. 177.

Zlobin, V. I., Demina, T. V., Belikov, S. I., Butina, T. V., Gorin, O. Z., Adel'shin, R. V., and Grachev, M. A. 2001. Genetic typing of tick-borne encephalitis virus based on an analysis of the levels of homology of a membrane protein gene fragment. *Vopr. Virusol.* 46(1), 17–22.

Zlobin, V. I., Demina, T. V., Mamaev, L. V., Butina, T. V., Belikov, S. I., Gorin, O. Z., Dzhioev, Iu. P., Verkhozina, M. M., Kozlova, I. V., Voronko, I. V., Adel'shin, R. V., and Grachev, M. A. 2001. Analysis of genetic variability of strains of tick-borne encephalitis virus by primary structure of a fragment of the membrane protein E gene. *Vopr. Virusol.* 46(1), 12–6.

11 St. Louis Encephalitis

Luis Adrian Diaz, Lorena I. Spinsanti,
and Marta S. Contigiani

CONTENTS

11.1 INTRODUCTION

St. Louis encephalitis virus (SLEV) was isolated for the first time during a human encephalitis outbreak in St. Louis, Missouri United States of America (USA) in 1933 (Lumsdem 1958). The viral isolation was carried out from a brain sample of a death patient. The outbreak took place during an exceptionally hot and dry summer. More than 1000 cases were reported; most of them localized near open storm drains, rain drainage and sewage channels, which worked as *Culex* mosquitoes breading sites (Reisen 2003). Further ecological studies carried out during a SLEV human encephalitis outbreak in Yakima Valley (Washington, USA) (1941–1942) incriminated peridomestics bird species as hosts and *Culex* mosquitoes as vectors (Hammon et al. 1945). Understanding the ecological and epidemiological behavior of SLEV and the development of new diagnostic techniques allowed a global vision regarding the public health importance of SLEV in the USA.

In the past decades the concern about SLEV for the public health has decreased in the USA. However, in our days, the epidemiological pattern of SLEV is changing. Since 2002, a reemergence scenario for this pathogen was observed in South America. Human encephalitis cases were reported in Argentina and Brazil

TABLE 11.1

Taxonomic Classification of St. Louis Encephalitis Virus

Family	Genus	Serocomplex	Species
Flaviviridae	*Flavivirus*	Japanese encephalitis	Cacipacoré virus
			Japanese encephalitis virus
			Koutango virus
			Murray Valley virus
			St. Louis encephalitis virus
			Usutu virus
			West Nile virus
			Yaounde virus

(López et al. 2011; Mondini et al. 2007; Rocco et al. 2005; Spinsanti et al. 2003, 2008).

11.2 TAXONOMIC CLASSIFICATION

SLEV belongs to the genus *Flavivirus*, *Flaviviridae* family (Table 11.1). The virus prototype of the genus is Yellow Fever. It is composed of 53 different viral species, most of them being pathogenic for humans and arthropod-borne viruses (ICTV 2009). According to their serologic relatedness, flaviviruses were divided into antigenic complexes (Heinz and Roehrig 1990). Based on its antigenic properties, SLEV belongs to the Japanese encephalitis serocomplex. This group includes other viruses with medical and veterinary concerns (West Nile (WNV), Japanese encephalitis (JEV), and Murray Valley (MVEV), among others) (Burke and Monath 2001) (Table 11.1).

11.3 VIRUS STRUCTURE

The *Flavivirus* virion is a small icosahedral enveloped particle of 40 to 60 nm diameter, which includes a 30-nm core (Mukhopadhyay et al. 2003). Structural analysis of mature Flavivirus virions revealed that the virus possesses an icosahedral envelope organization and a spherical nucleocapsid core (Kuhn et al. 2002) (Figure 11.1a). Mature virions contain three structural proteins; the capsid protein C, membrane protein M, and the envelope protein E. Multiple copies of the C protein (11 kDa) encapsulate the RNA genome to form the viral nucleocapsid (Jones et al. 2003). The nucleocapsid is surrounded by a host-cell-derived lipid bilayer, in which copies of M and E are anchored (Mukhopadhyay et al. 2003) (Figure 11.1a). The M protein is a small (approximately 8 kDa) proteolytic fragment of its precursor form prM. The E protein is approximately 50 kDa and is the main protein present in the virion envelope. The E protein is in charge of recognizing the host cell receptors and is the main target of neutralizing antibodies (Lindenbach and Rice 2001; Nybakken et al. 2006). Certain mutations in the E protein can cause the virion's lack of virulence (Beasley et al. 2004; Engel et al. 2010; Gritsun et al. 1995).

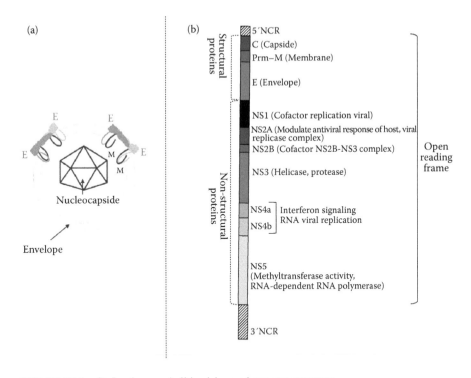

(a)

Nucleocapside

Envelope

(b)

Structural proteins
5′NCR
C (Capside)
Prm–M (Membrane)
E (Envelope)

Non-structural proteins
NS1 (Cofactor replication viral)
NS2A (Modulate antiviral response of host, viral replicase complex)
NS2B (Cofactor NS2B-NS3 complex)
NS3 (Helicase, protease)
NS4a } Interferon signaling RNA viral replication
NS4b
NS5 (Methyltransferase activity, RNA-dependent RNA polymerase)
3′NCR

Open reading frame

FIGURE 11.1 St. Louis encephalitis virion and genome structure.

11.4 GENOME ORGANIZATION AND PROTEIN FUNCTIONS

The SLEV genome consists of a single-stranded positive-sense RNA fragment of approximately 10,963 nt (nucleotides). The viral genome works as a single RNA messenger molecule, which possess an open reading frame (ORF) (Chambers et al. 1990a) (Figure 11.1b). The ORF encodes a 3429-aa polyprotein. The ORF is flanked by noncoding regions (NCR). The 5′NCR (125 nt) presents an m7G5′ppp5′cap. The 3′NCR is 551 nt long and lacks the polyA tail (Brinton 2002; Diaz et al. 2010). These NCR form RNA secondary structures, which could intervene directing the processes of amplification, translation, and packaging of genomes (Hahn et al. 1987; Proutski et al. 1997).

NS1 is a homodimer that participates in the replication process of viral RNA; it is one of the first viral proteins being secreted and induces a strong humoral immune response (Mackenzie et al. 1996; Schlesinger et al. 1986). NS2A is a small hydrophobic protein (22 kDa) thought to intervene in the RNA templates recovery associated with viral polymerase (Mackenzie et al. 1998), to module the host's antiviral response and cleavage of the NS1-NS2A junction after translation, and to play a functional role in the viral replicase complex (Leung et al. 2008). NS2B is a small membrane-associated protein, and acts as a cofactor necessary for the NS2B-NS3 complex serine-protease activity, which cleaves the viral poly-protein at the NS2A/NS2B, NS2B/NS3, NS3/NS4A and NS4B/NS5 junctions (Bera et al. 2007; Jan et al. 1995; Shiryaev et al. 2007). NS3 is a big cytoplasmic protein (70 kDa) that intervenes in several enzymatic activities (protease, helicase) involved in the poly-protein processing and viral RNA replication (Chambers et al. 1990b; Li et al. 1999; Luo et al. 2008). Interestingly, NS3 also appears to be involved in the virus assembly through mechanisms that are independent from the enzymatic functions outlined above (Patkar and Kuhn 2008). NS4A and NS4B are small hydrophobic membrane-associated proteins of 16 and 27 kDa, respectively. Based on its sub-cellular local-ization, both proteins may intervene in the viral RNA replication (Mackenzie et al. 1998; Westaway et al. 1997). NS5 is the biggest (103 kDa) and more conservative protein throughout the *Flavivirus* genus (Davidson 2009). It has a methyltransferase activity on its N-terminal region and a RNA-dependent RNA polymerase (RdRp) activity on the C-terminal motifs (Mukhopadhyay et al. 2003; Liu et al. 2010).

11.5   REPLICATION CYCLE

The virus enters into the cell through a mechanism known as receptor-mediated endocytosis, where the viral receptor for recognition and cell adsorption is protein E (Hung et al. 1999). Once the endocytic vesicle is formed, the endosome acid pH generates structural alterations in protein E, producing endosome-virion mem-brane's fusion and releasing the nucleocapsid to the cytoplasm (Stiasny et al. 2002); although direct fusion of the viral envelope with the cellular membrane has been observed too (Hase et al. 1989). After the viral uncoating process, the replication starts. Viral RNA replication occurs in perinuclear spots and implies the synthesis of a single complementary negative strand that works as a template for the positive strand molecule's synthesis (Lindenbach and Rice 2001). The genomic viral RNA is used directly as a messenger and is completely translated from its 5' end to produce a big precursor poly-protein that later is cleaved to generate each individual viral pro-tein (Clyde et al. 2006). The new viral particle's assembly occurs in the endoplasmic reticulum (ER), where immature particles are generated (containing prM) and then transported to the exterior through the exocytic pathway. Evidence was found that the acid pH in the trans Golgi network (TGN) produces conformational changes in the prM-E complex that are necessary for the particle's maturation. Once the cleav-age of the complex is produced by the action of cellular furins, the mature particles are released through exocytosis (Lindenbach and Rice 2001).

11.6   PATHOLOGY AND PATHOGENESIS

After the virus inoculation, it replicates in local tissue and regional lymph nodes. Afterward, the virus is carried away through the lymph pathway and is poured to the bloodstream through the thoracic duct, generating a secondary viraemia that trans-ports it to the extra-neural tissues where also occurs viral replication and release to circulation (Malkova 1960). The viraemia level is modulated by the clearance rate of macrophages and finishes with the humoral response appearance, usually one week after infection. In most of the cases, the viraemia curve presents a short-duration peak (2 to 3 days) followed by a quick dropping. The extra-neural tissues with greater replication are connective tissue, skeletal, cardiac and smooth muscle, lymphoreticular tissue, and endocrine and exocrine glands. In newborn hamsters infected with SLEV and Rocío virus, the pancreas and heart were the organs most severely affected (Harrison et al. 1980). Experimental research on mice infected with neurotropics Flavivirus has demonstrated the link among viraemia level, brain infection development, and appearance of multiple sites with viral antigens in neural tissue (Albretch 1998), supporting the concept of a hematogenous release to the central nervous system (CNS) (Johnson 1982). The mechanism used by Flavivirus to pass through the blood-brain barrier during the natural infection remains unclear. The viruses ability for replicating in endothelial vascular cells suggests they may pass through the brain capillaries. However, only a few times were viral antigens found *in vivo* on endothelial cells of brain capillaries, and also it was observed that Flavivirus do not replicate at high titers in brain endothelial cells *in vitro* either (Dropulic and Masters 1990). Some experimental studies suggest that CNS invasion occurs through the olfactory epithelium. The olfactory tract has been recognized as an alternative pathway to the CNS and an important release mode after nasal spray exposures. Intranasal inoculation with Flavivirus in murine animal models can result in lethal encephalitis, probably due to the direct infection of olfactory neurons and the posterior release in the brain, while peripheral inoculation with the same virus does not produce CNS invasion. Nevertheless, in experimental models using mice and hamsters, olfactory neurons were the access gateway to CNS after infection (Monath et al. 1983). On the other hand, pathologic studies on Japanese encephalitis cases indicate a widespread involvement of the brain stem, deep nuclei, and cortex, more consistent with a hematogenous infection.

The infection's starting point and development are influenced by viral and host specific factors. The intracerebral (i.c.) or intranasal (i.n.) infection with high viral doses predisposes to fatal encephalitis. The viral strains can differ in neuro-invasiveness, neuro-virulence or both. Among the factors involved in pathogenesis, the most important are age, gender, genetic susceptibility, preexistent infections, or immunity to heterologous agents. Newborn animals are more susceptible to lethal encephalitis than adult animals. Animals inoculated peripherally are susceptible in the first 3 to 4 weeks of life when they develop resistance, but can remain susceptible to lethal encephalitis if they are i.c. inoculated. Immature neurons are more sensible to infection (Ogata et al. 1991). In SLEV induced encephalitis, susceptibility in humans increases with advanced age. The mechanisms underlying this increase are unknown. Physiological factors leading to temporal immunosuppression may be responsible for a greater susceptibility. In this way, mice exposed to cold or stress and inoculated with WNV developed a bigger viral replication and mortality rate (Ben-Nathan and Feuerstein 1990). Sexually mature female mice showed a bigger resistance to Flavivirus infection (Andersen and Hanson 1974), while in humans this has not been demonstrated yet. Genetic markers play a central role in the Flavivirus infection pathogenesis (Sangster et al. 1998). A genetic resistance to Flavivirus infection has been observed in nonimmune inbred mice strains (Mashimo et al. 2008).

The recovery from flaviviral encephalitis depends on early intrathecal antibodies synthesis and viral clearance by macrophages. The inflammatory response in CNS-related infections consists of helper-inducer T cells and, to a lesser degree, B lymphocytes, infiltrating from the blood to the perivascular space and parenchyma.

Macrophages and activated microglial cells in the perivascular space and parenchyma, respectively, are responsible for viral clearance. The outcome is determined
by the comparative rates of viral spread and neuronal infection, migration of inflammatory cells into the CNS, and the rapidity of the antibody response. Interferon
production is elicited in the brain of human SLE patients, but its role in limiting the
virus spread in the CNS is unclear.

11.7   CLINICAL PRESENTATIONS

The clinical spectrum of a SLEV infection can comprise from an unspecific
febrile syndrome, alike to influenza, to a disease affecting the CNS. The clinical features of meningitis and encephalitis due to SLEV are not specific, and
other etiologies (bacterial, fungal, other viral, toxic, cerebrovascular), must be
considered.

Clinical manifestations of SLEV infection can be grouped in three syndromes
(Table 11.2): Encephalitis (including meningoencephalitis and encephalomyelitis),
meningitis, and febrile cephalea.

The incubation period can last from 4 to 21 days. The beginning of the symptoms
are characterized by general discomfort, fever, chills, cephalea, anorexia, nausea,
myalgia, and sore throat or cough, followed after 1–4 days by the neurological or
meningeal signs. Less than 1% of SLEV infections are clinically apparent (Tsai et al.
1987). The disease's severity increases with age, with people over 60 years old the

---

TABLE 11.2

Definitions of Clinical Syndromes Caused by St. Louis Encephalitis Virus

I. Encephalitis (including meningoencephalitis and encephalomyelitis)
  A. Acute febrile illness (oral temperature ≥37.8°C (≥100°F)
  B. One or more signs in either of the following categories:
    1. Altered level of consciousness (confusion, disorientation, delirium, lethargy, stupor, coma)
    2. Objective signs of neurologic dysfunction (convulsion, cranial nerve palsy, dysarthria,
       rigidity, paresis, paralysis, abnormal reflexes, tremor, etc.)
II. Aseptic meningitis[a]
  A. Acute febrile illness
  B. Sign(s) of meningeal irritation (stiff neck with or without positive Kernig's or Brudzinski's sign)
  C. No objective signs of neurologic dysfunction
III. Febrile headache[a]
  A. Acute febrile illness
  B. Headache (may also have other systemic symptoms, such as nausea or vomiting)
  C. No signs of meningeal irritation or neurologic dysfunction

Source: From Brinker, K.R.M. and Monath, T.P., The acute disease, in Monath, T.P. (ed.), *St. Louis
Encephalitis.* Washington, DC: American Public Health Association, 1980, pp. 503–534.

[a] Cerebrospinal fluid pleocytosis present in patients with encephalitis and aseptic meningitis; it may also
be found in patients with the syndrome of febrile headache.

ones having more frequent cases of encephalitis. Being elderly contributes to virus neuropathogenesis, brain damage, and severity in the clinical manifestation (Burke and Monath 2001).

Mortality rate increases with age (over 75 years) (Reisen 2003). Underlying diseases such as diabetes, hypertension, chronic alcoholism and arteriosclerosis predispose to severe infection accompanied by a tragic ending (Brinker and Monath 1980).

From clinical data obtained during the first SLEV outbreak in Cordoba (Argentina) stood out, in the preludes, cephalea, somnolence, and some degree of temporo-spatial disorientation in the first 72 h after the symptoms appeared (Spinsanti et al. 2008). Bradypsychia and temporo-spatial disorientation were the prevailing finding. In some patients the symptoms progressed with a significant depression of the sensory system, and some of them needed assisted mechanical ventilation. There were observed tremors in the face, hands, and feet with myoclonia episodes. Other patients presented holocranial cephalea accompanied by photophobia, some with mixed aphasia and others with episodes of tonic clonic seizures. The encephalitis frequency (including meningoencephalitis) varied from 80% of cases in persons under 20 years to 95% in those over 60 years. Figure 11.2 shows the age distribution for the most common clinical syndromes observed with SLEV infection.

Symptoms can spontaneously resolve during any stage of the disease with complete recovery. The acute disease can be followed by the "convalescent fatigue syndrome" in <50% of the patients, characterized by asthenia, irritability, tremors, somnolence, depression, memory loss, and cephalea, and can last up to three years. Approximately 20% of these patients can present symptoms that persist for long periods, such as speech and sensory-motor alterations and tremors. Elderly and severity of the acute disease seem to predispose to these sequels (Finley and Riggs 1980).

The cerebrospinal fluid (CSF) is usually under normal pressure and contains from ten to hundreds of mononuclear cells (≤500), mainly lymphocytes. However, at the beginning of the disease predominantly polymorphonuclear leucocytes can be present (Luby 1994). Protein concentration can be slightly high, while glucose levels

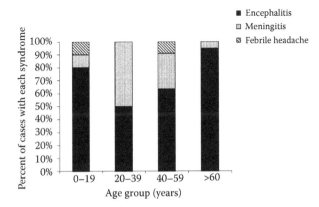

FIGURE 11.2 Frequency of clinical symptoms notified in St. Louis encephalitis cases. (Reproduced from Spinsanti et al. 2008.)

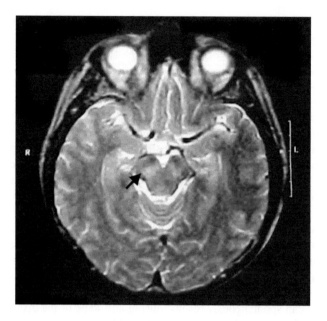

FIGURE 11.3 Magnetic resonance imaging (MRI) from a patient suffering from SLEV encephalitis. The cranial axial T2-weighted MRI shows hyperintense abnormalities in the substantia nigra with major compromise on the right side (arrows).

remain normal. In peripheral blood there is mainly a polymorphonuclear leucocytosis. The interval observed between the beginning of the disease and death has been consistent in all the studies. Approximately 50% of the fatal cases die during the first week of the disease's appearance and 80% during the following two weeks. It is difficult to assign mortality directly to SLEV or to secondary complications or underlying diseases. In general, death due to direct viral damage on CNS occurs without secondary complications appearing during the first 2 weeks, and death late is probably due to nonrelated causes (Brinker and Monath 1980).

The electroencephalogram shows a diffuse and generalized diminution and an amorphous and generalized delta wave activity (Brinker et al. 1979). Computed tomography scans may be normal, but magnetic resonance images have disclosed T2-weighted hyper-intense abnormalities in the substantia nigra, consistent with edema (Cerna 1999) (Figure 11.3).

11.8   DIAGNOSIS

Table 11.3 shows laboratory criteria for SLEV infection diagnosis. In the human infection with SLEV, patient's age, season of the year, place of residence and exposition, and information about similar cases occurring in the community are important epidemiologic data in the differential diagnostic compared with other infections. It is essential to discard other agents such as bacteria, mycobacteria, spirochetes, fungal and viral infections like herpes, enterovirus (that are spread also during summer),

TABLE 11.3
Laboratory Criteria for SLEV neurological Infection Diagnosis[a]

Suspicious case: Is every person presenting
- Compatible clinical symptoms (febrile illness, temperature >38°C, with neurological signs, aseptic meningitis, encephalitis, etc.).
- Symptoms onset during a known period of Flavivirus spreading.

Probable case: Probable illness that satisfies the anterior criteria and at least one of the following:
- Serum or CSF IgM without seroconversion by NT in serum paired samples.
- IgM and IgG in a single serum or CSF sample.

Confirmed case: Febrile illness associated to neurological manifestations and at least one of the following laboratory results:
- Viral isolation or antigen or viral genome demonstration in tissue, blood, CSF or other organic fluids.
- Specific IgM in CSF and/or serum and sero-conversion by NT technique in serum or CSF paired samples.

[a] The following diagnosis criteria were adapted from Moore et al. 1993.

and other arboviruses (WNV, Rocio Virus, or Eastern, Western, and Venezuelan Equine Encephalitis Viruses). In elder people it is possible to mistake a SLEV infection with a cerebrovascular accident (Burke and Monath 2001).

Viral isolation from serum or CSF is very difficult due to the shortness of the viraemia period; viraemia can precede the symptoms for a few days. SLEV has been frequently recovered in fatal cases from brain and also from spleen, liver, lung, and kidney (Calisher and Poland 1980). The specific molecular diagnosis has a high sensibility and specificity degree to detect SLEV when it is compared with traditional techniques such as cellular culture plates assay and enzyme immunoassay with antigen capture (Howe et al. 1992; Kramer et al. 2002). Several authors have developed different RT-PCR methods able to detect a high number of SLEV strains (Kramer et al. 2002; Lanciotti and Kerst 2001; Chiles et al. 2004). Recently, Re et al. (2008) have developed a SLEV specific RT-nested PCR more sensitive than RT-PCR, allowing a low detection limit (7 PFU-plaque forming unit). This method was able to amplify the genome of SLEV strains of different geographic origins and also to detect viral RNA from mosquito homogenates and from a cell culture infected with two SLEV strains recently isolated in Argentina (Diaz et al. 2006, 2012).

The definitive diagnosis in humans depends on the serology almost exclusively. The presumptive diagnosis of recent infection is based on the detection of immunoglobulin M (IgM) antibodies by the IgM capture technique enzyme-linked immunosorbent assay (MAC-ELISA) in CSF and/or serum (Martin et al. 2000). Serum antibodies type IgM specific appear in the first 4 days after the beginning of the disease, with a peak at 7–14 days and decline to extinguish generally at 60 days (Burke and Monath 2001). The rapidity of this test is of great utility on the early diagnosis and epidemiological surveillance. However, the persistence of IgM antibodies has been detected in some patients. Spinsanti et al. (2011) have detected specific SLEV

IgM antibodies in serum until more than a year after the beginning of the symptoms, indicating that the presence of IgM is not systematically associated with recent infections. On the other hand this test uses a conjugated monoclonal antibody (6B6C-1) that detects antibodies against different Flavivirus species (Monath et al. 1984).

Specific diagnosis usually relies on serological tests on appropriately timed acute and convalescent samples. The IgG-type antibodies can be detected by ELISA tests, Hemagglutination Inhibition (HI) and Neutralization (PRNT); the IgG-type antibodies titers increase from the week following to the beginning of the symptoms. The HI test detects mainly group-reactive antigens and is useful for screening studies due to its sensibility, but it has the disadvantage of being low-specific especially in geographic areas where more than one flavivirus is circulating. The PRNT is the most specific test, "gold standard" for arbovirus. Neutralizing antibodies (NTAbs) appear in first place and in higher number than HI antibodies; they reach a maximum titer at 7–21 days after the disease's onset and persist usually during the whole life. The PRNT is used to confirm results derived from serological surveys realized through HI and MAC-ELISA (Calisher and Poland 1980) (Figure 11.4).

Certain flaviviruses seem to share more antigens than others; antibodies against Flavivirus group members closely related are more difficult to differentiate with low-specificity techniques such as HI and MAC-ELISA (Martin et al. 2004). One of these groups is that integrated by SLEV, JEV WNV, and MVEV (Table 11.1). Other flaviviruses that share extensively with SLEV are Rocío virus, Ilheus virus, and DENV (Calisher and Poland 1980).

Spinsanti et al. (2011) provide data about the patterns of response of the subclasses IgG1, IgG2, IgG3, and IgG4 produced during a SLEV natural infection (acute and convalescent phases) and in humoral long-term immunity. They had demonstrated the persistence of the four IgG isotypes for more than one year in patients infected by SLEV. However, IgG1 isotype was present at the highest titers, with a peak between

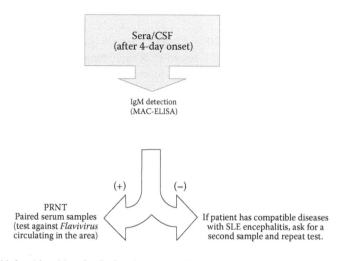

FIGURE 11.4   Algorithm for St. Louis encephalitis serological diagnosis.

day 8 and 30 after onset of the disease, coincident with the highest titer of NTAbs. IgG1 antibodies have been described as the main subclass in infections by WNV, as well as those with the highest neutralizing activity, which could be responsible for viral clearance (Hoffmeister et al. 2011).

11.9 ECOLOGY

SLEV presents an exclusive distribution in the American continent, where it is widely extended (Figure 11.5). In the mid-1980s, the demographic variation between the different SLEV strains through molecular studies of genetic and biological variability was demonstrated.

Based on the envelope's gen complete sequence, SLEV strains have been classified in 7 genotypes (I-VII), being genotypes I and II widely distributed in the USA and the others in Central and South American countries (Kramer and Chandler 2001) (Figure 11.5). Recent studies of SLEV molecular diversity characterization indicate a new genotype's presence (genotype VIII) exclusive of the Amazonia region

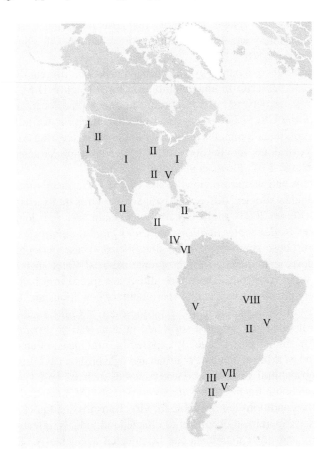

FIGURE 11.5   Geographic distribution of St. Louis encephalitis virus genotypes.

(Brazil) (Rodriguez et al. 2010). The phylogenetic analysis indicated that different viral strain isolations had created a monophyletic group in which most of the strains are grouped according to the geographic origin (Auguste et al. 2009; Kramer and Chandler 2001). In a recent phylogeographic study it has been postulated that SLEV would originate in South America and migrate to the northern countries, resulting in a limited interchange (Auguste et al. 2009). Recently, it was detected the presence of genotype V (abundant in South America) in the state of Florida (Ottendorfer et al. 2009), while genotype I was found in mosquitoes collected in Argentina (Diaz et al. 2012). This evidence would indicate an effective introduction of SLEV strains in regions between North and South America, probably through bird migration, as it was proposed for WNV by Diaz et al. (2008a).

In the US, SLEV has been one of the main causes of arbovirus encephalitis epidemics until the introduction of WNV in 1999. Most of the clinical cases have been reported by the states of Texas, Florida, southeastern states, and the Ohio River's basin (Reisen 2003). By the contrary, urban epidemics of encephalitis due to SLEV in other American countries are rare, focal, or of small magnitude or remain undetected. This low incidence in Central and South America may be due to an inadequate case notification system, laboratory diagnosis deficiencies, attenuated viral strains spreading, and/or enzootic cycles involving mosquitoes that do not often feed on humans (Spence 1980).

SLEV is maintained in nature by transmission between different *Culex* spp. mosquito species and passeriform and columbiform birds (Figure 11.6). The members in this transmission network vary according to geographic localization and time of the year. In the US, SLEV ecology is well characterized, while for the rest of the American continent it remains practically unknown. Excepting Argentina where research has been done, moving forward SLEV ecological characterization (Diaz 2006, 2008b, 2009, 2012; Flores et al. 2010).

In the eastern and western regions of the US, SLEV transmission networks are separated by epidemiological differences based on the virus transmission's ecological determinants (Reisen 2003). In the eastern states, main vectors belong to the *Culex pipiens* complex (*Culex pipiens pipiens* and *Culex pipiens quinquefasciatus*) and its main hosts are house sparrows (*Passer domesticus*). These peridomestic mosquitoes vectors develop frequently in rich organic material water such as sewers and peridomestic water reservoirs. These mosquitoes are spread in urban and suburban ambient densely populated, especially where sanitary conditions are deficient. In the western regions of the USA, the main vector mosquito is *Culex tarsalis*. This specie reproduces in flooded and irrigated soils, and in industrial or urban residual water (Mitchell 1980). Humans are frequently exposed in rural areas, often determined by recreational and working activities. Periurban and wild birds act as hosts, mainly those abundant in agricultural areas close to water sources such as house sparrows (*Passer domesticus*) and house finches (*Carpodacus mexicanus*) (McLean and Bowen 1980).

When all the conditions are favorable for viral transmission (quick amplification, with a progressive increment in number of infected individuals, infective vectors and hosts), humans and other mammals can be infected accidentally (dead-end host). At this point, other environmental and behavioral factors that determine human exposition to mosquitoes acquire epidemiologic relevance. Humans and domestic

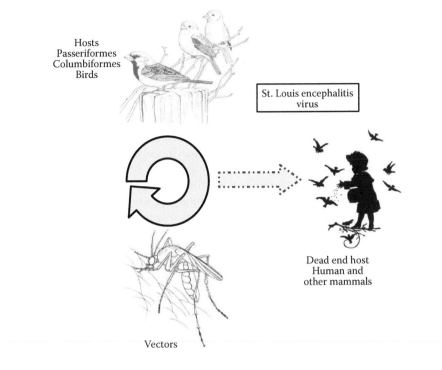

FIGURE 11.6 Transmission cycle of St. Louis encephalitis virus.

mammals are excluded from the basic transmission cycle because the viraemia titers are insufficient to infect vector mosquitoes (Monath 1980).

The "overwinter" mechanism by which the virus survives during winter, is unknown; however, studies suggest that the virus could persist locally in vertebrate hosts (birds, bats) with viraemia resurgence in springtime, contributing to the local transmission's re-initiation (Reisen et al. 2001). Other data suggest overwinter through vertical transmission in mosquitoes of the *Culex pipiens* complex or the overwinter hibernantion in adult mosquitoes (Flores et al. 2010; Monath and Tsai 1987).

In Central and South America, SLEV was isolated from humans in Argentina, Brazil, Panama, and Trinidad; from birds in Brazil, Haiti, Jamaica, Mexico, Panama, and Trinidad; and from arthropods in Argentina, Brazil, Ecuador, French Guyana, Guatemala, Jamaica, Mexico, Panama, and Trinidad (Diaz et al. 2006; Monath 1980; Rocco et al. 2007; Sabattini et al. 1998). In these regions, the virus has been isolated from 11 different mosquito's genera, including *Culex nigripalpus* and *Culex quinquefasciatus* (Spence 1980). Strong evidence support birds as hosts. Several viral strains have been isolated from 27 bird species (cormorants, egrets, pigeons, thrushes, celestines) in six different countries; the mocking birds (Mimidae Family) could be implicated in transmission in Jamaica, and certain formicaridos (*Formicarius canalis, Myrmotherula axillaris, Myrmotherula hauxwelli*) in forest regions of Brazil. Although, wild mammals (micro-rodents, sloths) and domestic mammals have been found infected, the evidence supporting their role as hosts are scarce (Spence 1980).

In Argentina the SLEV transmission cycles have been partially clarified. Even when antibodies against SLEV have been detected in domestic mammals such as horses, cows, sheep, and goats, they would only have relevance as dead-end hosts (Monath et al. 1985; Sabattini et al. 1998).

Serological studies have detected the presence of birds from families Furnaridae, Columbidae, Tyranidae, Fringilidae, Icteridae, Ardeide, and Phytotomidae infected with SLEV (Sabattini et al. 1998). Experimental inoculation studies had demonstrated that Eared Dove (*Zenaida auriculata*) and Picui Ground-dove (*Columbina picui*) develop viraemia sufficiently high to infect *Culex quinquefasciatus* mosquitoes (Diaz 2009; Diaz et al. 2008b). On the contrary, House Sparrows in Argentina, differently from the USA, do not play a significant role in transmission and maintenance of SLEV (Diaz 2009).

Regarding the vector, SLEV has been isolated from *Culex quinquefasciatus* and *Culex* spp. in Santa Fe province (Argentina) (Mitchell et al. 1985). In Cordoba City, several mosquitoes' species (*Aedes aeygpti, Aedes albifasciatus, Aedes scapularis, Anopheles albitarsis, Culex apicinus, Culex interfor, Culex quinquefasciatus*, and *Psorophora* sp.) have been detected infected by SLEV during enzootic periods (Diaz et al. 2012). Vector competence studies carried out in *Culex quinquefasciatus* collected in Esperanza (Santa Fe) and Cordoba showed this species' ability to infect and transmit SLEV strain 78V-6507 (Diaz 2009; Mitchell et al. 1980).

Activity patterns present characteristics of a temporal seasonal nature and spatial heterogeneous nature, coincident with the focal nature of the transmission cycles that arbovirus have in other regions such as the USA. The greater viral activity periods are concentrated in the summer season (February and March), starting the spreading in November and December (spring). According to recent studies by Diaz (2009), in Cordoba would be a primary transmission network formed by *Culex quinquefasciatus* and *Culex interfor* mosquitoes, acting as avian host Eared Dove (*Zenaida auriculata*) and Picui Ground-dove (*Columbina picui*), who can also be part of the transmission network in epidemic periods.

11.10 EPIDEMIOLOGY

SLEV epidemiological transmission patterns reflect the interactions between humans and the virus, its reservoirs, and vector mosquitoes (Day 2001; Reisen 2003). The sporadic appearance of cases in the USA has been documented since 1933. From 1964 through 2010, an average of 102 cases were reported annually (range 2–1967) (CDC 2011). In USA western states, SLEV has an endemic transmission pattern. Epidemics are limited due to the high immunity level in populations with long residence in the area, setting aside to a less sensitive part of the adult population; in consequence, cases occur frequently in children and young adults (Reisen 2003). Infections occur mainly in rural areas associated to the vector's habitat. In the central-eastern region, average outbreaks occur sporadically, followed by periods, sometimes long, without viral transmission's evidence. The intermittent occurrence of outbreaks has been associated with climatic factors, such as temperate winter, rainy spring, and hot and dry summer (Monath 1980). High temperatures are favorable to the virus replication in mosquito, while rains below normal levels allow the formation of small pools in drainage systems, leading to big mosquito populations of the complex *Culex pipiens*. Sometimes small warning outbreaks occurred followed by big outbreaks in the same place the next year, probably as a result of an elevated viral amplification in the second year. The virus intermittent activity produces that the human population may be immunologically susceptible, allowing the virus' introduction and outbreak occurrence. Epidemics have occurred frequently in urban areas or their periphery and were restricted to areas where environmental factors are associated to an increased reproduction or exposition of mosquitoes. In general, these areas are of low socioeconomical level, with precarious housing, or with sewage effluents (Luby 1979; Monath 1980; Tsai 1991). On the contrary, during the 1933 outbreak, the highest case rate was observed in the population with greater economical resources and low density housing, but with open drains, pools, creeks, and open spaces (Froeschle and Reeves 1965).

Culex pipiens and *Culex quinquefasciatus* are highly domestic mosquito species that prefer the interior of houses or their surroundings. A higher infection risk has been observed in houses without mosquito nets or air conditioning, with more cases in women, probably due to the latter's exposition to the peridomestic vector (Marfin et al. 1993; Monath 1980; Tsai et al. 1988). Nevertheless, in the epidemics that occurred in Florida in 1990, people with outdoor occupations had the highest risk of infection (Meehan et al. 2000). In the west of the USA, where the virus is transmitted by *Culex tarsalis*, rural work is a risk factor and the case rate is higher in men (Reisen and Chiles 1997). A serological survey performed during the Florida epidemic in the 1990s indicated that infection rates were highest in people with outdoor occupations. In that case, health warnings, closing recreational parks such as Walt Disney World at night, and the use of personal protection seemed to reduce infection rates (Meehan et al. 2000).

Since 2002, SLEV is experiencing a reemergence as a human encephalitis etiological agent in the south cone of South America, producing small outbreaks and epidemics in Argentina and Brazil (López et al. 2011; Mondini et al. 2007; Rocco et al. 2005; Spinsanti et al. 2008). Serological studies carried out in Argentina indicate a wide distribution and endemicity of SLEV in temperate and subtropical areas (central and northern Argentina) (seroprevalence from 10% to 68%) (Sabattini et al. 1998; Spinsanti et al. 2000, 2002). In two populations from Cordoba (Argentina), the risk of infection are associated with the presence of garbage dumps near dwellings, the practice of outdoor activities at night, and the place of residence (Spinsanti et al. 2007). The practice of outdoor activities at night increased the chance of infection, probably due to the nocturnal habits of the *Culex* mosquitoes. During summer–autumn of 2005, in this city, SLEV encephalitis epidemic occurred in humans, and it was the first one in South America (Spinsanti et al. 2008). There were 47 reported cases, of which most were hospitalized. The cases predominantly occurred among people 60 years and older. Nine deaths were reported. In this study, a correlation between age and disease severity was observed. Advanced age is associated with a greater severity of disease caused by several flavivirus (WNV, JEV) (Brinker and Monath 1980; Johnson 2002).

In the following years, there were only isolated cases registered, whereas between 2010 and 2011, there was an increase in notified cases with neurological compromise in several provinces of Argentina (Fabbri et al. 2011; Vergara Cid et al. 2011; Seijo et al. 2011).

Serological evidence of viral activity exists in other countries; some of them do not have records of isolations, such as Uruguay, Colombia, Venezuela, El Salvador, and Caribbean Islands. Many of the serological studies had been carried out with low specific techniques; in consequence, those results are uncertain because there may be serological cross reactions with other flaviviruses spread in the region as DENV (Monath 1980).

11.11 CONCLUSION

SLEV is an emerging flavivirus in the south cone of the American continent, in particular in Argentina and Brazil, where advances are being made for its eco-epidemiological characterization. Most of the bordering countries (Bolivia, Paraguay, Uruguay, Chile, Peru, Ecuador, and Colombia) do not have research programs of regional relevance focused in this viral infection.

The SLEV epidemiology is driven for climatic, entomological, viral, and host factors that form a complex network of interactions not completely understood.

From the explained above it is very important that the design and adjustment of cooperative research programs move forward in this viral infection study; sharing previous experiences with countries with more episodes and counseling to public health systems about prevention policies and detection of early febrile and neurological symptoms.

SLEV is a neglected diseases; however, knowing and understanding its eco-epidemiology are of concern. Other sympatric flavivirus cause similar symptoms in human population making diagnosis more difficult.

REFERENCES

Albrecht, P. 1998. Pathogenesis of neurotropic arbovirus infection. *Curr. Top. Microbiol. Immunol.* 43; 45–91.

Andersen, A. A., and Hanson, R. P. 1974. Influence of sex and age on natural resistance to St. Louis encephalitis virus infection in mice. *Infect. Immun.* 9; 1123–1125.

Auguste, A. J., Pybus, O. G. and Carrington, C. V. 2009. Evolution and dispersal of St. Louis encephalitis virus in the Americas. *Infect. Genet. Evol.* 9; 709–715.

Beasley, D. W., Davis, C. T., Whiteman, M., Granwehr, B., Kinney, R. M., and Barrett, A. D. 2004. Molecular determinants of virulence of West Nile virus in North America. *Arch Virol.* (Suppl 18); 35–41.

Ben-Nathan, D., and Feuerstein, G. 1990. The influence of cold or isolation stress on resistance of mice to West Nile virus encephalitis. *Experientia.* 46; 285–290.

Bera, A. K., Kuhn, R. J., and Smith, K. L. 2007. Functional characterization of cys and trans activity of the Flavivirus NS2B-NS3 protease. *J. Biol. Chem.* 282; 12883–12892.

Bowen, G. S., Monath, T. P., Kemp, G. E., Kerschner, J. H., and Kirk, L. J. 1980. Geographic variation among St. Louis encephalitis virus strains in the viremic responses of avian hosts. *Am. J. Trop. Med. Hyg.* 29; 1411–1419.

Brinker, K. R., and Monath, T. P. 1980. The acute disease, In: Monath, T. P. (Ed.), *St. Louis Encephalitis*. APHA, Washington, DC, pp. 503–534.

Brinker, K. R., Paulson, G., Monath, T. P., Wise, G., and Fass, R. J. 1979. St Louis encephalitis in Ohio, September 1975: clinical and EEG studies in 16 cases. *Arch. Intern. Med.* 139; 561–566.

Brinton, M. A. 2002. The molecular biology of West Nile Virus: a new invader of the western hemisphere. *Annu. Rev. Microbiol.* 56; 371–402.

Burke, D. S., and Monath, T. P. 2001. Flaviviruses, In: Knipe, D. M., and Howely, P. M. (Eds.), *Fields Virology*, fourth ed. Lippincott Williams & Wilkins, New York, pp. 1043–1126.

Calisher, C. H., and Poland, J. D. 1980. Laboratory diagnosis, In: Monath, T. P. (Ed.), *St.Louis Encephalitis.* APHA, Washington, DC, pp. 571–601.

Center for Diseases Control and Prevention. 2011. Saint Louis Encephalitis. Epidemiology and Geographic distribution. http://www.cdc.gov/sle/technical/epi.html.

Cerna, F., Mehrad, B., Luby, J. P., Burns, D., and Fleckenstein, J. L. 1999. St. Louis encephalitis and the substantia nigra: MR imaging evaluation. *Am. J. Neuroradiol.* 20; 1281–1283.

Chambers, T. J., Hahn, C. S., Galler, R., and Rice, C. M. 1990a. Flavivirus genome organization, expression, and replication. *Annu. Rev. Microbiol.* 44; 649–688.

Chambers, T. J., Weir, R. C., Grakoui, A., McCourt, D. W., Bazan, J. F., Fletterick, R. J., and Rice, C. M. 1990b. Evidence that the N-terminal domain of nonstructural protein NS3 from yellow fever virus is a serine protease responsible for site-specific cleavages in the viral polyprotein. *Proc. Natl. Acad. Sci. U S A.* 87; 8898–8902.

Chiles, R. E., Green, E. N., Fang, Y., Goddard, L., Roth, A., Reisen, W. K., and Scott, T. W. 2004. Blinded laboratory comparison of the *in situ* enzyme immunoassay, the VecTest wicking assay, and a reverse transcription-polymerase chain reaction assay to detect mosquitoes infected with West Nile and St. Louis encephalitis viruses. *J. Med. Entomol.* 41; 539–544.

Clyde, K., Kyle, J. L., and Harris, E. 2006. Recent advances in deciphering viral and host determinants of dengue virus replication and pathogenesis. *J. Virol.* 80; 11418–11431.

Davidson, A. D. 2009. Chapter 2. New insights into flavivirus nonstructural protein 5. *Adv. Virus Res.* 74; 41–101.

Day, J. F. 2001. Predicting St. Louis encephalitis virus epidemics: lessons from recent, and not so recent, outbreaks. *Annu Rev Entomol.* 46; 111–138.

Diaz, L. A. 2009. Patrones de actividad y estacionalidad del virus St. Louis encephalitis en Córdoba, Argentina. Tesis en Ciencias Biológicas. Facultad de Ciencias Exactas, Físicas y Naturales. Universidad Nacional de Córdoba. pp.167.

Diaz, L. A., Albrieu Llinás, G., Vázquez, A., Tenorio, A., and Contigiani, M. S. 2012. Silent circulation of St. Louis encephalitis virus prior to an encephalitis outbreak in Cordoba, Argentina (2005). *PLoS Negl. Trop. Dis.* 6(1); e1489.

Diaz, L. A., Goñi, S., Iserte, J., Logue, C., Singh, A., Powers, A., and Contigiani, M. S. 2010. Molecular characterization of epidemic and nonepidemic St. Louis encephalitis virus (SLEV) strains isolated in Argentina. *Am. J. Trop. Med. Hyg.* 83(S5); 4.

Diaz, L. A., Komar, N., Visintin, A., Dantur Juri, M. J., Stein, M., Lobo Allende, R., Spinsanti, L., Konigheim, B., Aguilar, J., Laurito, M., Almirón, W., and Contigiani, M. 2008a. West Nile virus in birds, Argentina. *Emerg. Infect. Dis.* 14; 689–691.

Diaz, L. A., Occelli, M., Almeida, F. L., Almirón, W. R., and Contigiani, M. S. 2008b. Eared dove (Zenaida auriculata, Columbidae) as host for St. Louis encephalitis virus (Flaviviridae, Flavivirus). *Vector Borne Zoonotic Dis.* 8; 277–282.

Diaz, L. A., Ré, V., Almirón, W. R., Farías, A., Vázquez, A., Sanchez-Seco, M. P., Aguilar, J., Spinsanti, L., Konigheim, B., Visintin, A., Garciá, J., Morales, M. A., Tenorio, A., and Contigiani, M. 2006. Genotype III Saint Louis encephalitis virus outbreak, Argentina, 2005. *Emerg. Infect. Dis.* 12; 1752–1754.

Dropulic, B., and Masters, C. L. 1990. Entry of neurotropic arboviruses into the central nervous system: an *in vitro* study using mouse brain endothelium. *J. Infect Dis.* 161; 685–691.

Engel, A. R., Rumyantsev, A. A., Maximova, O. A., Speicher J. M., Heiss, B., Murphy, B. R., and Pletnev, A. G. 2010. The neurovirulence and neuroinvasiveness of chimeric tick-borne encephalitis/dengue virus can be attenuated by introducing defined mutations into the envelope and NS5 protein genes and the 3' non-coding region of the genome. *Virology*. 405; 243–252.

Fabbri, C. M., Morales, M. A., Luppo, V. C., Cappato Berger, F., Salanitro, B., Manrique, M., and Enria, D. 2011. Brote de encefalitis de San Luis en la provincia de San Juan, Argentina, 2011. *Rev. Arg. Microb.* 43(S1); 89.

Finley, K., and Riggs, N. 1980. Convalescence and sequelae, In: Monath, T. P. (Ed.), *St. Louis Encephalitis*. APHA, Washington, DC, pp. 535–550.

Flores, F. S., Diaz, L. A., Batallán, G. P., Almirón, W. R., and Contigiani, M. S. 2010. Vertical transmission of St. Louis encephalitis virus in Culex quinquefasciatus (Diptera: Culicidae) in Córdoba, Argentina. *Vector Borne Zoonotic Dis.* 10; 999–1002.

Froeschle, J. E., and Reeves, W. C. 1965. Serologic epidemiology of Western Equine and St. Louis Encephalitis virus infection in California. II. Analysis of inapparent infections in residents of an endemic area. *Am. J. Epidemiol.* 81; 44–51.

Gritsun, T. S., Holmes, E. C., and Gould, E. A. 1995. Analysis of flavivirus envelope proteins reveals variable domains that reflect their antigenicity and may determine their pathogenesis. *Virus Res.* 35; 307–321.

Hahn, C. S., Hahn, Y. S., Rice, C. M., Lee, E., Dalgarno, L., Strauss, E. G., and Strauss, G. H. 1987. Conserved elements in the 3' untranslated region of flavivirus RNAs and potential cyclization sequences. *J. Mol. Biol.* 198; 33–41.

Hammon, W. M., Reeves, W. C., and Galindo, P. 1945. Epidemiologic studies of encephalitis in the San Joaquin Valley of California 1943, with the isolation of viruses from mosquitoes. *Am. J. Hyg.* 42; 299–306.

Harrison, A. K., Murphy, F. A., Gardner, J. J., and Bauer, S. P. 1980. Myocardial and pancreatic necrosis induced by Rocio virus, a new flavivirus. *Exp. Mol. Pathol.* 32; 102–113.

Hase, T., Summers, P. L., and Eckels, K. H. 1989. Flavivirus entry into cultured mosquito cells and human peripheral blood monocytes. *Arch. Virol.* 104; 129–143.

Heinz, F. X., and Roehrig, J. T. 1990. Flaviviruses, In: *"Immunochemistry of Viruses*, vol II." Elsevier, New York, pp. 289–305.

Hofmeister, Y., Planitzer, C. B., Farcet, M. R., Teschner, W., Butterweck, H. A., Weber, A., Holzer, G. W., and Kreil, T. R. 2011. Human IgG subclasses: *in vitro* neutralization of and *in vivo* protection against West Nile virus. *J. Virol.* 85; 1896–1899.

Howe, D. K., Vodkin, M. H., Novak, R. J., Shope, R. E., and McLaughlin, G. L. 1992. Use of the polymerase chain reaction for the sensitive detection of St. Louis encephalitis viral RNA. *J. Virol. Meth.* 36; 101–110.

Hung, S. L., Lee, P. L., Chen, H. W., Chen, L. K., Kao, C. L., and King, C. C. 1999. Analysis of the steps involved in Dengue virus entry into host cells. *Virology.* 257; 156–167.

International Committee on Taxonomy of Viruses (ICTV). Virus Taxonomy, 2009 Release. 2009. http://ictvonline.org/virusTaxonomy.asp?version=2009.

Jan, L. R., Yang, C. S., Trent, D. W., Falgout, B., and Lai, C. J. 1995. Processing of Japanese encephalitis virus non-structural proteins: NS2B-NS3 complex and heterologous proteases. *J. Gen. Virol.* 76; 573–580.

Johnson, R. T. 1982. *Viral Infections of the Nervous System*. Raven Press, New York.

Johnson, R. T., and Irani, D. N. 2002. West Nile virus encephalitis in the United States. *Curr. Neurol. Neurosci. Rep.* 2; 496–500.

Jones, C. T., Ma, L., Burgner, J. W., Groesch, T. D., Post, C. B., and Kuhn, R. J. 2003. Flavivirus capsid is a dimeric alpha-helical protein. *J. Virol.* 77; 7143–7149.

Kramer, L. D., and Chandler, L. J. 2001. Phylogenetic analysis of the envelope gene of St. Louis encephalitis virus. *Arch. Virol.* 146; 2341–2355.

Kramer, L. D., Wolfe, T. M., Green, E. N., Chiles, R. E., Fallah, H., Fang, Y., and Reisen, W. K. 2002. Detection of encephalitis viruses in mosquitoes (Diptera: Culicidae) and avian tissues. *J. Med. Entomol.* 39; 312–323.

Kuhn, R. J., Zhang, W., Rossmann, M. G., Pletnev, S. V., Corver, J., Lenches, E., Jones, C. T., Mukhopadhyay, S., Chipman, P. R., Strauss, E. G., Baker, T. S., and Strauss, J. H. 2002. Structure of dengue virus: implications for flavivirus organization, maturation, and fusion. *Cell.* 108; 717–725.

Lanciotti, R. S., and Kerst, A. J. 2001. Nucleic acid sequence-based amplification assays for rapid detection of West Nile and St. Louis encephalitis viruses. *J. Clin. Microbiol.* 39; 4506–4513.

Leung, J. Y., Pijlman, G. P., Kondratieva, N., Hyde, J., Mackenzie, J. M., and Khromykh, A. A. 2008. Role of nonstructural protein NS2A in flavivirus assembly. *J. Virol.* 82; 4731–4741.

Li, H., Clum, S., You, S., Ebner, K. E., and Padmanabhan, R. 1999. The serine protease and RNA-stimulated nucleoside triphosphatase and RNA helicase functional domains of dengue virus type 2 NS3 converge within a region of 20 amino acids. *J. Virol.* 73; 3108–3116.

Lindenbach, B. D., and Rice, C. M. 2001. Flaviviridae: The viruses and their replication, In: Knipe, D. M., and Howely, P. M. (Eds.), *Fields Virology*, fourth edition. Lippincott Williams & Wilkins, New York, pp. 991–1042.

Liu, L., Dong, H., Chen, H., Zhang, J., Ling, H., Li, Z., Shi, P. Y., and Li, H. 2010. Flavivirus RNA cap methyltransferase: structure, function, and inhibition. *Front Biol.* 5; 286–303.

López, H., Neira, J., Morales, M. A., Fabbri, C., D'Agostino, M. L., and Zitto, T. 2011. Saint Louis encephalitis virus in Buenos Aires city during the outbreak of dengue in 2009. *Medicina (B Aires).* 71; 247–250.

Luby, J. P. 1979. St. Louis encephalitis. *Epidemiol. Rev.* 1; 55–73.

Luby, J. P. 1994. St. Louis encephalitis, in: Beran, G. W., and Steele, J. H., (Eds.), *Handbook of Zoonoses. Section B: Viral.* Second edition. CRC Press, Boca Raton, Florida, pp. 47–58.

Lumsden, L. L. 1958. St. Louis encephalitis in 1933. Observations on epidemiological features. *Public Health Rep.* 73; 340–353.

Luo, D., Xu, T., Watson, R. P., Scherer-Becher, D., Sampath, A., Jahnke, W., Yeong, S. S., Wang, C. H., Lim, S. P., Strongin, A., Vasudevan, S. G., and Lescar, J. 2008. Insights into RNA unwinding and TP hydrolysis by the Flavivirus NS3 protein. *EMBO J.* 27; 3209–3219.

Mackenzie, J. M., Jones, M. K., and Young, P. R. 1996. Immunolocalization of the dengue virus nonstructural glycoprotein NS1 suggests a role in viral RNA replication. *Virology.* 220; 232–240.

Mackenzie, J. M., Khromykh, A. A., Jones, M. K., and Westaway, E. G. 1998. Subcellular localization and some biochemical properties of the flavivirus Kunjin nonstructural proteins NS2A and NS4A. *Virology.* 245; 203–215.

Malkova, D. 1960. The role of the lymphatic system in experimental infection with tick-borne encephalitis. 2. Neutralizing antibodies in the lymph and blood plasma of experimentally infected sheep. *Acta Virol.* 4; 283–289.

Marfin, A. A., Bleed, D. M., Lofgren, J. P., Olin, A. C., Savage, H. M., Smith, G. C., Moore, P. S., Karabatsos, N., and Tsai, T. F. 1993. Epidemiologic aspects of a St. Louis encephalitis epidemic in Jefferson County Arkansas, 1991. *Am. J. Trop. Med. Hyg.* 49; 30–37.

Martin, D. A., Muth, D. A., Brown, T., Johnson, A. J., Karabatsos, N., and Roehrig, J. T. 2000. Standarization of immunoglobulin M capture enzyme-linked immunosorbent assays for routine diagnosis of arboviral infections. *J. Clin. Microbiol.* 38; 1823–1826.

Martin, D. A., Noga, A., Kosoy, O., Johnson, A. J., Petersen, L. R., and Lanciotti, R. S. 2004. Evaluation of a diagnostic algorithm using immunoglobulin M enzyme-linked immunosorbent assay to differentiate human West Nile Virus and St. Louis Encephalitis virus infections during the 2002 West Nile Virus epidemic in the United States. *Clin. Diagn. Lab. Immunol.* 11; 1130–1132.

Mashimo, T., Simon-Chazottes, D., and Guénet, J. L. 2008. Innate resistance to flavivirus infections and the functions of 2'–5' oligoadenylate synthetases. *Curr. Top. Microbiol. Immunol.* 321; 85–100.

McLean, R. G., and Bowen, G. S. 1980. Vertebrate hosts, In: Monath, T. P. (Ed.), *St. Louis Encephalitis.* American Public Health Association, Washington, DC, pp. 381–450.

Meehan, P. J., Wells, D. L., Paul, W., Buff, E., Lewis, A., Muth, D., Hopkins, R., Karabatsos, N., and Tsai, T. F. 2000. Epidemiological features of and public health response to a St. Louis encephalitis epidemic in Florida, 1990–1. *Epidemiol. Infect.* 125; 181–188.

Mitchell, C. J., Francy, D. B., and Monath, T. P. 1980a. Arthropod vectors, In: Monath, T. P. (Ed.), *St. Louis Encephalitis.* American Public Health Association, Washington, DC, pp. 313–379.

Mitchell, C. J., Monath, T. P., and Sabattini, M. S. 1980. Transmission of St. Louis encephalitis virus from Argentina by mosquitoes of the Culex pipiens (Diptera: Culicidae) complex. *J. Med. Entomol.* 17; 282–287.

Mitchell, C. J., Monath, T. P., Sabattini, M. S., Cropp, C. B., Daffner, J. F., Calisher, C. H., Jakob, W. L., and Christensen, H. A. 1985. Arbovirus investigations in Argentina, 1977–1980. II. Arthropod collections and virus isolations from Argentine mosquitoes. *Am. J. Trop. Med. Hyg.* 3; 945–955.

Monath, T. P. 1980. Epidemiology, In: Monath, T. P. (Ed.), *St. Louis Encephalitis.* American Public Health Association, Washington, DC, pp. 239–312.

Monath, T. P., and Tsai, T. F. 1987. St. Louis encephalitis: lessons from the last decade. *Am. J. Trop. Med. Hyg.* 37; 40S–59S.

Monath, T. P., Cropp, C. B., and Harrison, A. K. 1983. Mode of entry of a neurotropic arbovirus into the central nervous system. Reinvestigation of an old controversy. *Lab. Invest.* 48; 399–410.

Monath, T. P., Cropp, C. B., Bowen, G. S., Kemp, G. E., Mitchell, C. J., and Gardner, J. J. 1980. Variation in virulence for mice and rhesus monkeys among St. Louis encephalitis virus strains of different orgin. *Am. J. Trop. Med. Hyg.* 29; 948–962.

Monath, T. P., Nystrom, R. R., Bailey, R. E., Calisher, C. H., and Muth, D. J. 1984. Immunoglobulin M antibody capture enzyme-linked immunosorbent assay for diagnosis of St. Louis encephalitis. *J. Clin. Microbiol.* 20; 784–790.

Monath, T. P., Sabattini, M. S., Pauli, R., Daffner, J. F., Mitchell, C. J., Bowen, G. S., and Cropp, C. B. 1985. Arbovirus investigations in Argentina, 1977–1980. IV Serological surveys and sentinel equine program. *Am. J. Trop. Med. Hyg.* 34; 966–975.

Mondini, A., Cardeal, I. L., Lázaro, E., Nunes, S. H., Moreira, C. C., Rahal, P., Maia, I. L., Franco, C., Góngora, D. V., Góngora-Rubio, F., Cabrera, E. M., Figueiredo, L. T., da Fonseca, F. G., Bronzoni, R. V., Chiaravalloti-Neto, F., and Nogueira, M. L. 2007. Saint Louis encephalitis virus, Brazil. *Emerg. Infect. Dis.* 13; 176–178.

Moore, C. G., Mc Lean, R. G., Mitchell, C. J., Nasci, R. S., Tsai, T. F., Calisher, C. H., Marfin, A. A., Moore, P. S., and Gubler, D. J. 1993. Guidelines for arbovirus surveillance programs in the United States. pp. 1–64.

Mukhopadhyay, S., Kim, B. S., Chipman, P. R., Rossmann, M. G., and Kuhn, R. J. 2003. Structure of West Nile virus. *Science.* 302; 248.

Nybakken, G. E., Nelson, C. A., Chen, B. R., Diamond, M. S., and Fremont, D. H. 2006. Crystal structure of the West Nile virus envelope glycoprotein. *J. Virol.* 80; 11467–11474.

Ogata, A., Nagashima, K., Hall, W. W., Ichikawa, M., Kimura-Kuroda, J., and Yasui, K. 1991. Japanese encephalitis virus neurotropism is dependent on the degree of neuronal maturity. *J. Virol.* 65; 880–886.

Ottendorfer, C. L., Ambrose, J. H., White, G. S., Unnasch, T. R., and Stark, L. M. 2009. Isolation of genotype V St. Louis encephalitis virus in Florida. *Emerg. Infect. Dis.* 15; 604–606.

Patkar, C. G., and Kuhn, R. J. 2008. Yellow Fever virus NS3 plays an essential role in virus assembly independent of its known enzymatic functions. *J. Virol.* 82; 3342–3352.

Proutski, V., Gould, E. A., and Holmes, E. C. 1997. Secondary structure of the 3′ untranslated region of flaviviruses: similarities and differences. *Nucleic Acids Res.* 25; 1194–1202.

Ré, V., Spinsanti, L., Farías, A., Díaz, A., Vázquez, A., Aguilar, J., Tenorio, A., and Contigiani, M. 2008. Reliable detection of St. Louis encephalitis virus by RT-nested PCR. *Enferm. Infecc. Microbiol. Clin.* 26; 10–15.

Reisen, W. K. 2003. Epidemiology of St. Louis encephalitis virus. *Adv. Virus Res.* 61; 139–183.

Reisen, W. K., and Chiles, R. E. 1997. Prevalence of antibodies to western equine encephalomyelitis and St. Louis encephalitis viruses in residents of California exposed to sporadic and consistent enzootic transmission *Am. J. Trop. Med. Hyg.* 57; 526–529.

Reisen, W. K., Kramer, L. D., Chiles, R. E., Green, E. G., and Martinez, V. M. 2001. Encephalitis virus persistence in California birds: preliminary studies with house finches. *J. Med. Entomol.* 38; 393–399.

Rocco, I. M., Santos, C. L., Bisordi, I., Petrella, S. M., Pereira, L. E., Souza, R. P., Coimbra, T. L., Bessa, T. A., Oshiro, F. M., Lima, L. B., Cerroni, M. P., Marti, A. T., Barbosa, V. M., Katz, G., and Suzuki, A. 2005. St. Louis encephalitis virus: first isolation from a human in São Paulo State, Brazil. *Rev. Inst. Med. Trop. Sao Paulo.* 47; 281–285.

Rodrigues, S. G., Nunes, M. R., Casseb, S. M., Prazeres, A. S., Rodrigues, D. S., Silva, M. O., Cruz, A. C., Tavares-Neto, J. C., and Vasconcelos, P. F. 2010. Molecular epidemiology of Saint Louis encephalitis virus in the Brazilian Amazon: genetic divergence and dispersal. *J. Gen. Virol.* 91; 2420–2427.

Sabattini, M. S., Avilés, G., and Monath, T. P. 1998. Historical, epidemiological and ecological aspects of arbovirus in Argentina: Flaviviridae, Bunyaviridae and Rhabdoviridae, In: Travassos da Rosa, A. P. A. (Ed.), *Overview of Arbovirology in Brazil and Neighboring Countries.* Instituto Evandro Chagas, Belen. Brazil, pp. 135–153.

Sangster, M. Y., Mackenzie, J. S., and Shellam, G. R. 1998. Genetically determined resistance to flavivirus infection in wild Mus musculus domesticus and other taxonomic groups in the genus Mus. *Arch. Virol.* 143; 697–715.

Schlesinger, J. J., Brandriss, M. W., Cropp, C. B., and Monath, T. P. 1986. Protection against yellow fever in monkeys by immunization with yellow fever virus nonstructural protein NS1. *J. Virol.* 60; 1153–1155.

Seijo, A., Morales, M. A., Poustis, G., Romer, Y., Efron, E., Vilora, G., Lloveras, S., Giamperetti, S., Puente, T., Monroig, J., Luppo, V., and Enría, D. 2011. Outbreak of St. Louis encephalitis in the Metropolitan Buenos Aires Area. *Medicina (B Aires).* 71; 211–217.

Shiryaev, S. A., Koslov, I. A., Ratnikov, B. I., Smith, J. W., Lebl, M., and Strongin, A. Y. 2007. Cleavage preference distinguishes the two-component NS2B-NS3 serine proteinases of Dengue and West Nile viruses. *Biochem. J.* 401; 743–752.

Spence, L. P. 1980. St. Louis encephalitis in tropical America, In: Monath, T. P. (Ed.), *St. Louis Encephalitis.* American Public Health Association, Washington, DC, pp. 451–471.

Spinsanti, L. I., Díaz, L. A., Glatstein, N., Arselán, S., Morales, M. A., Farías, A. A., Fabbri, C., Aguilar, J. J., Ré, V., Frías, M., Almirón, W. R., Hunsperger, E., Siirin, M., Da Rosa, A. T., Tesh, R. B., Enría, D., and Contigiani, M. 2008. Human outbreak of St. Louis encephalitis detected in Argentina, 2005. *J. Clin. Virol.* 42; 27–33.

Spinsanti, L. I., Farías, A. A., Aguilar, J. J., Del Pilar Díaz, M., and Contigiani, M. S. 2011. Immunoglobulin G subclasses in antibody responses to St. Louis encephalitis virus infections. *Arch. Virol.* 156; 1861–1864.

Spinsanti, L. I., Ré, V. E., Díaz, M. P., and Contigiani, M. S. 2002. Age-related seroprevalence study for St. Louis encephalitis in a population from Cordoba, Argentina. *Rev. Inst. Med. Trop. Sao Paulo* 44; 59–62.

Spinsanti, L. I., Ré, V., Bassualdo, M., Diaz, G., Yacci, M. R., and Contigiani, M. 2000. Seroprevalencia de infección por virus Encefalitis de San Luis en la provincia de Formosa. *Medicina (B Aires).* 60; 474–476.

Spinsanti, L., Basquiera, A. L., Bulacio, S., Somale, V., Kim, S. C., Ré, V., Rabbat, D., Zárate, A., Zlocowski, J. C., Mayor, C. Q., Contigiani, M., and Palacio, S. 2003. St. Louis encephalitis in Argentina: the first case reported in the last seventeen years. *Emerg. Infect. Dis.* 9; 271–273.

Spinsanti, L., Farías, A., Aguilar, J., Díaz, M. P., Ghisiglieri, S., Bustos, M. A., Vilches, N., González, B., and Contigiani, M. 2007. Risk factors associated with St. Louis encephalitis seroprevalence in two populations from Córdoba, Argentina. *Trans. R. Soc. Trop. Med. Hyg.* 101; 1248–1252.

Stiasny, K., Allison, S. L., Schalich, J., and Heinz, F. X. 2002. Membrane interactions of the tick-borne encephalitis virus fusion protein E at low pH. *J. Virol.* 76; 3784–3790.

Trent, D. W., Grant, J. A., Vorndam, A. V., and Monath, T. P. 1981. Genetic heterogeneity among Saint Louis encephalitis virus isolates of different geographic origin. *Virology.* 114; 319–332.

Trent, D. W., Monath, T. P., Bowen, G. S., Vorndam, A. V., Cropp, B. C., and Kemp, G. E. 1980. Variation among strains of St. Louis encephalitis virus: Basis for a genetic, pathogenetic and epidemiological classification. *Ann. NY Acad. Sci.* 354; 219–237.

Tsai, T. F. 1991. Arboviral infections in the United States. *Infect. Dis. Clin. North Am.* 5; 73–102.

Tsai, T. F., Canfield, M. A., Reed, C. M., Flannery, V. L., Sullivan, K. H., Reeve, G. R., Bailey, R. E., and Poland, J. D. 1988. Epidemiological aspects of a St. Louis encephalitis outbreak in Harris County, Texas, 1986. *J. Infect Dis.* 157; 351–356.

Tsai, T. F., Cobb, W. B., Bolin, R. A., Gilman, N. J., Smith, G. C., Bailey, R. E., Poland, J. D., Doran, J. J., Emerson, J. K., and Lampert, K. J. 1987. Epidemiologic aspects of a St. Louis encephalitis outbreak in Mesa County, Colorado. *Am. J. Epidemiol.* 126; 460–473.

Vergara Cid, C., Spinsanti, L. I., Rivarola, M. E., Beltran, N., Diaz, A., Cogo, G., Maders, J., Arri, V., Chancalay, O., and Contigiani, M. S. 2011. Detección de infecciones humanas por flavivirus en la ciudad de Córdoba durante el año 2010. *Rev. Arg. Microb.* 43(S1); 37.

Westaway, E. G., Khromykh, A. A., Kenney, M. T., Mackenzie, J. M., and Jones, M. K. 1997. Proteins C and NS4B of the flavivirus Kunjin translocate independently into the nucleus. *Virology.* 234; 31–41.

12 Powassan Virus

Laura D. Kramer, Alan P. Dupuis II,
and Norma P. Tavakoli

CONTENTS

12.1 INTRODUCTION

Powassan virus (POWV; family Flaviviridae, genus *Flavivirus*) is a member of the mammalian tick-borne virus group (Grard et al. 2007). The virus appears to be widely distributed in its enzootic hosts in North America and Far East Asia (Mandl et al. 1993). Remarkable disease is rare (Hoang Johnson et al. 2010), but encephalitis in humans may be associated with significant neurologic sequelae. The first case was identified in 1958 in Powassan, Ontario, Canada (McLean and Donahue 1959). The virus appears to be increasing in prevalence in the United States, possibly as a consequence of improved diagnostics leading to increased detection, but equally likely as a consequence of the proliferation of vector tick populations or increased contact between infected ticks and humans due to lifestyle changes. An increased incidence of the closely related TBEV has also been noted in Europe, more likely due to socio-economic factors than climate warming (Godfrey and Randolph 2011). POWV is comprised of two lineages, lineage I (POWV) and II (*Deer tick virus*; DTV), with distinct transmission cycles (Ebel et al. 2001). It has been speculated that DTV may lead to milder cases (Ebel et al. 1999); however, at least two recent cases of DTV that were fatal (Tavakoli et al. 2009) (and unpublished data) demonstrate this virus has the potential to be virulent. This chapter will address the biology, epidemiology and ecology, pathology, and diagnostics of these two viruses.

12.2 CLASSIFICATION AND DISTRIBUTION

Flaviviruses (family Flaviviridae, genus Flavivirus) fall into distinct ecologic groups, i.e., mosquito-borne (*Culex* or *Aedes*), tick-borne, those with no known vector, and agents that infect arthropods only (Gaunt et al. 2001). The genus was originally divided serologically into groups (Porterfield 1980; Calisher et al. 1989), with the tick-borne flaviviruses grouping together. Molecular genetic analyses have upheld the original antigenic and ecologic groupings. Further intensive analyses have indicated that the tick-borne flaviviruses can be divided into mammalian, seabird, and Kadam tick-borne flavivirus groups (Grard et al. 2007) (Figure 12.1). The mammalian tick-borne virus group was originally referred to as the tick-borne encephalitis serocomplex. It was suggested that ticks that feed on mammals and sea birds may constitute the evolutionary bridge among these three groups (Grard et al. 2007). Tick-borne viruses share a common ancestor with the other flaviviruses (Thiel et al. 2005), and while closely related overall to each other, they are genetically divergent (Figure 12.2), widespread (Gritsun et al. 2003), and epidemiologically important (Demina et al. 2010; Gritsun et al. 2003). Extensive phylogenetic analysis suggested that acquisition of tick-borne transmission is a derived trait within the flaviviruses (Cook and Holmes 2006). *Powassan virus* is the most genetically divergent member of the TBEV antigenic complex (Calisher et al. 1989). The virus exists as two lineages, POWV and DTV (Ebel et al. 2001; Kuno et al. 2001), in which the E protein nucleotide and amino acid sequences differ by 14.6% and 4%, respectively (Beasley et al. 2001), and the nucleotide sequence of the entire genome of DTV differs by 16% from POWV (Kuno et al. 2001). This was interpreted as indicating that they represent distinct genetic subtypes ("genotypes") of the same virus type. The genetic distance between these two viruses suggests they diverged and evolved independently into two distinct ecological niches from a single origin (Telford et al. 1997). DTV and POWV coexist, and DTV has been found throughout the historical range of POWV (Kuno et al. 2001). Viruses from both lineages have been responsible for human illness (Kuno et al. 2001; Tavakoli et al. 2009). POWV and DTV appear to be genetically stable over time suggesting evolutionary constraint (Pesko et al. 2010; Kuno et al. 2001) consistent with other arboviruses. The viruses are also conserved over distance, as demonstrated by POWV isolated from a human case in Primorsky krai, Russia, in 2006, which was 99.8% similar to the LB strain that was isolated in Canada in 1958 (Leonova et al. 1991). In this chapter, unless otherwise stated, POWV includes both lineage I and II.

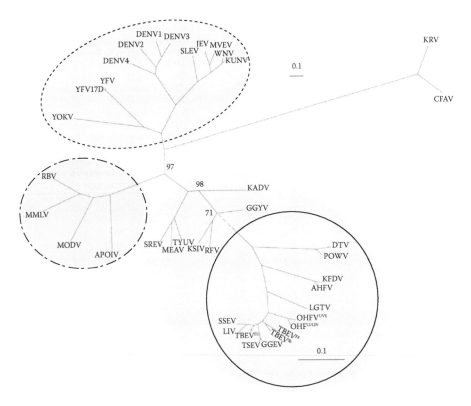

AHFV: Alkhurma hemorrhagic fever virus
APOIV: Apoi virus
CFAV: Cell fusing agent virus
DENV1–4: Dengue virus types 1–4
DTV: Deer tick virus
GGEV: Greek goat encephalitis virus
GGYV: Gadget gully virus
JEV: Japanese encephalitis virus
KADV: Kadam virus
KFDV: Kyasanur forest disease virus
KRV: Kamiti river virus
KSIV: Karshi virus
KUNV: Kunjin virus
LGTV: Langat virus
LIV: Louping ill virus
MEAV: Meaban virus

MODV: Modoc virus
MLV: Montana myotis leukoencephalitis virus
MVEV: Murray valley encephalitis virus
OHFV: Omsk hemorrhagic fever virus
POWV: Powassan virus
RBV: Rio bravo virus
RFV: Royal farm virus
SLEV: St. Louis encephalitis virus
SREV: Saumarez reef virus
SSEV: Spanish sheep encephalomyelitis virus
TBEV: Tick-borne encephalitis virus
TSEV: Turkish sheep encephalitis virus
TYUV: Tyulenly virus
WNV: West Nile virus
YFV: Yellow fever virus
YOKV: Yokose virus

FIGURE 12.1 Phylogenetic analysis based on complete polyprotein sequences. Phylogenetic reconstruction was performed using the maximum likelihood method. All branchings were supported by quartet puzzling frequencies at 99% or 100% except at the forks where a value is indicated. The tick-borne flavivirus group is enclosed in a circle with a solid line, the mosquito-borne flavivirus group in a circle with a dashed line, and the no-known vector flavivirus group in a circle with an intermittent dashed line. To improve the legibility of the tree, the distal part of the TBFV branch is presented with a 3.5× magnification. (From Grard, G. et al., *Virology*, 361, 80, 2007. With permission.)

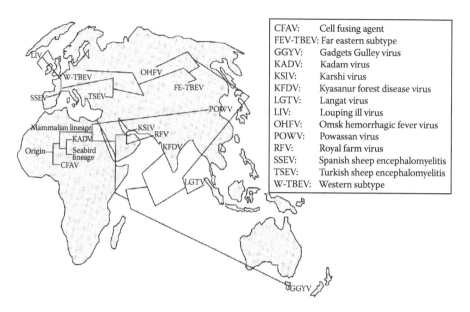

CFAV:	Cell fusing agent
FEV-TBEV:	Far eastern subtype
GGYV:	Gadgets Gulley virus
KADV:	Kadam virus
KSIV:	Karshi virus
KFDV:	Kyasanur forest disease virus
LGTV:	Langat virus
LIV:	Louping ill virus
OHFV:	Omsk hemorrhagic fever virus
POWV:	Powassan virus
RFV:	Royal farm virus
SSEV:	Spanish sheep encephalomyelitis
TSEV:	Turkish sheep encephalomyelitis
W-TBEV:	Western subtype

FIGURE 12.2 Evolution/dispersal of mammalian tick-borne viruses. (From Gritsun, T. S. et al., *Adv. Virus Res.*, 61, 317, 2003. With permission.)

POWV is the only tick-borne flavivirus detected in the Nearctic zoogeographic region including mainly Canada and the United States (Clarke 1964), and is distributed rather widely within this region. Serological evidence of the virus in wild mammals has been detected from the Pacific to the Atlantic coast, in British Columbia, Alberta, Ontario, Nova Scotia, and in southeastern Siberia. Details follow describing hosts in diverse locations.

12.2.1 CANADA

POWV has been isolated from ticks (*Ixodes cookei, Ix. marxi*) (Artsob et al. 1984, 1989; McLean et al. 1964, 1966, 1967; McLean and Larke 1963) and small mammals [woodchucks (*Marmota monax*), red squirrel (*Tamiasciurus hudsonicus*), striped skunk (*Mephitis mephitis*)] in Ontario (McLean et al. 1964; McLean and Larke 1963; Artsob et al. 1986). Serologic evidence from hemagglutination inhibition (HI), complement fixation (CF), and/or neutralization tests (NT) have been obtained from snowshoe hares (*Lepus americanus*) in Nova Scotia, from snowshoe hares and Richardson's ground squirrels (*Urocitellus richardsonii*) in Alberta (Zarnke and Yuill 1981a,b; Hoff Yuill et al. 1970), from chipmunks (*Tamias striatus*), Columbian ground squirrels (*Ur. columbianus*), golden-mantled ground squirrels (*Callospermophilus lateralis*), and marmots (*Marmota* sp.) in British Columbia (McLean et al. 1968, 1970), and from long-tailed ground squirrels (*Ur. undulates*) in the Yukon Territory (McLean et al. 1972). Human cases have been detected in Quebec as well as Ontario (Mahdy et al. 1979, 1982; McLean and Donahue 1959; McLean et al. 1960; Partington et al. 1980; Rossier et al. 1974).

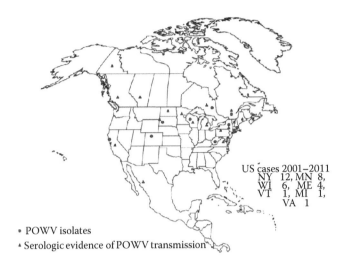

US cases 2001–2011
NY 12, MN 8,
WI 6, ME 4,
VT 1, MI 1,
VA 1

• POWV isolates
▲ Serologic evidence of POWV transmission

FIGURE 12.3 Map of North America indicating locations of viral isolates, serological evidence of virus activity, and human cases from 2001 to 2011.

12.2.2 UNITED STATES

POWV is distributed primarily throughout the northeastern and midwestern states. Virus has been isolated from ticks, humans, and/or small mammals in New York (Centers for Disease Control and Prevention 1972, 1975; Deibel et al. 1979; Embil et al. 1983; Hinten et al. 2008; Tavakoli et al. 2009; Srihongse et al. 1980; Whitney et al. 1968; Whitney 1963, 1965), Connecticut and Massachusetts (Telford et al. 1997; Main et al. 1979), West Virginia (Artsob 1989), Colorado (Thomas et al. 1960), California (Johnson 1987), Minnesota (Minnesota Department of Health 2011), Wisconsin (Brackney et al. 2008, 2010; Ebel et al. 2000), and South Dakota (Keirans and Clifford 1983). Additional serologic evidence has been detected in Maine, Vermont, Pennsylvania, and Michigan (Artsob 1989; Centers for Disease Control and Prevention 2001; Hoang Johnson et al. 2010; Main et al. 1979; Telford et al. 1997; Keirans and Clifford 1983) (Figure 12.3).

12.2.3 MEXICO

Reeves et al. found HI antibodies to POWV in sera collected from humans, rodents, and chickens in Hermosillo, Mexico (Sonora State) (Reeves et al. 1962). Reported seropositivity rates from this study were 4% in humans, 6% in chickens, and 11% in rodents. Confirmatory plaque reduction neutralization tests (PRNTs) were not performed, so the significance of these results may be diminished. HI tests, especially for flavivirus infections, are not specific (Srihongse et al. 1980).

12.2.4 RUSSIA

POWV was first isolated in Russia in 1972 from a pool of *Haemaphysalis longicornis (neumanni)* ticks (L'Vov et al. 1974) and apparently co-circulates with TBEV in Russia in the same locations (Leonova et al. 2009). Since the initial isolation, the virus has been found throughout the Far Eastern Russia region of Primorsky krai. Fourteen cases have been reported through 1987 (Leonova et al. 1987). POWV isolates have been reported from humans, ticks, small mammals, and mosquitoes (L'Vov et al. 1974; Leonova et al. 1987, 1991; Tkachenko et al. 1976; Kislenko et al. 1982). The identification of POWV-positive mosquitoes is interesting, but of questionable significance without accompanying vector competence experiments.

12.3 BIOLOGICAL PROPERTIES (VIRUS STRUCTURE, GENOME ORGANIZATION, PROTEIN FUNCTIONS, REPLICATION CYCLE)

Structurally, the POWV virion is similar to other members of the Flavivirus genus (Mandl 2005). The virion is enveloped, with polyhedral nucleocapsid symmetry. Virus particles are spherical, ~50 nm in diameter with a single envelope protein (E) and a membrane protein (M) on the surface surrounding a lipid bilayer derived from the host cell. The nucleocapsid core consists of single-stranded RNA complexed with multiple copies of the capsid protein. The ~11-kb nucleotide viral genome comprises 3415 amino acids in a single open reading frame encoding three structural proteins, capsid, prM/M, and E, and seven nonstructural proteins, NS1, 2a, 2b, 3, 4,

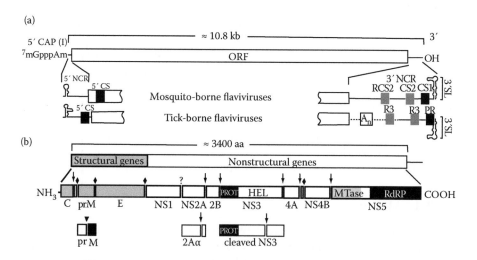

FIGURE 12.4 *Flavivirus* genome structure and expression. (a) Genome structure and RNA elements. NCR, noncoding region. Models of functionally important secondary and tertiary structures within the 5′ and 3′ NCR and the coding region are shown with predicted hairpin loops indicated. (b) Polyprotein processing and cleavage products. Structural proteins are C, prM, E, while nonstructural (NS) proteins are NS1, NS2A and 2B, NS3, NS4A and 4B, NS5. Cleavage sites for host signalase (♦), the viral serine protease (↓), furin or related protease (▼), or unknown proteases (?) are indicated. (From Lindenbach, B. D. et al., Flaviviridae: the viruses and their replication, in *Fields Virology*, eds. D. M. Knipe and P. M. Howley, Lippincott-Raven Publishers, Philadelphia, 2007, 1101. With permission.)

4a, 5. Untranslated regions of 100 and ~500 nt, respectively, are found at the 5′ and 3′ ends, respectively. A type I cap m7 GpppAmpN2 exists at the 5′ end. While the flavivirus genome generally lacks a 3′ polyadenylated tail (Westaway et al. 1985; Lindenbach et al. 2007), tick-borne viruses are an exception, as a poly-A structure is found in some strains. Cleavage of the polyprotein into individual proteins occurs co- and post-translationally through cellular and viral proteases. The differences in genome structure and expression between tick-borne and mosquito-borne flaviviruses are illustrated in Figure 12.4 (Lindenbach et al. 2007). The majority of differences are found in the 5′ and 3′ noncoding regions. The replication cycle of flaviviruses and TBEV specifically have been well described (Mandl 2005) and will not be discussed further here.

12.4 CLINICAL PRESENTATION

POWV is transmitted to humans by tick bite. DTV has been demonstrated to be transmitted to mice within 15 min of attachment by infected nymphal stage ticks (Ebel and Kramer 2004), although it is possible that transmission to humans may take longer. The first reported case of POW encephalitis occurred in Ontario, Canada, in 1958 (McLean and Donahue 1959). From 1958 to 1998, 27 cases of POWV disease were reported in North America, and from 1999 to 2005, an additional nine cases were reported in the United States (Hinten et al. 2008) and one in Canada (Ford-Jones et al. 2002). The first case of POW encephalitis was reported in Russia in 1973 and 14 additional cases were reported between 1974 and 1989 (Leonova et al. 1991). In 2007 alone, six cases were reported in New York State (Centers for Disease Control and Prevention 2009; Tavakoli et al. 2009), and from 2008 to June 2011, eight cases were reported in Minnesota; two of the cases were reported in 2011 with one fatality (Minnesota Department of Health 2011) (Table 12.1 and Figure 12.3), five cases reported in New York, four cases in Wisconsin (2010), and one case in Virginia (2009) (U.S. Geological Survey 2011). The number of POW cases reported to the CDC strongly suggests an increase in incidence of disease in recent years (Hinten et al. 2008; Ebel 2010). The clinical symptoms of some of the more recent reported cases in North America are listed in Table 12.1.

The incubation period of POWV ranges from 8 to 34 days (Smith et al. 1974; Rossier et al. 1974). The clinical syndromes most often associated with the infection are encephalitis, meningoencephalitis, and aseptic meningitis. A review of the earliest reported cases of POW encephalitis indicated that the disease is characterized by a sudden onset of fever with a temperature of up to 40°C and convulsions (Smith et al. 1974; Rossier et al. 1974). A prodrome of nonspecific syndromes lasting 1–3 days may include sore throat, drowsiness, generalized malaise, nausea, headache, myalgia, and disorientation (Smith et al. 1974). Patients showed signs of encephalitis with vomiting, respiratory distress, prolonged fever, stupor, and possible convulsions. Encephalopathy is common and in these cases includes such symptoms as generalized weakness, ataxia, tremor, and ocular symptoms (Table 12.1) (Hinten et al. 2008). In some cases, a fine macular erythematous rash has been reported (Wilson et al. 1979; Partington et al. 1980; Tavakoli et al. 2009; Rossier et al. 1974; Embil et al. 1983; Smith et al. 1974; Kolski et al. 1998). Muscle weakness or rigidity and some degree of paralysis have been observed in some patients (Table 12.1) (Hinten et al.

TABLE 12.1

Patient Symptoms and Outcomes in a Number of the Most Recent Reported Cases of POW Encephalitis

Age	Sex	State	Symptoms	Outcome	Reference
Child, age N/R	N/R	Ontario, Canada	Fever, generalized seizures, altered level of consciousness	Discharged with normal outcome	(Kolski et al. 1998)
64	M	Ontario, Canada	Drowsiness, mild right facial weakness, clumsy movement, right side weakness, decreased consciousness, respiratory distress	Died of massive pulmonary embolism	(Gholam et al. 1999)
70	M	ME	Muscle weakness, somnolence, anorexia, fever, leukocytosis, anemia, left sided hemiplegia, confusion	Discharged to rehabilitation facility	(Centers for Disease Control and Prevention 2001)
25	M	ME	Fever, headache, vomiting, somnolence, confusion, inability to walk, bilateral hand twitching, bilateral weakness in upper extremities, lip smacking	Discharged to rehabilitation facility	(Centers for Disease Control and Prevention 2001)
66	M	VT	Somnolence, severe headache, confusion, bilateral leg weakness, slow speech, short term memory loss	Discharged home with cognitive difficulties	(Centers for Disease Control and Prevention 2001)
53	F	ME	Loss of balance, vomiting, diarrhea, fever, ataxia, diplopia, bilateral lateral gaze palsy, dysarthria, agitation, muscle weakness, altered mental status, ophthalmoplegia	Persistent ophthalmoplegia	(Lessell and Collins 2003)
74	F	ME	Headache, fever, myalgia, confusion, inability to speak or walk, combative, tremulous	Outpatient rehabilitation	(Hinten et al. 2008)
69	M	WI	Abdominal pain, vomiting, fever, chills, lethargy, denied neurologic symptoms	No apparent neurologic symptoms	(Hinten et al. 2008)

(continued)

TABLE 12.1 (Continued)
Patient Symptoms and Outcomes in a Number of the Most Recent Reported Cases of POW Encephalitis

Age	Sex	State	Symptoms	Outcome	Reference
60	F	MI	Proximal muscle weakness in 4 extremities, diplopia, fever, paralysis, respiratory failure	Discharged to rehabilitation facility	(Hinten et al. 2008)
83	M	NY	Fever, headache, altered mental status, stiff neck, generalized muscle weakness	Discharged to nursing home	(Hinten et al. 2008)
91	F	NY	Fever, headache, altered mental status, stiff neck, generalized muscle pain and weakness	Discharged to nursing home	(Hinten et al. 2008)
62	M	NY	Fatigue, fever, bilateral maculopapular palmar rash, diplopia, dysarthria, weakness in right arm and leg	Fatal encephalitis	(Tavakoli et al. 2009)
Child age N/R	N/R	MN	Severe neurological symptoms	Required ongoing care	(ProMED Mail 2009)
Adult age N/R	N/R	MN	Severe neurological symptoms	Required ongoing care	(ProMED Mail 2009)
60s	M	MN	N/R	Recovering	(ProMED Mail 2011)
60s	F	MN	N/R	Fatal	(ProMED Mail 2011)

Note: N/R, not reported.

2008; Gholam et al. 1999; Tavakoli et al. 2009; Lessell and Collins 2003; Goldfield et al. 1973; Rossier et al. 1974; Jackson 1989; Partington et al. 1980). In one case, temporal lobe involvement including olfactory hallucinations and the localization of electroencephalogram (EEG) irregularity initially complicated the diagnosis as such clinical evidence is typical of herpes simplex encephalitis (Embil et al. 1983). Although definite focal features have been observed in some cases, specific temporal lobe involvement has not been reported as a common feature of POW encephalitis which is likely generalized throughout the brain (Embil et al. 1983). In the most severe cases patients become comatose and a fatality rate of approximately 10% has been reported (Artsob 1989; Ebel 2010).

The symptoms reported for POWV infections in Russia between 1974 and 1989 included fever, headache, nausea, vomiting, fatigue, drowsiness, neurological and meningeal symptoms, paralysis, seizures, cerebellar ataxia, and spastic hemiparesis

(Leonova et al. 1991). Only one fatality was reported, which may be attributed to a dual infection with TBEV (Leonova et al. 1991). In Russia, POWV co-circulates with TBEV, and therefore the incidence of encephalitis cases caused by POWV may be masked by those caused by TBEV. In addition, coinfections with both viruses have been shown to occur (Leonova et al. 1991). It should be noted that the Russian strains of POWV isolated between 1972 and 2006 are genetically highly homologous to strains belonging to lineage I POWV (Leonova et al. 2009). Dual infections with other tick-borne pathogens have also been noted in the United States, e.g., *Anaplasma phaghocytophilum* (Hoang Johnson et al. 2010).

Symptoms of POWV infection can be difficult to differentiate from those caused by other arboviruses. Furthermore, asymptomatic infections occur as evidenced by seroprevalence of up to 3% of the population in certain northern Ontario communities (McLean et al. 1962).

12.5 DIAGNOSIS

POWV is endemic in North America, and although the disease is rare, it should be part of the differential diagnosis when arboviral encephalitis is suspected. This is especially important in areas where tick activity has been reported. Obtaining an in-depth patient history is a first step toward performing a diagnosis. Information regarding travel history, contact with animals, vaccinations, and possible tick bites will help in determining the type of diagnostic tests that should be performed. In many cases patients do not recall being bitten by a tick. This is because ticks, in particular nymphal ticks, are small (1.5 mm in diameter) and are therefore difficult to see.

Some of the tests that are performed on an encephalitic patient include magnetic resonance imaging (MRI), computed tomography (CT) scan, and EEG. Results of MRI, in general, show changes consistent with microvascular ischemia or demyelinating disease in the parietal lobe in one case, temporal lobe in a second (Centers for Disease Control and Prevention 2001), and superior cerebellum in a third case (Tavakoli et al. 2009). CT scans are not as sensitive and therefore have not been as informative as MRI scans in detecting neurologic abnormalities (Partington et al. 1980; Lessell and Collins 2003). EEG reveals generalized slowing and diffuse encephalitis (Centers for Disease Control and Prevention 2001; Hinten et al. 2008). Blood and CSF also should be collected. CSF glucose is generally normal as expected for a viral infection. CSF protein is normal or mildly elevated (Hinten et al. 2008; Lessell and Collins 2003; Embil et al. 1983; Jackson 1989). The initial CSF cell count may be normal or will show a lymphocytic pleocytosis cell predominance which on repeat examination in most cases will reveal lymphocytic pleocytosis of less than 500/mm³ (Hinten et al. 2008; Lessell and Collins 2003; Embil et al. 1983; Wilson et al. 1979; Jackson 1989). During the early phase of the infection, viral RNA can be detected in CSF using molecular methods, more commonly, reverse transcription polymerase chain reaction (RT-PCR). In the course of the viremic phase, there is a window of opportunity during which the virus is present in the central nervous system, and in this period, it is possible to detect the viral nucleic acid by RT-PCR. A reasonable strategy would be to perform a flavivirus group-specific PCR to narrow the range of possible etiologic agents (Whitby et al. 1993; Fulop et al.

1993; Kuno 1998; Scaramozzino et al. 2001; Maher-Sturgess et al. 2008), and if that is reactive, then virus-specific PCR primers can be used in the second stage for virus identification (Scaramozzino et al. 2001; Tavakoli et al. 2009; Lanciotti 2003). In addition, PCR products can be sequenced. A modification of this method is to use group-specific PCR followed by restriction enzyme analysis (Gaunt and Gould 2005). An advantage of using group-specific PCR is that lower specimen volume is used and costs associated with PCR reactions are lower. Using this methodology, the group-specific PCR primers should be designed for sensitive detection of all viruses within the group and the virus-specific PCR primers should be designed for specific virus identification. Flavivirus group-specific PCR primers have in general targeted the NS5 gene or the 3' noncoding region as these regions possess a high degree of sequence conservation (Fulop et al. 1993; Kuno 1998; Scaramozzino et al. 2001; Lanciotti 2003; Maher-Sturgess et al. 2008).

An RT-PCR electrospray ionization mass spectrometry (RT-PCR/ESI-MS) method based on analysis of base composition of PCR amplicons has been reported (Grant-Klein et al. 2010). This assay couples an 8 primer broad-range flavivirus assay using RT-PCR to ESI-MS to detect pan-flavivirus, pan-dengue virus and WNV gene targets (Grant-Klein et al. 2010). The method is a high-throughput assay that can detect mosquito and tick-borne flaviviruses, including POWV, for diagnostic and epidemiologic surveillance. A mass-spectrometer, specialized software, and trained staff are required to perform this procedure.

RT-PCR is no longer useful once the immune system has cleared the virus. At this stage, serology is a more effective method for diagnosis. The principle diagnostic method is the detection of POWV-specific IgM and neutralizing antibodies in CSF or serum. IgM antibody capture enzyme-linked immunosorbent assay (MAC-ELISA) and indirect IgG ELISA are performed to detect encephalitis caused by flaviviruses including WNV (Johnson et al. 2000; Martin et al. 2000). Positive ELISA results are in general confirmed by PRNT in biosafety level three containment facilities (Lindsey et al. 1976; Beaty et al. 1995). Confirmation is required because the possibility of cross-reaction with other flaviviruses is fairly high. Indirect fluorescent antibody tests may also be used for detection of flaviviruses. However, IFA tests are less sensitive than ELISA and they are not suitable for high throughput testing (Gubler et al. 2000). In general, serologic confirmation consists of the following: (1) a fourfold or greater change in POWV-specific neutralizing antibody in the same specimen or later specimen or (2) detection of POWV-specific IgM in CSF or (3) detection of POWV-specific IgM in a serum specimen and POWV-specific neutralizing antibody in the same specimen or later specimen.

In recent years, fluorescent microsphere immunoassays (MIA) have been developed that measure antibodies induced by flavivirus infections (Wong et al. 2003; Johnson et al. 2005). Multiplex MIAs can simultaneously measure antibodies to several antigens at the same time and can therefore save time, reagents, and patient sample. An MIA is based on the conjugation of an antigen to a fluorescent microsphere. When patient serum is added to the suspension of microspheres, any antibody present in the serum that recognizes the antigen will bind. Washing will remove any nonspecifically bound molecules. The addition of a secondary reporter anti-human immunoglobulin antibody will allow the detection of the specific antibody-antigen complex. Measurement of the fluorescence extrinsic to the beads and fluorescence of the fluorophore conjugated to the secondary antibody will enable the identification of the antibody present in the patient sample. The measuring instrument is a simplified flow cytometer with lasers that identify and measure the fluorescence associated with the reaction. Since flavivirus proteins have a high degree of amino acid sequence similarity, significant cross-reaction is observed in many ELISA tests. For example, an MIA assay that was developed to detect antibodies to the E-protein of WNV also detects antibodies to E-proteins of related flaviviruses including St. Louis encephalitis, Japanese encephalitis, and dengue viruses (Wong et al. 2004). However, specificity can be added to the assay by multiplexing with additional antigens. For example, adding recombinant NS5 antigens can allow antibodies from WNV to be distinguished from SLE or dengue infection, and JE or yellow fever vaccination (Wong et al. 2003). An MIA assay to detect total antibodies (IgG, IgA, and IgM) to recombinant WNV E protein, recombinant NS5 and recombinant DTV E protein has been successfully used to detect cases of POWV in the state of New York (Hinten et al. 2008; Wong et al. 2003, 2004).

The results of antibody tests could well be negative during the early phase of infection as antibody production begins to increase to a detectable level. Therefore, serological tests should be repeated after 1–2 weeks. Serological tests are not genotype specific and therefore it is not possible to determine whether an infection is caused by POWV (lineage I) or DTV (lineage II). Furthermore, as previously discussed, flavivirus cross-reactivity can confound a diagnosis unless additional specificity is added to the testing strategy.

Historically, mouse inoculations have been used for isolation of arboviruses including POWV. When the first case of POW encephalitis was being investigated in 1958, portions of the brain were inoculated into newborn mice; those inoculated with suspensions of basal ganglia and cortex developed signs of acute encephalitis 5 days after inoculation (McLean and Donahue 1959). The second, third, and fourth suckling mouse brain passage also induced encephalitis (McLean and Donahue 1959). Subsequent to inoculation, virus can be typed using neutralization tests. Intracranial inoculation of suckling mice is a sensitive method of virus isolation, but its use has become uncommon, as most diagnostic laboratories no longer use mice for diagnostic purposes.

An alternative method that is no longer routinely used for diagnosis of POWV is cell culture. This method, however, remains in use in a limited number of specialized laboratories for diagnostic and research purposes. POWV produces cytopathic effects and/or plaques in several vertebrate cell lines including pig kidney embryo cells (PEK) (Leonova et al. 2009), rhesus monkey kidney cells (LLC-MK2) (Abdelwahab et al. 1964; Stim 1969), baby hamster kidney cells (BHK) (Karabatsos and Buckley 1967; Brackney et al. 2008), and African green monkey kidney cells (VERO) (Stim 1969), among others. POWV has been isolated from patient brain tissue (McLean and Donahue 1959; Centers for Disease Control and Prevention 1975; Deibel et al. 1979) and blood (Leonova et al. 2009).

The only laboratories that currently provide diagnostic testing for POWV are State Health laboratories and the CDC. Commercial laboratories do not at present offer serologic testing.

12.6 PATHOLOGY AND PATHOGENESIS

The first reported case of POW encephalitis occurred in 1958 and was fatal (McLean and Donahue 1959). An autopsy was performed and macroscopically the brain and meninges appeared normal. However, histological preparation and staining of various areas of the central nervous system including the cortex, basal ganglia, pons, and medulla showed an inflammatory process with characteristic perivascular infiltration and focal parenchymatous infiltration (McLean and Donahue 1959). The amount of perivascular infiltration varied and in general the inflammatory cells were composed of lymphocytes and monocytes and were confined to the perivascular space. The focal infiltrations were situated in the parenchyma, separated from the blood vessels and were varied in size. The main cells in these foci were macrophages or microglia and occasionally polymorphonuclear cells. In addition, a limited number of degenerating nerve cells with satellite inflammatory cells were also observed (McLean and Donahue 1959).

Neuropathological examination of a patient who died of a massive pulmonary embolism following POW encephalitis in 1997 revealed mild diffuse swelling of the cerebral hemispheres with diffuse meningeal congestion (Gholam et al. 1999). Histologic examination of the meninges and Virchow-Robin spaces showed severe chronic inflammatory infiltration in these areas and focal areas of infiltration into the brain parenchyma. Tissue necrosis was observed in the most involved areas: mediotemporal lobes, ventral midbrain, and basal ganglia (Gholam et al. 1999). Diffuse reactive astrocytic gliosis and microglial activation were observed throughout the gray matter. Occasionally brain stem neurons with an intranuclear eosinophilic inclusion consistent with a viral inclusion were also observed (Gholam et al. 1999). It should be noted that when the virus from this case was subsequently isolated and typed it was found to belong to the POWV lineage II/DTV (Kuno et al. 2001).

Histological findings at autopsy have also been reported for a third case of POW encephalitis (specifically, lineage II/DTV genotype) in which the patient presented with meningoencephalitis and succumbed to the infection (Figure 12.5) (Tavakoli et al. 2009). In this case multinodular mononuclear infiltrates and areas of necrosis were observed throughout the brain (Figure 12.5a and b). The predominant cells in the parenchyma were CD8$^+$ cytotoxic T cells (Figure 12.5c), while those in the leptomeninges and perivascular spaces were CD4$^+$ helper T cells. Extensive neuronal loss was observed in the substantia nigra (Figure 12.5d) and gray matter regions and to a lesser extent white matter tracts showed microglia-macrophage infiltration (Figure 12.5e). Virus antigen was detected by immunohistochemical staining in neuronal cell bodies, dendrites, and axons as well as within the few surviving Purkinje cells (Tavakoli et al. 2009). Perivascular and parenchymal infiltration of T cells, neuronal loss, and focal necrosis appear to be characteristics of POW encephalitis and may account for the significant neurological impairment observed in a substantial number of patients.

In animal models (monkey, rabbit, horse), POWV infection results in widespread encephalitis which is characterized by lymphoid perivascular cuffing, a lymphocytic meningitis, and choroiditis (Gritsun et al. 2003; Little et al. 1985). In experimentally infected horses, neuronophagia and zones of parenchymal necrosis were observed throughout the white and gray matter with the most severe lesions in the medulla and mesencephalon (Little et al. 1985). It has been postulated that the intense

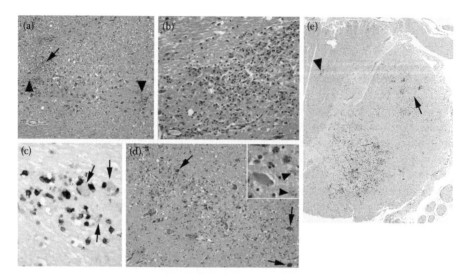

FIGURE 12.5   Histological findings of fatal case of POW encephalitis attributed to Lineage II, DTV. (a) Microglial nodules and lymphocytic infiltrates in the pons are visible in basal pontine nuclei (arrowheads). There is less involvement of descending fiber tracts (arrow) and pontocerebellar fibers. (b) In pontine basal nuclei, confluent foci of parenchymal necrosis is evident. (c) Upon CD8+ immunostaining of the basal pontis, a cytotoxic T-cell infiltrate with close association with surviving neurons (arrows) is observed. (d) Significant neuronal loss is apparent in the substantia nigra such that surviving neurons are rare (arrows). (inset) An eosinophilic dying neuron and remaining neuromelanin pigment are seen encased in macrophages or free in the parenchyma (arrowheads). (e) Phosphoglucomutase immunostaining of lumbar spinal cord shows prominent infiltration by microglia-macrophages and in the anterior horn and focal microglial nodules in the lateral corticospinal tract (arrow) and posterior column (arrowhead). Paraffin sections in panels a, b, and d were stained with hematoxylin and eosin. (From Tavakoli, N. P. et al., *N. Engl. J. Med.*, 360, 2099, 2009. With permission.)

inflammatory response and destruction of nervous tissue elements relates to antibody and sensitized lymphocyte interaction with POWV in the brain (Little et al. 1985).

A number of studies examining the pathogenesis of POWV in diverse animals have been published. Suckling mice demonstrate impaired movement and died by 5 days following intracranial (i.c.) inoculation of DTV (Telford et al. 1997). The LD_{50} for an adult CD mouse following subcutaneous injection of a 20% brain suspension was approximately $10^{4.8}$/mL, and death occurred within 14 days. In contrast, colonized adult *P. leucopus*, a natural host, survived similar infection without demonstrating any morbidity or mortality (Telford et al. 1997). A significantly lower concentration of POWV (10^4 adult mouse LD_{50}) was measured in SM brain following infection compared with Central European TBEV (10^8 adult mouse LD_{50}) (Telford et al. 1997). Ninety percent of larval ticks acquired POWV from mice that had been intraperitoneally inoculated with 10^5 PFU. Engorged larvae contained approximately 10 PFU. Transstadial transmission resulted in approximately 20% of nymphs infected following feeding as larvae on viremic mice. Titer increased approximately 100-fold during molting. Nymphal deer ticks efficiently transmitted POWV to naive mice after as few as 15 minutes of attachment (Ebel and Kramer 2004). Inflammatory degenerative changes were observed in the nerve tissue of white mice following intraperitoneal inoculation of $10^{7.5}$ LD_{50}/ml Russian strain of POWV. The mice developed convulsions by day 4–5 and often died suddenly. Virus was seen by EM in neurons, dendrites, glial cells, and intracellular spaces (Isachkova et al. 1979). Multilayered proliferation of membranes were observed in the cytoplasm of brain cells, similar to what has been observed with other neurotropic flaviviruses (Whitney et al. 1972; Isachkova et al. 1979). Intraperitoneal injection of Vero cell-derived DTV or POW virus into females, 5–6 weeks old, NIH Swiss mice yielded comparable LD_{50} values of $10^{2.7}$ and $10^{2.3}$ PFU, respectively. However, onset of illness was slightly delayed in DTV-infected mice (day 9 or 10 postinfection compared with day 7 or 8 in POWV-infected mice) (Telford et al. 1997). These results indicate virus strains from the two POWV lineages are equally pathogenic in mice.

When *Macaca rhesus* primates were infected by the i.c. route with Canadian and Russian strains of POWV, similar patterns of excitation and loss of movement were observed as with mice. The monkeys remained viremic from 3–21 days postinfection (pi) with a maximum titer of 10^5–10^6 LD_{50} 3–9 dpi. There were no differences in pathogenesis between the two viruses (Frolova et al. 1985). POWV replicates to lower levels in wild rodents in Russia when compared with TBEV (Leonova et al. 1987), suggesting decreased virulence. Yet in Far Eastern Russia, there appear to be more cases with mild symptoms compared with North America; this could be a consequence of strain differences or reflect differing ecological conditions (Gritsun et al. 2003).

Gray squirrels (*Sciurus carolinensis*) inoculated subcutaneously (sc) with 10^4 whole mouse (WM)icLD_{50} POWV demonstrated prolonged but low level viremia, suggesting this species may be a natural reservoir of the virus (Timoney 1971). POWV produced inapparent infection in chicks inoculated sc with 1–100 WMicLD50, and viremia peaked d 3–4 (McLean et al. 1960). The infection threshold for adult female *Dermacentor andersoni* feeding on viremic rabbits was approximately $10^{2.5}$/ml WMicLD_{50} (Chernesky 1969). Following feeding by experimentally infected *D. andersoni*, hamsters were found to circulate ~10^4 WMicLD_{50} POWV (Chernesky 1969), well above the threshold of infection.

There is a low public health risk of POWV transmission through raw goat's milk (Woodall and Roz 1977). Following intramuscular inoculation of 10^3 suckling mouse (SM)icLD_{50} virus, goats produced undetectable viremia, similar to TBEV which produces a low level viremia, but approximately 10^5 SMicLD_{50}/ml virus was detected in the milk 7–15 dpi. This was sufficient to infect kids, although no morbidity was observed. In contrast, transmission through unpasteurized milk appears to be unlikely in cows (Drozdov 1959).

12.7 ECOLOGY AND EPIDEMIOLOGY

Recent studies have focused on the virologic properties of POWV (Brackney et al. 2009; Brackney et al. 2010; Davis et al. 2005; Ebel et al. 2001; Pesko et al. 2010; Leonova et al. 2009; Kuno et al. 2001). The ecologic and epidemiologic-based investigations have been lacking since the POWV chapter published in *The Arboviruses*

(Artsob 1989) except for the reporting of human clinical cases (Hicar et al. 2011; Minnesota Department of Health 2011; Tavakoli et al. 2009; Centers for Disease Control and Prevention 2009; Hinten et al. 2008; Ford-Jones et al. 2002; Centers for Disease Control and Prevention 2001) and the identification and characterization of Lineage II, DTV (Telford et al. 1997; Ebel et al. 1999, 2000; Brackney et al. 2008). Intensive field studies are required to determine if the apparent increase in human cases is due to the emergence of DTV in the black-legged tick (*Ixodes scapularis*) population (majority of recent POWV cases are in areas with high *Ix. scapularis* populations), or the result of improved diagnostic capabilities. It is unclear if prototype POWV is still extant within the United States or if it has been displaced by DTV.

12.7.1 Transmission Cycle

Protoype POWV and DTV lineage strains are maintained in nature in a transmission cycle involving ixodid ticks and small mammals. A systemic viremia within the vertebrate host may not be necessary for efficient transmission. Co-feeding or non-viremic transmission, proposed and demonstrated in the laboratory with TBEV by Labuda et al. (1993), may be sufficient to maintain POWV in nature. This has been modeled for POWV for long-term maintenance in natural foci (Nonaka et al. 2010). Another mode of virus transmission, transovarial transmission (female to larvae via the egg), has been documented in the laboratory with *Ix. ricinus*, *Dermacentor reticulatus*, *H. longicornis* (*neumanni*), and other ticks and various strains of TBEV (Naumov et al. 1980; Danielova et al. 2002).

The ecological difference between POWV lineages appears to be the result of the invertebrate host responsible for transmission. Furthermore, as evidenced by mosquito isolates in Russia, transmission may involve nontraditional vectors (Tkachenko et al. 1976; Kislenko et al. 1982), although more studies are needed to ascertain the validity and/or importance of this alternative cycle.

12.7.2 Arthropod Hosts

12.7.2.1 *Ixodes cookei*

Ixodes cookei (woodchuck tick) has been incriminated as the principal vector of prototype POWV, especially in the northeast United States and eastern Canada (Artsob et al. 1986; McLean et al. 1960, 1962, 1964a,b, 1966, 1967; Whitney and Jamnback 1965). This tick is distributed from South Dakota to Texas northeasterly through the United States and eastern Canada. At least 22 virus isolates have been acquired from *Ix. cookei* ticks and a number of other isolates from the vertebrate hosts that these ticks feed upon (Artsob 1989; Karabatsos 1985; Ebel 2010). Somewhat surprising is the fact that experimental studies to assess vector competence of this species have not been conducted or have not been published, possibly a consequence of the difficulty of collecting sufficient numbers of individuals to conduct such studies.

Ix. cookei behaviorally resemble the nidicolus argasids (soft ticks) rather than other ixodids. This species is restricted to the burrows of its preferred hosts, woodchucks and other rodents, mustelids, raccoons, foxes, coyotes, etc. (Farkas and

Surgeoner 1990; Main et al. 1979; Ko 1972; Kollars and Oliver 2003) and may complete its life cycle on a single host or family group. Ticks are not routinely collected by the flagging method suggesting that dispersal of ticks is via movement of the host from burrow to burrow during male-female encounters in early spring and young of the year dispersals in late summer (Ko 1972).

Human encounters with *Ix. cookei* are infrequent as compared with other tick species (Cohen et al. 2010; Anderson and Magnarelli 1980; Campbell and Bowles 1994; Hall et al. 1991; NYS, unpublished data) possibly explaining the relatively low number of human cases of POW encephalitis, especially where *Ix. scapularis* abundance is low or nonexistent.

12.7.2.2   *Ixodes scapularis*

With the exception of a few historical isolates (fox brain from WV and *D. andersoni* ticks in CO), DTV has been isolated primarily from the Lyme disease vector, *Ix. scapularis* (black-legged tick or deer tick). *Ix. scapularis* is a three host tick. Each stage—larva, nymph, and adult female—will take a bloodmeal from a separate host (Barbour and Fish 1993). Larvae predominantly feed on white-footed mice (*Peromyscus leucopus*), although they have been recorded feeding on numerous other species (Keirans et al. 1996). Nymphs are more indiscriminate feeders, acquiring their bloodmeal from a wider host range including small mammals, birds, reptiles, and humans (Keirans et al. 1996; Smith et al. 1996; Cohen et al. 2010; Apperson et al. 1990, 1993; Levine et al. 1997). Adult females feed on larger mammals, particularly deer and livestock (Keirans et al. 1996; Smith et al. 1996; Cohen et al. 2010). The majority of tick-derived DTV isolates have been from the adult stage of *Ix. scapularis* (Brackney et al. 2008, 2010; Telford et al. 1997; Ebel et al. 1999, 2000; unpublished data from NYS).

In the laboratory, *Ix. scapularis* has been shown to be a competent vector of POWV. Costero and Grayson reported infection rates of 10%, 40%, and 57% for larvae, nymphs, and females, respectively, after feeding on viremic hosts (Costero and Grayson 1996). Transstadial (larva to nymph, nymph to adult) and transovarial transmission were also reported in this study. Another study demonstrated the transmission of Lineage II/DTV, by infected nymphal *Ix. scapularis* in as little as 15 minutes after feeding on naive *P. leucopus* (Ebel and Kramer 2004), suggesting that unlike other tick-borne diseases, such as Lyme, ehrlichiosis, and babesiosis, there is no grace period for removal of an attached tick to prevent POWV infection. The authors of this study also reported transstadial transmission.

Due to the indiscriminate feeding behavior and experimentally derived vector competence of *Ix. scapularis*, it is hypothesized that this species may have provided the bridge for POWV to escape from the focal, enzootic cycle, thus becoming a potential (re)emerging pathogen.

12.7.2.3   *Dermacentor andersoni*

As stated earlier, the first recorded POWV isolate, although unidentified until after POWV and described in the literature by McLean and Donahue (1959), was isolated from a pool of *D. andersoni* (Rocky Mountain wood tick) collected along North Cache la Poudre River, Colorado in 1952 (Thomas et al. 1960). *D. andersoni* larvae and nymphs primarily feed upon small mammals, including mice, chipmunks, and ground squirrels. Adults will feed on larger mammals including wild and domestic ungulates, rabbits, and porcupines (Scott and Brown 2011; Wilkinson 1984; Burgdorfer 1969; Burgdorfer 1975). *D. andersoni* is the principal vector of Colorado tick fever virus (Emmons 1988). POWV development in this species of tick following feeding on infected rabbits indicated virus multiplication in various tick organs leading to peroral transmission through salivary secretion of infected nymphs and adults, and transstadial transfer of virus, but no transovarial transmission (Chernesky 1969; Artsob 1989).

12.7.2.4   Other Species

POWV has been isolated from at least two other tick species in North America, *Ix. marxi* (McLean and Larke 1963) and *Ix. spinipalpis* (Keirans and Clifford 1983). *Ix. marxi* could be an important enzootic vector of POWV transmission particularly in arboreal squirrels of Canada as hypothesized by Main (Main 1977) based on virus isolation and serologic results from field investigations by McLean et al. (1963, 1964a,b, 1966, 1967). *Ix. spinipalpis* ticks are distributed from the Rocky Mountains westward with populations extending into the Badlands region of the Dakotas (Gregson 1956; Dolan et al. 1997). It is primarily nidicoulous and feeds on *Neotoma* rodent species (Dolan et al. 1997). Maupin et al. (1994) did not collect *Ix. spinipalpis* with standard dragging procedures, and therefore this species is likely an enzootic vector of POWV with little chance of infecting humans.

There is compelling evidence that the expansion of POWV into an *Ix. scapularis* driven cycle is responsible for the apparent increase in human cases. 1. Numerous POWV virus isolates (Lineage II DTV) have been obtained from *Ix. scapularis*, 2. DTV has been isolated from at least 2 recent fatal human infections, 3. *Ix. scapularis* ticks are competent vectors of POWV, 4. *Ix. scapularis* ticks are able to transmit virus in as little as 15 minutes, 5. Experiments have determined transstadial and transovarial transmission of POWV in *Ix. scapularis*, and 6. The majority of human cases occur during peak larval and nymphal *Ix. scapularis* activity and in areas where *Ix. scapularis* populations are abundant.

12.7.3   Disease Incidence

Since 1999, the majority (80%) of reported human POWV cases had onset dates between April–September. Another 15% had onset dates in October and November (Hinten et al. 2008; U.S. Geological Survey 2011). This is not surprising since most Lyme disease cases also occur during the summer months although vectored solely by *Ix. scapularis*, especially in the northeast and upper midwestern United States (Hinten et al. 2008), and McLean demonstrated POWV activity in the field during these months (McLean et al. 1964a,b, 1966, 1967; McLean and Larke 1963). Of interest, 2 cases in 2009, one each in NY (January) and VA (December), had onset dates in winter months (U.S. Geological Survey 2011). An additional case from Ontario had onset in December 1979 (Mahdy et al. 1982; Partington et al. 1980).

Of the first 19 POW cases reported only 2 were in individuals greater than 55 years old (57 and 82). Sixteen of the cases were in children less than 15 years old and a single case was in a 19 year old (Artsob 1989). Between 1999 and 2005, Hinten et al. reported only two POWV cases out of nine in individuals less than 55 years old (25 and 53). The remaining seven individuals were 60, 66, 69, 70, 74, 83, and 91 years old (Hinten et al. 2008). Of cases reported by NYS, in 2007–09, five cases were individuals between the ages of 74 and 84, while three cases were in children younger than 10 years old and another was in a young man aged 24 years (U.S. Geological Survey 2011; NYS, unpublished data). Of the 37 cases for which we have information, 13 were females and 24 were males (Artsob 1989; Hinten et al. 2008; NYS unpublished data).

12.8   PROGNOSIS AND TREATMENT

With a fatality rate of 10%, POW encephalitis is a serious disease (Artsob 1989). Furthermore, even among patients who survive, the long term affects can be severe. In up to 50% of cases, due to significant neurologic sequelae, prolonged inpatient rehabilitation is required subsequent to acute care hospitalization (Table 12.1) (Wilson et al. 1979; Mahdy et al. 1982; Hinten et al. 2008). In many patients, symptoms such as hemiplegia, quadriplegia, ophthalmoplegia, severe headaches, weakness, and memory loss can persist for months (Hinten et al. 2008; Wilson et al. 1979; Goldfield et al. 1973; Lessell and Collins 2003; Partington et al. 1980).

There are no vaccines or specific therapies available for prevention and treatment of POW encephalitis. However, prevention strategies including vector and vertebrate control can help reduce the incidence considerably. Avoidance of tick bites is the best strategy and can include reducing human contact with small and medium-sized mammals (woodchucks, mice, squirrels) in order to reduce the risk of exposure to infected ticks, avoiding bushy areas, wearing light colored clothing that fully covers the arms and legs, and using insect repellant. In addition, people should check themselves and their pets for ticks and if they detect any, they should remove them as soon as possible. Environmental controls such as removing rodent nests will also reduce the risk of contact with ticks.

It is doubtful that a substantial amount of effort and resources will be allocated to vaccine development as the numbers of POW encephalitis cases are too few to justify such an undertaking. However, there is a vaccine against TBEV, which demonstrates broad cross-protection against three subtypes of TBEV strains and a somewhat reduced but still protective neutralization capacity against more distantly related viruses, such as OHFV (Orlinger et al. 2011).

Although there is no specific therapy for the treatment of POW encephalitis, supportive therapy is used to treat some of the symptoms. Mechanical ventilation can be used to protect the airway and reduce the affects of apnea. As seizures are a common symptom of POW encephalitis in children (McLean and Donahue 1959; Rossier et al. 1974; Embil et al. 1983; Smith et al. 1974; Kolski et al. 1998), anticonvulsant therapy can be beneficial. In addition, it is important to control the temperature and nutritional status of the patient. The initiation of early physical and speech therapy to maintain various functions such as joint mobility and speech is key in minimizing the long term affects of the infection (Rossier et al. 1974; Hinten et al. 2008).

Six out of nine cases reported in the United States between 1999 and 2005 had significant neurological sequelae and required prolonged inpatient rehabilitation (Hinten et al. 2008). None of the nine cases were fatal during the acute phase of disease. However, as mentioned previously, death has been reported in a significant number of cases (Table 12.1) (McLean and Donahue 1959; Centers for Disease Control and Prevention 1975; Gholam et al. 1999; Tavakoli et al. 2009). In some cases death was due to acute encephalitis and occurred within days of symptom onset (McLean and Donahue 1959; Centers for Disease Control and Prevention 1975; Tavakoli et al. 2009), while in others it was due to sequelae directly related to disease and occurred many months later (Joshua 1979; Mahd et al. 1982; Artsob and Spence 1981; Artsob 1989).

12.9 CONCLUSION

POWV and DTV are emerging tick-borne pathogens. Neurologic sequelae following infection are common and require medical care. The lack of awareness of this tick-borne disease and the need for specialized laboratory tests to confirm diagnosis suggest the frequency of POW infections may be greater than previously suspected. Increased human surveillance following the introduction of West Nile virus into North America and improved diagnostic methods have demonstrated increased prevalence of POWV activity in the northeastern United States (New York, Massachusetts, Maine, Vermont, Connecticut) and north central United States (Michigan, Minnesota, Wisconsin). The number of human cases has nearly doubled since 1998. The population at risk is increasing as homes are built on the edges of wooded tracts of land that are occupied by tick hosts, bringing humans and potential POWV hosts and vectors in close proximity. As the northeastern range of *I. scapularis* continues to expand northward and westward, so does the likelihood of contact with new populations. Research on the ecology of this virus elucidating vertebrate hosts and environmental factors supporting efficient virus transmission should be conducted.

ACKNOWLEDGEMENT

We thank Betsy Kauffman and Mary Franke for their invaluable help with this chapter.

REFERENCES

Abdelwahab, K. S., Almeida, J. D., Doane, F. W., and McLean, D. M. 1964. Powassan virus: morphology and cytopathology 251. *Can. Med. Assoc. J.* 90, 1068–1072.
Anderson, J. F., and Magnarelli, L. A. 1980. Vertebrate host relationships and distribution of ixodid ticks (Acari: Ixodidae) in Connecticut, USA. *J. Med. Entomol.* 17, 314–323.
Apperson, C. S., Levine, J. F., and Nicholson, W. L. 1990. Geographic occurrence of Ixodes scapularis and Amblyomma americanum (Acari: Ixodidae) infesting white-tailed deer in North Carolina. *J. Wildl. Dis.* 26, 550–553.
Apperson, C. S., Levine, J. F., Evans, T. L., Braswell, A., and Heller, J. 1993. Relative utilization of reptiles and rodents as hosts by immature Ixodes scapularis (Acari: Ixodidae) in the coastal plain of North Carolina, USA. *Exp.Appl.Acarol.* 17, 719–731.

Artsob, H. 1989. Powassan encephalitis. In: T. P. Monath (Ed.), *The Arboviruses*. CRC Press, Boca Raton, pp. 29–49.

Artsob, H., and Spence, L. 1981. Human arboviral infections in Canada, 1980. *Can. Dis. Wkly. Rep.* 7, 194.

Artsob, H., Spence, L., Surgeoner, G., McCreadie, J., Thorsen, J., Th'ng, C., and Lampotang, V. 1984. Isolation of Francisella tularensis and Powassan virus from ticks (Acari: Ixodidae) in Ontario, Canada. *J. Med. Entomol.* 21, 165–168.

Artsob, H., Spence, L., Th'ng, C., Lampotang, V., Johnston, D., MacInnes, C., Matejka, F., Voigt, D., and Watt, I. 1986. Arbovirus infections in several Ontario mammals, 1975–1980. *Can. J. Vet. Res.* 50, 42–46.

Barbour, A. G., and Fish, D. 1993. The biological and social phenomenon of Lyme disease. *Science.* 260, 1610–1616.

Beasley, D. W., Suderman, M. T., Holbrook, M. R., and Barrett, A. D. 2001. Nucleotide sequencing and serological evidence that the recently recognized deer tick virus is a genotype of Powassan virus. *Virus Res.* 79, 81–89.

Beaty, B. J., Calisher, C. H., and Shope, R. E. 1995. Arboviruses. In: E. H. Lennette, E. H. Lennette, and E. T. Lennette (Eds.), *Diagnostic Procedures for Viral, Rickettsial and Chlamydial Infections.* American Public Health Association, Washington, D.C., pp. 189–212.

Brackney, D. E., Beane, J. E., and Ebel, G. D. 2009. RNAi targeting of West Nile virus in mosquito midguts promotes virus diversification. *PLoS Pathog.* 5, e1000502.

Brackney, D. E., Brown, I. K., Nofchissey, R. A., Fitzpatrick, K. A., and Ebel, G. D. 2010. Homogeneity of Powassan virus populations in naturally infected Ixodes scapularis. *Virology.* 402, 366–371.

Brackney, D. E., Nofchissey, R. A., Fitzpatrick, K. A., Brown, I. K., and Ebel, G. D. 2008. Stable prevalence of Powassan virus in Ixodes scapularis in a northern Wisconsin focus. *Am. J. Trop. Med. Hyg.* 79, 971–973.

Burgdorfer, W. 1969. Ecology of tick vectors of American spotted fever. *Bull. World Health Organ.* 40, 375–381.

Burgdorfer, W. 1975. A review of Rocky Mountain spotted fever (tick-borne typhus), its agent, and its tick vectors in the United States. *J. Med. Entomol.* 12, 269–278.

Calisher, C. H., Karabatsos, N., Dalrymple, J. M., Shope, R. E., Porterfield, J. S., Westaway, E. G., and Brandt, W. E. 1989. Antigenic relationships between flaviviruses as determined by cross- neutralization tests with polyclonal antisera. *J. Gen. Virol.* 70(Pt 1), 37–43.

Campbell, B. S., and Bowles, D. E. 1994. Human tick bite records in a United States Air Force population, 1989–1992: implications for tick-bornes disease risk. *J. Wild. Med.* 5, 405–412.

Centers for Disease Control and Prevention. 1972. Powassan encephalitis—New York. *Morb. Mortal. Wkly. Rep.* 21, 206–207.

Centers for Disease Control and Prevention, 1975. Powassan virus isolated from a patient with encephalitis—New York. *Morb. Mortal. Wkly. Rep.* 24, 379.

Centers for Disease Control and Prevention, 2001. Outbreak of Powassan encephalitis—Maine and Vermont, 1999–2001. *Morb. Mortal. Wkly. Rep.* 50, 761–764.

Centers for Disease Control and Prevention. Confirmed and Probable Powassan Neuroinvasive Disease Cases, Human, United States, 2001–2008, By State (as of 4/7/2009). Centers for Disease Control and Prevention. 2009. 7–12–2011.

Chernesky, M. A. 1969. Powassan virus transmission by ixodid ticks infected after feeding on viremic rabbits injected intravenously. *Can. J. Microbiol.* 15, 521–526.

Clarke, D. H. 1964. Further studies on antigenic relationships among the viruses of the group B tick-borne complex. *Bull. World Health Organ.* 31, 45–56.

Cohen, S. B., Freye, J. D., Dunlap, B. G., Dunn, J. R., Jones, T. F., and Moncayo, A. C. 2010. Host associations of Dermacentor, Amblyomma, and Ixodes (Acari: Ixodidae) ticks in Tennessee. *J. Med. Entomol.* 47, 415–420.

Cook, S., and Holmes, E. C. 2006. A multigene analysis of the phylogenetic relationships among the flaviviruses (Family: Flaviviridae) and the evolution of vector transmission. *Arch. Virol.* 151, 309–325.

Costero, A., Grayson, M. A. 1996. Experimental transmission of Powassan virus (Flaviviridae) by Ixodes scapularis ticks (Acari:Ixodidae). *Am. J. Trop. Med. Hyg.* 55, 536–546.

Danielova, V., Holubova, J., Pejcoch, M., and Daniel, M. 2002. Potential significance of trans-ovarial transmission in the circulation of tick-borne encephalitis virus. *Folia Parasitol. (Praha).* 49, 323–325.

Davis, C. T., Ebel, G. D., Lanciotti, R. S., Brault, A. C., Guzman, H., Siirin, M., Lambert, A., Parsons, R. E., Beasley, D. W., Novak, R. J., Elizondo-Quiroga, D., Green, E. N., Young, D. S., Stark, L. M., Drebot, M. A., Artsob, H., Tesh, R. B., Kramer, L. D., and Barrett, A. D. 2005. Phylogenetic analysis of North American West Nile virus isolates, 2001–2004: Evidence for the emergence of a dominant genotype. *Virology.* 342, 252–265.

Deibel, R., Srihongse, S., and Woodall, J. P. 1979. Arboviruses in New York State: an attempt to determine the role of arboviruses in patients with viral encephalitis and meningitis. *Am. J. Trop. Med. Hyg.* 28, 577–582.

Demina, T. V., Dzhioev, Y. P., Verkhozina, M. M., Kozlova, I. V., Tkachev, S. E., Plyusnin, A., Doroshchenko, E. K., Lisak, O. V., and Zlobin, V. I. 2010. Genotyping and characterization of the geographical distribution of tick-borne encephalitis virus variants with a set of molecular probes. *J. Med. Virol.* 82, 965–976.

Dolan, M. C., Maupin, G. O., Panella, N. A., Golde, W. T., and Piesman, J. 1997. Vector competence of Ixodes scapularis, I. spinipalpis, and Dermacentor andersoni (Acari: Ixodidae) in transmitting Borrelia burgdorferi, the etiologic agent of Lyme disease. *J. Med. Entomol.* 34, 128–135.

Drozdov, S. G. 1959. Role of domestic animals in epidemiology of diphasic milk fever (in Russian). *Zh. Mikrobiol. Epidemiol. Immunobiol.* 30, 102–108.

Ebel, G. D. 2010. Update on Powassan virus: emergence of a North American tick-borne flavivirus. *Annu. Rev. Entomol.* 55, 95–110.

Ebel, G. D., and Kramer, L. D. 2004. Short report: duration of tick attachment required for transmission of Powassan virus by deer ticks. *Am. J. Trop. Med. Hyg.* 71, 268–271.

Ebel, G. D., Campbell, E. N., Goethert, H. K., Spielman, A., and Telford, S. R., III, 2000. Enzootic transmission of deer tick virus in New England and Wisconsin sites. *Am. J. Trop. Med. Hyg.* 63, 36–42.

Ebel, G. D., Dupuis, A. P., II, Ngo, K. A., Nicholas, D. C., Kauffman, E. B., Jones, S. A., Young, D. M., Maffei, J. G., Shi, P.-Y., Bernard, K. A., and Kramer, L. D. 2001. Partial genetic characterization of West Nile virus strains, New York State. *Emerg. Infect. Dis.* 7, 650–653.

Ebel, G. D., Foppa, I., Spielman, A., and Telford, S. R. 1999. A focus of deer tick virus transmission in the northcentral United States. *Emerg. Infect. Dis.* 5, 570–574.

Ebel, G. D., Spielman, A., and Telford, S. R., III. 2001. Phylogeny of North American Powassan virus. *J. Gen. Virol.* 82, 1657–1665.

Embil, J. A., Camfield, P., Artsob, H., and Chase, D. P. 1983. Powassan virus encephalitis resembling herpes simplex encephalitis. *Arch. Intern. Med.* 143, 341–343.

Emmons, R. W. 1988. Ecology of Colorado tick fever. *Annu. Rev. Microbiol.* 42, 49–64.

Farkas, M. J., and Surgeoner, G. A. 1990. Incidence of Ixodes cookei (Acari: Ixodidae) on groundhogs, Marmota monax, in Southwestern Ontario. *Proc. Entomol. Soc. Ontario* 121, 105–110.

Ford-Jones, E. L., Fearon, M., Leber, C., Dwight, P., Myszak, M., Cole, B., Greene, P. B., Artes, S., McGeer, A., D'Cunha, C., and Naus, M. 2002. Human surveillance for West Nile virus infection in Ontario in 2000. *Can. Med. Assoc. J.* 166, 29–35.

Frolova, M. P., Isachkova, L. M., Shestopalova, N. M., and Pogodina, V. V. 1985. Experimental encephalitis in monkeys caused by the Powassan virus. *Neurosci. Behav. Physiol.* 15, 62–69.

Fulop, L., Barrett, A. D., Phillpotts, R., Martin, K., Leslie, D., and Titball, R. W. 1993. Rapid identification of flaviviruses based on conserved NS5 gene sequences. *J. Virol. Methods* 44, 179–188.

Gaunt, M. W., and Gould, E. A. 2005. Rapid subgroup identification of the flaviviruses using degenerate primer E-gene RT-PCR and site specific restriction enzyme analysis. *J. Virol. Methods* 128, 113–127.

Gaunt, M. W., Sall, A. A., de Lamballerie, X., Falconar, A. K., Dzhivanian, T. I., and Gould, E. A. 2001. Phylogenetic relationships of flaviviruses correlate with their epidemiology, disease association and biogeography. *J. Gen. Virol.* 82, 1867–1876.

Gholam, B. I., Puksa, S., and Provias, J. P. 1999. Powassan encephalitis: a case report with neuropathology and literature review. *Can. Med. Assoc. J.* 161, 1419–1422.

Godfrey, E. R., and Randolph, S. E. 2011. Economic downturn results in tick-borne disease upsurge. *Parasit. Vectors.* 4, 35.

Goldfield, M., Austin, S. M., Black, H. C., Taylor, B. F., and Altman, R. 1973. A non-fatal human case of Powassan virus encephalitis. *Am. J. Trop. Med. Hyg.* 22, 78–81.

Grant-Klein, R. J., Baldwin, C. D., Turell, M. J., Rossi, C. A., Li, F., Lovari, R., Crowder, C. D., Matthews, H. E., Rounds, M. A., Eshoo, M. W., Blyn, L. B., Ecker, D. J., Sampath, R., and Whitehouse, C. A. 2010. Rapid identification of vector-borne flaviviruses by mass spectrometry. *Mol. Cell. Probes.* 24, 219–228.

Grard, G., Moureau, G., Charrel, R. N., Lemasson, J. J., Gonzalez, J. P., Gallian, P., Gritsun, T. S., Holmes, E. C., Gould, E. A., and de Lamballerie, X. 2007. Genetic characterization of tick-borne flaviviruses: new insights into evolution, pathogenetic determinants and taxonomy. *Virology.* 361, 80–92.

Gregson, J. D. 1956. *The Ixodoidea of Canada.* Veterinary and Medical Entomology Section, Entomology Laboratory, Kamloops, British Columbia.

Gritsun, T. S., Nuttall, P. A., and Gould, E. A. 2003. Tick-borne flaviviruses. *Adv. Virus Res.* 61, 317–371.

Gubler, D. J., Campbell, G. L., Nasci, R., Komar, N., Petersen, L., and Roehrig, J. T. 2000. West Nile virus in the United States: guidelines for detection, prevention, and control. *Viral Immunol.* 13, 469–475.

Hall, J. E., Amrine, J. W., Jr., Gais, R. D., Kolanko, V. P., Hagenbuch, B. E., Gerencser, V. F., and Clark, S. M. 1991. Parasitization of humans in West Virginia by Ixodes cookei (Acari: Ixodidae), a potential vector of Lyme borreliosis. *J. Med. Entomol.* 28, 186–189.

Hicar, M. D., Edwards, K., and Bloch, K. 2011. Powassan virus infection presenting as acute disseminated encephalomyelitis in Tennessee. *Pediatr. Infect. Dis. J.* 30, 86–88.

Hinten, S. R., Beckett, G. A., Gensheimer, K. F., Pritchard, E., Courtney, T. M., Sears, S. D., Woytowicz, J. M., Preston, D. G., Smith, R. P., Jr., Rand, P. W., Lacombe, E. H., Holman, M. S., Lubelczyk, C. B., Kelso, P. T., Beelen, A. P., Stobierski, M. G., Sotir, M. J., Wong, S., Ebel, G., Kosoy, O., Piesman, J., Campbell, G. L., and Marfin, A. A. 2008. Increased recognition of Powassan encephalitis in the United States, 1999–2005. *Vector. Borne Zoonotic Dis.* 8, 733–740.

Hoang Johnson, D. K., Staples, J. E., Sotir, M. J., Warshauer, D. M., and Davis, J. P. 2010. Tick-borne Powassan virus infections among Wisconsin residents. *Wisc. Med. J.* 109, 91–97.

Hoff, G. L., Yuill, T. M., Iversen, J. O., and Hanson, R. P. 1970. Selected microbial agents in snowshoe hares and other vertebrates of Alberta. *J. Wildl. Dis.* 6, 472–478.

Isachkova, L. M., Shestopalova, N. M., Frolova, M. P., and Reingold, V. N. 1979. Light and electron microscope study of the neurotropism of Powassan virus strain P-40. *Acta Virol.* 23, 40–44.

Jackson, A. C. 1989. Leg weakness associated with Powassan virus infection—Ontario. *Can. Dis. Wkly. Rep.* 15, 123–124.

Johnson, A. J., Martin, D. A., Karabatsos, N., and Roehrig, J. T. 2000. Detection of anti-arboviral immunoglobulin G by using a monoclonal antibody-based capture enzyme-linked immunosorbent assay. *J. Clin. Microbiol.* 38, 1827–1831.

Johnson, A. J., Noga, A. J., Kosoy, O., Lanciotti, R. S., Johnson, A. A., and Biggerstaff, B. J. 2005. Duplex microsphere-based immunoassay for detection of anti-West Nile virus and anti-St. Louis encephalitis virus immunoglobulin M antibodies. *Clin. Diagn. Lab. Immunol.* 12, 566–574.

Johnson, H. N. 1987. Isolation of Powassan virus from a spotted skunk in California. *J. Wildl. Dis.* 23, 152–153.

Joshua, J. M. 1979. A case of Powassan virus encephalitis—Ontario. *Can. Dis. Wkly. Rep.* 5, 129–130.

Karabatsos, N. 1985. *International Catalogue of Arboviruses, 1985, Including Certain Other Viruses of Vertebrates.* American Society of Tropical Medicine and Hygeine, San Antonio.

Karabatsos, N., and Buckley, S. M. 1967. Susceptibility of the baby-hamster kidney-cell line (BHK-21) to infection with arboviruses. *Am J. Trop. Med. Hyg.* 16, 99–105.

Keirans, J. E., and Clifford, C. M. 1983. Ixodes (Pholeoixodes) eastoni N. Sp. (Acari: Ixodidae). A parasite of rodents and insectivores in the Black Hills of South Dakota, USA. *J. Med. Entomol.* 20, 90–98.

Keirans, J. E., Hutcheson, H. J., Durden, L. A., and Klompen, J. S. 1996. Ixodes (Ixodes) scapularis (Acari: Ixodidae): redescription of all active stages, distribution, hosts, geographical variation, and medical and veterinary importance. *J. Med. Entomol.* 33, 297–318.

Kislenko, G. S., Chunikhin, S. P., Rasnitsyn, S. P., Kurenkov, V. B., and Izotov, V. K. 1982. Reproduction of Powassan and West Nile viruses in Aedes aegypti mosquitoes and their cell culture (in Russian). *Med. Parazitol. (Mosk).* 51, 13–15.

Ko, R. C. 1972. Biology of Ixodes cookei Packard (Ixodidae) of groundhogs (Marmota monax Erxleben). *Can. J. Zool.* 50, 433–436.

Kollars, T. M., Jr., and Oliver, J. H., Jr. 2003. Host associations and seasonal occurrence of Haemaphysalis leporispalustris, Ixodes brunneus, I. cookei, I. dentatus, and I. texanus (Acari: Ixodidae) in Southeastern Missouri. *J. Med. Entomol.* 40, 103–107.

Kolski, H., Ford-Jones, E. L., Richardson, S., Petric, M., Nelson, S., Jamieson, F., Blaser, S., Gold, R., Otsubo, H., Heurter, H., and MacGregor, D. 1998. Etiology of acute childhood encephalitis at The Hospital for Sick Children, Toronto, 1994–1995. *Clin. Infect. Dis.* 26, 398–409.

Kuno, G. 1998. Universal diagnostic RT-PCR protocol for arboviruses. *J. Virol. Methods* 72, 27–41.

Kuno, G., Artsob, H., Karabatsos, N., Tsuchiya, K. R., and Chang, G. J. 2001. Genomic sequencing of deer tick virus and phylogeny of Powassan-related viruses of North America. *Am. J. Trop. Med. Hyg.* 65, 671–676.

Labuda, M., Nuttall, P. A., Kozuch, O., Eleckova, E., Williams, T., Zuffova, E., and Sabo, A. 1993. Non-viraemic transmission of tick-borne encephalitis virus: a mechanism for arbovirus survival in nature. *Experientia.* 49, 802–805.

Lanciotti, R. S. 2003. Molecular amplification assays for the detection of flaviviruses 34. *Adv. Virus Res.* 61, 67–99.

Leonova, G. N., Kondratov, I. G., Ternovoi, V. A., Romanova, E. V., Protopopova, E. V., Chausov, E. V., Pavlenko, E. V., Ryabchikova, E. I., Belikov, S. I., and Loktev, V. B. 2009. Characterization of Powassan viruses from Far Eastern Russia. *Arch. Virol.* 154, 811–820.

Leonova, G. N., Krugliak, S. P., Lozovskaia, S. A., and Rybachuk, V. N. 1987. The role of wild murine rodents in the selection of different strains of tick-borne encephalitis and Powassan viruses (in Russian). *Vopr. Virusol.* 32, 591–595.

Leonova, G. N., Sorokina, M. N., and Krugliak, S. P. 1991. The clinico-epidemiological characteristics of Powassan encephalitis in the southern Soviet Far East (in Russian). *Zh. Mikrobiol. Epidemiol. Immunobiol.* 35–39.

Lessell, S., and Collins, T. E. 2003. Ophthalmoplegia in Powassan encephalitis. *Neurology* 60, 1726–1727.

Levine, J. F., Apperson, C. S., Howard, P., Washburn, M., and Braswell, A. L. 1997. Lizards as hosts for immature Ixodes scapularis (Acari: Ixodidae) in North Carolina. *J. Med. Entomol.* 34, 594–598.

Lindenbach, B. D., Thiel, H. J., and Rice, C. M. 2007. Flaviviridae: The Viruses and Their Replication. In: D. M. Knipe, P. M. Howley (Eds.), *Fields Virology*. Lippincott-Raven Publishers, Philadelphia, pp. 1101–1152.

Lindsey, H. S., Calisher, C. H., and Matthews, J. H. 1976. Serum dilution neutralization test for California group virus identification and serology. *J. Clin. Microbiol.* 4, 503–510.

Little, P. B., Thorsen, J., Moore, W., and Weninger, N. 1985. Powassan viral encephalitis: a review and experimental studies in the horse and rabbit. *Vet. Pathol.* 22, 500–507.

L'Vov, D. K., Leonova, G. N., Gromashevskii, V. L., Belikova, N. P., and Berezina, L. K. 1974. Isolation of the Powassan virus from Haemaphysalis neumanni Donitz, 1905 ticks in the Maritime Territory (in Russian). *Vopr. Virusol.* 538–541.

Mahdy, M. S., Bansen, E., McLaughlin, B., Artsob, H., and Spence, L. 1982. California and Powassan virus disease in Ontario. *Can. Dis. Wkly. Rep.* 8, 185.

Mahdy, M. S., Wilson, M., Wherrett, B., and Dorland R. 1979. Powassan virus (POWV) encephalitis in Ontario. A case of meningoencephalitis attributed to infection with POWV in eastern Ontario. In: *Arboviral Encephalitis in Ontario With Special Reference to St. Louis Encephalitis*. A Report to the Ontario Ministry of Health from the Committee on Programs for the Prevention of Mosquito-Borne Encephalitis, pp. 48–69.

Maher-Sturgess, S. L., Forrester, N. L., Wayper, P. J., Gould, E. A., Hall, R. A., Barnard, R. T., and Gibbs, M. J. 2008. Universal primers that amplify RNA from all three flavivirus subgroups. *Virol. J.* 5, 16.

Main, A. J. J. 1977. The epizootiology of some tick-borne arboviral diseases. *J. N. Y. Entomol. Soc.* 85, 209–211.

Main, A. J., Carey, A. B., and Downs, W. G. 1979. Powassan virus in Ixodes cookei and Mustelidae in New England. *J. Wildl. Dis.* 15, 585–591.

Mandl, C. W. 2005. Steps of the tick-borne encephalitis virus replication cycle that affect neuropathogenesis. *Virus Res.* 111, 161–174.

Mandl, C. W., Holzmann, H., Kunz, C., and Heinz, F. X. 1993. Complete genomic sequence of Powassan virus: evaluation of genetic elements in tick-borne versus mosquito-borne flaviviruses. *Virology.* 194, 173–184.

Martin, D. A., Muth, D. A., Brown, T., Johnson, A. J., Karabatsos, N., and Roehrig, J. T. 2000. Standardization of immunoglobulin M capture enzyme-linked immunosorbent assays for routine diagnosis of arboviral infections. *J. Clin. Microbiol.* 38, 1823–1826.

Maupin, G. O., Gage, K. L., Piesman, J., Montenieri, J., Sviat, S. L., VanderZanden, L., Happ, C. M., Dolan, M., and Johnson, B. J. 1994. Discovery of an enzootic cycle of Borrelia burgdorferi in Neotoma mexicana and Ixodes spinipalpis from northern Colorado, an area where Lyme disease is nonendemic. *J. Infect. Dis.* 170, 636–643.

McLean, D. M., and Donahue, W. 1959. Powassan virus: isolation of virus from a fatal case of encephalitis. *Can. Med. Assoc. J.* 80, 708.

McLean, D. M., and Larke, R. P. 1963. Powassan and Silverwater viruses: ecology of two Ontario arboviruses. *Can. Med. Assoc. J.* 88, 182–185.

McLean, D. M., Best, J. M., Mahalingam, S., Chernesky, M. A., and Wilson, W. E. 1964a. Powassan virus: summer infection cycle, 1964. *Can. Med. Assoc. J.* 91, 1360–1362.

McLean, D. M., Cobb, C., Gooderham, S. E., Smart, C. A., Wilson, A. G., and Wilson, W. E. 1967. Powassan virus: persistence of virus activity during 1966. *Can. Med. Assoc. J.* 96, 660–664.

McLean, D. M., Crawford, M. A., Ladyman, S. R., Peers, R. R., and Purvin-Good, K. W. 1970. California encephalitis and Powassan virus activity in British Columbia, 1969. *Am. J. Epidemiol.* 92, 266–272.

McLean, D. M., Devos, A., and Quantz, E. J. 1964b. Powassan virus: field investigations during the summer of 1963. *Am. J. Trop. Med. Hyg.* 13, 747–753.

McLean, D. M., Goddard, E. J., Graham, E. A., Hardy, G. J., and Purvin-Good, K. W. 1972. California encephalitis virus isolations from Yukon mosquitoes, 1971. *Am. J. Epidemiol.* 95, 347–355.

McLean, D. M., Ladyman, S. R., and Purvin-Good, K. W. 1968. Westward extension of Powassan virus prevalence. *Can. Med. Assoc. J.* 98, 946–949.

McLean, D. M., Macpherson, L. W., Walker, S. J., and Funk, G. 1960. Powassan Virus: Surveys of Human and Animal Sera. *Am. J. Public Health Nations. Health.* 50, 1539–1544.

McLean, D. M., McQueen, E. J., Petite, H. E., Macpherson, L. W., Scholten, T. H., and Ronald, K. 1962. Powassan Virus: Field Investigations in Northern Ontario, 1959 to 1961. *Can. Med. Assoc. J.* 86, 971–974.

McLean, D. M., Smith, P. A., Livingstone, S. E., Wilson, W. E., and Wilson, A. G. 1966. Powassan virus: vernal spread during 1965. *Can. Med. Assoc. J.* 94, 532–536.

Minnesota Department of Health. Minnesota Records First Death from Tick-Borne Powassan Virus. Minnesota Department of Health. 7–12–2011. 7–12–2011.

Naumov, R. L., Gutova, V. P., and Chunikhin, S. P. 1980. Ixodid ticks and the causative agent of tick-borne encephalitis. 2. The genera Dermacentor and Haemaphysalis (in Russian). *Med. Parazitol. (Mosk)* 49, 66–69.

Nonaka, E., Ebel, G. D., and Wearing, H. J. 2010. Persistence of pathogens with short infectious periods in seasonal tick populations: the relative importance of three transmission routes. *PLoS One.* 5, e11745.

Orlinger, K. K., Hofmeister, Y., Fritz, R., Holzer, G. W., Falkner, F. G., Unger, B., Loew-Baselli, A., Poellabauer, E. M., Ehrlich, H. J., Barrett, P. N., and Kreil, T. R. 2011. A tick-borne encephalitis virus vaccine based on the european prototype strain induces broadly reactive cross-neutralizing antibodies in humans. *J. Infect. Dis.* 203, 1556–1564.

Partington, M. W., Thomson, V., and O'Shaughnessy, M. V. 1980. Powassan virus encephalitis in southeastern Ontario [letter]. *Can. Med. Assoc. J.* 123, 603–606.

Pesko, K., Torres-Perez, F., Hjelle, B., and Ebel, G. D. 2010. Molecular epidemiology of Powassan virus in North America. *J. Gen. Virol.* 91, 2698–2705.

Porterfield, J. S. 1980. Antigenic characteristics and classification of Togaviridae. In: R. W. Schlesinger (Ed.), *The Togaviruses: Biology, Structure, Replication.* Academic Press, New York, pp. 13–46.

ProMED Mail. Powassan Virus, Encephalitis—USA: (Minnesota) Fatal. ProMED Mail. 7–1–2011. 7–5–2011.

ProMED Mail. Powassan Virus, Encephalitis—USA: (Minnesota). ProMED Mail. 7–31–2009. 6–1–2011.

Reeves, W. C., Mariotte, C. O., Johnson, H. N., and Scrivani, R. E. 1962. Encuesta serologica sobre los virus transmitidos por artropodos en la zona de Hermosillo, Mexico. Reimpreso del Boletin de la Oficina Sanitaria Panamericana LII, 228–229.

Rossier, E., Harrison, R. J., and Lemieux, B. 1974. A case of Powassan virus encephalitis. *Can. Med. Assoc. J.* 110, 1173–1174.

Scaramozzino, N., Crance, J. M., Jouan, A., DeBriel, D. A., Stoll, F., and Garin, D. 2001. Comparison of flavivirus universal primer pairs and development of a rapid, highly sensitive hemi-nested reverse transcription-PCR assay for detection of flaviviruses targeted to a conserved region of the NS5 gene sequences. *J. Clin. Microbiol.* 39, 1922–1927.

Scott, T. W., and Brown, S. J. 2011. Differential attachment and blood-feeding by the tick Dermacentor andersoni (Acari ixodidae). *Acarologia.* 26, 241–245.

Smith, R. P., Jr., Rand, P. W., Lacombe, E. H., Morris, S. R., Holmes, D. W., and Caporale, D. A. 1996. Role of bird migration in the long-distance dispersal of Ixodes dammini, the vector of Lyme disease. *J. Infect. Dis.* 174, 221–224.

Smith, R., Woodall, J. P., Whitney, E., Deibel, R., Gross, M. A., Smith, V., and Bast, T. F. 1974. Powassan virus infection. A report of three human cases of encephalitis. *Am. J. Dis. Child.* 127, 691–693.

Srihongse, S., Woodall, J. P., Grayson, M. A., and Deibel, R. 1980. Arboviruses in New York State; surveillance in arthropods and nonhuman vertebrates, 1972–1977. *Mosq. News.* 40, 269–276.

Stim, T. B. 1969. Arborvirus plaquing in two simian kidney cell lines. *J. Gen. Virol.* 5, 329–338.

Tavakoli, N. P., Wang, H., Dupuis, M., Hull, R., Ebel, G. D., Gilmore, E. J., and Faust, P. L. 2009. Fatal case of deer tick virus encephalitis. *N. Engl. J. Med.* 360, 2099–2107.

Telford, S. R., III, Armstrong, P. M., Katavolos, P., Foppa, I., Garcia, A. S., Wilson, M. L., and Spielman, A. 1997. A new tick-borne encephalitis-like virus infecting New England deer ticks, Ixodes dammini. *Emerg. Infect. Dis.* 3, 165–170.

Thiel, H.-J., Collett, M. S., Gould, E. A., Heinz, F. X., Houghton, M. et al. 2005. *Flaviviridae.* In: C. M. Fauquet, M. A. Mayo, J. Maniloff, U. Desselberger, and L. A. Ball (Eds.), Virus *Taxonomy: Eighth Report of the International Committee on Taxonomy of Viruses.* Virol. Div., Int. Union Microbiol. Soc., San Diego, CA, pp. 981–998.

Thomas, L. A., Kennedy, R. C., and Eklund, C. M. 1960. Isolation of a virus closely related to Powassan virus from Dermacentor andersoni collected along North Cache la Poudre River, Colo. *Proc. Soc. Exp. Biol. Med.* 104, 355–359.

Timoney, P. 1971. Powassan virus infection in the grey squirrel. *Acta Virol.* 15, 429.

Tkachenko, E. A., Linev, M. B., Bashkirtsev, V. N., Berezin, V. V., Dzhagurova, T. K., Rubin, S. A., Chumakov, M. P., Dekonenko, E. P., Korotkov, Yu. S., Povalishina, T. P., Ivliev, V. V., Kharlamova, I. I., Maiorov, S. P., and Savel'eva, I. A. 1976. Isolation of Powassan virus from adult mosquitoes, Anopheles hycranus, in Khabarovsk region (from data of expedition in 1975). *Dokl. Simp. Transkont. Svyazi Pereletn. Ptits Rol' v Rasp. Arbovirus* 195–197.

U.S. Geological Survey. Disease Maps. U.S. Geological Survey. 2011. 7–14–2011.

Westaway, E. G., Brinton, M. A., Gaidamovich, S. Y., Horzinek, M. C., Igarashi, A., Kaariainen, L., Lvov, D. K., Porterfield, J. S., Russell, P. K., and Trent, D. W. 1985. Flaviviridae. *Intervirology.* 24, 183–192.

Whitby, J. E., Ni, H., Whitby, H. E., Jennings, A. D., Bradley, L. M., Lee, J. M., Lloyd, G., Stephenson, J. R., and Barrett, A. D. 1993. Rapid detection of viruses of the tick-borne encephalitis virus complex by RT-PCR of viral RNA. *J. Virol. Methods* 45, 103–114.

Whitney, E. 1963. Serologic evidence of group A and B arthropod-borne virus activity in New York State. *Am. J. Trop. Med. Hyg.* 12, 417–424.

Whitney, E. 1965. Arthropod-borne viruses in New York state: serologic evidence of groups A, B, and Bunyamwera viruses in dairy herds. *Am. J. Vet. Res.* 26, 914–919.

Whitney, E., and Jamnback, H. 1965. The first isolations of Powassan virus in New York State. *Proc. Soc. Exp. Biol. Med.* 119, 432–435.

Whitney, E., Deibel, R., and Edwards, M. R. 1972. Ultrastructural studies of Powassan virus. In: J. L. Melnick (Ed.), *International Virology 2. Proceedings of the Second International Congress for Virology Budapest 1971.* S. Karger, Basel, pp. 163–164.

Whitney, E., Jamnback, H., Means, R. G., and Watthews, T. H. 1968. Arthropod-borne-virus survey in St. Lawrence County, New York. Arbovirus reactivity in serum from amphibians, reptiles, birds, and mammals. *Am. J. Trop. Med. Hyg.* 17, 645–650.

Wilkinson, P. R. 1984. Hosts and distribution of Rocky Mountain wood ticks (Dermacentor andersoni) at a tick focus in British Columbia rangeland. *J. Entomol. Soc. Brit. Columbia* 81, 57–71.

Wilson, M. S., Wherrett, B. A., and Mahdy, M. S. 1979. Powassan virus meningoencephalitis: a case report. *Can. Med. Assoc. J.* 121, 320–323.

Wong, S. J., Boyle, R. H., Demarest, V. L., Woodmansee, A. N., Kramer, L. D., Li, H., Drebot, M., Koski, R. A., Fikrig, E., Martin, D. A., and Shi, P. Y. 2003. Immunoassay targeting nonstructural protein 5 to differentiate West Nile virus infection from dengue and St. Louis encephalitis virus infections and from flavivirus vaccination. *J. Clin. Microbiol.* 41, 4217–4223.

Wong, S. J., Demarest, V. L., Boyle, R. H., Wang, T., Ledizet, M., Kar, K., Kramer, L. D., Fikrig, E., and Koski, R. A. 2004. Detection of human anti-flavivirus antibodies with a West Nile virus recombinant antigen microsphere immunoassay. *J. Clin. Microbiol.* 42, 65–72.

Woodall, J. P., and Roz, A. 1977. Experimental milk-borne transmission of Powassan virus in the goat. *Am. J. Trop. Med. Hyg.* 26, 190–192.

Zarnke, R. L., and Yuill, T. M. 1981a. Powassan virus infection in snowshoe hares (Lepus americanus). *J. Wildl. Dis.* 17, 303–310.

Zarnke, R. L., and Yuill, T. M. 1981b. Serologic survey for selected microbial agents in mammals from Alberta, 1976. *J. Wildl. Dis.* 17, 453–461.

13 Neurological Dengue

Aravinthan Varatharaj

CONTENTS

13.1   INTRODUCTION

Dengue is a viral disease which poses a significant and increasing problem to global health. The World Health Organization (WHO) estimates that 2.5 billion people, 40% of the world's population, are at risk of dengue infection (WHO 2009). Fifty million infections occur each year, with an increasing incidence, and result in 24,000 deaths. The magnitude of the dengue problem demands action.

To act against the dengue virus, we must understand it. An increasing knowledge of viral interaction with the human body is revealing how dengue has the capacity to cause disease. The familiar form of dengue infection presents as an acute febrile illness, but it is better to think of a spectrum of clinical manifestations, where the features of infection range from asymptomatic carriage to a severe hemorrhagic disorder with multisystem involvement. The factors that determine where along the spectrum an infected individual will manifest illness are complex, but key toward developing an effective management strategy.

The public health implications are clear, but why is dengue of interest to neuroscientists? The broad spectrum of dengue infection does not spare the nervous system, peripheral or central. Neurological manifestations are well-reported, but poorly understood. For decades it has been a matter of debate as to how these manifestations are mediated, and whether dengue virus has the potential to directly infect the nervous system. An increasing body of evidence now places us in a position to develop an answer, and in doing so, advances our understanding of the clinical spectrum of dengue infection.

13.2 VIROLOGY

Dengue is a single-stranded positive-sense ribonucleic acid (RNA) virus of the *Flavivirus* genus, which includes among others yellow fever, West Nile, and Japanese encephalitis viruses. The flaviviruses are part of the (non-taxonomic) descriptive group of "viral hemorrhagic fevers," which includes Ebola, Marburg, and Lassa fever. The RNA genome of the dengue virus is protected by an icosahedral (20-sided) protein capsid and lipid outer envelope, forming a complete virion with a diameter of around 50 nm. There are four viral serotypes, named DEN-1 to DEN-4, that are genetically distinct although sharing a common phylogeny. Numerous strains of each serotype have also been discovered. The complete RNA genome has been sequenced for all four serotypes, and runs to a length of around 11,000 bases (Henchal and Putnak 2009). For comparison, the human genome contains 2.85 billion bases (IHGSC 2001). Contained within this "simple" genome are merely 10 individual genes; the human genome has 25,000. Three structural genes code for the capsid protein (C), the membrane-associated protein (M), and the envelope protein (E). The remaining seven nonstructural genes—numbered NS1, NS2A, NS2B, NS3, NS4A, NS4B, NS5—encode proteins with various roles in replication and infection. Together, these ten genes and their protein products are the causative agents of the dengue problem. Existing, as genes do, only to make more copies of themselves, one has to concede that they have developed a tremendously successful survival strategy.

13.3 HISTORICAL ASPECTS

13.3.1 ORIGINS

> I venture to submit the following propositions, which possibly may not be deemed very extravagant:—that dengue is a disease not yet thoroughly understood.
>
> **Charles C. Godding**
> *Staff surgeon aboard HMS Agamemnon, 1890*

It is likely that dengue has plagued humanity since antiquity, although the form in which it has done so has undergone considerable evolution in parallel with our own. Phylogenetic analyses suggest that dengue existed several millennia ago as a disease of forest-dwelling nonhuman primates (the "sylvatic cycle") (Wang et al. 2000).

The first major step in the dengue-human evolutionary relationship occurred when human civilization shifted from a hunter-gatherer society to one based in urban aggregations, in inadvertent concert with insect vectors of the genus *Aedes*. A few thousand years ago in Asia, these populations reached a critical mass of over 10,000 human individuals, which allowed dengue to make the leap into a form able to maintain itself in an endemic-epidemic human transmission cycle. Around this time, chroniclers of the Chinese dynasties began to make observations regarding a febrile illness with muscle aches that was associated with proximity to water and spread by insects. The causative agent was likely DEN-2, and the illness likely dengue fever (DF). Similar shifts occurred independently across the world, and the sylvatic cycle progenitor fell into the niche of endemic-epidemic cycling in geographically isolated human population centers, leading to the four distinct serotypes identified today.

13.3.2 DISCOVERIES

For centuries, dengue cycled endemic-epidemic in urban population centers, causing a self-limiting febrile illness, killing few, and attracting only occasional attention from the medical men of the time. Benjamin Rush, Pennsylvanian physician and 25th signatory of the Declaration of Independence, gave his now infamous description of "breakbone fever" in 1780. The Spanish-American War of 1898 meant that U.S. troops were stationed in dengue-endemic areas, and led to Ashburn and Craig's paper proving that the cause of dengue is an "ultramicroscopic agent" that is present in the blood (Ashburn and Craig 1907). In 1919, Cleland proved that the vector was *Aedes aegypti* (Cleland and Bradley 1919). Virus, insect, and man existed in balance. All this changed in the 20th century. Population upheaval in the aftermath of the World War II allowed unprecedented spread of the virus to pandemic levels. Rapid urbanization coupled with inadequate public sanitation, especially in the population centers of South-East Asia, provided ample breeding ground for *Aedes aegypti*, catalyzing a string of epidemics. Air travel exposed the virus to naive populations, ripe for infection. Something else changed too; dengue began to kill. The emergence of dengue hemorrhagic fever (DHF) heralded the second major step in the dengue-human relationship.

13.3.3 THE EMERGENCE OF DHF

DHF was first described in the Philippines in 1953 and soon spread throughout the region. China, the Maldives, India, Sri Lanka; one by one, DHF became endemic. During the 1960s and 1970s, DHF progressed through South-East Asia, setting up a pattern in each country which began with a few sporadic cases, a sudden outbreak in the rainy season, and then a stable cycle of yearly surges and bigger 3–5 yearly epidemics. For reasons that are now being understood, individuals in an area with an endemic serotype are vulnerable to secondary infection by another serotype, which results in a more fulminant disease and an increased likelihood of progression to DHF. Dengue-naive populations in areas infested with *Aedes aegypti* are highly vulnerable; for example, when DEN-1 was introduced to Cuba in 1977, over 44% of the population were infected, although the majority with mild disease only (Halstead

2007). Five years later, the 1981 DEN-2 epidemic was markedly more severe, with hundreds of thousands of cases of DF and around 10,000 cases of DHF. In this pattern, the worldwide spread of dengue has continued into the new millennium.

13.4 EPIDEMIOLOGY

13.4.1 GLOBAL PATTERNS

Today, dengue virus is endemic to human populations in over one hundred countries, and approximately 2.5 billion individuals, 40% of the global population, are at risk (WHO 2009). Tropical and subtropical areas are worst affected (shown in Figure 13.1). It is estimated that 50 million infections and 24,000 fatalities occur worldwide every year. The incidence has increased by a factor of 30 in the last 50 years and continues to climb. At the 2005 World Health Assembly in Geneva, WHO member states declared that the dengue phenomenon "may constitute a public health emergency of international concern" (Documentation of the World Health Assembly 2005).

13.4.2 SOUTH-EAST ASIA

South-East Asia bears the brunt of the dengue problem. Subdividing by the Köppen climate classification, the tropical rainforest (e.g., Indonesia, Philippines) and tropical monsoon (e.g., Sri Lanka, Thailand) areas are worst affected, with large populations of *Aedes aegypti* and multiple circulating viral serotypes. In these areas, dengue has an established foothold in the cities and is now spreading to rural areas. Meanwhile, the tropical savannah areas such Bangladesh and parts of India are experiencing epidemics of increasing range and frequency, and in the last decade, dengue has also begun to encroach on the temperate areas such as Nepal and Bhutan.

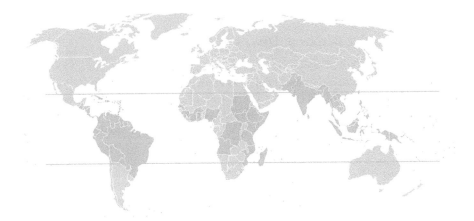

FIGURE 13.1 Global distribution of dengue. The Tropics of Cancer and Capricorn are marked. The southern United States, Mexico, Australian Queensland, and the Pacific Islands are also variably affected.

13.4.3 AMERICAS

In the Americas, dengue is endemic throughout large parts of South and Central America. From 2001 to 2007, there were nearly 4.5 million reported cases, occurring in regular outbreaks (WHO 2009). Brazil is particularly affected, with over 2.7 million cases during that period. DEN-1, DEN-2, and DEN-3 are in common circulation, although DEN-4 is also present, especially in the Andean countries. In a large study conducted between 2000 and 2007, enlisting 20,880 patients from Western South America, Forshey et al. (2010) reported that dengue was the most common cause of acute febrile illness in that region, responsible for 26% of cases.

13.4.4 AFRICA

Dengue in Africa is poorly understood, due to a lack of reliable surveillance and a greater focus on malaria and HIV. Nevertheless, dengue is clearly present on the continent, and what data there is suggests that outbreaks are occurring with increasing frequency (WHO 2009). East Africa is worst affected, with circulating DEN-1, DEN-2, and DEN-3. The WHO has called for attention to the dengue problem in Africa, especially the particular issue of dengue in majority HIV-positive populations and the potential implications for transmission.

13.4.5 NON-ENDEMIC AREAS AND INTERNATIONAL TRAVEL

Dengue does not commonly occur in Europe, North America, or Russia, but is an important differential diagnosis in the febrile traveler returning from the tropics. Analyzing global surveillance data of 17,353 patients, Freedman et al. (2006) showed that dengue is the most common identifiable cause of systemic febrile illness in travelers returning from South East Asia (58% of cases with identified causes), the Caribbean (52%), South America (31%), or South Central Asia (27%), even higher than malaria.

13.4.6 ECONOMIC BURDEN OF DENGUE

The economic impact of dengue in endemic areas is vast. Suaya et al. (2009) conducted a landmark study looking at the costs associated with dengue in 1695 patients in eight American and Asian countries. The average cost per patient (in international dollars) was I\$514 for cases managed in the community and I\$1394 for inpatients. The total cost for the study cohort was I\$587 million, a very conservative estimate given the degree of under-reporting.

13.5 VECTORS

13.5.1 INSECT VECTORS

The primary vector of the dengue virus is the mosquito *Aedes aegypti*, and hence dengue may be classed as an "arbovirus"—an "arthopod-borne virus." *Aedes* is found in abundance from latitudes 35°N to 35°S, reflecting locations in which winters are above 10°C, allowing the insect to survive year-round. Summer invasions have been recorded up to 45°N, but the mosquitoes perish in winter. Low temperatures also ensure that high-altitude areas within the Tropics are relatively spared.

Other vectors of the genus *Aedes* have also been implicated in dengue outbreaks. The 2001 Hawaiian outbreak was spread by *Aedes albopictus*, a less efficient forest-living vector which resulted in a slowly-spreading epidemic (Halstead 2007). The transport of *Aedes albopictus* from its Asian homeland was likely due to the global trade in tires, inadvertently containing viable eggs. *Aedes polynesiensis* and *scutellaris* have also been implicated.

13.5.2   LIFE CYCLE

The female of *Aedes aegypti* lays its eggs in stagnant water, which exists in nature but is provided in abundance wherever there is human habitation—discarded bottles, buckets, and tires are perfect locations. There is evidence that dengue virus can pass from a female mosquito to its eggs (transovarial spread) (Arunchalam et al. 2008), and this may be a useful strategy to ensure viral persistence out of season. The eggs are resistant to drying and may remain in a quiescent state for several months. Following a period of rainfall, the eggs hatch into larvae; after a week, the larvae pupate, and 2 days later, the mature mosquitoes emerge. The insect has a predilection for cool and dark areas, causing it to live indoors, in close contact with humans. The females feed on human blood, which provides a nutritious diet for egg production, and bite mainly during the day. To take up the virus, the mosquito must bite during the period of peak viremia, the start of which usually precedes symptoms. As the blood meal is digested the virus infects the gut and within 8–12 days undergoes massive replication and systemic spread, penetrating the salivary glands. Further feeding then transmits the virus to humans. *Aedes aegypti* itself lacks the ability to clear the virus and remains infected for the duration of its life, which may be a month or more. Individual insects have a relatively narrow range, usually confined to around the house in which they hatched. Humans serve to amplify the virus and transport it to fresh pastures.

13.5.3   OTHER METHODS OF TRANSMISSION

Spread between humans through infected blood transfusions and organ transplants is possible, and vertical transmission from human mother to fetus has also been reported (Chye et al. 1997). However, these represent a rare minority of cases.

13.6   PATHOGENESIS

13.6.1   INITIAL EVENTS

After the bite, dengue virus passes into the blood and infects and replicates within cells of the immune system, particularly macrophages and their precursor monocytes. Lymphocytes, mast cells, dendritic cells, endothelial cells—and many others—may also be targets for infection. Epidermal dendritic cells (Langerhans cells) around the bite area may well be the first targets, and infection down-regulates their production of the major histocompatibility complex (MHC) and induces apoptosis, compromising antigen presentation and delaying an effective immune response. After an incubation period of 7–10 days, large numbers of mature virions are released into the circulation, resulting in viremia and the variable development of symptoms (and infectivity). Blood-borne virus infiltrates organs (especially the spleen) and begins replication in tissue macrophages. It is likely that it is the immune response to viremia which determines the progression and clinical manifestations of dengue infection. It has long been observed that secondary dengue infections lead to a more severe phenotype than the primary infection, and much work has focused on aberrant immune responses in secondary dengue.

13.6.2   Humoral Immune Response

Viral proteins are immunogenic and elicit a neutralizing antibody response, especially the envelope proteins which serve as highly visible epitopes. Many antibodies are cross-reactive, however, and bind to endothelial cells and platelets resulting in their apoptosis (Lin et al. 2001, 2002). Also, antibodies (via the classical pathway) and viral proteins including NS1 (Avirutnan et al. 2006) trigger complement activation, which may contribute to vascular permeability and coagulopathy.

Antibody-dependant enhancement (ADE) occurs in secondary dengue infection when immunoglobulins persisting from the primary infection bind to circulating dengue virus (Dejnirattisai et al. 2010). Present at concentrations inadequate for effective viral neutralization, the immunoglobins form complexes with virions, bind to immune cells, and in doing so enhance the uptake of effective virions by their targets. ADE effectively subverts the immune response to the cause of viral replication. As IgG can cross the placenta, ADE may also contribute to the severity of dengue infection in infants born to dengue-exposed mothers.

13.6.3   Cell-Mediated Response

Presentation of dengue antigens initiates a clonal expansion of CD8+ (cytotoxic) and CD4+ (helper) T-lymphocytes. Following resolution a significant number remain and render lifelong immunity to that serotype. However, the serotypes are sufficiently heterogenous in their antigenicity that infection with one does not confer immunity to the others. Preferential activation of memory T-lymphocytes from the primary infection at the expense of generating a new and more specific cell-mediated response (a concept dubbed "original antigenic sin") delivers a sub-optimal response which may be at least partly responsible for the increased severity of secondary infections (Martina et al. 2009).

13.6.4   Cytokine Storm

Large amounts of inflammatory mediators produced by infected and activated immune cells create a "cytokine storm" that contributes to vascular endothelial breakdown (King et al. 2000). Both Th1 and Th2 responses are elicited. The Th1 response produces IFN-γ and IL-2 and is biased toward cell-mediated immunity, whereas the Th2 response produces IL-4, IL-5, IL-10, and TGF-β, and is biased toward antibody synthesis. There is evidence that the Th2 response is less effective and associated with more severe disease (Mustafa et al. 2001).

13.6.5 Viral-Host Interplay

The clinical outcome of dengue infection reflects the interplay of viral and host factors. On the one hand, it may be that certain viral strains are simply more virulent, and indeed, genotypic variation between strains has been implicated in differential pathogenesis (Leitmeyer et al. 1999). Numerous host factors are also at play, however. As previously mentioned, aberrant immune responses likely play a large part in mediating severe dengue infection, and these may be a predominant feature of the secondary response. Host genetic factors may also be involved, and numerous HLA polymorphisms associated with varied susceptibility have been identified (Loke et al. 2001). Females (Kabra et al. 1999) and infants (Guzman et al. 2002) are generally more susceptible to severe disease, as are individuals with preexisting chronic disease such as asthma (Guzman et al. 1992).

13.7 CLINICAL SPECTRUM OF DENGUE INFECTION

> Dengue is one disease entity with different clinical presentations and often with unpredictable clinical evolution and outcome. (WHO 2009)

For reasons that are now being understood, the clinical manifestations of dengue infection are highly variable. The outcome of the virus-host interaction may affect wide range of organ systems, with varying severity, and potential for systemic failure. The traditional WHO classification into distinct disease entities is widely used and is shown in Table 13.1. However, in the face of practical difficulties in applying this classification to patients who may straddle categories, a new classification has been produced which divides cases into severe dengue and nonsevere dengue (with or without warning signs).

TABLE 13.1
Traditional WHO Classification

Asymptomatic or subclinical
Dengue fever (DF)
Dengue hemorrhagic fever (DHF)
Dengue shock syndrome (DSS)
"Unusual manifestations"

13.7.1 ASYMPTOMATIC INFECTION

In some cases, detectable symptoms may fail to develop at all, resulting in an asymptomatic carrier state. During viremia, the patient is still infectious, however, and asymptomatic carriers likely play a significant role in disseminating the virus.

13.7.2 DENGUE FEVER

DF classically presents with a rapid onset of fever, malaise, headache, and retro-orbital pain, with severe myalgia and arthralgia ("breakbone fever"). Erythema of the face, neck, and chest is typical. A generalized maculopapular rash erupts 3 to 5 days after the onset of fever in 50%–82% of patients and is characteristically speck-led with petechiae and larger islands of spared skin (Pincus et al. 2008). In infants and younger children the presentation is nonspecific, with prominent coryza, and also diarrhea, rash, seizures (usually febrile convulsions), vomiting, and abdominal pain. In a minority of individuals with DF there may be some signs of a mild hemor-rhagic tendency ("DF with unusual bleeding").

DF may result from either primary or secondary dengue infection. The onset of symptoms is usually 7–10 days after the bite, although the incubation period can be as short as three or as long as fifteen days. As a rule, febrile illness in the traveler more than 2 weeks after return from the tropics is unlikely to be dengue. The fever lasts for 2–7 days and is in the majority of cases followed by a complete recovery.

13.7.3 DENGUE HEMORRHAGIC FEVER

DHF usually results from secondary infection, although may occur after primary infection in infants. DHF is largely indistinguishable from DF in the initial stages; after a few days, however, vascular leak and derangement of clotting become mani-fest. There is easy bruising, bleeding from injection sites, and widespread petechiae. The classic bedside investigation is the tourniquet test; a blood pressure cuff around the upper arm is inflated to halfway between systolic and diastolic pressure for 5 min, and the test is considered positive if more than 30 petechiae per square inch are observed on the underlying skin. There may also be gastrointestinal bleeding (especially if with existing peptic ulceration), epistaxis, hematuria, and menorrha-gia. Vascular leak results in hemoconcentration, serous effusions (mostly pleural and peritoneal), and hypoproteinemia. The liver is often enlarged and tender, and acute liver failure may occur.

Fever persists for 2–7 days, after which the disease may take one of two courses. Most patients experience sweating and some circulatory disturbance during defer-vescence, and in less severe cases this is followed by spontaneous resolution. In more severe cases, however, the disease progresses to a state of critical vascular leak and circulatory collapse, known as dengue shock syndrome (DSS). Thus, the critical window for modifying the course of disease is at and just before the time of defervescence. Worsening thrombocytopenia and elevation of the hematocrit herald impending DSS.

13.7.4 DENGUE SHOCK SYNDROME

DSS is both hypovolemic, due to blood loss, and distributive, due to vascular leak. Classical signs of shock are present; tachycardia, hypotension, and cool, clammy, poorly perfused peripheries. Complications include electrolyte and blood glucose abnormalities, metabolic acidosis, hemorrhage (including intracranial hemorrhage), disseminated intravascular coagulation (DIC), and large serous effusions. Eventually, there is multi-organ failure. Untreated, death usually occurs within 12–24 h from the onset of shock.

13.7.5 UNUSUAL MANIFESTATIONS

13.7.5.1 Hepatitis

Dengue virus and antigens have been isolated from the liver (Nogueira et al. 1988; Miagostovich et al. 1997). Some degree of hepatic involvement accompanies most dengue infection, probably reflecting a predilection for viral infiltration into liver macrophages (Kupffer cells) and hepatocytes. Direct liver tropism is not the only mechanism, however, and dengue hepatitis is likely to be multifactorial, and may involve liver hemorrhage and ischemic injury. Patients with preexisting hepatic impairment are likely to be at greater risk. Use of paracetamol to control fever may also contribute. The usual presentation of dengue hepatitis is as a rise in serum transaminases (alanine transaminase [ALT]; aspartate transaminase [AST]) which reflects the severity of infection, and there may be some right-upper quadrant pain. In a retrospective study of DHF and liver failure, Kuo et al. (1992) found that the transaminitis in dengue is usually AST-predominant. Progression to frank liver failure is uncommon but may occur together with hepatic encephalopathy. There is evidence that DEN-3 and DEN-4 serotypes may have a greater predisposition to liver involvement (Dengue Bulletin 24, 2000).

13.7.5.2 Myocarditis

Acute myocarditis with impaired left ventricular function has been reported (Wali et al. 1998), and may add a cardiogenic element to DSS and increase the likelihood of fluid overload with volume resuscitation. Cardiac rhythm abnormalities may also occur. It is unclear whether these manifestations are due to dengue viral invasion of cardiomyocytes or part of a systemic inflammatory process.

13.7.6 NEUROLOGICAL MANIFESTATIONS

Neurological manifestations of dengue infection have been recognized for some time, and are receiving increased attention in light of the continued spread of dengue. The latest WHO guidance specifically mentions neurological manifestations (encephalopathy and encephalitis), recommending that although these may occur in the absence of classical features, they should be considered markers of "severe dengue" (WHO 2009). Fever and exposure in an endemic area should be sufficient to raise suspicion.

Numerous neurological manifestations have been reported. They may be classified as primarily *central* (inside the meninges) or *peripheral* (outside the meninges), and are outlined in Table 13.2. These will be examined in detail in the following sections.

TABLE 13.2
Neurological Manifestations of Dengue Infection

"Central"	Encephalopathy (Section 13.8)
	Encephalitis (Section 13.9)
	Transverse myelitis (Section 13.10)
"Peripheral"	Guillain-Barré syndrome (Section 13.11.1)
	Mononeuropathy (Section 13.11.2)
	Myositis (Section 13.11.3)

13.8 DENGUE ENCEPHALOPATHY

Encephalopathy, a clinical picture of reduced consciousness with variable other features of central nervous system dysfunction, is the most frequently reported neurological complication of dengue infection. The incidence is variably reported as 0.5% (Cam et al. 2001) to 6.2% (Hendarto and Hadinegoro 1992) of DHF cases. There is evidence that DEN-2 and DEN-3 are most often implicated (Cam et al. 2001; Solomon et al. 2000).

Encephalopathy is often caused by infections, metabolic derangements, alcohol or drugs. Many extra-cranial infections result in encephalopathy, not through central nervous system penetration, but as a result of a systemic inflammatory response. In contrast, *encephalitis* is a histological diagnosis of inflammation of the brain parenchyma, commonly due to viral infection. Organisms with the capacity to infect neurons are described as *neurotropic*, and those causing disease are *neurovirulent*. The typical clinical features of encephalitis are fever (if infective), reduced consciousness, headache, seizures, and focal neurological signs. Thus, encephalitis is one of the causes of encephalopathy, albeit not the most common.

Although dengue encephalopathy has been recognized since the 1970s, there has been much controversy as to the underlying mechanism; in particular, whether the dengue virus is neurotropic and therefore has the potential to penetrate the blood–brain barrier (BBB) and cause encephalitis. For this reason, Solomon and Barrett (2003) have suggested the term "cerebral dengue," by analogy to "cerebral malaria," the term implies brain involvement without specifying a pathological mechanism. The traditional view has been that dengue is nonneurotropic and that dengue encephalopathy is mediated indirectly by the systemic effects of severe dengue infection. These are outlined in Table 13.3. Later research has challenged this understanding, and will be reviewed below.

TABLE 13.3
Possible Causes of Dengue Encephalopathy

Liver failure leading to hepatic encephalopathy
Vascular leak leading to cerebral edema
Bleeding tendency leading to intracranial hemorrhage
Hyponatremia
Direct viral infiltration leading to encephalitis

13.8.1   Hepatic Encephalopathy

In a study of dengue encephalopathy in Vietnam, 24% of cases were attributable to hepatic encephalopathy (Solomon et al. 2000). Dengue virus has a recognized tropism for liver macrophages (Kupffer cells) and hepatocytes, and hepatic involvement is common in severe dengue infection. Although this is usually manifest only as a slight increase in transaminases, reflecting a degree of hepatocellular injury, there may be progression to more severe forms of liver failure (Lawn et al. 2003). Mohan et al. (2000) estimate that jaundice occurs in 12–62% of patients with DSS, representing impaired hepatic function in the excretion of bilirubin. As the liver fails and excretory function is further impaired, neurotoxic products of cellular metabolism, including ammonia (which should undergo hepatic detoxification to urea), are retained in concentrations that result in complex and deleterious effects on cerebral function. The clinical consequences range from neuropsychiatric disturbances to coma. A classic clinical sign is asterixis, a flapping tremor of the outstretched hands that results from dysfunction of central motor areas controlling posture. In a study of 191 Thai children with various dengue grades, Wiwanitkit (2007) found that 35% had liver dysfunction, and 8% frank hepatic encephalopathy, while in Malaysia, Lum et al. (1996) found that hepatic encephalopathy occurred in 20% of children with DHF/DSS.

13.8.2   Cerebral Edema

An abnormal accumulation of water in the brain parenchyma may occur in a wide range of pathological states, reflecting the multifaceted control of intracranial homeostasis in normal physiology. *Vasogenic* edema occurs when there is disruption of tight junctions between endothelial cells that comprise the BBB, allowing uncontrolled fluid shift; whereas *cytotoxic* edema results from cellular injury and loss of intracellular contents.

Cerebral edema compromises brain function. First, extracellular water interrupts delicately maintained concentrations of ions and neurotransmitters. Second, the Monro-Kellie doctrine states that, since the cranium describes a fixed volume, the brain, blood, and cerebrospinal fluid (CSF) contained within it must maintain a state of volume equilibrium. Thus, the cerebral perfusion pressure, intracranial pressure, and volume of brain tissue are related, and if one is elevated there must be a compensation in the others. As parenchymal volume rises, cerebral perfusion is rapidly compromised, leading to neuronal death. The final consequence of cerebral edema is brain herniation, as the increased intracranial pressure is relieved by the evacuation of brain tissue through the foramen magnum, with fatal results.

Cerebral edema has been shown to occur widely in dengue encephalopathy, both at postmortem and on brain imaging (see Table 13.4). The pathophysiology is likely multifactorial. In part it may be a continuation of the widespread endothelial disruption and vascular leak that occurs in severe dengue, leading to vasogenic cerebral edema. Whether the effect on cerebral microvasculature reflects dengue infection of endothelial cells or a systemic cytokine storm remains to be seen. In part it may also occur secondary to hyponatremia, leading to fluid shift. Finally, if dengue is indeed neurotropic, cerebral edema may occur due to cytotoxic effects on neurons, as it may do in other

TABLE 13.4
Cerebral Edema in Dengue

Study	Patients	Cases with Cerebral Edema
Postmortem Diagnosis		
Nimmannitya et al. 1987	10 (DHF)	3
Janssen et al. 1998	1 (DF)	1
Chimelli et al. 1990	5 (DHF)	3
Radiological Diagnosis		
Lum et al. 1996	6 (DHF)	3 (on CT)
Kankirawatana et al. 2000	8 (DHF)	2 (on CT)
Cam et al. 2001	27 (DHF)	12 (on MRI)
Wasay et al. 2008	6 (DHF)	3 (on CT)

viral encephalitides. Interestingly, Solomon et al. (2000) identified a case of dengue encephalopathy with associated cerebral edema on CT in which no diagnostic features of DF or DHF were apparent—this was likely edema secondary to dengue encephalitis.

13.8.3 INTRACRANIAL HEMORRHAGE

The hemorrhagic diathesis and vasculopathy of severe dengue infection predisposes to intracranial hemorrhage which may result in encephalopathy. This has been demonstrated in several postmortem and neuroimaging studies (see Table 13.5). The

TABLE 13.5
Intracranial Hemorrhage in Dengue

Study	Patients with Encephalopathy	Cases with Intracranial Hemorrhage
Postmortem Diagnosis		
Burke 1968	12 (DHF)	2 intracerebral
		1 subarachnoid
		1 subdural
Nimmannitya et al. 1987	10 (DHF)	6 intracerebral
Janssen et al. 1998	1 (DF)	1 brainstem
Radiological Diagnosis		
Patey et al. 1993	1 (DHF)	1 subarachnoid (on CT and MRI)
Cam et al. 2001	27 (DHF)	1 unspecified (on MRI)
De Souza et al. 2005	1 (DSS)	1 brainstem (on CT and MRI)
Kumar et al. 2007	1 (DHF)	1 basal ganglia and intracerebral (on CT)
Kumar et al. 2009	5 (DHF)	3 basal ganglia (on CT)
		2 intracerebral and subdural (on CT)

distinction between postmortem and radiological diagnoses is important, as clinically significant microscopic and petechial brain hemorrhage may occur without obvious correlation on brain imaging; especially as much of the literature has utilized computed tomography (CT), which provides suboptimal images of the posterior fossa and could potentially miss small but significant hemorrhages in the brainstem.

13.8.4   DERANGED ELECTROLYTES

Several studies have reported an association between dengue infection and hyponatremia (Mekmullica 2005), with a recent study of 150 patients by Lumpaopong et al. (2010) showing that 61% of DF and 72% of DHF cases are mildly hyponatremic. Again, this is likely multifactorial, but is probably a result of intravascular volume depletion in severe dengue infection leading to pituitary release of anti-diuretic hormone (ADH) and plasma dilution. It is worth noting that viral encephalitis is a recognized cause of the syndrome of inappropriate ADH secretion (siADH).

Severe hyponatremia is generally taken as a serum sodium concentration below 125 mmol/L, the level below which cerebral edema occurs. When developing rapidly, a hyponatremic encephalopathy results. A more moderate and insidious decline in serum sodium is better-tolerated, and chronic hyponatremia is common and often asymptomatic. It appears that the hyponatremia in dengue infection tends to be fairly mild, and is unlikely to be the sole cause of encephalopathy.

13.8.5   CEREBRAL HYPOPERFUSION

Profound hypotension in DSS may result in hypoxic-ischemic encephalopathy, and Limonta et al. (2007) have demonstrated cell apoptoses in the brain tissue of fatal cases of DSS. Below a mean arterial pressure of approximately 50 mmHg, there is a failure of cerebral autoregulation and blood flow to the brain is compromised. There is a spectrum of presentation related to the severity of the ischemic insult and reflecting the selective vulnerability of various cell types. Neurons have a high metabolic activity and are highly vulnerable; following a period of global cerebral ischemia cellular dysfunction and death ensues, resulting in encephalopathy. The spatial distribution of ischemia and infarction is typically in the "watershed area," found in the border zone between the anterior and the middle cerebral arteries where perfusion has little physiological reserve. Widespread infarction is largely irreversible and carries a poor prognosis.

13.9   DENGUE ENCEPHALITIS

13.9.1   LITERATURE REVIEW

When you have eliminated the impossible, whatever remains, however improbable, must be the truth. Sherlock Holmes, *The Sign of the Four* (A. Conan Doyle 1988).

Dengue virus was previously believed to be nonneurotropic. It was thought that dengue encephalopathy must be a result of the systemic disruption that occurs in severe infection. Individual cases in which the encephalopathy was attributable to one or

TABLE 13.6
Isolating Dengue Encephalitis

Key Studies			
Study	Location	Patients	Exclusion Criteria
Kankirawatana et al. 2000	Bangkok, Thailand	8	All studies excluded:
Solomon et al. 2000	Ho Chi Minh City, Vietnam	9	Hepatic encephalopathy
Misra et al. 2006	Lucknow, India	11	Intracranial hemorrhage
Kularatne et al. 2008	Peradeniya, Sri Lanka	6	Electrolyte derangement
			Cerebral hypoperfusion

more of the causes outlined above (hepatic encephalopathy, cerebral edema, intra-cranial hemorrhage, deranged electrolytes, or cerebral hypoperfusion) lent credence to this view. However, with the increasing prevalence of dengue encephalopathy there has been a growing body of literature which identifies a subset of patients in which one of these causes cannot be identified. A parallel strand of evidence has emerged from the discovery of dengue virus and anti-dengue immunoglobulins in the CSF of these patients. Together, these findings strongly suggest that dengue virus is indeed neurotropic; it is capable of infection and replication within the central nervous system, and that therefore there exists a separate clinical entity which is correctly called *dengue encephalitis*.

Many of the early studies in this area were unable to adequately exclude other causes of encephalopathy and hence it is difficult to draw conclusions from them regarding encephalitis *per se*. Much of the literature is limited to case reports, which although instructive, are of limited statistical value. However, four studies with exhaustive exclusion criteria have provided the preliminary evidence. Table 13.6 outlines the key clinical studies supporting the hypothesis of dengue viral neurotropism. As discussed previously, cerebral edema is compatible with true viral encephalitis so is not included as an exclusion criterion.

13.9.2 CLINICAL FEATURES

The core clinical features of dengue encephalitis are fever, reduced consciousness, headache, and seizures (Varatharaj 2010)—the core features of any viral encephalitis. These are listed in Table 13.7. Numerous other features have been associated with dengue encephalitis and are outlined in Table 13.8.

The presence of classical features of dengue infection such as rash and arthralgia is variable. In two studies, 50% (Soares 2006) and 78% (Solomon 2000) of cases of dengue encephalitis did not have typical features of dengue infection. Thus, the absence of these features should not bar the consideration of dengue encephalitis as the diagnosis in a suitable patient.

Dengue encephalitis is more often a consequence of secondary than primary dengue infection (Varatharaj 2010). This likely reflects the role of the immune response (or lack thereof) in determining disease phenotype. In the key studies identified

TABLE 13.7
Core Clinical Features of Presumptive Dengue Encephalitis

Feature	Percentage of Cases
Fever	100
Reduced consciousness	100
Headache	65
Seizures	47

Source: Adapted from Varatharaj, A., 2010, *Neurol. India* 58(4), 585–91.

TABLE 13.8
Other Clinical Features Associated with Dengue Encephalitis

Feature	Study	Comments
Abnormal posturing	Solomon et al. 2000	Bilateral hippocampal hyperintensities on MRI.
Amnesia	Yeo et al. 2005	
Epilepsia partialis continua	Verma et al. 2010	Possibility of focal involvement of primary motor area.
Extensor plantars	Solomon et al. 2000	
Facial nerve palsy	Kankirawatana et al. 2000 Verma et al. 2010	
Frontal release signs	Solomon et al. 2000	Frontal lobe involvement.
Tetraparesis	Misra et al. 2006	Brainstem or spinal cord involvement.
Meningism	Solomon et al. 2000 Kankirawatana et al. 2000 Kularatne et al. 2008	Likely co-existent meningo-encephalitis.

above, the mean time of onset of neurological symptoms ranged from three to seven days from the start of fever. Consensus suggests that the clinical course of dengue encephalitis is relatively self-limiting, and that with intensive care most patients make a full recovery in days-weeks, with little or no residual deficits. The Lucknow patients were atypical in this regard, as out of 11, 3 died and 3 were left with residual deficits (Misra 2006). It is difficult to determine what interplay of viral, host, or medical factors were at play, but it would not be surprising to discover that different strains possess varying properties of neurovirulence, nor to find that certain hosts are more vulnerable. Clearly, this will be an important avenue of future research.

13.9.3 LABORATORY FEATURES

CSF lymphocytosis may occur and suggests a meningoencephalitic process. Reported frequencies range from 12.5% (Kankirawatana 2000) to 73% (Misra

2006). Although dengue virus or antibody is reliably isolated from the serum, evidence of dengue in the CSF (either antigen or antibody) is found in only a minority of patients, 17% in the four key studies. In another study dengue antibody was found in the CSF of only 2 out of 7 (29%) patients with dengue encephalitis (Soares 2006).

Is the presence of dengue virus and/or antibody in the CSF evidence of encephalitis? It could be argued that disruption of cerebral vascular endothelium allows serum contents to passively leak into the CSF, without active viral CNS invasion. This hypothesis is unsatisfying for three reasons. First, these patients with evidence of dengue in the CSF have an encephalopathy which cannot otherwise be explained, and it is parsimonious to conclude that viral neurotropism is the explanation. Second, virus may be present in the CSF while simultaneously absent in the serum, a finding which does not correspond with the suggestion of passive viral leak during the viremic phase (Domingues 2008). Third, histological studies have confirmed the presence of viral components in brain tissue, directly supporting the hypothesis of neurotropism (Miagostovich 1997; Ramos 2008).

It then remains to be explained why only a minority of patients with dengue encephalitis has detectable evidence of virus in the CSF. For comparison, detection of virus in the CSF by PCR has a sensitivity of >95% for herpes simplex encephalitis (Cinque 1996). Perhaps the apparent low sensitivity is due to a low CSF viral load, because even though PCR has a sensitivity of 93%–100% for serum dengue virus, this level of reliability requires a viral load of at least 100 genome copies (Lanciotti 1992). Kao et al. (2005) have commented that this problem applies to dengue antibody detection in the CSF. An additional problem is that the temporal fluctuations in CSF viral load and antibody titer are not known, and hence it is difficult to time sample collection to maximize sensitivity. These problems will need to be addressed by future studies.

13.9.4 RADIOLOGICAL FEATURES

Computed tomography (CT), magnetic resonance imaging (MRI), and other brain imaging modalities aid in the diagnosis of viral encephalitis. MRI provides more information than CT by delivering greater definition of brain parenchyma and improved views of the posterior fossa. Imaging helps with the exclusion of differential diagnoses and may also identify signs suggestive of viral encephalitis, such as cerebral edema, white matter changes, and localized necrosis. The addition of a gadolinium-based contrast agent identifies areas of BBB breakdown. Focal and asymmetrical abnormalities are suggestive of encephalitis over encephalopathy, the latter tending to produce more global and symmetrical changes.

Many viral encephalitides display a tropism for particular brain structures, which results in typical imaging patterns. The predilection of herpes simplex virus for the temporal lobes or that of Japanese encephalitis virus for the basal ganglia, is well-established. Is there is a similar tropism for dengue encephalitis, and corresponding features on brain imaging? A summary of reported brain imaging findings in dengue encephalitis is shown in Table 13.9. No stereotypical pattern of involvement has yet emerged, although the focal nature of abnormalities supports the diagnosis of encephalitis.

TABLE 13.9
Brain Imaging Findings in Dengue Encephalitis

Study	Imaging	Findings	Comments
Cam et al. 2001	MRI	Focal "encephalitis-like" changes	Authors did not specify location
Yeo et al. 2005	MRI	Bilateral hippocampal hyperintensity	Patient had retrograde amnesia
Misra et al. 2006	MRI	Largely normal, one showed hyperintensity in globus pallidus	
Muzaffar et al. 2006	MRI	Temporal lobe hyperintensity	
Kamble et al. 2007	CT	Thalamic hyperintensity	JE serology negative
Wasay et al. 2008	CT/MRI	Cerebral edema Focal changes in temporal, occipital, frontal lobes, and pons and upper spinal cord.	

13.9.5   DENGUE ENCEPHALITIS IN PERSPECTIVE

Sufficient evidence has now emerged to support the hypothesis of dengue viral neurotropism and establish the existence of dengue encephalitis as a distinct clinical entity. A case definition is outlined in Table 13.10. As several authors have pointed out, the validation and adoption of a uniform case definition will greatly aid the further recognition and study of this condition (Varatharaj 2011; Soares and Puccioni-Sohler 2011).

What is the impact of dengue encephalitis? Rather than taking patients with dengue and narrowing down to those with encephalitis, several studies have taken patients with encephalitis and filtered out those with dengue (see Table 13.11). Just as the clinician's thought-process works from presentation to etiology rather than vice-versa, these studies provide a very interesting picture of the real impact of dengue encephalitis. The results show that dengue is not just "on the list" of causes of viral encephalitis; in endemic areas it is an important agent and needs to be actively considered.

TABLE 13.10
Case Definition for Dengue Encephalitis

Dengue Virus or IgM in Serum		
Core Features	**Not Explained by**	**Corroborating Evidence**
Fever	Acute liver failure	CSF lymphocytic pleocytosis
Reduced consciousness	Shock	Dengue virus or IgM in CSF
Headache	Electrolyte derangement	Suggestive brain imaging
Seizures	Intracranial hemorrhage	

TABLE 13.11

Dengue as a Cause of Encephalitis in Endemic Areas

Study	Location	Patients	Frequency of Dengue (%)
Kankirawatana 2000	Thailand	Children with suspected viral encephalitis	18
Solomon et al. 2000	Vietnam	Children with suspected CNS infection	4.2
Horm Srey et al. 2002	Cambodia	Children and adults with suspected encephalitis	5
Van Tan et al. 2010	Vietnam	Children with suspected viral encephalitis	4.6
Soares et al. 2011	Brazil	Adults with suspected viral encephalitis	47

13.9.6 NEUROPATHOGENESIS

How does dengue defeat the BBB, and how does it damage neurons? Clearly, not all dengue infections result in encephalitis, so some interplay of host and viral factors is likely at work. Understanding these factors will be key in future efforts for prevention, detection, and treatment.

In general, viral entry to the central nervous system occurs via transmission through nerve axons or by spread across the BBB during viremia. There is no evidence to suggest that the former occurs with dengue, although retrograde spread through the olfactory nerve has been shown to occur with the related flaviviruses St. Louis encephalitis virus (Monath 1983) and Japanese encephalitis virus (Yamada 2009). In contrast, there is evidence to suggest that dengue may be able to weaken the BBB. Chaturvedi et al. (1991) showed that dengue virus causes BBB breakdown via a histamine-dependent pathway. This is notable given that mast cells are targets of dengue infection and are vulnerable to antibody-dependent enhancement in secondary infection (Brown et al. 2006). Mast cell infection results in the release of various vasoactive and immunologically active cytokines (King et al. 2002; St John et al. 2011), and it is known that products of mast cell degranulation, including histamine, result in BBB breakdown (Abbott 2000). Thus, it seems reasonable to postulate that a defective immune response in secondary dengue infection coupled with the ability of infected mast cells to open the BBB may a play a role in dengue neurovirulence.

Little is known about the specific effects of dengue on neurons. In general, neurotropic viruses cause neuronal cell death either by direct cytopathic effects or by inducing a fatal immune response against infected cells. Amaral et al. (2011) have shown that dengue virus (DEN-3) injected directly into the brains of mice results in behavioral changes, seizures, and death (an encephalitis-like syndrome). Viral load within the brain increased with time, suggesting active infection and replication, and a CNS inflammatory response was stimulated, resulting in inflammatory cell infiltration and the release of cytokines.

13.10 DENGUE TRANSVERSE MYELITIS

Transverse myelitis is an inflammatory condition of the spinal cord. Presentation depends on the level of involvement but typically there is initial flaccid paraparesis

TABLE 13.12
Dengue Transverse Myelitis

Author	Time to Onset of Paraparesis	Recovery Period
Solomon et al. 2000	4–5 days	Improvement after 7–15 days with some residual symptoms
Leao et al. 2002	12 days (although urinary retention developed after 2 days)	Improvement after 35 days, full recovery after 6 months
Chanthamat and Sathirapanya 2010	6 days	Improvement after 10 days, full recovery after 1 year

which evolves into spasticity, reflecting interruption of descending corticospinal fibers. Sphincters are often involved, and a sensory level is characteristic. The cause is typically either demyelinating disease, such as multiple sclerosis, neuromyelitis optica or acute disseminated encephalomyelitis; systemic inflammatory disease such as lupus or sarcoidosis; or related to infections such as with herpesviruses, flaviviruses, and bacteria such as *Borrelia burgdorferi*. In infectious transverse myelitis, cord involvement typically occurs contemporaneously with the febrile phase of illness, and there is usually a CSF reaction with cells and protein.

Transverse myelitis occurring in the acute phase of dengue infection has been recorded in the literature (see Table 13.12). In these cases the onset of paraparesis coincided with the febrile phase of illness, so it is reasonable to suppose the etiology is para-infectious rather than postinfectious. However, it remains to be seen whether the underlying mechanism is direct viral infiltration or an immune phenomenon.

13.11 PERIPHERAL NERVOUS SYSTEM MANIFESTATIONS

13.11.1 Guillain-Barré Syndrome

The term "Guillain-Barré syndrome" describes the clinical picture of an acute inflammatory demyelinating polyradiculoneuropathy, with variable motor, sensory, and autonomic involvement. The typical presentation is with ascending symmetrical paralysis and areflexia, which may progress to respiratory weakness and failure. The majority of cases are preceded by an infection, often *Campylobacter jejuni*, although numerous antecedent infections have been associated. The etiology is thought to be molecular mimicry leading to immunological cross-reactivity against nerve components.

Several authors have reported cases of Guillain-Barré syndrome associated with dengue infection (Chew et al. 1998; Esack et al. 1999; Leão et al. 2002; Santo et al. 2004; Sulekha et al. 2004; Kumar et al. 2005; Soares et al. 2006; Chen and Lee 2007; Soares et al. 2008; Gupta et al. 2009; Chanthamat and Sathirapanya 2010). In all cases typical features of DF/DHF were initially present, followed by a delay ranging from 7 to 30 days before the onset of paralysis. CSF analysis and nerve conduction studies have yielded results consistent with classical Guillain-Barré,

namely cytoalbuminemic dissociation (high protein and low cells) with demyelination and/or denervation. Intravenous immunoglobulin has been used with good
outcomes.

13.11.2 Mononeuropathy

Post-infectious mononeuropathies have also been reported in association with dengue. Case reports describe involvement of phrenic (Chien et al. 2008; Ansari et al.
2010), long thoracic (Chappuis et al. 2004), optic (Sanjay et al. 2008), facial (Patey
et al. 1993), and ulnar and peroneal (Kaplan and Lindgren 1945) nerves. As with
postinfectious Guillain-Barré syndrome, there is a delay of days or weeks between
the initial infection and the development of neurological symptoms, reflecting the
presumed immunological etiology. Immunosuppressive therapies have been used in
a range of dengue mononeuropathies with variable success.

13.11.3 Myositis

Myalgia has long been recognized as a characteristic feature of dengue infection,
even more so than with other viral illnesses. Muscle biopsies in uncomplicated dengue have shown inflammatory cell infiltrates, with rare myonecrosis (Malheiros
1993). In some cases, however, the disease may progress to frank myositis with
variable degrees of muscle breakdown, weakness, and elevation of serum creatine
kinase (CK). These patients have tender muscles, flaccid weakness, and typically
no evidence of CNS involvement. CSF analysis and neuro-imaging are normal, and
evidence of dengue infection is obtained from the serum but not the CSF. Muscle
biopsies in these cases shown dense inflammatory cell infiltrates (Kalita et al. 2005;
Paliwal et al. 2011). Interestingly, Paliwal et al. (2011) have identified two distinct
presentations of dengue myositis, which likely represent points on a spectrum of
underlying immune responses. In primary infections, myositis featuring predominantly lower limb weakness developed 3–15 days after dengue symptoms, and was
associated with a moderate rise in CK. These patients gradually recovered over
weeks, with a good outcome. In secondary infections, however, patients experienced
a delay of several weeks before the onset of a rapidly progressive myositis, with generalized skeletal muscle dysfunction and respiratory failure, massively elevated CK,
and poor outcome.

Management of dengue myositis is supportive, with an emphasis on early
respiratory support for patients at risk of ventilatory failure. Some groups have
found benefit from immunosuppression (Finsterer and Kongchan 2006), a strategy that has been used with some success in HIV-associated myositis (Johnson
et al. 2003). A rhabdomyolysis-like picture may occur in conjunction with renal
failure due to glomerular deposition of myoglobin, which can be prevented by
vigorous hydration (Davis and Bourke 2004; Lim and Goh 2005; Acharya et
al. 2010). Transvere myelitis and Guillain-Barré syndrome should be excluded
as other causes of a dengue-associated weakness, as these may have different
therapeutic options.

Thus, muscle involvement in dengue infection runs along a spectrum from myalgia and benign self-limiting myositis to fulminant myositis. The pathology is unclear and may variably reflect direct viral infiltration of myocytes (Salgado et al. 2010) or an immune-mediated insult. The increased severity associated with secondary infections is in keeping with other manifestations and does suggest a degree of immunopathogenesis.

13.12 LABORATORY DIAGNOSIS OF DENGUE INFECTION

13.12.1 GENERAL INVESTIGATIONS

In uncomplicated DF, routine blood tests are usually normal. In DHF/DSS, however, the full blood count invariably shows thrombocytopenia and elevated hematocrit. The white cell count (WCC) is variable, and there may be a reactive lymphocytosis; however, a neutropenia and fall in total WCC at the end of the febrile phase is almost universal. Clotting analysis shows a coagulopathy with an increase in APTT (activated partial thromboplastin time) and PT (prothrombin time). Plasma albumin is low due to vascular leak, and liver enzymes may be deranged in the presence or absence of apparent hepatic failure. Additionally, in DSS metabolic acidosis, hyponatremia, and deranged renal function may be seen.

13.12.2 CONFIRMING DENGUE INFECTION

It is a general principle in the laboratory diagnosis of viral infections that one may aim to detect either the virus or the host immune response (Table 13.13). Which strategy to pursue is a decision that is based on timing. The initial febrile stage of infection corresponds with the viremic phase, so it is sensible to aim to detect the virus. In an immunocompetent individual, after about 5 days, there is an immune response that abolishes detectable viremia and defervesence ensues. Hence, in these patients, it is more suitable to aim to detect the host immune response.

TABLE 13.13
Laboratory Methods of Confirming Dengue Infection

Detection of Virus

Viral culture
PCR amplification of viral RNA
Immunochemistry for viral antigens

Detection of Host Immune Response

MAC-ELISA for anti-dengue IgM
Hemagglutination-inhibition (HI) test

13.12.3 DETECTION OF VIRUS

Detection of the virus has traditionally been achieved by viral culture, and this remains the gold-standard test, though it is time-consuming and costly. Specimens must be collected before defervescence or soon after, as the humoral response interferes with culture. Excessive heat may inactivate the virus, and specimens must be transported chilled. The sample is then inoculated into larval or adult mosquitoes of the genus *Toxorhynchites*. After a few days, in which almost all tissues of the inoculated mosquito become infiltrated by virus, a tissue smear is prepared from the head of the mosquito and examined by immunofluorescence. Alternatively, samples may be inoculated into mosquito cell culture (typically the C6/36 clone from *Aedes albopictus*) with comparable results, and this method is now widely used.

The second option is detection of viral RNA by PCR (polymerase chain reaction) assay. PCR is quicker, more widely available, can detect viremia regardless of disease phase, and can be used to differentiate serotypes based on distinct genetic sequences. Viral RNA is extracted and purified from the sample and the desired sequences are rapidly amplified using a combination of specific primers. The amplified product which results is separated and identified by agarose gel electrophoresis. A well-validated PCR assay developed by Lanciotti et al. (1992) demonstrates sensitivities of 94% (DEN-1), 93% (DEN-2), and 100% (DEN-3 and -4). However, the disadvantage of PCR is that it is susceptible to sample contamination and false-positives, which may result from nonspecific primer binding or binding to conserved sequences of other flaviviruses.

The third option now emerging is detection of viral antigens by immunochemistry. An interesting candidate currently being investigated is the NS1 antigen. In a recent multicenter trial with 1385 patients, one commercially available assay kit had a reported sensitivity and specificity of 64% and 100%, respectively (Guzman et al. 2010). In a smaller trial, another group achieved a sensitivity of 89% (Dussart et al. 2006). This test has the advantage of being easier and quicker than culture, cheaper than PCR, and can be used in the acute phase unlike serology. The poor sensitivity is a problem, however, and further work is needed.

13.12.4 DETECTION OF HOST IMMUNE RESPONSE

Detection of the host immune response (serology) has numerous advantages. Specimen collection is not time-critical, as antibodies persist for several weeks, and there is little risk of inactivation by heat. Serological assays are also fairly simple to use, and widely available as self-contained kits. The commonly used technique is MAC-ELISA (IgM antibody-capture enzyme-linked immunosorbent assay) which measures "dengue-specific" IgM. The presence of IgM antibodies indicates recent infection (within 24 weeks), and it is possible to confirm acute infection by demonstrating rising antibody titers in paired acute and convalescent samples. The main disadvantage of serological tests is that they have a poor sensitivity in the acute phase of infection, before the development of an immune response. There also have a limited specificity as there is an element of cross-reactivity with antibodies against other flaviviruses, especially in areas where dengue and Japanese encephalitis co-circulate. In an evaluation of one commonly-used proprietary MAC-ELISA kit, the initial sensitivity was 69% rising to 90% on convalescent testing, while specificity was 80% (Singh et al. 2006).

IgG antibody-capture ELISA (GAC-ELISA) is also available. Low titers of IgG become detectable after the first week and continue to rise for months. These likely persist for life, though eventually at concentrations which may become undetectable. By paired ELISA, the ratio of IgM to IgG can be calculated and this allows the differentiation of primary (predominantly IgM) from secondary (predominantly IgG) infections.

The hemagglutination-inhibition test has been largely superseded by newer methods. The serum sample is added to a fixed dose of dengue antigens. When red blood cells are added the antigens normally cause hemagglutination. In the presence of anti-dengue antibodies this hemagglutination is inhibited to a degree which is quantifiable and corresponds to antibody titer.

13.13 MANAGEMENT

13.13.1 Dengue Fever

No specific treatment exists for dengue infection. Treatment is supportive and aimed toward the early detection and management of complications. In DF, control of fever may be achieved with cautious use of paracetamol. Aspirin is best avoided due to the antiplatelet effect and the risk of precipitating Reye's syndrome. Adequate nutrition should be ensured and, if necessary, oral rehydration therapy considered. Close monitoring for signs of conversion to DHF/DSS is essential, especially around the period of defervescence. It must be remembered that in the early stage it is difficult to accurately predict which patients will go on to develop severe infection; regular monitoring is the only sure strategy. In practice, this means that after an initial assessment (see Table 13.14) most cases with nonsevere infection and no warning

TABLE 13.14
Initial Assessment

History	Examination	Investigation
Time of onset of fever	Hydration	Full blood count
Oral intake	Hemodynamic stability	Urea and electrolytes
Warning signs	Respiratory distress, pleural effusion	Baseline hematocrit
Diarrhea	Abdominal tenderness, hepatomegaly,	Confirmation of dengue infection
Urine output	ascites	(not usually necessary in
Dengue in family or	Rash, bleeding	uncomplicated cases)
neighborhood	Tourniquet test	
Travel history	Neurological manifestations	
Medical history		

signs may be managed as outpatients, with daily examination and monitoring of platelet count and hematocrit.

13.13.2 DENGUE HEMORRHAGIC FEVER AND SHOCK

Management of DHF rests upon the careful replacement of intravascular fluid and electrolyte losses. Early fluid resuscitation avoids complications. In mild cases fluid replacement may be oral; if so oral rehydration solutions as used for diarrhea are ideal. Again, close monitoring is required, especially during defervescence. Signs of hemodynamic compromise or fall in platelet count and elevation of hematocrit are indications for parenteral therapy. Isotonic solutions of crystalloid may be infused at a rate of 5–7ml/kg/hr, adjusted according to response. Fluid replacement should be carefully titrated to hemodynamic status and urine output (aiming for above 0.5ml/kg/hr), to avoid the risk of overload. In patients with warning signs, further laboratory tests including blood glucose, renal function, liver function, and clotting should also be monitored.

DSS is a medical emergency and the aim should be to urgently expand plasma volume. Crystalloid or colloid should be given in a bolus of 10–20 ml/kg in order to support effective circulation and organ perfusion. According to response the rate of infusion may be gradually reduced to a maintenance regime. Again, strict fluid balance is required to optimize intravascular filling and avoid overload. If there are signs of bleeding or a falling hematocrit then urgent tranfusion should be arranged along with, if appropriate, specific interventions to arrest the bleeding point (e.g., urgent endoscopy in the case of upper gastrointestinal tract hemorrhage). Ideally the patient should be managed in an intensive care setting, with invasive monitoring of physiological parameters.

13.13.3 DENGUE ENCEPHALOPATHY

As has been discussed previously, the term "dengue encephalopathy" covers a range of mechanisms which may cause cerebral insult. The etiological distinction is of critical importance if effective management is to be delivered, and hence these patients require a detailed diagnostic work-up (see Table 13.15).

If a nonencephalitic etiology is established, it may be managed according to established protocols. All are best handled in an intensive care or high dependency unit.

Current strategies to manage *hepatic encephalopathy* focus on control of the raised serum ammonia levels which result from impaired hepatic detoxification (Bernal et al. 2010). Lactulose is commonly given for this reason as it reduces the number of ammonia-forming gut bacteria, as well as acidifying the contents so as to convert NH_4^- to NH_3 and potentiate the excretion of ammonia. Antibiotics such as neomycin may also be given with the same purpose of reducing gut bacterial load. If these methods fail, serum ammonia concentrations may be reduced directly by hemofiltration. There is some evidence that therapeutic hypothermia slows cellular metabolism and production of ammonia, though this strategy is not yet widely used

TABLE 13.15
Investigation of Dengue Encephalopathy

Test	Findings
Hemodynamic monitoring	Prolonged hypotension suggests hypoxic-ischemic encephalopathy
Electrolytes	Low sodium suggests hyponatremic encephalopathy
	Raised creatinine suggests acute renal failure and uremic encephalopathy
Liver function tests	Raised bilirubin, transaminases, and prothrombin time suggest acute liver
Clotting tests	failure and hepatic encephalopathy
Lumbar puncture	Lymphocytosis and evidence of dengue in CSF suggests encephalitis
	Red cells and xanthrochromia suggests hemorrhage
Brain imaging	Intracranial hemorrhage
	Cerebral edema
	Focal changes suggestive of encephalitis
EEG	Generalized changes of encephalopathy (e.g., slowing)
	Focal changes suggestive of encephalitis (e.g., periodic lateralized epileptiform discharges)
	Seizure activity

(Vaquero et al. 2005). Ultimately, however, the only effective treatment for severe hepatic encephalopathy is liver transplantation.

Cerebral edema requires the careful control of several physiological parameters, and it may be necessary to surgically implant an intracranial pressure (ICP) monitoring device to better guide the fine adjustment of these variables. Management can then be instigated in a step-wise fashion. Nursing in a head-up position is a starting point; this aims to reduce ICP, however, and care must be taken not to compromise cerebral perfusion. As hypoxia and hypercapnia both result in cerebral vasodilation, it is important to ensure good oxygenation and carbon dioxide clearance. If necessary, this may be achieved by therapeutic hyperventilation. Careful fluid balance is needed to maintain cerebral perfusion pressure without exacerbating fluid overload. Electrolyte levels should be corrected to maintain serum osmolarity, as hypo-osmolarity worsens cerebral edema. If these holding measures fail then mannitol, an osmotically active diuretic, may be used to draw water from the brain parenchyma into the intravascular space. Hypertonic saline solutions may be used in a similar way. In more desperate situations it may be possible to induce a therapeutic coma using drugs such as phenobarbital, which suppress cerebral metabolism and reduce ICP. Finally, in the case of catastrophic brain swelling and impending herniation the only option is decompressive craniectomy.

General medical management of *intracranial hemorrhage* is largely supportive. Cerebral autoregulation is impaired in the acute phase so adjustments to blood pressure (which is often high) should be avoided for fear of compromising perfusion. As to specific data on the management of intracranial hemorrhage in dengue, there is little available evidence. It is unclear to what extent dengue hemorrhagic encephalopathy reflects damage to cerebral vascular endothelium, bleeding diathesis, or exacerbation of preexisting cerebrovascular disease. However, as the bleeding diathesis likely plays at least some role, it would seem reasonable to correct the clotting abnormalities, and some groups have used platelet transfusion for this purpose (Kumar et al. 2009). In some cases it may be appropriate to use fresh frozen plasma (FFP), prothrombin complex concentrate (PCC), or even activated factor VII (fVIIa). A large hemorrhage may cause a significant mass effect, especially in the confined space of the posterior fossa, and if there are signs of raised intracranial pressure it may be necessary to perform a decompressive craniectomy or urgent CSF shunting.

Hyponatremic encephalopathy is managed by correcting the serum sodium. In dengue the patient is likely to be intravascularly volume deplete so this may be achieved by the judicious use of intravenous 0.9% saline. Too-rapid (more than 8mmol/L/day) correction of the serum sodium should be avoided, as this carries a risk of precipitating central pontine myelinolysis.

Hypoxic–ischemic encephalopathy carries a poor prognosis. The initial priority of management is to stabilize hemodynamic status and secure cerebral perfusion. As fever and seizure activity both increase brain metabolic activity, these should be suppressed. There is great interest in the application of therapeutic hypothermia for reducing brain metabolism, and early results have been promising.

13.13.4 DENGUE ENCEPHALITIS

General management of viral encephalitis requires close support in an intensive care setting, with meticulous attention to the airway, to oxygenation, hydration, and nutrition (Solomon et al. 2007). Seizure activity should be suppressed with anti-epileptic drugs, and intracranial pressure should be carefully monitored and controlled. Until bacterial infection and HSV encephalitis have been positively excluded by analysis of the CSF, empirical treatment with a third-generation cephalosporin and acyclovir should be continued. As an inhibitor of viral DNA polymerase, however, acyclovir has no effect on the RNA replication of dengue virus. With no specific antiviral yet available, management of a confirmed case of dengue encephalitis must focus on intensive organ support. If the illness is indeed self-limiting, as has been suggested, then this approach may buy enough time to allow recovery.

13.13.5 FUTURE TREATMENTS

There is currently no clinically available antiviral effective against dengue, though an increasing understanding of the molecular basis of dengue pathogenesis has provided an array of potential drug targets. A combination of high-throughput screening with intelligent drug design has yielded various agents which have shown promise for future use (see Table 13.16). All are currently in laboratory stages of development and much further work is needed before large-scale clinical trials can be conducted. From a CNS standpoint, one must also consider the question of drug delivery across the BBB if a viable treatment for dengue encephalitis is to be developed.

TABLE 13.16
Potential Dengue Antivirals

Agent	Putative Targets	Studies
Amantadine	Viral entry	(*in vitro*) Koff et al. 1980
Zosteric acid	Viral entry	(*in vitro*) Rees et al. 2008
Ribavirin	RNA synthesis	(*in vitro*) Koff et al. 1982
		(in mice) Koff et al. 1983
Interferon	RNA synthesis	(*in vitro*) Diamond et al. 2000
		(in monkeys) Ajariyakhajorn et al. 2005
Triaryl pyrazoline	RNA synthesis	(*in vitro*) Puig-Basagoiti et al. 2006
Morpholino oligomers	RNA synthesis	(in mice) Stein et al. 2006
Geneticin	RNA synthesis	(*in vitro*) Zhang et al. 2009
	Translation	
Protease inhibitors	Viral protease	(*in vitro*) Tomlinson et al. 2009

13.14   VACCINATION

There is currently no effective vaccine against dengue. However, recent decades have seen great leaps forward in vaccine development, and promising candidates are now nearing clinical reality.

As our current understanding of dengue pathogenesis suggests that the primary protective host response is the initiation of specific neutralizing antibodies, the ideal dengue vaccine should generate high and long-lasting antibody titers to cover all four viral serotypes (tetravalence). Given the suspected role of antibody-dependent enhancement in severe dengue infection, full tetravalency is crucial to avoid the theoretical risk that an incomplete dengue vaccine may predispose toward enhanced infection by an omitted serotype, especially as all four serotypes are now in widespread co-circulation. This requirement has proved to be a significant challenge.

TABLE 13.17
Dengue Vaccine Candidates

Vaccine	Type	Comments
ChimeriVax	Chimeric live attenuated virus on yellow fever backbone	Safe, immunogenic, but requires extended multiple-dose course
DEN4Δ30	Live virus attenuated by gene deletion	Effective monovalent vaccine, tetravalent formulation currently in trials
DENVax	Chimeric live attenuated dengue virus	
DEN-80E	Recombinant envelope protein	Less interference between serotypes
D1ME-VR-P	DNA vaccine of envelope and membrane genes	

Source: Adapted from Webster, D. P. et al., 2009, *Lancet Infect. Dis.* 9, 678–87; Coller, B. G., and Clements, D. E., 2011, *Curr. Opin. Immunol.* 23, 1–8.

Creating a tetravalent vaccine which generates a balanced immune response requires overcoming interference between the separate components. Promising candidate vaccines currently in development are shown in Table 13.17.

13.15   VECTOR CONTROL

An integrated strategy for the management of dengue will necessarily require control of the insect vectors. The highly resistant eggs of *Aedes aegypti* mean that it is insufficient to attempt eradication of the mosquitoes, their larvae, and pupae alone, as following rain the population will be regenerated from quiescent eggs. Thus, a many-pronged approach is required, involving the eradication of adult and larval forms with insecticides coupled with the clearing out and elimination of suitable nesting locations. Clearly, this process is related to economic development and increasing standards of public health and sanitation. The World Health Organization has developed detailed guidelines for Integrated Vector Management (IVM), which promote a multidisciplinary strategy operating at a range of levels from individual to government (Table 13.18).

13.16   CONCLUSION

Dengue infections are common worldwide and represent a significant burden to global health. The individual clinical manifestations of infection encompass a broad spectrum of disease states, and represent the outcome of complex human-viral interactions. The virus has the capacity to disrupt all major organ systems with results that range from benign to fatal. Neurological manifestations of dengue infection have long been appreciated as part of this spectrum. Although relatively infrequent, the vast scale of the dengue problem means that the absolute incidence is significant. Whereas these presentations were previously thought to be indirectly mediated, decades of research now suggest that the dengue virus is truly neurovirulent, and that dengue encephalitis is a significant entity in endemic areas. An increasing appreciation of the neurological manifestations of dengue infection will advance our understanding of dengue viral-human interactions in general. Some future research questions are outlined in Table 13.18. In particular, understanding the interplay of host and viral factors that determine the clinical outcome of infection in any given

---

TABLE 13.18

Future Research in Neurological Dengue

What is the temporal pattern of CSF viral load and antibody titer?

What is the sensitivity of PCR and ELISA in CSF?

What are imaging features that characterise dengue encephalitis?

What is the role of mast cells in CNS penetration?

What viral and host factors influence dengue neurotropism?

What is the efficacy of novel antiviral agents in the treatment of dengue encephalitis?

What is the mortality, morbidity, and economic impact of neurological dengue?

individual will be an important step forward that will aid the search for an effective management strategy. The worldwide public health and economic ramifications of the dengue problem are vast, and have driven efforts to achieve a sustainable solution. Aggressive vector control, widespread deployment of an effective vaccine, and development of specific antiviral agents will all help to reduce the burden of this pernicious disease. The next decades will show if these efforts are successful in halting the continued spread of the dengue virus.

ACKNOWLEDGEMENT

I thank A. J. Phillips (University of Cambridge) for assistance with obtaining references.

REFERENCES

Abbott, N. J. 2000. Inflammatory mediators and modulation of blood-brain barrier permeability. *Cell. Mol. Neurobiol* 20(2), 131–47.

Acharya, S., Shukla, S., Mahajan, S. N., and Diwan, S. K. 2010. Acute dengue myositis with rhabdomyolysis and acute renal failure. *Ann. Indian Acad. Neurol.* 13(3), 221–2.

Ajariyakhajorn, C., Mammen Jr., M. P., Endy, T. P., Gettayacamin, M., Nisalak, A., Nimmannitya, S., and Libraty, D. H. 2005. Randomized, placebo-controlled trial of non-pegylated and pegylated forms of recombinant human alpha interferon 2a for suppression of dengue virus viremia in rhesus monkeys. *Antimicrob. Agents Chemother.* 49, 4508–14.

Amaral, D. C., Rachid, M. A., Vilela, M. C., Campos, R. D., Ferreira, G. P., Rodrigues, D. H. et al. 2011. Intracerebral infection with dengue-3 virus induces meningoencephalitis and behavioural changes that precede lethality in mice. *J. Neuroinflam.* 8, 23.

Ansari, M. K., Jha, S., and Nath, A. 2010. Unilateral diaphragmatic paralysis following dengue infection. *Neurol. India.* 58, 596–8.

Arunachalam, N., Tewari, S. C., Thenmozhi, V., Rajendran, R., Paramasivan, R., Manavalan, R. et al. 2008. Natural vertical transmission of dengue viruses by Aedes aegypti in Chennai, Tamil Nadu, India. *Indian J. Med. Res.* 127, 395–7.

Ashburn, P. M., and Craig, C. F. 1907. Experimental Investigations Regarding the Etiology of Dengue. *J. Infect. Dis.* 4, 440–75.

Avirutnan, P., Punyadee, N., and Noisakran, S. 2006. Vascular leakage in severe dengue virus infections: a potential role for the nonstructural viral protein NS1 and complement. *J. Infect. Dis.* 193, 1078–88.

Bernal, W., Auzinger, G., Dhawan, A., and Wendon, J. 2010. Acute liver failure. *Lancet.* 376, 190–201.

Brown, M. G., King, C. A., Sherren, C., Marshall, J. S., and Anderson, R. 2006. A dominant role for FcgammaRII in antibody-enhanced dengue virus infection of human mast cells and associated CCL5 release. *J. Leukoc. Biol.* 80(6), 1242–50.

Burke, T. 1968. Dengue haemorrhagic fever: a pathological study. *Trans. R. Soc. Trop. Med. Hyg.* 62(5), 682–92.

Cam, B. V., Fonsmark, L., Hue, N. B., Phuong, N. T., Poulsen, A., and Heegaard, E. D. 2001. Prospective case-control study of encephalopathy in children with dengue hemorrhagic fever. *Am. J. Trop. Med. Hyg.* 65, 848–51.

Chanthamat, N., and Sathirapanya, P. 2010. Acute transverse myelitis associated with dengue viral infection. *J. Spinal Cord Med.* 33(4), 425–7.

Chappuis, F., Justafré, J. C., Duchunstang, L., Loutan, L., and Taylor, W. R. 2004. Dengue fever and long thoracic nerve palsy in a traveller returning from Thailand. *J. Travel. Med.* 11(2), 112–4.

Chaturvedi, U. C., Dhawan, R., Khanna, M., and Mathur, A. 1991. Breakdown of the blood-brain barrier during dengue virus infection of mice. *J. Gen. Virol.* 72, 859–66.

Chen,. T. Y., and Lee, C. T. 2007. Guillain-Barré syndrome following dengue fever. *Ann. Emerg. Med.* 50, 94–5.

Chew, N. K., Goh, K. J., Omar, S., and Tan, C. T. 1998. Guillain-Barré syndrome with antecedent dengue infection—a report of two cases. *Neurol. J. Southeast Asia.* 3, 85–6.

Chien, J., Ong, A., and Low, S. Y. 2008. An unusual complication of dengue infection. *Singapore Med. J.* 49, e340.

Chimelli, L., Hahn, M. D., Netto, M. B., Ramos, R. G., Dias, M., and Gray, F. 1990. Dengue: neuropathological findings in 5 fatal cases from Brazil. *Clin. Neuropathol.* 9(3), 157–62.

Chye, J. K., Lim, C. T., Ng, K. B., Lim, J. M., George, R., and Lam, S. K. 1997. Vertical transmission of dengue. *Clin. Infect. Dis.* 25(6), 1374–7.

Cinque, P., Cleator, G. M., Weber, T., Monteyne, P., Sindic, C. J., and van Loon, A. M. 1996. The role of laboratory investigation in the diagnosis and management of patients with suspected herpes simplex encephalitis: a consensus report. The EU concerted action on virus meningitis and encephalitis. *J. Neurol. Neurosurg. Psychiatry.* 61(4), 339–45.

Cleland, J. B., and Bradley, B. 1919. Further Experiments in the etiology of dengue fever. *J. Hyg.* 18(3), 217–54.

Coller, B. G., and Clements, D. E. 2011. Dengue vaccines: progress and challenges. *Curr. Opin. Immunol.* 23, 1–8.

Conan Doyle, A. 1988. The sign of the four, In: *The Penguin Complete Sherlock Holmes.* Penguin, London.

Davis, J. S., and Bourke, P. 2004. Rhabdomyolysis associated with dengue virus infection. *Clin. Infect. Dis.* 38, e109–11.

de Souza, L. J., Martins, A. L., Paravidini, P. C., Nogueira, R. M., Gicovate Neto, C., Bastos, D. A. et al. 2005. Hemorrhagic encephalopathy in dengue shock syndrome: a case report. *Braz. J. Infect. Dis.* 9(3), 257–61.

Dejnirattisai, W., Jumnainsong, A., Onsirisakul, N., Fitton, P., Vasanawathana, S., Limpitikul, W. et al. 2010. Cross-reacting antibodies enhance dengue virus infection in humans. *Science.* 328(5979), 745–8.

Dengue Bulletin Volume 24, 2000. Retrieved October 1, 2011 from http://www.searo.who.int/en/Section10/Section332/Section522_2513.htm.

Diamond, M. S., Roberts, T. G., Edgil, D., Lu, B., Ernst, J., and Harris, E. 2000. Modulation of dengue virus infection in human cells by alpha, beta, and gamma interferons. *J. Virol.* 74, 4957–66.

Documentation of the 2005 World Health Assembly. Retrieved October 1, 2011 from http://apps.who.int/gb/e/e_wha58.html.

Domingues, R. B., Kuster, G. W., Onuki-Castro, F. L., Souza, V. A., Levi, J. E., and Pannuti, C. S. 2008. Involvement of the central nervous system in patients with dengue virus infection. *J. Neurol. Sci.* 267, 36–40.

Dussart, P., Labeau, B., Lagathu, G., Louis, P., Nunes, M. R. T., and Rodrigues, S. G. et al. 2006. Evaluation of an enzyme immunoassay for detection of dengue virus NS1 antigen in human serum. *Clin. Vacc. Immunol.* 13(11), 1185–9.

Esack, A., Teelucksingh, S., and Singh, N. 1999. The Guillain-Barré syndrome following dengue fever. *West Indian Med J.* 48, 36–7.

Finsterer, J., and Kongchan, K. 2006. Severe, persisting, steroid-responsive dengue myositis. *J. Clin. Virol.* 35, 426–8.

Forshey, B. M., Guevara, C., Laguna-Torres, V. A., Cespedes, M., Vargas, J. et al. 2010. Arboviral Etiologies of Acute Febrile Illnesses in Western South America, 2000–2007. *PLoS. Negl. Trop. Dis.* 4(8), e787.

Freedman, D. O., Weld, L. H., Kozarsky, P. E., Fisk, T., Robins, R., von Sonnenburg, F. et al. 2006. Spectrum of Disease and Relation to Place of Exposure among Ill Returned Travelers. *NEJM.* 354, 119–30.

Godding, C. C. 1890. An account of an obscure outbreak of dengue occurring aboard HMS Agamemmnon while stationed at Zanzibar between November, 1888, and September, 1889. *BMJ.* 1(1520), 352–354.

Gupta, P., Jain, V., Chatterjee, S., and Agarwal, A. K. 2009. Acute inflammatory motor axonopathy associated with dengue fever. *J. Indian Academy Clin. Med.* 10, 58–9.

Guzman, M. G., Kouri, G., and Soler, M. 1992. Dengue 2 virus enhancement in asthmatic and nonasthmatic individuals. *Mem. Inst. Oswaldo. Cruz.* 87, 559–64.

Guzman, M. G., Kouri, G., Bravo, J. et al. 2002. Effect of age on outcome of secondary dengue 2 infections. *Int. J. Infect. Dis.* 6, 118–24.

Guzman, M. G., Jaenisch, T., Gaczkowski, R., Ty Hang, V. T., Sekaran, S. D., Kroeger, A. et al. 2010. Multi-country evaluation of the sensitivity and specificity of two commercially-available NS1 ELISA assays for dengue diagnosis. *PLoS. Negl. Trop. Dis.* 4(8), e811.

Halstead, S. B. 2007. Dengue. *Lancet.* 370, 1644–52.

Henchal, E. A., and Putnak, J. R. 1990. The dengue viruses. *Clin. Microbiol. Rev.* 3(4), 376–396.

Hendarto, S. K., and Hadinegoro, S. R. 1992. Dengue encephalopathy. *Acta Paediatr. Jpn.* 34(3), 350–7.

Horm Srey, V., Sadones, H., Ong, S., Mam, M., Yim, C., Sor, S. et al. 2002. Etiology of encephalitis syndrome among hospitalized children and adults in Takeo, Cambodia, 1999–2000. *Am. J. Trop. Med. Hyg.* 66(2), 200–207.

International Human Genome Sequencing Consortium (IHGSC). 2001. Initial sequencing and analysis of the human genome. *Nature* 409, 860–921.

Janssen, H. L., Bienfait, H. P., Jansen, C. L., van Duinen, S. G., Vriesendorp, R., Schimsheimer, R. J. et al. 1998. Fatal cerebral edema associated with primary dengue infection. *J. Infect.* 36(3), 344–6.

Johnson, R. W., Williams, F. M., Kazi, S., Dimachkie, M. M., and Reveille, J. D. 2003. Human immunodeficiency virus-associated polymyositis: a longitudinal study of outcome. *Arthritis Rheum.* 49(2), 172–8.

Kabra, S. K., Jain, Y., Pandey, R. M. et al. 1999. Dengue haemorrhagic fever in children in the 1996 Delhi epidemic. *Trans. R. Soc. Trop. Med. Hyg.* 93, 294–8.

Kalita, J., Misra, U. K., Mahadevan, A., and Shankar, S. K. 2005. Acute pure motor quadriplegia: is it dengue myositis? *Electromyogr. Clin. Neurophysiol.* 45, 357–61.

Kamble, R., Peruvamba, J. N., Kovoor, J., Ravishankar, S., and Kolar, B. S. 2007. Bilateral thalamic involvement in dengue infection. *Neurol. India.* 55, 418–9.

Kankirawatana, P., Chokephaibulkit, K., Puthavathana, P., Yoksan, S., Somchai, A., and Pongthapisit, V. 2000. Dengue infection presenting with central nervous system manifestation. *J. Child. Neurol.* 15, 544–7.

Kao, C. L., King, C. C., Chao, D. Y., Wu, H. L., and Chang, G. J. 2005. Laboratory diagnosis of dengue virus infection: current and future perspectives in clinical diagnosis and public health. *J. Microbiol. Immunol. Infect.* 38(1), 5–16.

Kaplan, A., and Lindgren, A. 1945. Neurological complications following dengue. *US Navy Med. Bull.* 3, 506–10.

King, C. A., Anderson, R., and Marshall, J. S. 2002. Dengue virus selectively induces human mast cell chemokine production. *J. Virol.* 76(16), 8408–19.

King, C. A., Marshall, J. S., Alshurafa, H. et al. 2000. Release of vasoactive cytokines by antibody enhanced dengue virus infection of a human mast cell/basophil line. *J. Virol.* 74, 7146–50.

Koff, W. C., Elm Jr., J. L., and Halstead, S. B. 1980. Inhibition of dengue virus replication by amantadine hydrochloride. *Antimicrob. Agents. Chemother.* 18, 125–9.

Koff, W. C., Elm Jr., J. L., and Halstead, S. B. 1982. Antiviral effects if ribavirin and 6-mer-capto-9-tetrahydro-2-furylpurine against dengue viruses *in vitro*. *Antiviral Res.* 2, 69–79.

Koff, W. C., Pratt, R. D., Elm Jr., J. L., Vekatseshan, C. N., and Halstead, S. B. 1983. Treatment of intracranial dengue virus infections in mice with a lipophilic derivative of ribavirin. *Antimicrob. Agents Chemother.* 24, 134–6.

Kularatne, S. A. M., Pathirage, M. M. K., Gunasena, S. 2008. A case series of dengue fever with altered consciousness and electroencephalogram changes in Sri Lanka. *Trans. Royal Soc. Trop. Med. Hyg.* 102, 1053–4.

Kumar, S., and Prabhakar, S. 2005. Guillain-Barré syndrome occurring in the course of dengue fever. *Neurol. India.* 53, 250–1.

Kumar, J., Kumar, A., Gupta, S., and Jain, D. 2007. Neurological picture. Dengue haemor-rhagic fever: an unusual cause of intracranial haemorrhage. *J. Neurol. Neurosurg. Psychiatry.* 78(3), 253.

Kumar, R., Prakash, O., and Sharma, B. S. 2009. Intracranial hemorrhage in dengue fever: management and outcome: a series of 5 cases and review of literature. *Surg. Neurol.* 72(4), 429–33.

Kuo, C. H., Tai, D. I., Chang-Chien, C. S., Lan, C. K., Chiou, S. S., and Liaw, Y. F. 1992. Liver biochemical tests and dengue fever. *Am. J. Trop. Med. Hyg.* 47(3), 265–70.

Lanciotti, R. S., Calisher, C. H., Gubler, D. J., Chang, G. J., and Vorndam, A. V. 1992. Rapid detection and typing of dengue viruses from clinical samples by using reverse transcrip-tase-polymerase chain reaction. *J. Clin. Microbiol.* 30(3), 545–51.

Lawn, S. D., Tilley, R., Lloyd, G. et al. 2003. Dengue hemorrhagic fever with fulminant hepatic failure in an immigrant returning to Bangladesh. *Clin. Infect. Dis.* 37, e1–4.

Le, V. T., Phan, T. Q., Do, Q. H., Nguyen, B. H., Lam, Q. B., Bach, V. C. et al. 2010. Viral eti-ology of encephalitis in children in southern Vietnam: results of a one-year prospective descriptive study. *PLoS. Negl. Trop. Dis.* 4(10), e854.

Leão, R. N., Oikawa, T., Rosa, E. S., Yamaki, J. T., Rodrigues, S. G., Vasconcelos, H. B. et al. 2022. Isolation of dengue 2 virus from a patient with central nervous system involve-ment (transverse myelitis). *Rev. Soc. Bras. Med. Trop.* 35(4), 401–4.

Leitmeyer, K. C., Vaughn, D. W., Watts, D. M., Salas, R,. Villalobos, I., Ramos, C. et al. 1999. Dengue virus structural differences that correlate with pathogenesis. *J. Virol.* 73, 4738–47.

Lim, M., and Goh, H. K. 2005. Rhabdomyolysis following dengue virus infection. *Singapore Med. J.* 46, 645–6.

Limonta, D., Capó, V., Torres, G., Pérez, A. B., and Guzmán, M. G. 2007. Apoptosis in tissues from fatal dengue shock syndrome. *J. Clin. Virol.* 40(1), 50–4.

Lin, C. F., Lei, H. Y., and Liu, C. C. 2001. Generation of IgM anti-platelet autoantibody in dengue patients. *J. Med. Virol.* 63, 143–9.

Lin, C. F., Lei, H. Y., and Shiau, A. L. 2002. Endothelial cell apoptosis induced by antibodies against dengue virus nonstructural protein 1 via production of nitric oxide. *J. Immunol.* 169, 657–64.

Loke, H., Bethell, D. B., and Phuong, C. X. T. et al. 2011. Strong HLA class I restricted responses in dengue haemorrhagic fever: a double edged sword? *J. Infect. Dis.* 184, 1369–73.

Lum, L. C., Lam, S. K., Choy, Y. S., George, R., and Harun, F. 1996. Dengue encephalitis: a true entity? *Am. J. Trop. Med. Hyg.* 54, 256–9.

Lumpaopong, A., Kaewplang, P., Watanaveeradej, V., Thirakhupt, P., Chamnanvanakij, S., Srisuwan, K. et al. 2010. Electrolyte disturbances and abnormal urine analysis in chil-dren with dengue infection. *Southeast Asian J. Trop. Med. Public Health.* 41(1), 72–6.

Malheiros, S. M., Oliveira, A. S., Schmidt, B., Lima, J. G., and Gabbai, A. A. 1993. Dengue. Muscle biopsy findings in 15 patients. *Arq. Neuropsiquiatr.* 51, 159–64.

Martina, B. E., Koraka, P., and Osterhaus, A. D. 2009. Dengue virus pathogenesis: an inte-grated view. *Clin. Microbiol. Rev.* 22(4), 564–81.

Mekmullica, J., Suwanphatra, A., Thienpaitoon, H., Chansongsakul, T., Cherdkiatkul, T., Pancharoen, C. et al. 2005. Serum and urine sodium levels in dengue patients. *Southeast Asian J. Trop. Med. Public Health.* 36(1), 197–9.

Miagostovich, M. P., Ramos, R. G., Nicol, A. F., Nogueira, R. M., Cuzzi-Maya, T., Oliveira, A. V., Marchevsky, R. S. et al. 1997. Retrospective study on dengue fatal cases. *Clin. Neuropathol.* 16, 204–8.

Misra, U. K., Kalita, J., Syam, U. K., and Dhole, T. N. 2006. Neurological manifestations of dengue virus infection. *J. Neurol. Sci.* 244, 117–22.

Mohan, B., Patwari, A. K., and Anand, V. K. et al. 2000. Hepatic dysfunction in childhood dengue infection. *J. Trop. Pediatrics.* 46, 40–3.

Monath, T. P., Cropp, C. B., and Harrison, A. K. 1983. Mode of entry of a neurotropic arbovirus into the central nervous system. Reinvestigation of an old controversy. *Lab. Invest.* 48(4), 399–410.

Mustafa, A. S., Elbishbishi, E. A., Agarwal, R. et al. 2001. Elevated levels of interleukin-13 and IL-18 in patients with dengue hemorrhagic fever. *FEMS Immunol. Med. Microbiol.* 30, 229–33.

Muzaffar, J., Venkata Krishnan, P., Gupta, N., and Kar, P. 2006. Dengue encephalitis: why we need to identify this entity in a dengue-prone region. *Singapore Med. J.* 47(11), 975–7.

Nimmannitya, S., Thisyakorn, U., and Hemsrichart, V. 1987. Dengue haemorrhagic fever with unusual manifestations. *Southeast Asian J. Trop. Med. Public Health.* 18(3), 398–406.

Nogueira, R. M. R., Miagostovich, M. P., Schatzmayr, H. G. et al. 1988. Virological study of a dengue type 1 epidemic in Rio de Janeiro. *Mem. Inst. Oswaldo. Cruz.* 83, 219–25.

Paliwal, V. K., Garg, R. K., Juyal, R., Husain, N., Verma, R., Sharma, P. K. et al. 2011. Acute dengue virus myositis: a report of seven patients of varying clinical severity including two cases with severe fulminant myositis. *J. Neurol. Sci.* 300(1–2), 14–18.

Patey, O., Ollivaud, L., Breuil, J., and Lafaix, C. 1993. Unusual neurologic manifestations occurring during dengue fever infection. *Am. J. Trop. Med. Hyg.* 48(6), 793–802.

Pincus, L. B., Grossmann, M. E., and Fox, L. P. 2008. The exanthem of dengue fever: Clinical features of two US tourists traveling abroad. *J. Am. Acad. Dermatol.* 58, 308–16.

Puig-Basagoiti, F., Tilgner, M., Forshey, B. M., Philpott, S. M., Espina, N. G., Wentworth, D. E. et al. 2006. Triaryl pyrazoline compound inhibits flavivirus RNA replication. *Antimicrob. Agents Chemother.* 50, 1320–9.

Ramos, C., Sanchez, G., Pando, R. H., Baguera, J., Hernández, D., Mota, J. et al. 2008. Dengue virus in the brain of a fatal case of haemorrhagic dengue fever. *J. Neurovirol.* 4, 465–8.

Rees, C. R., Costin, J. M., Fink, R. C., McMichael, M., Fontaine, K. A., Isern, S., and Michael, S. F. 2008. *In vitro* inhibition of dengue virus entry by p-sulfoxy-cinnamic acid and structurally related combinatorial chemistries. *Antiviral Res.* 80, 135–42.

Salgado, D. M., Eltit, J. M., Mansfield, K., Panqueba, C., Castro, D., Vega, M. R. et al. 2010. Heart and skeletal muscle are targets of dengue virus infection. *Pediatr. Infect. Dis. J.* 29, 238–42.

Sanjay, S., Wagle, A. M., and Au Eong, K. G. 2008. Optic neuropathy associated with dengue fever. *Eye (Lond).* 22(5), 7224.

Santo, N. Q., Azoubel, A. C., Lopes, A. A., Costa, G., and Bacellar, A. 2004. Guillain-Barré syndrome in the course of dengue: Case report. *Arq. Neuropsiquiatr.* 62, 144–6.

Singh, K., Lale, A., Ooi, E. E., Chiu, L.-L., Chow, V. T. K., Tambyah, P. E., and Koay, E. S. C. 2006. A prospective clinical study on the use of reverse transcription-polymerase chain reaction for the early diagnosis of dengue fever. *J. Mol. Diagnost.* 8(5), 613–6.

Soares, C. N., Faria, L. C., Peralta, J. M., and de Freitas, M. R. G., and Puccioni-Sohler, M. 2006. Dengue infection: neurological manifestations and cerebrospinal fluid (CSF) analysis. *J. Neurol. Sci.* 249, 19–24.

Soares, C. N., Cabral-Castro, M., Oliveira, C., Faria, L. C., Peralta, J. M., Freitas, M. R., and Puccioni-Sohler, M. 2008. Oligosymptomatic dengue infection: a potential cause of Guillain Barré syndrome. *Arq. Neuropsiquiatr.* 66(2A), 234–7.

Soares, C. N., Cabral-Castro, M. J., Peralta, J. M., de Freitas, M. R., Zalis, M., and Puccioni-Sohler, M. 2011. Review of the etiologies of viral meningitis and encephalitis in a dengue endemic region. *J. Neurol. Sci.* 303(1–2), 75–9.

Soares, C. N., and Puccioni-Sohler, M. 2011. Dengue encephalitis: Suggestion for case definition. *J. Neurol. Sci.* 306, 164.

Solomon, T., Dung, N. M., Vaughn, D. W., Kneen, R., Thao, L. T., Raengsakulrach, B. et al. 2000. Neurological manifestations of dengue infection. *Lancet.* 355, 1053–9.

Solomon, T., and Barrett, A. 2003. Dengue, In: Nath, A. (Ed.), *Clinical Neurovirology.* Marcel Dekker, New York, pp. 528–581.

Solomon, T., Hart, I. J., and Beeching, N. J. 2007. Viral encephalitis: a clinician's guide. *Pract. Neurol.* 7, 285–302.

St John, A. L., Rathore, A. P., Yap, H., Ng, M. L., Metcalfe, D. D., Vasudevan, S. G. et al. 2011. Immune surveillance by mast cells during dengue infection promotes natural killer (NK) and NKT-cell recruitment and viral clearance. *PNAS* 108(22), 9190–5.

Stein, D. A., Huang, C. Y., Silengo, S., Amantana, A., Crumley, S., Blouch, R. E. et al. 2008. Treatment of AG129 mice with antisense morpholino oligomers increases survival time following challenge with dengue 2 virus. *J. Antimicrob. Chemother.* 62, 555–65.

Suaya, J. A., Shepard, D. S., Siqueira, J. B., Martelli, C. T., Lum, L. C. S., Tan, L. H. et al. 2009. Cost of Dengue Cases in Eight Countries in the Americas and Asia: A Prospective Study. *Am. J. Trop. Med. Hyg.* 80(5), 846–55.

Sulekha, C., Kumar, S., and Philip, J. 2004. Guillain-Barré syndrome following dengue fever. *Indian Pediatr.* 41, 948–50.

Tomlinson, S. M., Malmstrom, R. D., Russo, A., Mueller, N., Pang, Y. P., and Watowich, S. J. 2009. Structure-based discovery of dengue virus protease inhibitors. *Antiviral Res.* 82(3), 110–4.

Vaquero, J., Rose, C., and Butterworth, R. F. 2005. Keeping cool in acute liver failure: rationale for the use of mild hypothermia. *J. Hepatol.* 43, 1067–77.

Varatharaj, A. 2010. Encephalitis in the clinical spectrum of dengue infection. *Neurol. India.* 58(4), 585–91.

Varatharaj, A. 2011. A case definition is needed for dengue encephalitis. *J. Neurol. Sci.* 306, 164.

Verma, R., and Varatharaj, A. 2011. Epilepsia partialis continua as a manifestation of dengue encephalitis. *Epilepsy Behav.* 20(2), 395–7.

Wali, J. P., Biswas, A., Chandra, S. et al. 1998. Cardiac involvement in dengue haemorrhagic fever. *Int. J. Cardiol.* 64, 31–6.

Wang, E., Ni, H., Xu, R., Barrett, A. D. T., Watowich, S. J., and Gubler, D. J. 2000. Evolutionary relationships of endemic/epidemic and sylvatic dengue viruses. *J. Virol.* 74(7), 3227–34.

Wasay, M., Channa, R., Jumani, M., Shabbir, G., Azeemuddin, M., and Zafar, A. 2008. Encephalitis and myelitis associated with dengue viral infection: Clinical and neuroimaging features. *Clin. Neurol. and Neurosurg.* 110, 635–40.

Webster, D. P., Farrar, J., and Rowland-Jones, S. 2009. Progress towards a dengue vaccine. *Lancet Infect. Dis.* 9, 678–87.

Wiwantkit, V. 2007. Liver dysfunction in dengue infection: an analysis of the previously published Thai cases. *J. Ayub. Med. Coll. Abbottabad.* 19(1), 10–2.

World Health Organisation, 2009. *Dengue: Guidelines for Diagnosis, Treatment, Prevention, and Control.* WHO, Geneva.

Yamada, M., Nakamura, K., Yoshii, M., Kaku, Y., and Narita, M. 2009. Brain lesions induced by experimental intranasal infection of Japanese encephalitis virus in piglets. *J. Comp. Pathol.* 141(2–3), 156–62.

Yeo, P. S. D., Pinheiro, L., Tong, P., Lim, P. L., and Sitoh, Y. Y. 2005. Hippocampal involvement in dengue fever. *Singapore Med. J.* 46(11), 647.

Zhang, X. G., Mason, P. W., Dubovi, E. J., Xu, X., Bourne, N., Renshaw, R. W., Block, T. M., and Birk, A. V. 2009. Antiviral activity of geneticin against dengue virus. *Antiviral Res.* 83, 21–7.

14 Influenza Virus and CNS Infections

Jun Zeng, Gefei Wang, and Kang-Sheng Li

CONTENTS

14.1 INTRODUCTION

Influenza, commonly referred to as the flu, is an infectious disease caused by influenza virus, a group of single-stranded minus-sense RNA viruses, which affects birds and mammals. There are three types of influenza virus, influenza A, B, and C. Influenza virus A or B causes the flu syndrome, including chills, fever, headache, and sore throat and muscle pains. Although it is often confused with other influenza-like illnesses, especially the common cold, influenza is a more severe disease than the common cold. In adults, complications may follow the primary viral infection of the respiratory tract, such as bronchitis and pneumonia (Sessa et al. 2001). In children less than 5 years of age, the most common infective complication is acute otitis media (Tsolia et al. 2006). Influenza C infection is usually asymptomatic.

Since the time of the Spanish flu during 1917–1919, influenza has been recognized as a virus that might cause neurological complications (Hayase and Tobita 1997; Ravenholt and Foege 1982). Influenza virus has been observed as the cause of central nervous system (CNS) dysfunction. Influenza virus is associated with various CNS lesions that have poor prognosis, including influenza-associated encephalitis/ encephalopathy (IAE), Reye's syndrome, and acute necrotizing encephalopathy (ANE; Wang et al. 2010). Influenza A infection was a common cause of febrile seizure admissions (Chiu et al. 2001), and encephalitis/encephalopathy (Morishima et al. 2002).

14.2 BIOLOGICAL PROPERTIES OF INFLUENZA VIRUS

14.2.1 Virus Structure

The influenza virus is about 80–120 nm in diameter; the virion is enveloped and can be either spherical or filamentous in form. The envelope of the virus is a lipid bilayer membrane which originates from the virus-producing cell and which contains prominent projections formed by hemagglutinin (HA) and neuraminidase (NA), as well as the M2 protein. The lipid layer covers the matrix formed by the M1 protein.

14.2.2 Genome Organization

Influenza A and B virus genomes consist of 8 separate segments covered by the nucleocapsid protein. Together, these build the ribonucleoprotein (RNP), and each segment codes for a functionally important protein (Figure 14.1). Influenza C virus harbors only 7 genome segments, and its surface carries only one glycoprotein. Type A viruses are divided into subtypes based on differences of two surface proteins called hemagglutinin (HA) and neuraminidase (NA). There are 16 different HA subtypes and 9 NA subtypes.

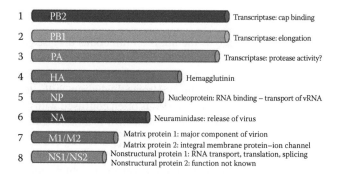

FIGURE 14.1 The relative sizes of the eight influenza segments as well as the genes that are specified by each. (From PatentLens (2011). The influenza genome comprises eight segments. In *Figure 1: The Eight RNA Segments of the Influenza Genome*, vol. 2011, patentlens. With permission.)

14.2.2.1 Protein Functions

14.2.2.1.1 Hemagglutinin (HA)

Hemagglutinin (HA) is a glycoprotein that binds the virus to the cell being infected. The HA molecule is a combination of three homogeneous proteins which are bound together to form an elongated cylindrical shape. HA is also the main viral target of protective humoral immunity by neutralizing antibody. The binding affinity of HA to the sialic acid residues partly accounts for the host specificity of the various influenza A virus subtypes. Human viruses preferentially bind to sialic acid linked to galactose by α-2,6 linkages that are the main type found on the epithelial cells of the human respiratory tract, while avian viruses tend to bind to α-2,3 linkages that are found on duck intestinal epithelium (Couceiro et al. 1993; Ito et al. 1998). The specificity for different receptors has been one of the interpretations for the species barrier between human and avian influenza viruses. The presence of both α-2,6 and α-2,3 linkages on epithelium of the pig trachea is the reason why pigs may serve as the "mixing vessel" for the genesis of new viral subtypes through co-infection (Ito et al. 1998; Liu et al. 2009). Chickens may have a similar role, since their lung and intestinal epithelia have both types of linkages (Gambaryan et al. 2002). In the human respiratory epithelium in nasal mucosa, pharynx, trachea, and bronchi express high amounts of α-2,6 linkage, whereas the α-2,3 linkage is the major receptor on type II pneumocytes cells and nonciliated cuboidal bronchiolar cells at the junction between respiratory bronchiole and alveolus (Shinya et al. 2006), thereby allowing human infection by avian influenza viruses (Ge and Wang 2011; Suzuki 2011). A mutation that changes just one amino acid in hemagglutinin can alter the antigenic properties significantly. Thus, the barrier to interspecies infection can be overcome easily.

14.2.2.1.2 Neuraminidase

Neuraminidase (NA) is an enzyme that helps the virus to breach cell walls. NA is also known as sialidase, since it breaks the linkages between sialic acid and cellular glycoproteins and glycolipids found in cell walls. There are 9 NA antigenic subtypes. NA forms mushroom-like projections on the surface of the influenza virus. The top consists of four identical proteins with a roughly spherical shape.

14.2.2.1.3 M2

M2 is an ion channel crucial for the pH-dependent dissociation of matrix proteins from the nucleocapsid during viral uncoating and pH changes across the trans-Golgi network during maturation of hemagglutinin molecules. M2 is the target of the adamantanes (amantadine and rimantadine).

14.2.2.1.4 PB1

PB1 gene encodes protein, termed PB1-F2, a mitochondrial protein that causes cellular apoptosis may be related to it permeabilizes the mitochondrial membranes by forming an apoptotic pore with lipids (Chanturiya et al. 2004; Gibbs et al. 2003). The hemagglutinin and PB2 proteins appear to be important in determining host specificity and virulence.

The active RNA-RNA polymerase is responsible for replication and transcription. The polymerase contains the PB2, PB1, and PA proteins. PB1 has an endonuclease activity and holds active site (Poch et al. 1989), whereas PB2 is responsible for cap binding. The NS1 and NS2 proteins have a regulatory function to promote the synthesis of viral components in the infected cell.

14.3 EPIDEMIOLOGY

Thousands of deaths attributable to influenza infections occur annually in the United States. According to the Centers for Disease Control and Prevention (CDC) report, during 1976–2007, estimates of annual influenza-associated deaths from respiratory and circulatory causes ranged from 3349 in 1986–1987 to 48,614 in 2003–2004. The annual rate of influenza-associated death overall ranged from 1.4 to 16.7 deaths per 100,000 persons in the United States (CDC 2010).

The various subtypes of influenza present with new combinations of the surface glycoproteins HA (H1–H15) and NA (N1–N9). Historically, these antigenic shifts have resulted in pandemics every 10–40 years (Webster et al. 1992). Epidemics on a smaller scale occur yearly or every few years and are caused by minor changes in antigenicity of influenza virus (antigenic drift) by amino acid changes in the surface antigen (HA and NA) due to point mutations of the genome.

The cases of febrile seizures have accumulated in Asia, especially in Japan (Waruiru and Appleton 2004). The incidence of influenza-associated encephalopathy has been reported much higher in Asia than in Europe and the America (Bhat et al. 2005; Morishima et al. 2002; Okabe et al. 2000; Togashi et al. 2004). Based on these reports, a genetic background might be involved in the pathogenesis of these diseases.

14.4 CLINICAL PRESENTATIONS

The spectrum of influenza may range from subclinical illness to severe respiratory tract infection that affects multiple organs with abrupt onset of fever. The incubation period is one day to a week. The illness, with fever and cough, sore throat, and headache may last for 1–5 days. Children often present with nonspecific symptoms such as vomiting, diarrhea in addition to high fever, cough, and rhinorrhea. Pediatric influenza may provoke febrile convulsions, and give rise to otitis media and pneumonia (Peltola et al. 2003). Symptoms in neonates are lethargy, anorexia, apnea, and interstitial pneumonia (Yuen et al. 1998). Viral and bacterial pneumonia are frequent complications, whereas myositis, renal failure, myocarditis, and CNS symptoms develop more rarely. The certain risk groups, such as patients with chronic heart and lung disease, the elderly, transplant recipients, smokers, children with underlying medical conditions, and pregnant women are more common to show these complications of influenza infection. The most common causes of death are respiratory complications or cardiovascular diseases.

CNS involvement during influenza infection contains plenty of syndromes, more often described in children than in adults (Studahl 2003). The major clinical entities are encephalitis or encephalopathy. In etiological studies of encephalitis, influenza

A and/or B have been identified in up to 8.5% of adult patients with positive virological findings and in up to 10% of pediatric cases (Koskiniemi et al. 2001). Reye's syndrome and ANE are special forms of encephalopathies with high mortality and sequelae. Rare conditions are myelitis caused by influenza virus (Salonen et al. 1997), and even more seldom, autoimmune diseases elicited by influenza such as Guillain-Barré's syndrome (Tam et al. 2007).

Encephalitis and encephalopathy are not always distinguishable from each other, and there is probably a continuum and/or an overlap between these clinical symptoms, including the more severe condition acute nectrotizing encephalopathy. Although the clinical entity of influenza-associated encephalopathy has not gained universal recognition, it has been reported frequently as a complication of influenza in Japanese children (Sugaya 2002). Influenza A is most frequently reported, especially H3N2 and H1N1, although influenza B is associated with encephalitis/encephalopathy as well. A national survey, conducted in Japan during 1998–1999, reported that 148 out of 202 cases were diagnosed as influenza-associated encephalitis/encephalopathy on the basis of virologic analysis. According to their report, 87.8% (130/148) was type A influenza and 11.5% (17/148) was type B (Morishima et al. 2002). The onset of neurological symptoms is usually within a few days to a week after the first signs of influenza infection. Fever, decreased consciousness, and seizures are common symptoms, and among the less common are focal neurological signs such as paresis, cranial nerve palsies, and choreoathetosis. Encephalitis/encephalopathy is more common in children, although adult cases are described (Hakoda and Nakatani 2000; Kurita et al. 2001). Reports of influenza virus-associated encephalitis/encephalopathy with high fatality rate, especially among children, have increased in Japan with estimates of about 200 patients during 1998–1999 and 100 during 1999–2000 (Kasai et al. 2000). The mortality is approximately 30%, and 80.6% reported cases were children younger than 4 years of age. The risk of neurological sequelae is high (Sugaya 2002).

14.4.1 Febrile Seizures

Febrile seizures occur in approximately 20% of hospitalized infants and adolescents with influenza. In Hong Kong, it has been reported that 19.9% (54/272) and 18.8% (27/144) of children aged 6 months to 5 years hospitalized with influenza A infection in 1997 and 1998, respectively, had one or more febrile seizures (Chiu et al. 2001). There are two types of febrile seizures, simple febrile seizure and complex febrile seizure. The simple one is typical and characterized by single seizures that manifest as generalized tonic–clonic or clonic convulsions lasting no longer than 15 min and does not recur in 24 hours. The complex febrile seizure is characterized by longer duration, with recurrence or focus on only part of the body (Toovey 2008).

The risk of febrile seizure is associated with many factors, including age, gender, and family history. Febrile seizures occur more frequently in boys than in girls. A genetic predisposition to febrile seizure may also exist (Kwong et al. 2006). Influenza A viruses have been implicatively involve in the pathogenesis of febrile seizures (Chiu et al. 2001; Hara et al. 2007; Stricker and Sennhauser 2004), although their action has yet to be fully determined. Indirect involvement via the initiation of fever appears most likely, because fever is an established trigger event for febrile seizure (Toovey 2008), but direct neurological effects cannot be discounted, since some influenza A virus subtypes are probably neurotropic viruses. Few studies have demonstrated the presence of viral antigens in the CSF or CNS tissue (Schlesinger et al. 1998; Steininger et al. 2003). Furthermore, high levels of cytokines in patients who developed febrile seizures in influenza A virus infection have been reported (Ichiyama et al. 2008). Febrile seizure appears to resolve without neurological sequelae (Kolfen et al. 1998). Neurological complications of influenza infection may be partly related to the exaggerated cytokine response.

14.4.2 REYE'S SYNDROME

Reye's syndrome is a potentially fatal disease that causes numerous detrimental effects to many organs, especially the brain and the liver. The syndrome is characterized by a rapidly progressive noninflammatory encephalopathy and hepatic failure, largely affecting children and adolescents. Signs include vomiting, disorientation, loss of consciousness, and seizures. Signs of hepatomegaly and cerebral edema are often present (Gosalakkal and Kamoji 2008). The disorder commonly occurs during recovery from a viral infection, although it can also develop 3 to 5 days after the onset of the viral illness. Influenza viruses, especially influenza B virus infections, may precede Reye's syndrome (Studahl 2003). Reye's syndrome is often misdiagnosed as encephalitis, meningitis, diabetes, drug overdose, poisoning, sudden infant death syndrome, or psychiatric illness. Because manifestations of Reye's syndrome are not unique to Reye's syndrome but also are seen in other conditions and given that no test is specific for Reye's syndrome, the diagnosis must be one of exclusion. Early recognition and treatment are essential to prevent death and to optimize the likelihood of recovery without neurological impairment. The serious symptoms of Reye's syndrome appear to result from damage to cellular mitochondria.

14.4.3 ENCEPHALITIS LETHARGICA

Encephalitis lethargica was a devastating, mysterious, epidemic disease that killed as many as 500,000 people in early part of the twentieth century (Ravenholt and Foege 1982). Encephalitis lethargic could occur at any stage of life, but the incidence was greatest in those between ages 10 and 30 years. Encephalitis lethargic is characterized by high fever, headache, delayed physical, sleep inversion, and lethargy (Dale et al. 2004). In acute cases, patients may enter a coma-like state (Vilensky et al. 2006). The mechanism of causing encephalitis lethargica is not known for certain. Dale et al. (2004) suggested that the disease is mediated by the poststreptococcal immune response, and autoimmune origin with IgG against human basal ganglia antigens.

14.4.4 ACUTE NECROTIZING ENCEPHALOPATHY

ANE is characterized by multifocal symmetric brain lesions involving the bilateral thalami, putamen, and brainstem tegmentum. ANE is a rare disease first described in Japan by Mizuguchi in 1995 (Mizuguchi et al. 1995). The disease affects young children of both genders. ANE manifests as acute encephalopathy following 2–4 days of fever and minor symptoms of respiratory tract infection. The clinical course of ANE is rapidly progressive, including constitutional symptoms of emesis, cough, and diarrhea in combination with neurological dysfunction such as rapid consciousness and seizures. The hallmark of this encephalopathy consists of multifocal, symmetric brain lesions affecting the bilateral thalami and/or cerebellar medulla (Lyon et al. 2010; Ormitti et al. 2010; Weitkamp et al. 2004; Yadav et al. 2010). The prognosis is usually poor and associated with severe neurological sequelae in survivors (Mizuguchi 1997).

14.5 DIAGNOSIS

Typically, neurological examinations are performed on the patient who presents with signs and symptoms of encephalitis; several types of examination may aid in the diagnosis, such as a lumbar puncture may be performed to assess for evidence of infection in the CNS and help to exclude other potential causes of symptoms like meningitis. To ascertain the CNS infection, neuroimaging with MRI/CT can be available. Neuroimaging findings on CT or MRI may be normal initially, but pathological changes can develop after a few days of neurological symptoms. The pathogenesis of brain damage induced by influenza infection was quite variable. The results from MRI were divided into five categories: normal, diffuse involvement of the cerebral cortex, diffuse brain edema, symmetrical involvement of the thalamus, and postinfectious focal encephalitis (Kimura et al. 1998). MRI is particularly useful for detecting metabolic derangements in the brain, although electroencephalogram (EEG) is usually nonspecific with pathological changes, it can reflect brain function. High voltage amplitude slow waves and the occurrence of theta oscillation have been shown consistent with encephalitis/encephalopathy (Cisse et al. 2010; Fukumoto et al. 2007; Okumura et al. 2005). Whereas the brain MRI, CT, and EEG are nonspecific tests for the CNS infection, it may also help to rule out other causes and narrow down the diagnosis.

In influenza virus-associated encephalopathy or encephalitis, CSF analyses will often reveal a lack of pleocytosis or merely a discrete elevation of mononuclear leukocytes. Protein and glucose content are usually normal, although a slightly increased protein level may be present.

Determinations of white blood cell counts and serum C-reactive protein level may be helpful in the detection of bacterial coinfections because these values are low in patients with uncomplicated influenza. Leukopenia observed in association with influenza infection should not prompt any further evaluation, because influenza is known to cause lymphopenia. It has been shown that influenza B was more clearly associated with leukopenia than was influenza A (Peltola et al. 2003).

The diagnosis of influenza infection is based on viral isolation, the viral antigen test or RT-PCR. It has been reported that influenza A (Fujimoto et al. 1998) and influenza B (McCullers et al. 1999) may directly cause CNS infections by PCR analyses of CSF. Peltola et al. identified 11 children with encephalitis, encephalopathy, or status epilepticus associated with influenza infection (Peltola et al. 2003). Morishima et al. (2002) reported a high incidence of influenza associated encephalitis and encephalopathy in Japan, whereas they consider that direct invasion of the CNS by influenza virus is unlikely in most of their cases. Since it can be hard to find definitive evidence of influenza, brain biopsy is rarely performed to sample the infected brain tissue.

14.6 PATHOLOGY AND PATHOGENESIS

The pathogenic mechanisms of the various neurological syndromes during influenza infection in humans are largely unknown. In etiology, human encephalitis/encephalopathies that are associated with or connected with influenza virus infection are composed of two groups. The first group is necrotic encephalopathy of the cerebrum, and consists of ANE of childhood (Campistol et al. 1998; Huang et al. 2004; Khan et al. 2011), hemorrhagic shock and encephalopathy (Levin et al. 1983), and Reye's syndrome (Gosalakkal and Kamoji 2008). The pathogenesis of ANE is unknown but necropsy findings in fatal cases of ANE reveal diffuse cerebral edema and perivascular hemorrhage in the bilateral thalami and putamen (Mizuguchi et al. 2002). In these encephalopathies, the breakdown of the blood–brain barrier (BBB) was suggested to be the direct cause of the brain lesions (Hayase and Tobita 1997; Takahashi et al. 2000), but the mechanism leading to the breakdown is unknown. Encephalitis lethargica (van Toorn and Schoeman 2009) and postencephalitic Parkinson's disease (Hayase and Tobita 1997) constitute the second group, and the CNS lesion common to them is nonpurulent encephalitis of the brain stem. There has been no clear-cut explanation of the predilection of encephalitis for the brain stem.

Influenza replicates in the respiratory tract and is seldom isolated from the brain (Frankova et al. 1977). However, detection of influenza virus (Okabe et al. 2000) or viral RNA in the CSF (de Jong et al. 2005; Fujimoto et al. 1998; Gu et al. 2007) has indicated penetration of virus into the CNS. Although most viral infections are thought to spread to the brain hematogenously, this route has been doubted in influenza encephalitis/encephalopathy since viremia is sparsely reported in humans, where it has been found only during the incubation period and initial stage of disease (Xu et al. 1998). The neuronal pathway, shown in animal models via the olfactory and trigeminal nerve system (Park et al. 2002; Reinacher et al. 1983), may be favored by the free nerve endings near the influenza-infected epithelial cells in the upper respiratory tract (Mori and Kimura 2001). Different routes of virus entry to the brain, studied experimentally in mice, are linked to infection of different cells and regions of the CNS (Park et al. 2002) and might result in diverse clinical pictures and neuroimaging findings. Wang et al. reported that human H1N1 and avian H5N1 influenza viruses were replicative and productive in mouse microglia and astrocyte (Wang et al. 2008). Influenza infection in ependymal cells has been shown in an autopsy study of immunosuppressed patients (Frankova et al. 1977). The hypothesis of a vascular endothelial infection is supported by studies on mice. In the study, influenza strains replicate primarily in ependymal cells in the CNS (Ito et al. 1999). However, a limited direct invasion of neurons is not excluded. Virus-antigen positivity has been shown in Purkinje cells in the cerebellum and in several neurons in the pons of a 2-year-old girl who died from influenza encephalopathy (Takahashi et al. 2000).

Influenza virus RNA has been detected in CSF and brain tissues of patients who develop acute encephalitis/encephalopathy (Fujimoto et al. 1998). Influenza virus antigens have also been detected in glial cells and neurocytes in mouse models of encephalitis (Gao et al. 1999; Shinya et al. 1998). Besides, proinflammatory cytokines are reportedly increased in the CSF and plasma of patients with influenza encephalopathy and encephalitis (Ito et al. 1999; Shinya et al. 1998). These observations suggest the involvement of direct viral damage and immunopathological injury in influenza-associated encephalopathy and encephalitis.

Another hypothesis has suggested that cytokine release from virus-stimulated glial cells may be responsible for a neurotoxic effect on the brain (Wang et al. 2008) and a rapid breakdown of the BBB (Yokota et al. 2000). Autopsy studies of patients with CNS complications associated with influenza are generally scarce. Fatal cases with brain pathology have shown congestion and hyperemia of the brain without inflammatory cell infiltration, and in rare cases demyelination (Studahl 2003).

However, other researchers considered that the clinical significance of the presence of influenza virus genome in the CSF is questionable (Lee et al. 2010; Steininger et al. 2003). Reports found an increased permeability of the BBB in the only influenza virus-positive patient, indicating passive diffusion of viral genome from the periphery into the CSF (Fujimoto et al. 1998; Morishima et al. 2002; Steininger et al. 2003). According to the national survey conducted in Japan, it has been suggested that direct invasion by influenza virus and inflammation is unlikely to be the cause of encephalopathy, and despite the occurrence of brain edema, no influenza antigen has been detected in the brains of patients with influenza-associated encephalopathy (Morishima et al. 2002).

Cytokines such as IL-6 and TNF-alpha were markedly elevated in cerebrospinal fluid and in serum of patients with influenza-associated encephalopathy and encephalitis (Ichiyama et al. 2003, 2004; Kawada et al. 2003). The leakage of plasma protein was found in the brain of the patient who died with a rapid and fulminant course suggestive of damage of vascular endothelial cells, which is presumably caused by highly activated cytokines (Togashi et al. 2004).

Proinflammatory cytokines, such as IL-6 and TNF-a, can induce apoptosis, which may give rise to aggravated encephalopathy. In addition, chemokines including CCL2/MCP1, CXCL8/IL-8, and CXCL10/IP-10 were greatly increased both in CSF and serum (Mizuguchi et al. 2007). These chemokines induce injury of vascular endothelium, glial cells, and neurons, cause vascular lesions and breakdown of the BBB, and thereby induce brain edema and damage, CNS disorders, and/or systemic symptoms (Nakai et al. 2003; Wang et al. 2010).

14.7 PROGNOSIS AND TREATMENT

The prognosis of encephalitis/encephalopathy depends mainly on age and presence of MRI or CT pathology. Compared with patients with normal MRI or CT, patients with pathological MRI or CT are significantly younger and have more severe sequelae or fatal disease. Neuroimaging studies in influenza encephalitis/encephalopathy suggest that the majority of those who recover or have mild sequelae are the patients with nonpathological MRI or CT (Ormitti et al. 2010; Studahl 2003). However, severe sequelae such as choreoathetosis, altered personality, spastic quadriparesis, and persistent vegetative state may occur also in cases with normal imaging findings (Hakoda and Nakatani 2000; Ryan et al. 1999). A diffuse severe brain edema is associated with severe brain damage or death (Yokota et al. 2000).

For most viral infections such as influenza, there are no specific medications to treat the disease. In mild cases patients are generally instructed to eat well, drink plenty of fluids, and to rest. In more serious cases patients may be hospitalized. Methylprednisolone pulse therapy and large doses of IgG reduced the mortality from influenza-associated encephalopathy (Weitkamp et al. 2004). If the patient experiences seizures, anti-seizure medication may be prescribed. Anti-inflammatory drugs and high dosage corticosteroid therapy may be useful to reduce brain edema (Aiba et al. 2001).

Vaccines are the principal defense against influenza, but because it takes time to produce an antigenically appropriate and immunogenic product and deliver it to entire populations, antiviral drugs will be a principal countermeasure to reduce the impact of a new pandemic (Monto 2006). The current armamentarium of licensed anti-influenza medications include influenza M2 ion channel blockers (adamantadine and rimantadine), and NA inhibitors (oseltamivir and zanamivir). Nucleoside analogues that interfere with influenza virus RNA polymerase function (ribavirin and viramidine) were used to treat severe infections in a very limited extent (Beigel and Bray 2008).

The main advantages of neuraminidase inhibitors, compared with amantadine and rimantadine, are fewer adverse effects, activity against both influenza A and B, and rare resistance (Gubareva et al. 2000). In field trials, the greatest benefit from anti-influenza drugs is gained if therapy is started early, within 48 h after onset of symptoms (Bridges et al. 2002). Antiviral therapy for influenza generally should be based on detection of the virus. The primary care level cannot be based on data from hospitalized patients. In addition to treatment, antiviral drugs can be used prophylactically in specific situations when vaccination is not possible or effective (Bridges et al. 2002).

14.8 CONCLUSIONS AND FUTURE PERSPECTIVES

Avian influenza is very common, but crossing the species barrier to mammalian is a rare event. However, recent decade incidences of direct passage of highly pathogenic influenza A virus strains of the H5N1 and H1N1 subtypes from birds and pigs to humans have become a major public concern. Although presence of virus in the human brain has a wide discrepancy, certain avian influenza virus strains can invade the brain of experimental animals (Reinacher et al. 1983). These avian influenza subtypes have the propensity to invade the brain along cranial nerves to target brainstem and diencephalic nuclei following intranasal instillation in mice and ferrets (Maines et al. 2005; Zitzow et al. 2002). Unfortunately, the etiology and pathogenesis of influenza-associated CNS infections remain largely unknown. Although the pathogenesis remains unclear, the rapidity of the onset of symptoms and the negative presentation of viral antigen in brain tissue suggest that a cytokine-mediated process may be the mechanism rather than direct invasion of brain parenchyma and resulting direct cytopathic effect.

Since no specific diagnosis for influenza-associated nervous system dysfunctions such as encephalitis/encephalopathy, febrile seizures, Reye's syndrome, encephalitis lethargic, and ANE, the importance of imaging techniques (MRI/CT) should be advocated to aid clinicians to formulate a presumptive diagnosis.

So far, rare report influenza spread to the brain in humans and any association between influenza and neuropsychiatric disorders remains to be established. However, because neurotropic variants of influenza can rapidly be selected in other mammalians such as mice and ferrets, this virus may be a threat imposed by nature also to the human brain. A fight against this terror should therefore be a concern for clinicians, virologists, and neuroscientists.

REFERENCES

Aiba, H., Mochizuki, M., Kimura, M., and Hojo, H. (2001). Predictive value of serum interleukin-6 level in influenza virus-associated encephalopathy. *Neurology* 57(2), 295–9.

Beigel, J., and Bray, M. (2008). Current and future antiviral therapy of severe seasonal and avian influenza. *Antiviral Res* 78(1), 91–102.

Bhat, N., Wright, J. G., Broder, K. R., Murray, E. L., Greenberg, M. E., Glover, M. J., Likos, A. M., Posey, D. L., Klimov, A., Lindstrom, S. E., Balish, A., Medina, M. J., Wallis, T. R., Guarner, J., Paddock, C. D., Shieh, W. J., Zaki, S. R., Sejvar, J. J., Shay, D. K., Harper, S. A., Cox, N. J., Fukuda, K., and Uyeki, T. M. (2005). Influenza-associated deaths among children in the United States 2003–2004. *N Engl J Med* 353(24), 2559–67.

Bridges, C. B., Fukuda, K., Uyeki, T. M., Cox, N. J., and Singleton, J. A. (2002). Prevention and control of influenza. Recommendations of the Advisory Committee on Immunization Practices (ACIP). *MMWR Recomm Rep* 51(RR-3), 1–31.

Campistol, J., Gassio, R., Pineda, M., and Fernandez-Alvarez, E. (1998). Acute necrotizing encephalopathy of childhood (infantile bilateral thalamic necrosis): two non-Japanese cases. *Dev Med Child Neurol* 40(11), 771–4.

CDC, C. f. D. C. a. P. (2010). Estimates of deaths associated with seasonal influenza—United States 1976–2007. *MMWR Morb Mortal Wkly Rep* 59(33), 1057–62.

Chanturiya, A. N., Basanez, G., Schubert, U., Henklein, P., Yewdell, J. W., and Zimmerberg, J. (2004). PB1-F2, an influenza A virus-encoded proapoptotic mitochondrial protein, creates variably sized pores in planar lipid membranes. *J Virol* 78(12), 6304–12.

Chiu, S. S., Tse, C. Y., Lau, Y. L., and Peiris, M. (2001). Influenza A infection is an important cause of febrile seizures. *Pediatrics* 108(4), E63.

Cisse, Y., Wang, S., Inoue, I., and Kido, H. (2010). Rat model of influenza-associated encephalopathy (IAE): studies of electroencephalogram (EEG) *in vivo*. *Neuroscience* 165(4), 1127–37.

Couceiro, J. N., Paulson, J. C., and Baum, L. G. (1993). Influenza virus strains selectively recognize sialyloligosaccharides on human respiratory epithelium; the role of the host cell in selection of hemagglutinin receptor specificity. *Virus Res* 29(2), 155–65.

Dale, R. C., Church, A. J., Surtees, R. A., Lees, A. J., Adcock, J. E., Harding, B., Neville, B. G., and Giovannoni, G. (2004). Encephalitis lethargica syndrome: 20 new cases and evidence of basal ganglia autoimmunity. *Brain* 127(Pt 1), 21–33.

de Jong, M. D., Bach, V. C., Phan, T. Q., Vo, M. H., Tran, T. T., Nguyen, B. H., Beld, M., Le, T. P., Truong, H. K., Nguyen, V. V., Tran, T. H., Do, Q. H., and Farrar, J. (2005). Fatal avian influenza A (H5N1) in a child presenting with diarrhea followed by coma. *N Engl J Med* 352(7), 686–91.

Frankova, V., Jirasek, A., and Tumova, B. (1977). Type A influenza: postmortem virus isolations from different organs in human lethal cases. *Arch Virol* 53(3), 265–8.

Fujimoto, S., Kobayashi, M., Uemura, O., Iwasa, M., Ando, T., Katoh, T., Nakamura, C., Maki, N., Togari, H., and Wada, Y. (1998). PCR on cerebrospinal fluid to show influenza-associated acute encephalopathy or encephalitis. *Lancet* 352(9131), 873–5.

Fukumoto, Y., Okumura, A., Hayakawa, F., Suzuki, M., Kato, T., Watanabe, K., and Morishima, T. (2007). Serum levels of cytokines and EEG findings in children with influenza associated with mild neurological complications. *Brain Dev* 29(7), 425–30.

Gambaryan, A., Webster, R., and Matrosovich, M. (2002). Differences between influenza virus receptors on target cells of duck and chicken. *Arch Virol* 147(6), 1197–208.

Gao, P., Watanabe, S., Ito, T., Goto, H., Wells, K., McGregor, M., Cooley, A. J., and Kawaoka, Y. (1999). Biological heterogeneity, including systemic replication in mice, of H5N1 influenza A virus isolates from humans in Hong Kong. *J Virol* 73(4), 3184–9.

Ge, S., and Wang, Z. (2011). An overview of influenza A virus receptors. *Crit Rev Microbiol* 37(2), 157–65.

Gibbs, J. S., Malide, D., Hornung, F., Bennink, J. R., and Yewdell, J. W. (2003). The influenza A virus PB1-F2 protein targets the inner mitochondrial membrane via a predicted basic amphipathic helix that disrupts mitochondrial function. *J Virol* 77(13), 7214–24.

Gosalakkal, J. A., and Kamoji, V. (2008). Reye syndrome and Reye-like syndrome. *Pediatr Neurol* 39(3), 198–200.

Gu, J., Xie, Z., Gao, Z., Liu, J., Korteweg, C., Ye, J., Lau, L. T., Lu, J., Zhang, B., McNutt, M. A., Lu, M., Anderson, V. M., Gong, E., Yu, A. C., and Lipkin, W. I. (2007). H5N1 infection of the respiratory tract and beyond: a molecular pathology study. *Lancet* 370(9593), 1137–45.

Gubareva, L. V., Kaiser, L., and Hayden, F. G. (2000). Influenza virus neuraminidase inhibitors. *Lancet* 355(9206), 827–35.

Hakoda, S., and Nakatani, T. (2000). A pregnant woman with influenza A encephalopathy in whom influenza A/Hong Kong virus (H3) was isolated from cerebrospinal fluid. *Arch Intern Med* 160(7), 1041, 1045.

Hara, K., Tanabe, T., Aomatsu, T., Inoue, N., Tamaki, H., Okamoto, N., Okasora, K., Morimoto, T., and Tamai, H. (2007). Febrile seizures associated with influenza A. *Brain Dev* 29(1), 30–8.

Hayase, Y., and Tobita, K. (1997). Influenza virus and neurological diseases. *Psychiatry Clin Neurosci* 51(4), 181–4.

Huang, S. M., Chen, C. C., Chiu, P. C., Cheng, M. F., Lai, P. H., and Hsieh, K. S. (2004). Acute necrotizing encephalopathy of childhood associated with influenza type B virus infection in a 3-year-old girl. *J Child Neurol* 19(1), 64–7.

Ichiyama, T., Endo, S., Kaneko, M., Isumi, H., Matsubara, T., and Furukawa, S. (2003). Serum cytokine concentrations of influenza-associated acute necrotizing encephalopathy. *Pediatr Int* 45(6), 734–6.

Ichiyama, T., Morishima, T., Isumi, H., Matsufuji, H., Matsubara, T., and Furukawa, S. (2004). Analysis of cytokine levels and NF-kappaB activation in peripheral blood mononuclear cells in influenza virus-associated encephalopathy. *Cytokine* 27(1), 31–7.

Ichiyama, T., Suenaga, N., Kajimoto, M., Tohyama, J., Isumi, H., Kubota, M., Mori, M., and Furukawa, S. (2008). Serum and CSF levels of cytokines in acute encephalopathy following prolonged febrile seizures. *Brain Dev* 30(1), 47–52.

Ito, T., Couceiro, J. N., Kelm, S., Baum, L. G., Krauss, S., Castrucci, M. R., Donatelli, I., Kida, H., Paulson, J. C., Webster, R. G., and Kawaoka, Y. (1998). Molecular basis for the generation in pigs of influenza A viruses with pandemic potential. *J Virol* 72(9), 7367–73.

Ito, Y., Ichiyama, T., Kimura, H., Shibata, M., Ishiwada, N., Kuroki, H., Furukawa, S., and Morishima, T. (1999). Detection of influenza virus RNA by reverse transcription-PCR and proinflammatory cytokines in influenza-virus-associated encephalopathy. *J Med Virol* 58(4), 420–5.

Kasai, T., Togashi, T., and Morishima, T. (2000). Encephalopathy associated with influenza epidemics. *Lancet* 355(9214), 1558–9.

Kawada, J., Kimura, H., Ito, Y., Hara, S., Iriyama, M., Yoshikawa, T., and Morishima, T. (2003). Systemic cytokine responses in patients with influenza-associated encephalopathy. *J Infect Dis* 188(5), 690–8.

Khan, M. R., Maheshwari, P. K., Ali, S. A., and Anwarul, H. (2011). Acute necrotizing encephalopathy of childhood: a fatal complication of swine flu. *J Coll Physicians Surg Pak* 21(2), 119–20.

Kimura, S., Ohtuki, N., Nezu, A., Tanaka, M., and Takeshita, S. (1998). Clinical and radiological variability of influenza-related encephalopathy or encephalitis. *Acta Paediatr Jpn* 40(3), 264–70.

Kolfen, W., Pehle, K., and Konig, S. (1998). Is the long-term outcome of children following febrile convulsions favorable? *Dev Med Child Neurol* 40(10), 667–71.

Koskiniemi, M., Rantalaiho, T., Piiparinen, H., von Bonsdorff, C. H., Farkkila, M., Jarvinen, A., Kinnunen, E., Koskiniemi, S., Mannonen, L., Muttilainen, M., Linnavuori, K., Porras, J., Puolakkainen, M., Raiha, K., Salonen, E. M., Ukkonen, P., Vaheri, A., and Valtonen, V. (2001). Infections of the central nervous system of suspected viral origin: a collaborative study from Finland. *J Neurovirol* 7(5), 400–8.

Kurita, A., Furushima, H., Yamada, H., and Inoue, K. (2001). Periodic lateralized epileptiform discharges in influenza B-associated encephalopathy. *Intern Med* 40(8), 813–6.

Kwong, K. L., Lam, S. Y., Que, T. L., and Wong, S. N. (2006). Influenza A and febrile seizures in childhood. *Pediatr Neurol* 35(6), 395–9.

Lee, N., Wong, C. K., Chan, P. K., Lindegardh, N., White, N. J., Hayden, F. G., Wong, E. H., Wong, K. S., Cockram, C. S., Sung, J. J., and Hui, D. S. (2010). Acute encephalopathy associated with influenza A infection in adults. *Emerg Infect Dis* 16(1), 139–42.

Levin, M., Hjelm, M., Kay, J. D., Pincott, J. R., Gould, J. D., Dinwiddie, R., and Matthew, D. J. (1983). Haemorrhagic shock and encephalopathy: a new syndrome with a high mortality in young children. *Lancet* 2(8341), 64–7.

Liu, Y., Han, C., Wang, X., Lin, J., Ma, M., Shu, Y., Zhou, J., Yang, H., Liang, Q., Guo, C., Zhu, J., Wei, H., Zhao, J., Ma, Z., and Pan, J. (2009). Influenza A virus receptors in the respiratory and intestinal tracts of pigeons. *Avian Pathol* 38(4), 263–6.

Lyon, J. B., Remigio, C., Milligan, T., and Deline, C. (2010). Acute necrotizing encephalopathy in a child with H1N1 influenza infection. *Pediatr Radiol* 40(2), 200–5.

Maines, T. R., Lu, X. H., Erb, S. M., Edwards, L., Guarner, J., Greer, P. W., Nguyen, D. C., Szretter, K. J., Chen, L. M., Thawatsupha, P., Chittaganpitch, M., Waicharoen, S., Nguyen, D. T., Nguyen, T., Nguyen, H. H., Kim, J. H., Hoang, L. T., Kang, C., Phuong, L. S., Lim, W., Zaki, S., Donis, R. O., Cox, N. J., Katz, J. M., and Tumpey, T. M. (2005). Avian influenza (H5N1) viruses isolated from humans in Asia in 2004 exhibit increased virulence in mammals. *J Virol* 79(18), 11788–800.

McCullers, J. A., Facchini, S., Chesney, P. J., and Webster, R. G. (1999). Influenza B virus encephalitis. *Clin Infect Dis* 28(4), 898–900.

Mizuguchi, M. (1997). Acute necrotizing encephalopathy of childhood: a novel form of acute encephalopathy prevalent in Japan and Taiwan. *Brain Dev* 19(2), 81–92.

Mizuguchi, M., Abe, J., Mikkaichi, K., Noma, S., Yoshida, K., Yamanaka, T., and Kamoshita, S. (1995). Acute necrotising encephalopathy of childhood: a new syndrome presenting with multifocal, symmetric brain lesions. *J Neurol Neurosurg Psychiatry* 58(5), 555–61.

Mizuguchi, M., Hayashi, M., Nakano, I., Kuwashima, M., Yoshida, K., Nakai, Y., Itoh, M., and Takashima, S. (2002). Concentric structure of thalamic lesions in acute necrotizing encephalopathy. *Neuroradiology* 44(6), 489–93.

Mizuguchi, M., Yamanouchi, H., Ichiyama, T., and Shiomi, M. (2007). Acute encephalopathy associated with influenza and other viral infections. *Acta Neurol Scand Suppl* 186, 45–56.

Monto, A. S. (2006). Vaccines and antiviral drugs in pandemic preparedness. *Emerg Infect Dis* 12(1), 55–60.

Mori, I., and Kimura, Y. (2001). Neuropathogenesis of influenza virus infection in mice. *Microbes Infect* 3(6), 475–9.

Morishima, T., Togashi, T., Yokota, S., Okuno, Y., Miyazaki, C., Tashiro, M., and Okabe, N. (2002). Encephalitis and encephalopathy associated with an influenza epidemic in Japan. *Clin Infect Dis* 35(5), 512–7.

Nakai, Y., Itoh, M., Mizuguchi, M., Ozawa, H., Okazaki, E., Kobayashi, Y., Takahashi, M., Ohtani, K., Ogawa, A., Narita, M., Togashi, T., and Takashima, S. (2003). Apoptosis and microglial activation in influenza encephalopathy. *Acta Neuropathol* 105(3), 233–9.

Okabe, N., Yamashita, K., Taniguchi, K., and Inouye, S. (2000). Influenza surveillance system of Japan and acute encephalitis and encephalopathy in the influenza season. *Pediatr Int* 42(2), 187–91.

Okumura, A., Nakano, T., Fukumoto, Y., Higuchi, K., Kamiya, H., Watanabe, K., and Morishima, T. (2005). Delirious behavior in children with influenza: its clinical features and EEG findings. *Brain Dev* 27(4), 271–4.

Ormitti, F., Ventura, E., Summa, A., Picetti, E., and Crisi, G. (2010). Acute necrotizing encephalopathy in a child during the 2009 influenza A(H1N1) pandemia: MR imaging in diagnosis and follow-up. *AJNR Am J Neuroradiol* 31(3), 396–400.

Park, C. H., Ishinaka, M., Takada, A., Kida, H., Kimura, T., Ochiai, K., and Umemura, T. (2002). The invasion routes of neurovirulent A/Hong Kong/483/97 (H5N1) influenza virus into the central nervous system after respiratory infection in mice. *Arch Virol* 147(7), 1425–36.

PatentLens (2011). The influenza genome comprises eight segments. In *Figure 1: The Eight RNA Segments of the Influenza Genome*, vol. 2011. patentlens.

Peltola, V., Ziegler, T., and Ruuskanen, O. (2003). Influenza A and B virus infections in children. *Clin Infect Dis* 36(3), 299–305.

Poch, O., Sauvaget, I., Delarue, M., and Tordo, N. (1989). Identification of four conserved motifs among the RNA-dependent polymerase encoding elements. *EMBO J* 8(12), 3867–74.

Ravenholt, R. T., and Foege, W. H. (1982). 1918 influenza, encephalitis lethargica, parkinsonism. *Lancet* 2(8303), 860–4.

Reinacher, M., Bonin, J., Narayan, O., and Scholtissek, C. (1983). Pathogenesis of neurovirulent influenza A virus infection in mice. Route of entry of virus into brain determines infection of different populations of cells. *Lab Invest* 49(6), 686–92.

Ryan, M. M., Procopis, P. G., and Ouvrier, R. A. (1999). Influenza A encephalitis with movement disorder. *Pediatr Neurol* 21(3), 669–73.

Salonen, O., Koshkiniemi, M., Saari, A., Myllyla, V., Pyhala, R., Airaksinen, L., and Vaheri, A. (1997). Myelitis associated with influenza A virus infection. *J Neurovirol* 3(1), 83–5.

Schlesinger, R. W., Husak, P. J., Bradshaw, G. L., and Panayotov, P. P. (1998). Mechanisms involved in natural and experimental neuropathogenicity of influenza viruses: evidence and speculation. *Adv Virus Res* 50, 289–379.

Sessa, A., Costa, B., Bamfi, F., Bettoncelli, G., and D'Ambrosio, G. (2001). The incidence, natural history and associated outcomes of influenza-like illness and clinical influenza in Italy. *Fam Pract* 18(6), 629–34.

Shinya, K., Ebina, M., Yamada, S., Ono, M., Kasai, N., and Kawaoka, Y. (2006). Avian flu: influenza virus receptors in the human airway. *Nature* 440(7083), 435–6.

Shinya, K., Silvano, F. D., Morita, T., Shimada, A., Nakajima, M., Ito, T., Otsuki, K., and Umemura, T. (1998). Encephalitis in mice inoculated intranasally with an influenza virus strain originated from a water bird. *J Vet Med Sci* 60(5), 627–9.

Steininger, C., Popow-Kraupp, T., Laferl, H., Seiser, A., Godl, I., Djamshidian, S., and Puchhammer-Stockl, E. (2003). Acute encephalopathy associated with influenza A virus infection. *Clin Infect Dis* 36(5), 567–74.

Stricker, T., and Sennhauser, F. H. (2004). Complex febrile seizures associated with influenza A. *Pediatr Infect Dis J* 23(5), 480.

Studahl, M. (2003). Influenza virus and CNS manifestations. *J Clinical Virol* 28(3), 225–32.

Sugaya, N. (2002). Influenza-associated encephalopathy in Japan. *Semin Pediatr Infect Dis* 13(2), 79–84.

Suzuki, Y. (2011). Avian and human influenza virus receptors and their distribution. *Adv Exp Med Biol* 705, 443–52.

Takahashi, M., Yamada, T., Nakashita, Y., Saikusa, H., Deguchi, M., Kida, H., Tashiro, M., and Toyoda, T. (2000). Influenza virus-induced encephalopathy: clinicopathologic study of an autopsied case. *Pediatr Int* 42(2), 204–14.

Tam, C. C., O'Brien, S. J., Petersen, I., Islam, A., Hayward, A., and Rodrigues, L. C. (2007). Guillain-Barré syndrome and preceding infection with campylobacter, influenza and Epstein-Barr virus in the general practice research database. *PLoS One* 2(4), e344.

Togashi, T., Matsuzono, Y., Narita, M., and Morishima, T. (2004). Influenza-associated acute encephalopathy in Japanese children in 1994–2002. *Virus Res* 103(1–2), 75–8.

Toovey, S. (2008). Influenza-associated central nervous system dysfunction: a literature review. *Travel Med Infectious Dis* 6(3), 114–24.

Tsolia, M. N., Logotheti, I., Papadopoulos, N. G., Mavrikou, M., Spyridis, N. P., Drossatou, P., Kafetzis, D., and Konstantopoulos, A. (2006). Impact of influenza infection in healthy children examined as outpatients and their families. *Vaccine* 24(33–34), 5970–6.

van Toorn, R., and Schoeman, J. F. (2009). Encephalitis lethargica in 5 South African children. *Eur J Paediatr Neurol* 13(1), 41–6.

Vilensky, J. A., Goetz, C. G., and Gilman, S. (2006). Movement disorders associated with encephalitis lethargica: a video compilation. *Mov Disord* 21(1), 1–8.

Wang, G., Zhang, J., Li, W., Xin, G., Su, Y., Gao, Y., Zhang, H., Lin, G., Jiao, X., and Li, K. (2008). Apoptosis and proinflammatory cytokine responses of primary mouse microglia and astrocytes induced by human H1N1 and avian H5N1 influenza viruses. *Cell Mol Immunol* 5(2), 113–20.

Wang, G. F., Li, W., and Li, K. (2010). Acute encephalopathy and encephalitis caused by influenza virus infection. *Curr Opin Neurol* 23(3), 305–11.

Waruiru, C., and Appleton, R. (2004). Febrile seizures: an update. *Arch Dis Child* 89(8), 751–6.

Webster, R. G., Bean, W. J., Gorman, O. T., Chambers, T. M., and Kawaoka, Y. (1992). Evolution and ecology of influenza A viruses. *Microbiol Rev* 56(1), 152–79.

Weitkamp, J. H., Spring, M. D., Brogan, T., Moses, H., Bloch, K. C., and Wright, P. F. (2004). Influenza A virus-associated acute necrotizing encephalopathy in the United States. *Pediatr Infect Dis J* 23(3), 259–63.

Xu, H., Yasui, O., Tsuruoka, H., Kuroda, K., Hayashi, K., Yamada, A., Ishizaki, T., Yamada, Y., Watanabe, T., and Hosaka, Y. (1998). Isolation of type B influenza virus from the blood of children. *Clin Infect Dis* 27(3), 654–5.

Yadav, S., Das, C. J., Kumar, V., and Lodha, R. (2010). Acute necrotizing encephalopathy. *Indian J Pediatr* 77(3), 307–9.

Yokota, S., Imagawa, T., Miyamae, T., Ito, S., Nakajima, S., Nezu, A., and Mori, M. (2000). Hypothetical pathophysiology of acute encephalopathy and encephalitis related to influenza virus infection and hypothermia therapy. *Pediatr Int* 42(2), 197–203.

Yuen, K. Y., Chan, P. K., Peiris, M., Tsang, D. N., Que, T. L., Shortridge, K. F., Cheung, P. T., To, W. K., Ho, E. T., Sung, R., and Cheng, A. F. (1998). Clinical features and rapid viral diagnosis of human disease associated with avian influenza A H5N1 virus. *Lancet* 351(9101), 467–71.

Zitzow, L. A., Rowe, T., Morken, T., Shieh, W. J., Zaki, S., and Katz, J. M. (2002). Pathogenesis of avian influenza A (H5N1) viruses in ferrets. *J Virol* 76(9), 4420–9.

15 Human Paramyxoviruses and Infections of the Central Nervous System

Michael R. Wilson, Martin Ludlow, and W. Paul Duprex

CONTENTS

15.1 INTRODUCTION

Paramyxoviruses represent a diverse family of human and animal pathogens which, to a greater or lesser extent, have a propensity to infect the central nervous system (CNS).

Common pathological themes unite paramyxovirus infections and many of the viruses are capable of spreading to the CNS where acute encephalitis and reactivation following long-term persistence are prominent clinical features. Indeed, the prototypic morbillivirus measles virus (MV) provides a paradigm for the long-term persistent RNA virus infection in humans. Sub-acute sclerosing panencephalitis (SSPE) is an invariably fatal rare sequela of measles occurring months to years after the initial infection. Likewise the recently identified, and highly pathogenic, biosafety level 4 (BSL-4) agent Nipah virus (NiV) has been shown to reactivate in the CNS of a number of patients months after the acute infection. Here we seek to compare and contrast the symptoms presented when these human paramyxoviruses infect the CNS underpinning this by highlighting their common molecular biological and virological properties (Table 15.1).

Although outside the scope of this chapter, much has been learned from natural and experimental infections using animal models of paramyxovirus diseases (von Messling et al. 2003). Such approaches are all the more important given the zoonotic potential of some of these viruses. In fact, only two of the four neurotropic paramyxoviruses we discuss in detail, MV and mumps virus (MuV), are exclusively human pathogens. Zoonotic infections by hitherto unrecognized animal viruses are typically associated with higher levels of pathogenicity than is observed following infection with viruses which only circulate in a single species as co-evolution of the virus and host tends to diminish pathogenicity over time. Thus the 40–75% mortality rates observed in NiV and Hendra virus (HeV) infections are in striking contrast to the 0.01–0.03% mortality rates observed for MuV and MV in the developed world. It is tempting to speculate that much higher levels of mortality were observed when MV and MuV initially jumped species from their animal reservoirs into humans. The high levels of morbidity and mortality resulting from NiV and HeV infections in the 21st century may reflect what occurred several thousand years ago when human populations reached the size and density necessary to sustain endemic MV and MuV transmission. Given the current interest in emerging and re-emerging pathogens, the fact that MuV recently infected thousands of college students in the United Kingdom and the United States and with the regular importation of MV into Europe and the United States from the developing world, it is timely to compare, contrast, and review these neurotropic paramyxoviruses.

Given the similarities in virion structure, genome organization, replication, transcription, and how paramyxovirus proteins generally function within the cell, it is logical to address the biological aspects for MV, MuV, NiV, and HeV together. The pertinent historical perspectives and key aspects of paramyxovirus biology will be covered first to set the scene and allow the reader to appreciate the unifying molecular biological features of this family of viruses. However, there are tremendous differences among the four viruses in terms of clinical presentation, pathogenesis, epidemiology, and neurotropism, and therefore these aspects will be treated separately. For those who wish to gain a greater understanding of the molecular biological properties of the paramyxoviruses we refer the reader to the recently published book, *The Biology of Paramyxoviruses* (Samal 2011), which covers many of the viruses in greater detail as well as the relevant chapters in Fields Virology (Carbone and Rubin 2007; Eaton et al. 2007; Griffin 2007).

15.2 PARAMYXOVIRUSES: THE HISTORICAL PERSPECTIVE

As the prototypic morbillivirus, and probably the most well-known paramyxovirus, more is understood about the molecular and cell biology of MV than any of the other viruses we will discuss. Following the eradication of smallpox, MV is probably the most transmissible human virus having an R_0 between 12 and 18 (Moss and Griffin 2006). The virus causes a systemic disease primarily of the immune system and is associated with high levels of morbidity and mortality in the developing world, largely as a consequence of the profound immune suppression induced in infected individuals (Avota et al. 2010). The first written account of MV infection dates from the 9th century and is ascribed to the Arabian physician Abu Becr, also known as Rhazes of Baghdad, who dated the first description of measles to the 6th century (Hirsch 1883). Phylogenetic analysis indicates that MV probably evolved from the ancestor of the closely related rinderpest virus (RPV) which predominately infects cattle (Furuse et al. 2010). However, the strict tropism displayed by current circulating wild-type MV strains for humans and some species of monkey is indicative of the typical evolution of a virus following zoonotic infection whereby the virus becomes ever more adapted to the new host. It is assumed that MV only became permanently established in human populations after the development of cities in India and the Middle East of sufficient size to fulfill the requirement of 250,000 to 500,000 people necessary to maintain endemic MV transmission (Keeling and Grenfell 1997). Consequently MV has been termed a disease of civilization due to the requirement for a sufficiently large population of naive susceptible hosts to maintain an endemic infection.

The first scientific investigation into measles occurred in 1757 when the Scottish physician Francis Home transmitted the disease to uninfected individuals by injecting blood from individuals who were beginning to display the characteristic rash produced (Plotkin 1967). This crude approach provided the first demonstration that measles is caused by an infectious agent. Characterization of MV and vaccine development was facilitated by the introduction of sterile mammalian cell culture techniques in the mid-20th century, the use of which enabled Enders and Peebles to isolate MV from a child named David Edmonston in 1954 (Enders and Peebles 1954). The subsequent generation of a closely related collection of live attenuated measles virus vaccines which are used to this day can be traced back to this discovery.

TABLE 15.1

Virological and Clinical Features of Neurovirulent Human Paramyxoviruses

	Measles Virus	Mumps Virus	Nipah and Hendra Viruses
Molecular Biology			
Genome length	15,894 nucleotides	15,384 nucleotides	18,246 and 18,234 nucleotides
Transcription units	6	7	6
Proteins	N-P/V/C-M-F_0-H-L (2 nonstructural)	N-V/W/P-M-SH-F_0-HN-L (3 nonstructural)	N-P/V/W/C-M-F_0-G-L (3 nonstructural)
Pathogenesis			
Cellular receptor[a]	CD150 and Nectin-4	Unidentified sialylated glycoproteins and/or glycolipids	EphrinB2 (NiV and HeV) and ephrinB3 (NiV)
Target cells	Alveolar macrophages, dendritic cells, activated B and T cells, epithelial cells, neurons, oligodendrocytes, astrocytes (rarely), and endothelial cells (rarely)	Unknown[b]	Capillary and arterial endothelial cells, smooth muscle, and neurons
Systems targeted	Immune (circulating lymphocytes and lymphoid tissues), respiratory and CNS	Endocrine (e.g., salivary, thyroid, pancreas, testes, and ovaries) and CNS	Circulatory and CNS
Natural host range	Human[c]	Human[c]	Bat, human, pig, dog, cat, and horse
Mortality rate	0.03%[d]	0.03%[d]	40%–75%

CNS Manifestations	APME	MIBE	SSPE	Meningoencephalitis	Acute Encephalitis	Delayed or Recurrent
Disease onset after primary infection	1 to 4 weeks	1 to 6 months	5 to 10 years	0 to 2 weeks	0 to 8 days	9 days to 2 years
Neurologic signs and symptoms	Fever, headache, irritability, focal neurologic deficits, malaise, and seizures	Malaise, seizures (e.g., epilepsia partialis continua), cortical deficits progressing to coma	Behavioral and intellectual impairment progressing to ataxic-myoclonic dementia	Fever, meningismus, focal neurologic deficits, malaise, seizures, and papilledema (rarely)	Fever, meningismus, brainstem signs, malaise, and seizures	Fever (less common), headache, focal neurologic deficits, malaise, and seizures

MRI findings	Numerous, ill-defined T2-signal hyperintensities predominantly at the gray-white junction, uniform gadolinium enhancement	Focal T2-signal hyperintensities (few reports)	Diffuse subcortical white matter T2-signal hyperintensities	Frequently normal; diffuse T2-signal hyperintensities; hydrocephalus (very rarely)	Diffuse, punctate (2–7 mm) T2-signal hyperintensities (microinfarcts)	Confluent gray and white matter T2-signal hyperintensities
Diagnosis	CSF pleocytosis and elevated protein, MRI and history or recent infection or vaccination	CSF normal or with mild pleocytosis and elevated protein, MRI, history or recent infection and immunosuppression, absence of intrathecal MV-specific antibodies	EEG with periodic spike and wave complexes, MRI, elevated CSF gamma globulins and oligoclonal bands, elevated serum and intrathecal production of IgG MV-specific antibodies	CSF pleocytosis and elevated protein, MuV-specific antibodies	CSF pleocytosis and elevated protein, HeV- or NiV-specific antibodies	CSF pleocytosis, IgG HeV- or NiV-specific antibodies, history of NiV or HeV infection
Treatment	High-dose corticosteroids	Supportive	Combination of inosiplex and IFN-α (noncurative)	Supportive	Ribavarin (controversial)	Supportive
Prognosis	Excellent (<10% mortality)	Fatal over days to weeks	Fatal (95%) over months to years	Excellent	Fatal (40–75%) over days; Long-term neurologic sequelae (20–30%)	Fatal (20%) over days to weeks; Long-term neurologic sequelae (60%)

a For clinical isolates.

b As a respiratory infection, it is presumed, although not proven, that MuV infects epithelial cells in the URT and local lymph modes. As a neurotropic infection, ependymal cells and neurons are infected.

c Nonhuman primates can act as incidental hosts but are mainly used in voluntary laboratory infections.

d In the developed world.

MuV is a member of the *Rubulavirus* genus in the family *Paramyxoviridae*. Like MV, MuV is one of the earliest recorded diseases being described by Hippocrates in 400 BC in his treatise "Of the Epidemics." In 1790, Robert Hamilton provided the first detailed clinical description of mumps, including a case of fulminant mumps encephalitis (Hamilton 1790). The clinical manifestations were first demonstrated to be viral in etiology in 1934 by Johnson and Goodpasture when they successfully transferred the disease from children to monkeys (Johnson and Goodpasture 1934). However, it took until 1968 for the first live attenuated MuV vaccine to be developed (Hilleman et al. 1968). Before widespread vaccination, MuV was the leading cause of virus-induced aseptic meningitis and encephalitis in the US and Europe, causing meningitis in up to 65% of patients (Bang and Bang 1943). Indeed, meningoencephalitis is the most common extra-salivary gland manifestation of a MuV infection, although other neurological complications include transverse myelitis, sensorineural deafness, cerebellar ataxia, seizures, and cranial nerve palsies (Nussinovitch et al. 1995). Interestingly, MuV has recently reemerged in the developed world having infected over 6000 college students in the United States in 2006 (Barskey et al. 2009). The virus was imported from the UK, and there have been discussions as to whether or not it might be necessary to instigate a third round of vaccination to break transmission (Rubin 2011).

Vaccination strategies have been complicated by the fact that a number of MuV vaccines caused aseptic meningitis in vaccinees (Balraj and Miller 1995; da Cunha et al. 2002; Dourado et al. 2000; Sugiura and Yamada 1991). This resulted in withdrawal of the vaccines, public resistance to MuV vaccination, and, in some countries, complete cessation of national vaccination programs for mumps (Colville et al. 1994; Furesz and Contreras 1990; Hashimoto et al. 2009; Sasaki and Tsunoda 2009). As a consequence of the withdrawal of mumps vaccines from Japan's national vaccination program, over 2 million cases of mumps are reported annually which are accompanied by significant numbers of MuV-induced aseptic meningitis and deafness (Nagai et al. 2007).

Unlike MV and MuV, the henipaviruses are relative newcomers into the paramyxovirus arena. In fact, the *Henipavirus* genus was only created in 2002 after the identification and molecular characterization of NiV and HeV. In September 1994, 21 horses and 2 handlers in the Brisbane suburb of Hendra, Queensland, developed a severe respiratory illness that killed 14 of the horses and 1 person within 2 weeks (Murray et al. 1995; Selvey et al. 1995). Initially, the agent was called equine morbillivirus, although HeV was renamed after flying foxes of the genus *Pteropus* and not horses were identified as the reservoir (Chua et al. 2002; Halpin et al. 2000). Following the initial outbreak, HeV infections have continued to occur in horses once or twice a year, although unusually there have been at least 17 outbreaks in 2011 thus far (Ksiazek et al. 2011). Four of the seven infected people have died, including one person who died from encephalitis a year after a likely HeV exposure (O'Sullivan et al. 1997). NiV was first identified in 1998–1999 after an outbreak of viral encephalitis in Malaysian pig farmers. Interestingly this unidentified zoonotic agent was initially thought to be Japanese encephalitis virus, illustrating how a very similar clinical presentation presents significant challenges in the timely diagnosis of novel emerging viruses (Chua et al. 1999). The mortality rate was nearly

40% among the almost 300 people infected. After spreading to Singapore, the outbreak was stopped only after the slaughter of over one million swine (Ksiazek et al. 2011). NiV continues to expand its geographical range and virulence having caused large outbreaks in India, Bangladesh, Australia, Singapore, and Malaysia. The most recent outbreaks in India and Bangladesh have demonstrated increasing mortality rates approaching 75% as well as multiple cases of person-to-person transmission (Blum et al. 2009; Chadha et al. 2006; Homaira et al. 2010; Hsu et al. 2004). Due to their incredibly wide host range (horses, cats, dogs, rabbits, laboratory rodents), geographical-range, high mortality, transmissibility, and ease of culture *in vitro*, NiV and HeV were assigned as BSL-4 agents soon after their discovery. Two key features of these infections are their zoonotic potential and their propensity to establish persistent infection. Indeed, what we observe for NiV and HeV in the 21st century might well have been what was observed in ancient history for the BSL-2 agents, MV, and MuV (see above). This highlights the benefit and utility in studying emerging viruses alongside more established and closely related pathogens as the knowledge gained for one can be leveraged into the treatment of those which continue to emerge from unknown reservoirs.

15.3 PARAMYXOVIRUSES: THE BIOLOGICAL PROPERTIES

15.3.1 Virus Structure

Paramyxovirus virions are enveloped particles varying in shape from spherical to filamentous to pleomorphic. Spherical viruses, such as MV and MuV, have average diameters of 200 nm and are indistinguishable by electron microscopy (EM). Likewise, the filamentous virions of HeV and NiV are similar by EM and are morphologically similar to other members of the subfamily *Paramyxovirinae* (Chua et al. 2000b). However, NiV virions are typically larger on average than other paramyxoviruses (500 nm) having a broader variation in diameter (180–1900 nm) (Goldsmith et al. 2003). Paramyxoviruses are highly cell-associated and cell-to-cell spread may be very important *in vivo*. All of the viruses have a glycoprotein fringe of spikes which protrude from the cell-derived lipid envelope. Ultrastructurally, HeV surface projections have a double-fringed appearance while NiV surface projections have a single fringe (Hyatt et al. 2001). Two glycoproteins (see below) comprise the biologically active fusion complex which interacts with cell surface molecules to initiate the infection.

15.3.2 Genome Organization

The basic unit of infectivity for all paramyxoviruses is a negative (–) sensed RNA molecule which co-exists with an encapsidated helical ribonucleoprotein (RNP) complex, the (–)RNP (Eaton et al. 2006; Samal 2011). These helical structures protect the genome from nucleases, increasing the stability of the virus. Normally only a single (–)RNP is encapsidated, although interestingly measles virions can contain more than one copy of the genome and be functionally polyploid (Rager et al. 2002). Reverse genetics approaches have been used to split the MV genome and illustrate that the virus can encapsidate two (–)RNPs (Takeda et al. 2006). Although paramyxoviruses have differing numbers of transcription units (MV, NiV, and HeV have six whereas MuV has seven), the genomic organization is similar (Table 15.1). A gene start (GS) sequence contains the necessary signals for the initiation of transcription and a 5′ untranslated region (UTR) prior to each open reading frame (ORF). The ORF is followed by a gene-end (GE) sequence that contains a 3′UTR and sequences which mediate the template-independent polyadenylation of the resulting messenger RNA (mRNA). Transcription is mediated by a virus encoded RNA-dependent RNA polymerase (RdRp) which is associated with the (–)RNP and must be packaged into a virion to ensure infectivity (Samal 2011). Transcription units are separated by nontranscribed intergenic (Ig) spacers. These Ig spacers are ignored by the RdRp during primary and secondary transcription and are only copied during replication of the complete genome (see below). The genome is flanked by a leader (Le) sequence at the 5′ end which contains a single genomic promoter (GP) where the RdRp initiates transcription and genome replication. A trailer (Tr) sequence is present at the 5′ end of the genome. This contains a stronger anti-genomic promoter (AGP) from which the RdRp synthesizes nascent copies of the genome which are encapsidated into budding virions. Genome sizes vary with MuV (15,384 nt) being smaller than MV (15,894 nt) which in turn is smaller than HeV (18,234 nt) and NiV (18,246 nt) making these henipaviruses approximately 15% larger than others in the same family. Notably, each genome length obeys the "rule of six" adhered to by all paramyxoviruses. The helical nucleocapsid core is structured for each nucleocapsid (N) protein to be associated with precisely six nucleotides. Despite the varied genome lengths, most of the viral proteins are quite similar in size and the additional genome length of NiV and HeV is due to the presence of longer 5′ and 3′UTRs. MuV has an extra transcription unit that encodes the small hydrophobic (SH) protein which again adds to the length of the genome. Genes are arranged linearly and, for the most part, there is a common order for the four viruses (Table 15.1). From the 5′ end to the 3′ end six ORFs encode the N protein, phospho- (P) protein, matrix (M) protein, fusion (F) glycoprotein, an attachment glycoprotein, and the large (L) protein. Three types of attachment proteins are encoded depending on the virus, a standard glycoprotein (G), a hemagglutinin (H) glycoprotein, or a hemagglutinin-neuraminidase (HN) glycoprotein. The SH protein in MuV is located between the F and HN glycoproteins and is the fifth transcription unit. The P gene encodes multiple proteins and is more correctly termed the P/C/V gene for MV, HeV, and NiV and the V/W/P gene for MuV (see below).

15.3.3 PROTEIN FUNCTIONS

Proteins are defined as either structural (N, P, M, F, G, H, HN, and L) or nonstructural (C, V, SH, and W). The (–)RNP complex is composed primarily of the N protein with the P and L proteins comprising the RdRp (see below). Depending on the virus, three or four proteins form the virions. The type I F and the type II G/H/HN glycoproteins are integral membrane proteins which form the EM visible fusion spike complexes. Most of the proteins are externalized, and their short cytoplasmic tails interact with the membrane associated M protein which is the key bridge between the lipid envelope and the (–)RNP. Although normally considered to be a nonstructural protein, the MuV SH protein may act as a viroporin embedded in the virus envelope. The protein is not required for replication *in vitro* (Takeuchi et al. 1996), and it is unclear to what degree it plays a role in pathogenesis *in vivo* (Malik et al. 2011).

Virulence, host range, and cell tropism are determined largely by the two attachment proteins which are both required for entry of virus into target cells (Bossart et al. 2001; Samal 2011; Tamin 2002). The G proteins of HeV and NiV possess neither hemagglutination nor neuraminidase activities (Tamin 2002). Early studies suggested that the similar *in vivo* tropism made it possible that HeV and NiV shared a common cellular receptor and that the molecule should be highly expressed on endothelial cells. Furthermore, given the propensity of the viruses to infect a range of species it was likely that the receptor would be highly conserved (Bossart et al. 2002). Identification of ephrinB2 as the receptor (Bonaparte 2005; Negrete et al. 2005) was consistent with these hypotheses as it is expressed on arterial and capillary endothelial cells, smooth muscle of the tunica media, and neurons. The molecule is the membrane-bound ligand for the ephrinB class of receptor tyrosine kinases and is important for regulating axon pathfinding, neuronal cell migration, and vasculogenesis (Poliakov et al. 2004). EphrinB3 serves as an alternate receptor for NiV, although with lower affinity (Bossart et al. 2008; Negrete et al. 2006). The highly lymphotropic and immune suppressive nature of MV made it likely that the wild-type virus would bind a cellular receptor which is highly expressed on immune cells. Identification of CD150 as the primary MV receptor (Tatsuo et al. 2000) was consistent with primary pathogenesis as the molecule is expressed on activated T and B lymphocytes and regulate several leukocyte functions (Romero et al. 2004; Veillette 2006). However, MV also infects epithelial and neuronal cells which do not express CD150. Identification of PVRL4 as an epithelial receptor for MV (Noyce et al. 2011) has helped to explain the means by which MV infects epithelial cells, but the receptor used to infect neurons remains unclear. PVRL4 is present in adherent junctions of epithelial cells and binding is essential for virus release and probably transmission (Leonard et al. 2010; Shirogane et al. 2010). As an HN glycoprotein, the MuV attachment protein binds sialic acid moieties conjugated to glycoproteins and glycolipids (Samal 2011). Therefore it is unsurprising that the virus infects a wide range of cell types *in vitro*. However, this is not the case *in vivo*. Although basically nothing is known about the first cells targeted by MuV, it has been suggested it initially infects the upper respiratory tract (URT). Therefore it is probable that sialic acid molecules attached to particular molecules are used preferentially, although this has not been demonstrated. The HN protein has two apparently opposing activities, adsorption to sialic acid-containing cell surface molecules (hemagglutination) and enzymatic cleavage of sialic acid (neuraminidase activity). Recent studies have indicated that both functions are located in a single sialic acid recognition site. A recent crystal structure study of the HN glycoprotein of a closely related paramyxovirus, Newcastle disease virus, indicates that amino acid position 466 may be at or near this active site (Yuan et al. 2011). Paramyxovirus F glycoproteins are generated as an inactive precursor (F_0) which is cleaved by cellular proteases into a disulfide-linked F_1 and F_2 complex. The ubiquitous intracellular protease furin activates the MV F_0 glycoprotein in the Golgi or post-Golgi apparatus (Navaratnarajah et al.

2011; Watanabe et al. 1995). This is the same site where the MuV F_0 glycoprotein is cleaved into F_1 and F_2, although the specific protease has not formally been identified. Henipavirus F_0 glycoproteins are activated in a unique manner by endocytosis and cleavage following initial surface expression (Vogt et al. 2005). Cathepsin I cleaves the HeV F glycoprotein whereas cathepsin L cleaves NiV F glycoprotein (Diederich et al. 2009).

When observed by EM the M protein appears as a shell of electron dense material just below the surface of virions. Recent image reconstruction of MV particles has shown that the M protein forms helices coating the helical (–)RNP rather than coating the inner leaflet of the membrane, as previously thought (Liljeroos et al. 2011). Although not proven, this structural organization may well extend to other paramyxoviruses. The M protein provides structure to the virion by interacting with the cytoplasmic tail of the F and H/HN/G glycoproteins, the (–)RNP complex and the inner leaflet of the lipid bilayer (Eaton et al. 2006; Samal 2011). Above and beyond its structural role within the virion, the MV M protein also acts as a repressor of transcription and viral RNA synthesis (Suryanarayana et al. 1994).

The second transcription unit of the four human neurotropic paramyxoviruses is particular for a number of reasons. First, for MV, NiV, and HeV the primary transcript encodes the structural P protein whereas for MuV it encodes the nonstructural V protein. Additional coding capacity for all of the viruses is obtained by a novel co-transcriptional process in which one or more nontemplated G nucleotides are inserted at a conserved editing site in the gene, resulting in an altered mRNA in which there is a shift in the ORF. This leads to the generation of V proteins for MV, HeV, and MuV or the P protein for MuV. Second, an additional nonstructural protein is encoded in an overlapping reading frame which is accessed when the ribosome fails to initiate at the first AUG codon and scans to the subsequent start codon. Therefore it is formally correct to refer to the second gene of MV, NiV, and MuV as the P/C/V transcription unit and for MuV it is the V/W/P.

Regardless of how they are generated during transcription the nonstructural V proteins have similar functions in abrogating the antiviral type I interferon (IFN) response by interfering with dsRNA and IFN signaling, reviewed by Gerlier and Valentin (2009). The amino terminus of V, and consequently P, binds to signal transducers and activators of transcription (STAT) 1 proteins which inhibits IFN signaling. Unlike MuV, which inhibits STAT signaling by eliminating STAT 1 and STAT 3, henipaviruses sequester STAT proteins in high molecular weight complexes, preventing their dimerization and translocation into the nucleus. This activity is shared to varying degrees by the V, W, and P proteins. All three proteins also inhibit phosphorylation of tyrosine residues in STAT (Rodriguez and Horvath 2004; Samal 2011). The accessory W protein also blocks activation of IFN-regulatory factor 3 (IRF-3)-responsive promoters in response to intracellular dsRNA signaling and signaling through Toll-like receptor 3. The carboxyl terminus of the V protein is used to inhibit dsRNA by inhibiting oligomerization the helicase encoded by the melanoma differentiation-associated gene 5. This, in turn, restricts signaling and inhibits IFN production (Childs et al. 2009).

15.3.4   REPLICATION AND TRANSCRIPTION

An essential component of every virion is the RdRp which is comprised of the L and P proteins. RNA initiation, elongation and termination, mRNA capping, and methylation along with polyadenylation functions all reside with the L protein which acts both as a replicase and as a transcriptase (see above). Primary transcription is carried out by the incoming RdRp to produce a set of mRNAs which accumulate in the infected cell and are translated in the cytoplasm. When sufficient levels of virus proteins accumulate, some replication commences to produce (+)RNPs which, in turn, act as templates for the generation of (–)RNPs. These are used in secondary transcription and are packaged into nascent virions (see below). All RNA synthesis takes place in the cytoplasm, and intracytoplasmic inclusions which stain positive for the N, P, and L proteins are common. It has been suggested but not proven that these are the sites of transcription and replication.

15.3.5   REPLICATION CYCLE

Paramyxoviruses enter the cell by fusion at the plasma membrane following binding to cell surface receptors. Deposition of the (–)RNP into the cytoplasm initiates primary transcription, and the RdRp accesses the template at the single promoter in the 3′ end of the genome. At each Ig junction, there is the possibility that the RdRp will detach from the (–)RNP. This start-stop mechanism leads to the generation of a transcription gradient in which more mRNA transcripts encoding the N protein are present in the cell compared with proteins encoded from the downstream transcription units. This provides an elegant means to regulate gene expression. When sufficient levels of the N, P, and L proteins are produced, replication of the negative-sensed genome ensues (see above). Synthesis of the M protein and F_0 and G, H, or HN glycoproteins occurs in the cytoplasm with H and F_0 being trafficked to the cell surface through the endoplasmic reticulum and Golgi apparatus. MV budding occurs from lipid rafts at the plasma membrane (Manie et al. 2000). Neuraminidase activity of the MuV HN glycoprotein facilitates release from the infected cell by cleaving sialic acids moieties from the glycoproteins and glycolipids. This activity is not required for MV, NiV, and NiV, although CD150 is down-regulated from the surface of MV-infected cells (Erlenhoefer et al. 2001).

15.4   MEASLES VIRUS

15.4.1   CLINICAL PRESENTATION

Symptoms first become apparent during the viremic phase of the disease. The development of a cough, fever, and conjunctivitis typically precedes the appearance of the hallmark maculopapular rash which spreads from the trunk to the extremities. Although MV is not highly neurovirulent, three distinct neurological complications can occur following a natural MV infection.

15.4.1.1 Acute Postinfectious Measles Encephalomyelitis

Acute postinfectious measles encephalomyelitis (APME) or acute demyelinating encephalomyelitis (ADEM) usually presents within 1 to 3 weeks after rash onset and is characterized by malaise, recrudescence of fever, seizures, and a mortality rate less than 10% (Norrby and Kristensson 1997). CSF may be normal, although a mononuclear pleocytosis and a moderate elevation in protein levels is typically present. Intracranial pressure can be mildly elevated. Antibodies to MV and increased intrathecal production of IgG are not found (Johnson et al. 1984). MRI demonstrates diffuse, ill-defined white matter disease most prominently at the gray-white junction as evidenced by T2-signal hyperintensities along with uniform gadolinium contrast enhancement.

15.4.1.2 Measles Inclusion Body Encephalitis

Measles inclusion body encephalitis (MIBE) is characterized by progressive neurological deterioration, seizures (commonly epilepsia partialis continua), and coma over days to weeks in individuals who are unable to mount a CD4$^+$ or CD8$^+$ T-cell mediated immune response (Mustafa et al. 1993; Wolinsky et al. 1977). This may be due to a congenital immunodeficiency or a result of the immunosuppressive effects of infections such as HIV-1 (Budka et al. 1996). Clinical symptoms become apparent one to six months after primary infection (Kaplan et al. 1992). Unlike patients with subacute sclerosing panencephalitis (SSPE) (see below), levels of MV antibodies do not increase. MRI and pathological findings are also similar to what are observed for SSPE patients, except that inflammatory changes are absent.

15.4.1.3 Subacute Sclerosing Panencephalitis

The term SSPE was first used on the recommendation of Greenfield to describe a sporadic encephalitis occurring in Europe in the middle of the 20th century (Greenfield 1950) although the first pathological description of an "inclusion body encephalitis" was made by Dawson in 1933. SSPE occurs on average after a 5- to 10-year incubation period in the presence of elevated MV-specific antibody titers in both the serum and CSF (Bouteille et al. 1965; Connolly et al. 1967). Although adults can be affected (Prashanth et al. 2006), SSPE largely presents in immunocompetent children whose primary MV infection occurred before age two and is one of the few causes of progressive ataxic-myoclonic chronic dementia in children. Children typically present with intellectual decline along with psychiatric and behavioral problems (stage I) followed months to years later by the development of myoclonic jerks, ataxia, and seizures (stage II). The electroencephalography (EEG) in SSPE demonstrates characteristic periodic complexes that are stereotyped, bilaterally synchronous and symmetrical 100–1000 mV, 1–3 Hz waves lasting 1–3 seconds separated by a 2–20 second interval (Praveen-kumar et al. 2007). Coma ensues (stage III) months to years later. Stage IV of SSPE is characterized by akinetic mutism. Pseudobulbar affect and startle myoclonus are common. Death due to infection or vasomotor collapse typically occurs 2–3 years after disease onset. Although more fulminant courses have been reported as have spontaneous remissions in approximately 5% of cases (Freeman 1969; Gutierrez et al. 2010; Risk and Haddad 1979). MRI demonstrates T2 hyperintense lesions that progress from the subcortical white matter to the periventricular regions along with progressive cerebral atrophy (Anlar et al. 1996; Murata et al. 1987). There is little or no pleocytosis in the CSF, although total protein concentration is elevated. The gamma globulin fraction in particular is elevated with the presence of IgG oligoclonal bands. Neuro-ophthalmologic complications are also common and include retinal pigmentation, optic atrophy, chorioretinitis, optic neuritis and papilledema (Robb and Watters 1970). SSPE is viewed as the paradigm of a persistent RNA virus infection in the human.

15.4.2 Diagnosis

Prior to molecular diagnostic approaches, observing the presence of the pathognomonic prodromal Koplik spots around the buccal mucosa was the primary means of making the diagnosis of measles. Currently, serological assays to detect MV-specific IgG and IgM antibodies are typically used. APME is primarily a clinical diagnosis (see above). A presumptive diagnosis of SSPE can be made by a combination of the clinical presentation in a young patient, the presence of the characteristic periodic complexes on EEG, elevated gamma globulins and the presence of oligoclonal bands in the CSF, characteristic MRI findings and elevated measles antibody titers in the serum and CSF. Similarly, MIBE is primarily a clinical diagnosis, although for all three neurological complications of MV infection, neuropathology provides the ultimate confirmation of the diagnosis.

15.4.3 Pathology and Pathogenesis

MV is highly contagious, spreads by the aerosol route and infects alveolar macrophages and dendritic cells in the lower respiratory tract (Lemon et al. 2011). The virus spreads rapidly to bronchial associated lymphoid tissues and then local lymph nodes, where the infection is amplified. Viremia is primarily mediated by MV-infected lymphocytes and dendritic cells (de Swart et al. 2007), and this enables spread to many organs throughout the body (Esolen et al. 1993). Although some of the target organs such as the spleen or tonsils are primarily lymphoid in origin, numerous other organs and tissues are infected (e.g., kidney, lung, liver, and skin). Nebulization of recombinant MVs expressing enhanced green fluorescent protein (EGFP) into the macaque, the only animal model which recapitulates the natural, systemic infection, has facilitated the identification of the primary target cells (Lemon et al. 2011).

The three neurological complications of measles display differing pathology. Examination of fatal APME cases reveals perivascular inflammation and demyelination with a corresponding loss of myelin basic protein (Johnson et al. 1984). This is presumed to be due to an autoimmune response as virus has not been isolated or detected in brain tissue obtained from APME patients who succumbed to the infection (Gendelman et al. 1984). In contrast to APME, examination of brain tissues obtained from MIBE patients shows evidence of gliosis and both intranuclear and intracytoplasmic viral inclusion bodies but little evidence of inflammation (Aicardi et al. 1977). Therefore MIBE appears to share many common features with SSPE (see below) but has a more rapid disease progression due to the absence of a viable cell mediated immune response. SSPE is characterized by inflammatory infiltrates in both the gray and white matter, hence the term "panencephalitis." Diffuse demyelination, astroglial sclerosis, and viral antigen contained in inclusion bodies in neurons and oligodendrocytes are also observed (Herndon and Rubinstein 1968).

The route of entry used by MV to infect the CNS is unknown, but it may involve passage through the blood-brain-barrier in infected leukocytes or direct infection of cerebral endothelial cells at the blood-brain-barrier (Kirk et al. 1991). Examination of the anatomical distribution of MV antigen in the CNS of SSPE patients has shown that MV is present in the frontal cortex, basal ganglia, cerebellum, thalamus, medulla, and parietal cortex (McQuaid et al. 1998). EM analysis of brain tissues obtained from SSPE patients shows cell-to-cell fusion, albeit in rare instances. Virus budding is typically absent from infected cells (Iwasaki and Koprowski 1974). *In vitro* studies have shown that laboratory-adapted MV can spread between primary hippocampal neurons in the absence of CD46 (Lawrence et al. 2000). Examination of SSPE brain tissue sections by immunohistochemistry shows that CD150 cannot be detected on neurons or oligodendrocytes (McQuaid and Cosby 2002) and that CD46 cannot be detected in MV infected brain lesions (McQuaid et al. 1997). These observations have given credence to the idea that MV may spread within the CNS through localized fusion events at lateral cell-to-cell contacts, thus negating the need for a specific virus receptor (Allen et al. 1996). The interconnectivity between neurons is readily visible when indirect immunocytochemistry is used to detect viral antigen (Figure 15.1a). It remains to be determined if the recently identified wild-type MV receptor PVRL4 (Noyce et al. 2011) has a role in the cell-to-cell spread of MV within the CNS.

MV was first isolated from SSPE brain tissue by co-cultivation of explants with immortalized cells *in vitro* (Chen et al. 1969). The lack of virus budding *in vivo* was mirrored *in vitro* and consequently contributed to the development of cell lines persistently infected with "SSPE" viruses. Advances in molecular biology resulted in PCR amplification, cloning, and sequencing of MV genes directly from SSPE brain tissue, removing the need to generate persistently infected cell lines where the effect of the host cell environment on the virus could be a complicating factor. Sequence analysis showed that the N, P, and L genes are relatively well conserved in comparison to wild-type progenitor strains (Jin et al. 2002). However, the M, F, and H genes contain many alterations from the wild-type sequence and the M gene is particularly prone to mutations (Hall et al. 1979). The M gene can be disrupted in two main ways, first by biased hypermutations due to the action of the cellular dsRNA-dependent unwinding enzyme (Cattaneo et al. 1988). This results in frequent U to C substitutions, some of which prevent the generation of a functional M protein. Second, single point mutations or deletions in the P GE sequence are common (Ayata et al. 2002). This leads to read through transcription at the P-M Ig junction by the RdRp which generates bicistronic P-M mRNAs in which the second ORF cannot be accessed by the ribosome; this in turn decreases the levels of M protein in the cell (Cattaneo et al. 1987). Analysis of the F gene sequences has consistently shown the presence of single nucleotide substitutions or deletions which produce premature stop codons leading to the production of glycoproteins with truncated cytoplasmic

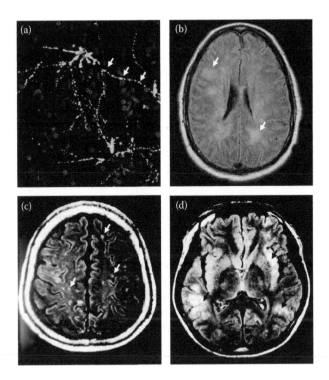

FIGURE 15.1   (See color insert.) (a) Detection of the N protein of MV in a 7-μm section obtained from an SSPE case by indirect immunofluorescence (green). Nuclei from uninfected neurons are counterstained with propidium iodide (red). Interconnecting neuronal processes (arrows) and cell bodies (asterisk) are indicated. (b) T2-weighted MRI sequence of a patient with MuV encephalitis. T2-signal hyperintensities are indicated (arrows). (Copyright © MedReviews®, LLC. Adapted and reprinted with permission of MedReviews, LLC. Cooper A.D. et al. Mumps encephalitis: return with a vengeance. *Rev Neurol Dis.* 2007; 4:100–102. *Reviews in Neurological Diseases* is a copyrighted publication of MedReviews, LLC. All rights reserved.) (c) T2-weighted MRI sequence of a patient with acute NiV encephalitis. Selected punctate T2-signal hyperintensities are indicated (arrows). (d) T2-weighted MRI sequence of a patient with relapsed NiV encephalitis. Selected confluent T2-signal hyperintensities are indicated (arrows). (Adapted and reprinted from Goh, K. J. et al., 2000, *N. Engl. J. Med.* 342, 1229–1235.)

tails (Schmid et al. 1992). Although the presence of truncated F glycoproteins hinders efficient virus budding from the cell surface, cell-to-cell fusion functions are not affected (Cathomen et al. 1998). Collectively these mutations keep the virus highly cell-associated which in turn probably facilitates transneuronal spread and keeps the virus "hidden" from the immune system.

   Although small animal models have been used to examine acute encephalitis and persistence of MV in the CNS, these require the use of either rodent-brain adapted strains or transgenic animals which express a MV receptor and typically are interferon incompetent (Duprex et al. 1999; Schubert et al. 2006). The disadvantage of these models is that the virus is injected via the intracerebral route and there is currently no model in which the virus reaches the CNS from the periphery. Unpublished studies from our group identified wild-type MV in the brain of a macaque shortly after infection, although these observations remain to be corroborated in additional animals. Whether this was a unique finding remains to be seen (Duprex et al., unpublished).

15.4.4 Epidemiology

MV only naturally infects humans and some species of monkey and is one of the most infectious human pathogens in current circulation. This has enabled the disruption of endemic MV transmission in many parts of the developed world, although the virus continues to cause significant levels of morbidity and mortality in the developing world, with 164,000 deaths being attributed to measles in 2008 (Bellini and Rota 2011). Importation of the virus from the developed world is common and is especially problematic in countries which have low levels of vaccination. Currently there are large outbreaks of measles in France where 14,000 people have been infected and six have died (2011). APME is the most common neurological complication resulting from natural MV infection occurring in approximately 1:1000 cases (Miller 1964) with MIBE cases only observed as a complication of MV infection of immunodeficient individuals. A re-evaluation of the incidence of SSPE in recent years revealed approximately 4 to 11 cases per 100,000 cases of measles (Campbell et al. 2007), and a recent analysis of neurological complications resulting from measles outbreaks in Papua New Guinea has reported rates as high a 1 in 10,000 children (Manning et al. 2011).

15.4.5 Prognosis and Treatment

Live attenuated MV vaccines were developed in the 1960s from a clinical isolate obtained from a patient, David Edmonston (Enders and Peebles 1954). APME is typically treated with high dose corticosteroids together with supportive care, although the benefit of steroids or other means of immunosuppression like plasma exchange or intravenous immunoglobulins have not been proven in prospective trials (Tenembaum et al. 2007). In addition to the 10% mortality rate, survivors of APME can be left with neurological sequelae including behavioral disorders, mental retardation and epilepsy (Johnson et al. 1984). As discussed above, MIBE and SSPE are almost invariably fatal, and treatment is largely supportive. Clinical trials have evaluated drug candidates for SSPE. The best results have been seen with different combinations of weekly intrathecal INF-alpha and daily oral isoprinosine either as monotherapy or in combination resulting in slowed disease progression in approximately one-third of patients as compared with the 5% spontaneous remission rate seen with historical controls (Dyken et al. 1982; Gascon 2003).

15.5 MUMPS VIRUS

15.5.1 Clinical Presentation

The classic clinical presentation of MuV infection is parotitis, which is typically preceded by a short prodromal phase of low-grade fever, anorexia, malaise, and headache. One third of cases are asymptomatic. Between 15% and 30% of infected adult men develop orchitis, and oophoritis can occur in women. Pancreatitis and deafness are other potential complications. One of the largest studies examining the neurological involvement of MuV by both clinical and laboratory criteria reported an epidemic which took place from 1941 to 1942 (Bang and Bang 1943). Evidence of neurological involvement, as defined by symptoms consistent with aseptic meningitis and/or evidence of inflammation in the CSF (lymphocytic predominance), was found in 65% of patients. In this study, lumbar puncture was routine for all patients at the time of presentation whether they had neurological symptoms or not. In other studies, there was no temporal association between when the parotitis presents, if it occurs at all, and the development of meningitis (Russell and Donald 1958).

An MuV infection can lead to encephalitis in 0.1%–0.2% of cases (Bjorvatn and Wolontis 1973; Cohen et al. 1992). Encephalitis complications include paresis (ocular, facial, hemiplegia, monoplegia) as well as seizures, ataxia, convulsions, coma, mental disturbance, and transverse myelitis (Cohen et al. 1992; Nussinovitch et al. 1992; Venketasubramanian 1997). Some cases of MuV, encephalitis can be quite severe, with a 1.5% mortality rate (Cooper et al. 2007; Kumar and Kuruvilla 2009). MRI demonstrates diffuse T2 signal hyperintensities (Figure 15.1b). Whether these more severe presentations are due to host or specific characteristics of the virus strain remains unclear. A 1983 study of 41 children with MuV encephalitis collected over a 12-year period found that a third of patients were ataxic, one quarter developed seizures, 20% had psychiatric complications, 20% had a depressed level of consciousness, and 13% suffered from vertigo (Koskiniemi et al. 1983). At long-term follow-up, a minority of patients was still ataxic and/or had psychiatric disturbances. The male to female ratio was 4:1. One third of patients had salivary gland swelling, which preceded the encephalitis by 1 week.

In 1967, Johnson and Johnson reported an experimental model of mumps-induced hydrocephalus in a hamster (Johnson et al. 1967). Since that time, a number of human cases of both acute and late onset, mumps-induced hydrocephalus in people have been reported (Aydemir et al. 2009; Bray 1972; Cinalli et al. 2004; Lahat et al. 1993; Ogata et al. 1992; Timmons and Johnson 1970). Transient sensorineural hearing loss occurs at a rate of 4% in adult men, although permanent deafness is much less common (Bitnun et al. 1986; Everberg 1957; Vuori et al. 1962).

15.5.2 Diagnosis

Clinical diagnosis of mumps is based on the presence of painful, unilateral, or bilateral (70%) parotitis. However, since not all mumps cases involve the parotid gland and because there are other infectious (e.g., influenza A virus, parainfluenza virus, Coxsackie virus, and lymphocytic choriomeningitis virus, *Staphylococcus aureus*), and noninfectious (e.g., Sjögren's syndrome, sarcoidosis, tumor, salivary gland obstruction, etc.) causes of parotitis. Laboratory diagnosis is based on isolation of virus, for example from urine, detection of viral nucleic acid or serological confirmation via detection of IgM mumps antibodies with enzyme linked immunosorbent assay (ELISA).

15.5.3 Pathology and Pathogenesis

MuV is restricted to humans, and transmission is via direct contact, droplet spread, or contaminated fomites. The primary cells targeted have not been identified, and the mechanism or route by which MuV enters the CNS is also unknown. Although the virus does not use a single receptor and the HN glycoprotein binds sialic acid moieties, the *in vivo* distribution of virus in the salivary glands, CNS, testes, ovaries, breasts, pancreas, thyroid gland, myocardium, and the joints suggests that there must be some predilection for particular cell types (Samal 2011).

Much of what is known about the neuropathogenesis of MuV has been gleaned from small animal models including rats, Syrian hamsters, and mice which are infected directly via the intracerebral route. There is some evidence for peripheral spread of MuV from the periphery to the CNS in a marmoset animal model (Saika et al. 2002). As discussed above, a hamster model of CNS MuV infection first demonstrated evidence of obstructive hydrocephalus caused by both wild-type and vaccine strains (Ennis et al. 1969; Herndon et al. 1974; Johnson and Johnson 1968; Johnson et al. 1967; Takano et al. 1993). These and subsequent studies demonstrated the presence of viral particles and intracytoplasmic viral-like inclusions in ependymal cells during the acute phase of infection and enlarged and distorted ependymal cells lining the ventricles during the chronic phase (Takano et al. 1993; Takano et al. 1999; Wolinsky et al. 1974).

Follow-up studies in humans confirmed the presence of ependymal cells in CSF in six out of six patients with acute MuV infection, lending weight to the notion that MuV causes an ependymitis (Herndon et al. 1974). While not all human cases of MuV-induced hydrocephalus fit this model, these data suggest that hydrocephalus is the result of accumulation of virus-infected cell debris in the aqueduct of Sylvius, blocking CSF egress. There is evidence that neuroadapted strains in particular are able to spread beyond the ependyma and choroid plexus and infect neuronal elements resulting in cortical microhemorrhages, perivascular inflammatory infiltrates, and limited neuronal necrosis. There is no evidence of endothelial cell infection (Johnson and Johnson 1968; Wolinsky et al. 1974).

15.5.4 Epidemiology

The institution of national vaccination programs led to a dramatic decline in mumps cases with a concordant drop in MuV meningitis and encephalitis (Modlin et al. 1975). In 1967, MuV accounted for 35.9% of encephalitis cases in the United States but only 12.5% in 1972 when national vaccine coverage had reached 40% of children. Overall, U.S. cases have declined from >100/100,000 to <1/100,000 (McNabb et al. 2007). Recently the virus has reemerged in the US and UK (see above) and there have been discussions as to whether it might be necessary to administer three doses of the MMR vaccine. However, there is no evidence that waning immunity plays a part in reinfections (Rubin et al. 2012).

15.5.5 Prognosis and Treatment

The mainstay of MuV treatment remains preventative using live attenuated vaccines which were developed in the 1960s. Despite the success of MuV vaccination, the neurotropism of MuV has complicated these efforts, as multiple cases of MuV vaccine-induced aseptic meningitis and encephalitis have resulted in widespread fear and even cessation of national vaccine programs (Arruda and Kondageski 2001; da Silveira et al. 2002; Furesz and Contreras 1990; Odisseev and Gacheva 1994). This highlights a key difficulty with regard to vaccine safety in that the vaccines which had to be withdrawn had passed the monkey neurovirulence (MNVT) test, which is the primary method by which the neurovirulence of candidate mumps vaccines is assessed. Given that the MNVT assay is not wholly reliable, this has prompted research into other animal models such as the (Rubin et al. 2000). Promising results have been obtained, although it is not clear as yet whether or not such rat neurovirulence tests (RNVT) will readily replace the MNVT which is integral in the vaccine licensing process. There are no proven anti-viral strategies for MuV. Fortunately, as discussed above, the prognosis for most neurological complications of MuV is excellent.

15.6   HENIPAVIRUSES

15.6.1   CLINICAL PRESENTATION

While HeV causes encephalitis in horses and humans, severe pulmonary symptoms are more common. After a 7–10 day incubation period, people develop an influenza-like illness characterized by fever, myalgia, headache, lethargy, sore throat, nausea, and vomiting with some patients recovering over a few weeks and others progressing to respiratory failure and/or fatal encephalitis.

NiV causes respiratory symptoms in up to 25% of patients, but the more prominent feature is the severe acute encephalitis that typically develops within a week of infection. Signs and symptoms include reduced levels of consciousness and signs consistent with brainstem involvement including segmental myoclonus, areflexia, hypertension, and tachycardia. MRI demonstrates many small (2–7 mm) T2 hyperintensities in the subcortical and deep white matter likely representing microinfarctions as a consequence of the severe vasculitis (Figure 15.1c). Laboratory abnormalities include thrombocytopenia, leukopenia, and transaminitis as well as pleocytosis and elevated protein levels in the CSF (Goh et al. 2000). Death typically ensues within ten days after illness onset likely secondary to brainstem involvement and respiratory failure (Goh et al. 2000). Twelve survivors from the initial outbreak in Malaysia and Singapore (7.5% of survivors) had recurrent encephalitis by 24 months while ten people (3.4%) who had either a nonencephalitic or asymptomatic primary infection, developed late-onset acute encephalitis. The mean interval between the first neurological episode and the time of initial infection was 8.4 months. The onset of the relapsed or late-onset encephalitis was usually acute and clinical features included fever, headache, seizures, and focal neurological signs. MRI in these cases demonstrates patchy areas of cortically based T2-weighted hyperintensities that are much more confluent than the T2-weighted hyperintensities seen in acute NiV encephalitis (Figure 15.1d). Eighteen percent of relapsed/late-onset patients died and 61% of late/relapsed patients had residual neurological deficits versus 22% who survived after acute Nipah encephalitis (Chong 2003; Tan et al. 2002; Wong et al. 2001). Interestingly, a single patient presented with fatal HeV encephalitis more than a year after a self-limited episode of meningitis in retrospect attributed to HeV. The neuro-pathology was similar to the relapsed NiV encephalitis cases (O'Sullivan et al. 1997).

15.6.2 DIAGNOSIS

RT-PCR can be used to detect henipavirus nucleic acids in nasopharyngeal secretions, urine, and internal organs including lung and brain (Goh et al. 2000; Harcourt et al. 2005). Given that NiV and HeV are classified as BSL-4 viruses, molecular-based assays represent the optimal means to make a rapid and sensitive diagnosis without having to culture a virus. Serologic diagnosis is made by detection of IgM antibody in serum using an ELISA. All patients have IgG antibodies by 17–18 days after infection. Since seroconversion occurs 7–15 days postinfection (10–15 days in the CSF), and patients die on average 9 days after infection, seroconversion is not required in some case study definitions (Goh et al. 2000; Ramasundrum 2000). There is no difference in outcome between patients with or without a positive serology, although there is a poorer prognosis for patients in whom virus was isolated from the CSF (Chua et al. 2000b).

15.6.3 PATHOLOGY AND PATHOGENESIS

Henipaviruses primarily infect neurons and endothelial cells of blood and lymphatic vessels, submandibular and bronchiolar lymph nodes, tonsil, and spleen. Both viruses induce a systemic vasculitis with microthromboses resulting in ischemic damage, most prominently in the CNS (Chua et al. 2000a; Wong et al. 2002a). Multifocal, necrotic plaques in the brain parenchyma likely correspond to the microinfarcts visualized on MRI. The primary receptor for both viruses is ephrinB2 which explains the majority, although not all, of the tropism *in vivo*.

NiV is present in cerebral vascular endothelial cells as well as the CNS of both symptomatic and asymptomatic animals. Unusual syncytial multinucleated endothelial cells are seen in both NiV and HeV infections (O'Sullivan et al. 1997). Viral antigens and RNP containing intracytoplasmic inclusion bodies are detectable in the brain by immunohistochemistry (Hooper et al. 2001; Wong et al. 2002b). Interestingly, no mature viral particles are observed (Goldsmith et al. 2003; Hyatt et al. 2001). It is not clear whether the henipaviruses enter the CNS via the cranial nerves and/or whether free or cell-associated virus is able to cross the blood brain barrier from the bloodstream via endothelial cells.

The delayed or relapsed encephalitis seen in NiV-infected patients presumably develops through direct neuronal infection (Chua et al. 2000b). While NiV cannot be cultured from autopsy material, the pathology is remarkable for encephalitis with immunolocalization for NiV antigen in neurons primarily but also in glial and ependymal cells without evidence of demyelination. The recurrent and delayed encephalitis cases do not demonstrate the vasculitis and the associated necrotic plaques seen in the acute encephalitis cases. Given the gray matter predominance of the pathology, the presence of viral antigen and the much delayed onset of recurrent illness, the etiology is very likely secondary to direct viral attack rather than a postinfectious demyelination syndrome like APME. Similarities in pathology and disease course between the single delayed case of HeV encephalitis and the numerous NiV cases have spurred comparisons to SSPE (Ksiazek et al. 2011; Wong et al. 2001). However, hypermutation of particular genes or "signature mutations" in, for example, the cytoplasmic tails of the F and G glycoproteins or the GE sequences have not been identified.

15.6.4 Epidemiology

The broad geographical range of the henipaviruses is in large part a result of the widespread distribution of the flying fox (order *Chiroptera*, genus *Pteropus* in the family *Pteropodidae*) which serves as the animal reservoir (Chua et al. 2002; Halpin et al. 2000; Yob et al. 2001). Its habitat extends from the western Indian Ocean to Southeast Asia and from Australia and the southwest Pacific islands (Olson et al. 2002; Reynes et al. 2005). Moreover, the virus naturally infects six species from five mammalian orders (pigs, horses, cats, dogs, and humans) and can be used to infect guinea pigs and hamsters experimentally (Eaton et al. 2006; Hooper et al. 2001; Williamson et al. 2001; Wong et al. 2003). Viral transmission typically occurs as a result of contact with pigs or horses, although recent outbreaks in Bangladesh and India were probably initiated by direct transmission from bats (Chadha et al. 2006; Luby et al. 2006).

While only one HeV strain has been reported, two distinct strains of NiV are currently circulating. The more recent strain reemerged from 2001 to 2004 across a wide area of central and western Bangladesh with the case fatality rate increasing from 38.5% to 75% (Blum et al. 2009; Chadha et al. 2006; Homaira et al. 2010; Hsu et al. 2004). Human to human transmission was not documented in the initial Malaysian outbreak (Mounts et al. 2001) but is thought to have occurred in subsequent outbreaks in 2001, 2003, and 2007 in Bangladesh (Blum et al. 2009; Homaira et al. 2010; Hsu et al. 2004) and India (Chadha et al. 2006).

15.6.5 Prognosis and Treatment

While there are no approved treatments for henipavirus infection, there have been some exciting recent advances. The only medication tested in humans remains ribavirin due to its broad-spectrum of antiviral activity. An open-label trial of ribavirin in 140 NiV-infected patients was conducted in 2001 (Chong et al. 2001). Compared with 54 patients who either refused ribavirin or for whom ribavirin was not available, ribavirin appeared to have a marginal but positive impact on mortality. The relative risk reduction was 36% with 32% mortality in the treatment group compared with 54% in the control group. However, an alternative analysis of these data from the same outbreak and subsequent animal studies has not borne out with these findings (Georges-Courbot et al. 2006; Goh et al. 2000).

While the efficacy of ribavirin is controversial, a recent study demonstrated the ability of a peripherally administered recombinant human neutralizing monoclonal antibody to completely prevent disease in African green monkeys 24 h postintrathecal infusion of HeV (Bossart et al. 2011). Monkeys given the MAb 72 h post-infection suffered some neurological sequelae, but they all survived as opposed to the 100%

mortality in the untreated group. Virus-to-cell fusion can be inhibited using peptides that may be exploitable as a potential therapy (Rey et al. 2010). Recombinant subunit vaccine formulation protects against lethal NiV challenge in cats (McEachern et al. 2008).

15.7 OTHER PARAMYXOVIRUSES NOT TRADITIONALLY ASSOCIATED WITH CNS MANIFESTATIONS

Although it primarily causes a pediatric respiratory disease difficult to distinguish from the phenotype caused by human respiratory syncytial virus (HRSV), human metapneumovirus (HMPV) has recently been associated with a number of viral encephalitis cases in children, including two fatalities (Arnold et al. 2009; Hata et al. 2007; Kaida et al. 2006; Schildgen et al. 2005). HRSV has also been associated with encephalitis in young children (Glaser et al. 2003; Hanna et al. 2003; Hirayama et al. 1999; Kawashima et al. 2009; Kho et al. 2004; Millichap and Wainwright 2009; Ng et al. 2001). Lastly, CNS manifestations have also been reported in a number of children with human parainfluenza virus type 3 (HPIV3) infections (Glaser et al. 2003; McCarthy et al. 1990). Clearly, these are unusual cases, although they illustrate the unusual propensity paramyxoviruses have for the CNS.

15.8 CONCLUSIONS AND FUTURE PERSPECTIVES

Much can be learned by comparing and contrasting the clinical manifestations caused by viruses which are united in their molecular biology and virology but divided, for example, by their levels of pathogenicity and the degree of mortality they cause. Such an analysis provokes questions such as:

1. Is CNS entry the key determinant of neurovirulence?
2. How do viral proteins, which specifically target intrinsic barriers in the host cell or modulate the efficacy of the adaptive immune response, enhance disease?
3. What makes one virus marginally epitheliotropic/endotheliotropic, highly lymphotropic, and quite neurotropic (MV) and another highly specific for the circulatory and central nervous systems (NiV)?
4. Why do some viruses readily infect a wide range of species (NiV and HeV) whereas others are exquisitely human specific (MV, MuV, HRSV, HMPV, and hPIV3)?
5. How can this knowledge help in the development of novel targeted therapeutics and the treatment and prevention of neurotropic paramyxoviruses in particular and neurotropic viruses in general?

Advances in molecular virology which permit the recovery of recombinant paramyxoviruses will help to answer such questions but only if the systems are generated from clinical and not laboratory-adapted isolates. Growth of these viruses in disease-relevant cell lines for example B cells (MV) or human salivary cells (MuV) is also vital as it must always be remembered that paramyxoviruses are products of the cells in which they are grown. Only when these two strands complement one another and optimal animal models are used, it will be possible to recapitulate many aspects of the disease and shed light on viral neuropathogenesis. Generation of chimeric viruses expressing the envelope glycoproteins of one virus and the internal proteins of another will be useful in dissecting the contribution virus receptors have in tropism. This is critically important as it will help to increase our understanding of the barriers to cross species infection which is highly relevant given that MV has been targeted for eradication by the World Health Organization. Given the fact that RNA viruses readily evolve to fill an empty niche, much thought needs to be given to cessation of MV vaccination campaigns as other morbilliviruses show much higher levels of neurotropism.

REFERENCES

2011. Increased transmission and outbreaks of measles—European region, 2011. *MMWR Morb. Mortal Wkly. Rep.* 60, 1605–1610.

Aicardi, J., Goutieres, F., Arsenio-Nunes, M. L., and Lebon, P. 1977. Acute measles encephalitis in children with immunosuppression. *Pediatrics* 59, 232–239.

Allen, I. V., McQuaid, S., McMahon, J., Kirk, J., and McConnell, R. 1996. The significance of measles virus antigen and genome distribution in the CNS in SSPE for mechanisms of viral spread and demyelination. *J. Neuropathol. Exp. Neurol.* 55, 471–480.

Anlar, B., Saatci, I., Kose, G., and Yalaz, K. 1996. MRI findings in subacute sclerosing panencephalitis. *Neurology* 47, 1278–1283.

Arnold, J. C., Singh, K. K., Milder, E., Spector, S. A., Sawyer, M. H., Gavali, S., and Glaser, C. 2009. Human metapneumovirus associated with central nervous system infection in children. *Pediatr. Infect. Dis. J.* 28, 1057–1060.

Arruda, W. O., and Kondageski, C. 2001. Aseptic meningitis in a large MMR vaccine campaign (590,609 people) in Curitiba, Parana, Brazil, 1998. *Rev. Inst. Med. Trop. Sao Paulo.* 43, 301–302.

Avota, E., Gassert, E., and Schneider-Schaulies, S. 2010. Measles virus-induced immunosuppression: from effectors to mechanisms. *Med. Microbiol. Immunol.* 199, 227–237.

Ayata, M., Komase, K., Shingai, M., Matsunaga, I., Katayama, Y., and Ogura, H. 2002. Mutations affecting transcriptional termination in the p gene end of subacute sclerosing panencephalitis viruses. *J. Virol.* 76, 13062–13068.

Aydemir, C., Eldes, N., Kolsal, E., Ustundag, G., Gul, S., and Erdem, Z. 2009. Acute tetraventricular hydrocephalus caused by mumps meningoencephalitis in a child. *Pediatr. Neurosurg.* 45, 419–421.

Balraj, V., and Miller, E. 1995. Complications of mumps vaccines. *Rev. Med. Virol.* 5, 219–227.

Bang, H. O., and Bang, J. 1943. Involvement of the central nervous system in mumps. *Acta Med. Scand.* 113, 487–505.

Barskey, A. E., Glasser, J. W., and LeBaron, C. W. 2009. Mumps resurgences in the United States: A historical perspective on unexpected elements. *Vaccine* 27, 6186–6195.

Bellini, W. J., and Rota, P. A. 2011. Biological feasibility of measles eradication. *Virus Res.* 162, 72–79.

Bitnun, S., Rakover, Y., and Rosen, G. 1986. Acute bilateral total deafness complicating mumps. *J. Laryngol. Otol.* 100, 943–945.

Bjorvatn, B., and Wolontis, S. 1973. Mumps Meningoencephalitis in Stockholm November 1964–July 1971. 1. Analysis of a Hospitalized Study Group—Questions of Selection and Representativity. *Scand. J. Infect Dis.* 5, 253–260.

Blum, L. S., Khan, R., Nahar, N., and Breiman, R. F. 2009. In-depth assessment of an outbreak of Nipah encephalitis with person-to-person transmission in Bangladesh: implications for prevention and control strategies. *Am. J. Trop. Med. Hyg.* 80, 96–102.

Bonaparte, M. I. 2005. From The Cover: Ephrin-B2 ligand is a functional receptor for Hendra virus and Nipah virus. *Proc. Natl. Acad. Sci.* 102, 10652–10657.

Bossart, K. N., Geisbert, T. W., Feldmann, H., Zhu, Z., Feldmann, F., Geisbert, J. B., Yan, L., Feng, Y. R., Brining, D., Scott, D., Wang, Y., Dimitrov, A. S., Callison, J., Chan, Y. P., Hickey, A. C., Dimitrov, D. S., Broder, C. C., and Rockx, B. 2011. A neutralizing human monoclonal antibody protects african green monkeys from hendra virus challenge. *Sci. Transl. Med.* 3, 105–103.

Bossart, K. N., Tachedjian, M., McEachern, J. A., Crameri, G., Zhu, Z., Dimitrov, D. S., Broder, C. C., and Wang, L. F. 2008. Functional studies of host-specific ephrin-B ligands as Henipavirus receptors. *Virology* 372, 357–371.

Bossart, K. N., Wang, L. F., Eaton, B. T., and Broder, C. C. 2001. Functional expression and membrane fusion tropism of the envelope glycoproteins of Hendra virus. *Virology* 290, 121–135.

Bossart, K. N., Wang, L. F., Flora, M. N., Chua, K. B., Lam, S. K., Eaton, B. T., and Broder, C. C. 2002. Membrane fusion tropism and heterotypic functional activities of the nipah virus and hendra virus envelope glycoproteins. *J. Virol.* 76, 11186–11198.

Bouteille, M., Fontaine, C., Vedrenne, C. L., and Delarue, J. 1965. Sur un cas d'encephalite subaigue a inclusions. Etude anatomclinique et ultrastructurelle. *Rev Neurol (Paris)* 118, 454–458.

Bray, P. F. 1972. Mumps—a cause of hydrocephalus? *Pediatrics* 49, 446–449.

Budka, H., Urbanits, S., Liberski, P. P., Eichinger, S., and Popow-Kraupp, T. 1996. Subacute measles virus encephalitis: a new and fatal opportunistic infection in a patient with AIDS. *Neurology* 46, 586–587.

Campbell, H., Andrews, N., Brown, K. E., and Miller, E. 2007. Review of the effect of measles vaccination on the epidemiology of SSPE. *Int. J. Epidemiol.* 36, 1334–1348.

Carbone, K. M., and Rubin, S. A. 2007. Mumps virus, In: Knipe, D. M., and Howley, P. M. (Eds.), *Fields Virology*, 5th ed. Lippincott Williams & Wilkins, Philadelphia, PA, pp. 1527–1542.

Cathomen, T., Naim, H. Y., and Cattaneo, R. 1998. Measles viruses with altered envelope protein cytoplasmic tails gain cell fusion competence. *J. Virol.* 72, 1224–1234.

Cattaneo, R., Rebmann, G., Schmid, A., Baczko, K., ter Meulen, V., and Billeter, M. A. 1987. Altered transcription of a defective measles virus genome derived from a diseased human brain. *EMBO J.* 6, 681–688.

Cattaneo, R., Schmid, A., Eschle, D., Baczko, K., ter, M., V, and Billeter, M. A. 1988. Biased hypermutation and other genetic changes in defective measles viruses in human brain infections. *Cell* 55, 255–265.

Chadha, M. S., Comer, J. A., Lowe, L., Rota, P. A., Rollin, P. E., Bellini, W. J., Ksiazek, T. G., and Mishra, A. 2006. Nipah virus-associated encephalitis outbreak, Siliguri, India. *Emerg. Infect. Dis.* 12, 235–240.

Chen, T. T., Watanabe, I., Zeman, W., Mealey, J., Jr. 1969. Subacute sclerosing panencephalitis: propagation of measles virus from brain biopsy in tissue culture. *Science* 163, 1193–1194.

Childs, K. S., Andrejeva, J., Randall, R. E., and Goodbourn, S. 2009. Mechanism of mda-5 inhibition by paramyxovirus V proteins. *J. Virol.* 83, 1465–1473.

Chong, H. T., Kamarulzaman, A., Tan, C. T., Goh, K. J., Thayaparan, T., Kunjapan, S. R., Chew, N. K., Chua, K. B., and Lam, S. K. 2001. Treatment of acute Nipah encephalitis with ribavirin. *Ann. Neurol.* 49, 810–813.

Chong, H. T., and T. C. 2003. Relapsed and late-onset Nipah encephalitis, a report of three cases. *Neurol. J. Sutheast Asia* 8, 109–112.

Chua, K. B., Bellini, W. J., Rota, P. A., Harcourt, B. H., Tamin, A., Lam, S. K., Ksiazek, T. G., Rollin, P. E., Zaki, S. R., Shieh, W., Goldsmith, C. S., Gubler, D. J., Roehrig, J. T., Eaton, B., Gould, A. R., Olson, J., Field, H., Daniels, P., Ling, A. E., Peters, C. J., Anderson, L. J., and Mahy, B. W. 2000a. Nipah virus: a recently emergent deadly paramyxovirus. *Science* 288, 1432–1435.

Chua, K. B., Goh, K. J., Wong, K. T., Kamarulzaman, A., Tan, P. S., Ksiazek, T. G., Zaki, S. R., Paul, G., Lam, S. K., and Tan, C. T. 1999. Fatal encephalitis due to Nipah virus among pig-farmers in Malaysia. *Lancet* 354, 1257–1259.

Chua, K. B., Koh, C. L., Hooi, P. S., Wee, K. F., Khong, J. H., Chua, B. H., Chan, Y. P., Lim, M. E., and Lam, S. K. 2002. Isolation of Nipah virus from Malaysian Island flying-foxes. *Microbes Infect.* 4, 145–151.

Chua, K. B., Lam, S. K., Tan, C. T., Hooi, P. S., Goh, K. J., Chew, N. K., Tan, K. S., Kamarulzaman, A., and Wong, K. T. 2000b. High mortality in Nipah encephalitis is associated with presence of virus in cerebrospinal fluid. *Ann. Neurol.* 48, 802–805.

Cinalli, G., Spennato, P., Ruggiero, C., Aliberti, F., and Maggi, G. 2004. Aqueductal stenosis 9 years after mumps meningoencephalitis: treatment by endoscopic third ventriculostomy. *Child's Nervous Syst.* 20, 61–64.

Cohen, H. A., Ashkenazi, A., Nussinovitch, M., Amir, J., Hart, J., and Frydman, M. 1992. Mumps-associated acute cerebellar ataxia. *Am. J. Dis. Child* 146, 930–931.

Colville, A., Pugh, S., and Miller, E. 1994. Withdrawal of a mumps vaccine. *Eur. J. Pediat.* 153, 467–468.

Connolly, J. H., Allen, I. V., Hurwitz, L. J., and Millar, J. H. D. 1967. Measles virus antibody and antigen in subacute sclerosing panencephalitis. *Lancet* 1, 542–544.

Cooper, A. D., Wijdicks, E. F., and Sampathkumar, P. 2007. Mumps encephalitis: return with a vengeance. *Rev. Neurol. Dis.* 4, 100–102.

da Cunha, S. S., Rodrigues, L. C., Barreto, M. L., and Dourado, I. 2002. Outbreak of aseptic meningitis and mumps after mass vaccination with MMR vaccine using the Leningrad-Zagreb mumps strain. *Vaccine* 20, 1106–1112.

da Silveira, C. M., Kmetzsch, C. I., Mohrdieck, R., Sperb, A. F., and Prevots, D. R. 2002. The risk of aseptic meningitis associated with the Leningrad-Zagreb mumps vaccine strain following mass vaccination with measles-mumps-rubella vaccine, Rio Grande do Sul, Brazil, 1997. *Int. J. Epidemiol.* 31, 978–982.

Dawson, J. R. 1933. Cellular inclusions in cerebral lesions of lethargic encephalitis. *Am. J. Pathol.* 9, 7–16.3.

de Swart, R. L., Ludlow, M., de Witte, L., Yanagi, Y., van Amerongen, G., McQuaid, S., Yuksel, S., Geijtenbeek, T. B., Duprex, W. P., and Osterhaus, A. D. 2007. Predominant infection of CD150+ lymphocytes and dendritic cells during measles virus infection of macaques. *PLoS. Pathog.* 3, e178.

Diederich, S., Dietzel, E., and Maisner, A. 2009. Nipah virus fusion protein: influence of cleavage site mutations on the cleavability by cathepsin L, trypsin and furin. *Virus Res.* 145, 300–306.

Dourado, I., Cunha, S., Teixeira, M. G., Farrington, C. P., Melo, A., Lucena, R., and Barreto, M. L. 2000. Outbreak of aseptic meningitis associated with mass vaccination with a urabe-containing measles-mumps-rubella vaccine: implications for immunization programs. *Amer. J. Epidemiol.* 151, 524–530.

Duprex, W. P., Duffy, I., McQuaid, S., Hamill, L., Cosby, S. L., Billeter, M. A., Schneider-Schaulies, J., ter Meulen, V., and Rima, B. K. 1999. The H gene of rodent brain-adapted measles virus confers neurovirulence to the Edmonston vaccine strain. *J. Virol.* 73, 6916–6922.

Dyken, P. R., Swift, A., and DuRant, R. H. 1982. Long-term follow-up of patients with subacute sclerosing panencephalitis treated with inosiplex. *Ann. Neurol.* 11, 359–364.

Eaton, B. T., Broder, C. C., Middleton, D., and Wang, L.-F. 2006. Hendra and Nipah viruses: different and dangerous. *Nat. Rev. Microbiol.* 4, 23–35.

Eaton, B. T., Mackenzie, J. S., and Wang, L. F. 2007. Henipaviruses, In: Knipe, D. M., and Howley, P. M. (Eds.), *Fields Virology*, 5th ed. Lippincott Williams & Wilkins, Philadelphia, PA, pp. 1587–1600.

Enders, J. F., and Peebles, T. C. 1954. Propagation in tissue cultures of cytopathogenic agents from patients with measles. *Proc. Soc. Exp. Biol. Med.* 86, 277–286.

Ennis, F. A., Hopps, H. E., Douglas, R. D., and Meyer, H. M., Jr. 1969. Hydrocephalus in hamsters: induction by natural and attenuated mumps viruses. *J. Infect. Dis.* 119, 75–79.

Erlenhoefer, C., Wurzer, W. J., Loffler, S., Schneider-Schaulies, S., Ter, M., V, and Schneider-Schaulies, J. 2001. CD150 (SLAM) is a receptor for measles virus but is not involved in viral contact-mediated proliferation inhibition. *J. Virol.* 75, 4499–4505.

Esolen, L. M., Ward, B. J., Moench, T. R., and Griffin, D. E. 1993. Infection of monocytes during measles. *J. Infect. Dis.* 168, 47–52.

Everberg, G. 1957. Deafness following mumps. *Acta Otolaryngol.* 48, 397–403.

Freeman, J. M. 1969. The clinical spectrum and early diagnosis of Dawson's encephalitis, with preliminary notes on treatment. *J. Pediat.* 75, 590–603.

Furesz, J., and Contreras, G. 1990. Vaccine-related mumps meningitis—Canada. *Can. Dis. Wkly. Rep.* 16, 253–254.

Furuse, Y., Suzuki, A., and Oshitani, H. 2010. Origin of measles virus: divergence from rinderpest virus between the 11th and 12th centuries. *Virol. J.* 7, 52.

Gascon, G. G. 2003. Randomized treatment study of inosiplex versus combined inosiplex and intraventricular interferon-alpha in subacute sclerosing panencephalitis (SSPE): international multicenter study. *J. Child. Neurol.* 18, 819–827.

Gendelman, H. E., Wolinsky, J. S., Johnson, R. T., Pressman, N. J., Pezeshkpour, G. H., and Boisset, G. F. 1984. Measles encephalomyelitis: lack of evidence of viral invasion of the central nervous system and quantitative study of the nature of demyelination. *Ann. Neurol.* 15, 353–360.

Georges-Courbot, M. C., Contamin, H., Faure, C., Loth, P., Baize, S., Leyssen, P., Neyts, J., and Deubel, V. 2006. Poly(I)-poly(C12U) but not ribavirin prevents death in a hamster model of Nipah virus infection. *Antimicrob. Agents Chemother.* 50, 1768–1772.

Gerlier, D., and Valentin, H. 2009. Measles virus interaction with host cells and impact on innate immunity. *Curr. Top. Microbiol. Immunol.* 329, 163–191.

Glaser, C. A., Gilliam, S., Schnurr, D., Forghani, B., Honarmand, S., Khetsuriani, N., Fischer, M., Cossen, C. K., and Anderson, L. J. 2003. In search of encephalitis etiologies: diagnostic challenges in the California Encephalitis Project, 1998–2000. *Clin. Infect. Dis.* 36, 731–742.

Goh, K. J., Tan, C. T., Chew, N. K., Tan, P. S., Kamarulzaman, A., Sarji, S. A., Wong, K. T., Abdullah, B. J., Chua, K. B., and Lam, S. K. 2000. Clinical features of Nipah virus encephalitis among pig farmers in Malaysia. *N. Engl. J. Med.* 342, 1229–1235.

Goldsmith, C. S., Whistler, T., Rollin, P. E., Ksiazek, T. G., Rota, P. A., Bellini, W. J., Daszak, P., Wong, K. T., Shieh, W. J., and Zaki, S. R. 2003. Elucidation of Nipah virus morphogenesis and replication using ultrastructural and molecular approaches. *Virus Res.* 92, 89–98.

Greenfield, J. G. 1950. Encephalitis and encephalomyelitis in England and Wales during the last decade. *Brain: J. Neurol.* 73, 141–166.

Griffin, D. E. 2007. Measles virus, In: Knipe, D. M., Howley, P. M. (Eds.), *Fields Virology*, 5th ed. Lippincott, Williams & Wilkins, Philadelphia, PA, pp. 1551–1585.

Gutierrez, J., Issacson, R. S., and Koppel, B. S. 2010. Subacute sclerosing panencephalitis: an update. *Dev. Med. Child. Neurol.* 52, 901–907.

Hall, W. W., Lamb, R. A., and Choppin, P. W. 1979. Measles and subacute sclerosing panencephalitis virus proteins: lack of antibodies to the M protein in patients with subacute sclerosing panencephalitis. *Proc. Natl. Acad. Sci. U S A* 76, 2047–2051.

Halpin, K., Young, P. L., Field, H. E., and Mackenzie, J. S. 2000. Isolation of Hendra virus from pteropid bats: a natural reservoir of Hendra virus. *J. Gen. Virol.* 81, 1927–1932.

Hamilton, R., 1790. An account of a distemper, by the common people in England vulgarly called mumps. *Trans. Roy. Soc. Edinburgh* 2, 59.

Hanna, S., Tibby, S. M., Durward, A., and Murdoch, I. A. 2003. Incidence of hyponatraemia and hyponatraemic seizures in severe respiratory syncytial virus bronchiolitis. *Acta Paediatr.* 92, 430–434.

Harcourt, B. H., Lowe, L., Tamin, A., Liu, X., Bankamp, B., Bowden, N., Rollin, P. E., Comer, J. A., Ksiazek, T. G., Hossain, M. J., Gurley, E. S., Breiman, R. F., Bellini, W. J., and Rota, P. A. 2005. Genetic characterization of Nipah virus, Bangladesh, 2004. *Emerg. Infect. Dis.* 11, 1594–1597.

Hashimoto, H., Fujioka, M., and Kinumaki, H. 2009. An office-based prospective study of deafness in mumps. *Pediatr. Infect. Dis. J.* 28, 173–175.

Hata, M., Ito, M., Kiyosawa, S., Kimpara, Y., Tanaka, S., Yamashita, T., Hasegawa, A., Kobayashi, S., Koyama, N., and Minagawa, H. 2007. A fatal case of encephalopathy possibly associated with human metapneumovirus infection. *Jpn. J. Infect Dis.* 60, 328–329.

Herndon, R. M., Johnson, R. T., Davis, L. E., and Descalzi, L. R. 1974. Ependymitis in mumps virus meningitis. Electron microscopical studies of cerebrospinal fluid. *Arch. Neurol.* 30, 475–479.

Herndon, R. M., and Rubinstein, L. J. 1968. Light and electron microscopy observations on the development of viral particles in the inclusions of Dawson's encephalitis (subacute sclerosing panencephalitis). *Neurology* 18, 8–20.

Hilleman, M. R., Buynak, E. B., Weibel, R. E., Stokes, J., Jr. 1968. Live, attenuated mumpsvirus vaccine. *N. England J. Med.* 278, 227–232.

Hirayama, K., Sakazaki, H., Murakami, S., Yonezawa, S., Fujimoto, K., Seto, T., Tanaka, K., Hattori, H., Matsuoka, O., and Murata, R. 1999. Sequential MRI, SPECT and PET in respiratory syncytial virus encephalitis. *Pediatr. Radiol.* 29, 282–286.

Hirsch, A. 1883. *Handbook of Geographical and Historical Pathology: Acute Infective Diseases*. New Syndenham Society, London.

Homaira, N., Rahman, M., Hossain, M. J., Epstein, J. H., Sultana, R., Khan, M. S., Podder, G., Nahar, K., Ahmed, B., Gurley, E. S., Daszak, P., Lipkin, W. I., Rollin, P. E., Comer, J. A., Ksiazek, T. G., and Luby, S. P. 2010. Nipah virus outbreak with person-to-person transmission in a district of Bangladesh, 2007. *Epidemiol. Infect.* 138, 1630–1636.

Hooper, P., Zaki, S., Daniels, P., and Middleton, D. 2001. Comparative pathology of the diseases caused by Hendra and Nipah viruses. *Microbes Infect.* 3, 315–322.

Hsu, V. P., Hossain, M. J., Parashar, U. D., Ali, M. M., Ksiazek, T. G., Kuzmin, I., Niezgoda, M., Rupprecht, C., Bresee, J., and Breiman, R. F. 2004. Nipah virus encephalitis reemergence, Bangladesh. *Emerg. Infect. Dis.* 10, 2082–2087.

Hyatt, A. D., Zaki, S. R., Goldsmith, C. S., Wise, T. G., and Hengstberger, S. G. 2001. Ultrastructure of Hendra virus and Nipah virus within cultured cells and host animals. *Microbes Infect.* 3, 297–306.

Iwasaki, Y., and Koprowski, H. 1974. Cell to cell transmission of virus in the central nervous system. I. Subacute sclerosing panencephalitis. *Lab. Investig. J. Tech. Methods Pathol.* 31, 187–196.

Jin, L., Beard, S., Hunjan, R., Brown, D. W., and Miller, E. 2002. Characterization of measles virus strains causing SSPE: a study of 11 cases. *J. Neurovirol.* 8, 335–344.

Johnson, C. D., and Goodpasture, E. W. 1934. An investigation of the etiology of mumps. *J. Exp. Med.* 59, 1–19.

Johnson, R. T., Griffin, D. E., Hirsch, R. L., Wolinsky, J. S., Roedenbeck, S., De Soriano, L., and Vaisberg, A. 1984. Measles encephalomyelitis-clinical and immunologic studies. *N. Engl. J. Med.* 310, 137–141.

Johnson, R. T., and Johnson, K. P. 1968. Hydrocephalus following viral infection: the pathology of aqueductal stenosis developing after experimental mumps virus infection. *J. Neuropathol. Exp. Neurol.* 27, 591–606.

Johnson, R. T., Johnson, K. P., and Edmonds, C. J. 1967. Virus-induced hydrocephalus: development of aqueductal stenosis in hamsters after mumps infection. *Science* 157, 1066–1067.

Kaida, A., Iritani, N., Kubo, H., Shiomi, M., Kohdera, U., and Murakami, T. 2006. Seasonal distribution and phylogenetic analysis of human metapneumovirus among children in Osaka City, Japan. *J. Clin. Virol.* 35, 394–399.

Kaplan, L. J., Daum, R. S., Smaron, M., and McCarthy, C. A. 1992. Severe measles in immunocompromised patients. *JAMA: J. Am. Med. Assoc.* 267, 1237–1241.

Kawashima, H., Ioi, H., Ushio, M., Yamanaka, G., Matsumoto, S., and Nakayama, T. 2009. Cerebrospinal fluid analysis in children with seizures from respiratory syncytial virus infection. *Scand. J. Infect Dis.* 41, 228–231.

Keeling, M. J., and Grenfell, B. T. 1997. Disease extinction and community size: modeling the persistence of measles. *Science* 275, 65–67.

Kho, N., Kerrigan, J. F., Tong, T., Browne, R., and Knilans, J. 2004. Respiratory syncytial virus infection and neurologic abnormalities: retrospective cohort study. *J. Child. Neurol.* 19, 859–864.

Kirk, J., Zhou, A. L., McQuaid, S., Cosby, S. L., and Allen, I. V. 1991. Cerebral endothelial cell infection by measles virus in subacute sclerosing panencephalitis: ultrastructural and *in situ* hybridization evidence. *Neuropathol. Appl. Neurobiol.* 17, 289–297.

Koskiniemi, M., Donner, M., and Pettay, O. 1983. Clinical appearance and outcome in mumps encephalitis in children. *Acta Paediatr. Scand.* 72, 603–609.

Ksiazek, T. G., Rota, P. A., and Rollin, P. E. 2011. A review of Nipah and Hendra viruses with an historical aside. *Virus Res.* 162, 173–183.

Kumar, S., and Kuruvilla, A. 2009. Teaching NeuroImages: acute hemorrhagic leukoencephalitis after mumps. *Neurology* 73, E98–E98.

Lahat, E., Aladjem, M., Schiffer, J., and Starinsky, R. 1993. Hydrocephalus due to bilateral obstruction of the foramen of Monro: a "possible" late complication of mumps encephalitis. *Clin. Neurol. Neurosurg.* 95, 151–154.

Lawrence, D. M., Patterson, C. E., Gales, T. L., D'Orazio, J. L., Vaughn, M. M., and Rall, G. F. 2000. Measles virus spread between neurons requires cell contact but not CD46 expression, syncytium formation or extracellular virus production. *J. Virol.* 74, 1908–1918.

Lemon, K., de Vries, R. D., Mesman, A. W., McQuaid, S., van Amerongen, G., Yuksel, S., Ludlow, M., Rennick, L. J., Kuiken, T., Rima, B. K., Geijtenbeek, T. B., Osterhaus, A. D., Duprex, W. P., and de Swart, R. L. 2011. Early target cells of measles virus after aerosol infection of non-human primates. *PLoS Pathog.* 7, e1001263.

Leonard, V. H., Hodge, G., Reyes-del, V. J., McChesney, M. B., and Cattaneo, R. 2010. Measles virus selectively blind to signaling lymphocytic activation molecule (SLAM; CD150) is attenuated and induces strong adaptive immune responses in rhesus monkeys. *J. Virol.* 84, 3413–3420.

Liljeroos, L., Huiskonen, J. T., Ora, A., Susi, P., and Butcher, S. J. 2011. Electron cryotomography of measles virus reveals how matrix protein coats the ribonucleocapsid within intact virions. *Proc. Natl. Acad. Sci. U S A* 108, 18085–18090.

Luby, S. P., Rahman, M., Hossain, M. J., Blum, L. S., Husain, M. M., Gurley, E., Khan, R., Ahmed, B. N., Rahman, S., Nahar, N., Kenah, E., Comer, J. A., and Ksiazek, T. G. 2006. Foodborne transmission of Nipah virus, Bangladesh. *Emerg. Infect. Dis.* 12, 1888–1894.

Malik, T., Shegogue, C. W., Werner, K., Ngo, L., Sauder, C., Zhang, C., Duprex, W. P., and Rubin, S. 2011. Discrimination of mumps virus small hydrophobic gene deletion effects from gene translation effects on virus virulence. *J. Virol.* 85, 6082–6085.

Manie, S. N., Debreyne, S., Vincent, S., and Gerlier, D. 2000. Measles virus structural components are enriched into lipid raft microdomains: a potential cellular location for virus assembly. *J. Virol.* 74, 305–311.

Manning, L., Laman, M., Edoni, H., Mueller, I., Karunajeewa, H. A., Smith, D., Hwaiwhanje, I., Siba, P. M., and Davis, T. M. 2011. Subacute sclerosing panencephalitis in Papua New Guinean children: the cost of continuing inadequate measles vaccine coverage. *PLoS Negl. Trop. Dis.* 5, e932.

McCarthy, V. P., Zimmerman, A. W., and Miller, C. A. 1990. Central nervous system manifestations of parainfluenza virus type 3 infections in childhood. *Pediatr. Neurol.* 6, 197–201.

McEachern, J. A., Bingham, J., Crameri, G., Green, D. J., Hancock, T. J., Middleton, D., Feng, Y.-R., Broder, C. C., Wang, L.-F., and Bossart, K. N. 2008. A recombinant subunit vaccine formulation protects against lethal Nipah virus challenge in cats. *Vaccine* 26, 3842–3852.

McNabb, S. J., Jajosky, R. A., Hall-Baker, P. A., Adams, D. A., Sharp, P., Anderson, W. J., Javier, A. J., Jones, G. J., Nitschke, D. A., Worshams, C. A., and Richard, R. A., Jr. 2007. Summary of notifiable diseases United States, 2005. *MMWR Morb. Mortal Wkly. Rep.* 54, 1–92.

McQuaid, S., Campbell, S., Wallace, I. J., Kirk, J., and Cosby, S. L. 1998. Measles virus infection and replication in undifferentiated and differentiated human neuronal cells in culture. *J. Virol.* 72, 5245–5250.

McQuaid, S., and Cosby, S. L. 2002. An immunohistochemical study of the distribution of the measles virus receptors, CD46 and SLAM, in normal human tissues and subacute sclerosing panencephalitis. *Lab. Invest.* 82, 403–409.

McQuaid, S., McMahon, J., Herron, B., and Cosby, S. L. 1997. Apoptosis in measles virus-infected human central nervous system tissues. *Neuropathol. Appl. Neurobiol.* 23, 218–224.

Miller, D. L. 1964. Frequency of Complications of Measles, 1963. Report on a national inquiry by the public health laboratory service in collaboration with the society of medical officers of health. *Brit. Med. J.* 2, 75–78.

Millichap, J. J., and Wainwright, M. S. 2009. Neurological complications of respiratory syncytial virus infection: case series and review of literature. *J. Child. Neurol.* 24, 1499–1503.

Modlin, J., Orenstein, W. A., and Brandling-Bennett, A. D. 1975. Current status of mumps in the United States. *J. Infect Dis.* 132, 106–109.

Moss, W. J., and Griffin, D. E. 2006. Global measles elimination. *Nat. Rev. Microbiol.* 4, 900–908.

Mounts, A. W., Kaur, H., Parashar, U. D., Ksiazek, T. G., Cannon, D., Arokiasamy, J. T., Anderson, L. J., and Lye, M. S. 2001. A cohort study of health care workers to assess nosocomial transmissibility of Nipah virus, Malaysia, 1999. *J. Infect. Dis.* 183, 810–813.

Murata, R., Matsuoka, O., Nakajima, S., Kawawaki, H., Hattori, H., Isshiki, G., Inoue, Y., and Maekubo, K. 1987. Serial magnetic resonance imaging in subacute sclerosing panencephalitis. *Jpn. J. Psychiat. Neurol.* 41, 277–281.

Murray, K., Selleck, P., Hooper, P., Hyatt, A., Gould, A., Gleeson, L., Westbury, H., Hiley, L., Selvey, L., Rodwell, B. et al. 1995. A morbillivirus that caused fatal disease in horses and humans. *Science* 268, 94–97.

Mustafa, M. M., Weitman, S. D., Winick, N. J., Bellini, W. J., Timmons, C. F., and Siegel, J. D. 1993. Subacute measles encephalitis in the young immunocompromised host: report of two cases diagnosed by polymerase chain reaction and treated with ribavirin and review of the literature. *Clin. Infect. Dis.* 16, 654–660.

Nagai, T., Okafuji, T., Miyazaki, C., Ito, Y., Kamada, M., Kumagai, T., Yuri, K., Sakiyama, H., Miyata, A., Ihara, T., Ochiai, H., Shimomura, K., Suzuki, E., Torigoe, S., Igarashi, M., Kase, T., Okuno, Y., and Nakayama, T. 2007. A comparative study of the incidence of aseptic meningitis in symptomatic natural mumps patients and monovalent mumps vaccine recipients in Japan. *Vaccine* 25, 2742–2747.

Navaratnarajah, C. K., Oezguen, N., Rupp, L., Kay, L., Leonard, V. H., Braun, W., and Cattaneo, R. 2011. The heads of the measles virus attachment protein move to transmit the fusion-triggering signal. *Nat. Struct. Mol. Biol.* 18, 128–134.

Negrete, O. A., Levroney, E. L., Aguilar, H. C., Bertolotti-Ciarlet, A., Nazarian, R., Tajyar, S., and Lee, B. 2005. EphrinB2 is the entry receptor for Nipah virus, an emergent deadly paramyxovirus. *Nature* 436, 401–405.

Negrete, O. A., Wolf, M. C., Aguilar, H. C., Enterlein, S., Wang, W., Muhlberger, E., Su, S. V., Bertolotti-Ciarlet, A., Flick, R., and Lee, B. 2006. Two key residues in ephrinB3 are critical for its use as an alternative receptor for Nipah virus. *PLoS Pathog.* 2, e7.

Ng, Y. T., Cox, C., Atkins, J., and Butler, I. J. 2001. Encephalopathy associated with respiratory syncytial virus bronchiolitis. *J. Child. Neurol.* 16, 105–108.

Norrby, E., and Kristensson, K. 1997. Measles virus in the brain. *Brain Res. Bull.* 44, 213–220.

Noyce, R. S., Bondre, D. G., Ha, M. N., Lin, L. T., Sisson, G., Tsao, M. S., and Richardson, C. D. 2011. Tumor cell marker PVRL4 (Nectin 4) is an epithelial cell receptor for measles virus. *PLoS Pathog.* 7, e1002240.

Nussinovitch, M., Brand, N., Frydman, M., and Varsano, I. 1992. Transverse myelitis following mumps in children. *Acta Paediatr.* 81, 183–184.

Nussinovitch, M., Volovitz, B., and Varsano, I. 1995. Complications of mumps requiring hospitalization in children. *Eur. J. Pediatr.* 154, 732–734.

O'Sullivan, J. D., Allworth, A. M., Paterson, D. L., Snow, T. M., Boots, R., Gleeson, L. J., Gould, A. R., Hyatt, A. D., and Bradfield, J. 1997. Fatal encephalitis due to novel paramyxovirus transmitted from horses. *Lancet* 349, 93–95.

Odisseev, H., and Gacheva, N. 1994. Vaccinoprophylaxis of mumps using mumps vaccine, strain Sofia 6, in Bulgaria. *Vaccine* 12, 1251–1254.

Ogata, H., Oka, K., and Mitsudome, A. 1992. Hydrocephalus due to acute aqueductal stenosis following mumps infection: report of a case and review of the literature. *Brain Dev.* 14, 417–419.

Olson, J. G., Rupprecht, C., Rollin, P. E., An, U. S., Niezgoda, M., Clemins, T., Walston, J., and Ksiazek, T. G. 2002. Antibodies to Nipah-like virus in bats (*Pteropus lylei*), Cambodia. *Emerg. Infect. Dis.* 8, 987–988.

Plotkin, S. A. 1967. Vaccination against measles in the 18th century. *Clin. Pediatr. (Phila.)* 6, 312–315.

Poliakov, A., Cotrina, M., and Wilkinson, D. G. 2004. Diverse roles of eph receptors and ephrins in the regulation of cell migration and tissue assembly. *Dev. Cell* 7, 465–480.

Prashanth, L. K., Taly, A. B., Ravi, V., Sinha, S., and Arunodaya, G. R. 2006. Adult onset subacute sclerosing panencephalitis: clinical profile of 39 patients from a tertiary care centre. *J. Neurol. Neurosurg. Psychiat.* 77, 630–633.

Praveen-kumar, S., Sinha, S., Taly, A. B., Jayasree, S., Ravi, V., Vijayan, J., and Ravishankar, S. 2007. Electroencephalographic and imaging profile in a subacute sclerosing panencephalitis (SSPE) cohort: a correlative study. *Clin. Neurophysiol.* 118, 1947–1954.

Rager, M., Vongpunsawad, S., Duprex, W. P., and Cattaneo, R. 2002. Polyploid measles virus with hexameric genome length. *EMBO J.* 21, 2364–2372.

Ramasundrum, V., T. C., Chua, K. B. et al. 2000. Kinetics of IgM and IgG seroconversion in Nipah virus infection. *Neurol. J. Southeast Asia* 5, 23–28.

Rey, F. A., Porotto, M., Rockx, B., Yokoyama, C. C., Talekar, A., DeVito, I., Palermo, L. M., Liu, J., Cortese, R., Lu, M., Feldmann, H., Pessi, A., and Moscona, A. 2010. Inhibition of Nipah virus infection *in vivo*: targeting an early stage of paramyxovirus fusion activation during viral entry. *PLoS Pathog.* 6, e1001168.

Reynes, J. M., Counor, D., Ong, S., Faure, C., Seng, V., Molia, S., Walston, J., Georges-Courbot, M. C., Deubel, V., and Sarthou, J. L. 2005. Nipah virus in Lyle's flying foxes, Cambodia. *Emerg. Infect. Dis.* 11, 1042–1047.

Risk, W. S., and Haddad, F. S. 1979. The variable natural history of subacute sclerosing panencephalitis: a study of 118 cases from the Middle East. *Arch. Neurol.* 36, 610–614.

Robb, R. M., and Watters, G. V. 1970. Ophthalmic manifestations of subacute sclerosing pan-encephalitis. *Arch. Ophthalmol.* 83, 426–435.

Rodriguez, J. J., and Horvath, C. M. 2004. Host evasion by emerging paramyxoviruses: Hendra virus and Nipah virus v proteins inhibit interferon signaling. *Viral Immunol.* 17, 210–219.

Romero, X., Benitez, D., March, S., Vilella, R., Miralpeix, M., and Engel, P. 2004. Differential expression of SAP and EAT-2-binding leukocyte cell-surface molecules CD84, CD150 (SLAM), CD229 (Ly9) and CD244 (2B4). *Tissue Antigens* 64, 132–144.

Rubin, S. A., Link, M. A., Sauder, C. J., Zhang, C., Ngo, L., Rima, B. K., and Duprex, W. P. 2012. Recent mumps outbreaks in vaccinated populations: no evidence of immune escape. *J. Virol.* 86, 615–620.

Rubin, S. A., Pletnikov, M., Taffs, R., Snoy, P. J., Kobasa, D., Brown, E. G., Wright, K. E., and Carbone, K. M. 2000. Evaluation of a neonatal rat model for prediction of mumps virus neurovirulence in humans. *J. Virol.* 74, 5382–5384.

Russell, R. R., and Donald, J. C. 1958. The neurological complications of mumps. *Br. Med. J.* 2, 27–30.

Saika, S., Kidokoro, M., Ohkawa, T., Aoki, A., and Suzuki, K. 2002. Pathogenicity of mumps virus in the marmoset. *J. Med. Virol.* 66, 115–122.

Samal, S. K. 2011. *The Biology of Paramyxoviruses.* Caister Academic Press, Norfolk, UK.

Sasaki, T., and Tsunoda, K. 2009. Time to revisit mumps vaccination in Japan? *Lancet* 374, 1722.

Schildgen, O., Glatzel, T., Geikowski, T., Scheibner, B., Matz, B., Bindl, L., Born, M., Viazov, S., Wilkesmann, A., Knopfle, G., Roggendorf, M., and Simon, A. 2005. Human meta-pneumovirus RNA in encephalitis patient. *Emerg. Infect. Dis.* 11, 467–470.

Schmid, A., Spielhofer, P., Cattaneo, R., Baczko, K., Ter, M., V, and Billeter, M. A. 1992. Subacute sclerosing panencephalitis is typically characterized by alterations in the fusion protein cytoplasmic domain of the persisting measles virus. *Virology* 188, 910–915.

Schubert, S., Moller-Ehrlich, K., Singethan, K., Wiese, S., Duprex, W. P., Rima, B. K., Niewiesk, S., and Schneider-Schaulies, J. 2006. A mouse model of persistent brain infection with recombinant measles virus. *J. Gen. Virol.* 87, 2011–2019.

Selvey, L. A., Wells, R. M., McCormack, J. G., Ansford, A. J., Murray, K., Rogers, R. J., Lavercombe, P. S., Selleck, P., and Sheridan, J. W. 1995. Infection of humans and horses by a newly described morbillivirus. *Med. J. Aust.* 162, 642–645.

Shirogane, Y., Takeda, M., Tahara, M., Ikegame, S., Nakamura, T., and Yanagi, Y. 2010. Epithelial-mesenchymal transition abolishes the susceptibility of polarized epithelial cell lines to measles virus. *J. Biol. Chem.* 285, 20882–20890.

Sugiura, A., and Yamada, A. 1991. Aseptic meningitis as a complication of mumps vaccina-tion. *Pediatr. Infect. Dis. J.* 10, 209–213.

Suryanarayana, K., Baczko, K., Ter, M., V, and Wagner, R. R. 1994. Transcription inhibi-tion and other properties of matrix proteins expressed by M genes cloned from measles viruses and diseased human brain tissue. *J. Virol.* 68, 1532–1543.

Takano, T., Mekata, Y., Yamano, T., and Shimada, M. 1993. Early ependymal changes in exper-imental hydrocephalus after mumps virus inoculation in hamsters. *Acta Neuropathol.* 85, 521–525.

Takano, T., Takikita, S., and Shimada, M. 1999. Experimental mumps virus-induced hydro-cephalus: viral neurotropism and neuronal maturity. *Neuroreport* 10, 2215–2221.

Takeda, M., Nakatsu, Y., Ohno, S., Seki, F., Tahara, M., Hashiguchi, T., and Yanagi, Y. 2006. Generation of measles virus with a segmented RNA genome. *J. Virol.* 80, 4242–4248.

Takeuchi, K., Tanabayashi, K., Hishiyama, M., and Yamada, A. 1996. The mumps virus SH protein is a membrane protein and not essential for virus growth. *Virology* 225, 156–162.

Tamin, A. 2002. Functional properties of the fusion and attachment glycoproteins of Nipah virus. *Virology* 296, 190–200.

Tan, C. T., Goh, K. J., Wong, K. T., Sarji, S. A., Chua, K. B., Chew, N. K., Murugasu, P., Loh, Y. L., Chong, H. T., Tan, K. S., Thayaparan, T., Kumar, S., and Jusoh, M. R. 2002. Relapsed and late-onset Nipah encephalitis. *Ann. Neurol.* 51, 703–708.

Tatsuo, H., Ono, N., Tanaka, K., and Yanagi, Y. 2000. SLAM (CDw150) is a cellular receptor for measles virus. *Nature* 406, 893–897.

Tenembaum, S., Chitnis, T., Ness, J., and Hahn, J. S. 2007. Acute disseminated encephalomyelitis. *Neurology* 68, S23–S36.

Timmons, G. D., and Johnson, K. P. 1970. Aqueductal stenosis and hydrocephalus after mumps encephalitis. *N. Engl. J. Med.* 283, 1505–1507.

Veillette, A. 2006. Immune regulation by SLAM family receptors and SAP-related adaptors. *Nat. Rev. Immunol.* 6, 56–66.

Venketasubramanian, N. 1997. Transverse myelitis following mumps in an adult—a case report with MRI correlation. *Acta Neurol. Scand.* 96, 328–331.

Vogt, C., Eickmann, M., Diederich, S., Moll, M., and Maisner, A. 2005. Endocytosis of the Nipah virus glycoproteins. *J. Virol.* 79, 3865–3872.

von Messling, V., Springfeld, C., Devaux, P., and Cattaneo, R. 2003. A ferret model of canine distemper virus virulence and immunosuppression. *J. Virol.* 77, 12579–12591.

Vuori, M., Lahikainen, E. A., and Peltonen, T. 1962. Perceptive deafness in connection-with mumps. A study of 298 servicemen suffering from mumps. *Acta Otolaryngol.* 55, 231–236.

Watanabe, M., Hirano, A., Stenglein, S., Nelson, J., Thomas, G., and Wong, T. C. 1995. Engineered serine protease inhibitor prevents furin-catalyzed activation of the fusion glycoprotein and production of infectious measles virus. *J. Virol.* 69, 3206–3210.

Williamson, M. M., Hooper, P. T., Selleck, P. W., Westbury, H. A., and Slocombe, R. F. 2001. A guinea-pig model of Hendra virus encephalitis. *J. Comp. Pathol.* 124, 273–279.

Wolinsky, J. S., Baringer, J. R., Margolis, G., and Kilham, L. 1974. Ultrastructure of mumps virus replication in newborn hamster central nervous system. *Lab. Invest.* 31, 403–412.

Wolinsky, J. S., Swoveland, P., Johnson, K. P., and Baringer, J. R. 1977. Subacute measles encephalitis complicating Hodgkin's disease in an adult. *Ann. Neurol.* 1, 452–457.

Wong, K. T., Grosjean, I., Brisson, C., Blanquier, B., Fevre-Montange, M., Bernard, A., Loth, P., Georges-Courbot, M. C., Chevallier, M., Akaoka, H., Marianneau, P., Lam, S. K., Wild, T. F., and Deubel, V. 2003. A golden hamster model for human acute Nipah virus infection. *Am. J. Pathol.* 163, 2127–2137.

Wong, K. T., Shieh, W. J., Kumar, S., Norain, K., Abdullah, W., Guarner, J., Goldsmith, C. S., Chua, K. B., Lam, S. K., Tan, C. T., Goh, K. J., Chong, H. T., Jusoh, R., Rollin, P. E., Ksiazek, T. G., and Zaki, S. R. 2002a. Nipah virus infection: pathology and pathogenesis of an emerging paramyxoviral zoonosis. *Am. J. Pathol.* 161, 2153–2167.

Wong, K. T., Shieh, W. J., Zaki, S. R., and Tan, C. T. 2002b. Nipah virus infection, an emerging paramyxoviral zoonosis. *Springer Semin. Immunopathol.* 24, 215–228.

Wong, S. C., Ooi, M. H., Wong, M. N., Tio, P. H., Solomon, T., and Cardosa, M. J. 2001. Late presentation of Nipah virus encephalitis and kinetics of the humoral immune response. *J. Neurol. Neurosurg. Psychiat.* 71, 552–554.

Yob, J. M., Field, H., Rashdi, A. M., Morrissy, C., van der Heide, B., Rota, P., bin Adzhar, A., White, J., Daniels, P., Jamaluddin, A., and Ksiazek, T. 2001. Nipah virus infection in bats (order *Chiroptera*) in peninsular Malaysia. *Emerg. Infect. Dis.* 7, 439–441.

Yuan, P., Swanson, K. A., Leser, G. P., Paterson, R. G., Lamb, R. A., and Jardetzky, T. S. 2011. Structure of the Newcastle disease virus hemagglutinin-neuraminidase (HN) ectodomain reveals a four-helix bundle stalk. *Proc. Natl. Acad. Sci. U S A* 108, 14920–14925.

16 Rabies Virus Neurovirulence

Claire L. Jeffries, Ashley C. Banyard,
Derek M. Healy, Daniel L. Horton,
Nicholas Johnson, and Anthony R. Fooks

CONTENTS

16.1 INTRODUCTION

16.1.1 RABIES

Rabies is an infectious encephalitic disease of mammals, caused by viruses of the genus *Lyssavirus* (Family *Rhabdoviridae*). Exposure to rabies virus, in the absence of timely medical intervention, almost invariably results in a fatal outcome. The term "rabies" comes from the Latin word *rabere*, which means "to rage or rave" and refers to the clinical disease progression seen following infection. This condition has been known, and feared, by people across the globe for thousands of years (Neville

2004). It is only within the last few centuries, however, that progress has been made in understanding the disease, and in the development of successful prevention and treatment strategies (Baer 2007). In the 1880s, Louis Pasteur developed the first successful postexposure prophylaxis (PEP) (Pasteur 1885). From this early innovation, scientific and technological advances during subsequent decades have provided the safe and efficacious vaccines available today (World Health Organization [WHO] 2005). Despite the existence of these tools, rabies continues to kill thousands of people every year, mostly in countries where people live on less than US$1 each day. The disease occurs in more than 75% of the world's countries, causing innumerable animal deaths and an estimated 55,000 human deaths per year, the majority of which are children younger than 15 years (WHO 2010). It is likely that the predicted annual figure for human rabies fatalities is a gross under-estimate due to the lack of infrastructure and reporting systems in developing countries (Fooks 2007).

Viral neurovirulence (the capacity to infect the nervous system) is a feature of rabies virus infection, and all lyssaviruses are known to be highly neurotropic (Schnell et al. 2010). The ability of the virus to spread throughout the nervous system of the host (neuroinvasiveness) and into the brain is a major contributing factor to the pathogenesis observed following rabies virus infection (Dietzschold et al. 2008).

16.1.2 CLINICAL COURSE

Once an individual has been exposed to rabies virus, it is essential that medical attention is rapidly sought, as it is at this first crucial stage where effective PEP can alter the outcome of infection and save lives. Following infection, there is a variable incubation period before the onset of clinical symptoms. This period generally lasts between 20 and 90 days in humans but may vary considerably, in some rare cases lasting several years (Jackson 2007a; Johnson et al. 2008a). Following incubation, the infected individual will begin to exhibit non-specific clinical symptoms, which may include but are not limited to malaise, weakness, loss of appetite, paresthesia, and fever (Hunter et al. 2010; Rupprecht et al. 2002). The disease then rapidly progresses to manifest as an acute central nervous system (CNS) disorder that produces a broad spectrum of clinical symptoms (Nicholson 1994). There are two clinical outcomes: furious and paralytic (Schnell et al. 2010). A large proportion (approximately 80%) of human cases demonstrate symptoms associated with the furious form including aggression, hyperexcitability, muscular spasms, and hydrophobia (Dacheux et al. 2008; Schnell et al. 2010). However, the remainder of cases generally follow a different clinical course typified by paralytic symptoms such as incoordination, lethargy, and flaccid muscle weakness that progress to paralysis and death (Hunter et al. 2010; Solomon et al. 2005). The two forms (furious and paralytic) are not distinct or mutually exclusive and many infections develop with clinical features from both. The factors that influence the differences in disease presentation are not fully understood (Hemachudha et al. 2003). Obtaining a differential diagnosis of rabies infection can often be problematic due to variations in length of incubation period and clinical presentation. Several of the symptoms that can be observed during rabies infection also resemble those observed in other neurological disorders.

For example, the clinical symptoms observed in human paralytic cases can often be confused with Guillain-Barré syndrome, but the two diseases can be differentiated when there is sphincter involvement, particularly urinary incontinence, as this only occurs during rabies infection (Asbury and Cornblath 1990; Jackson 2007a; Solomon et al. 2005).

Regardless of differences in disease presentation, the ultimate outcome for infected individuals is almost always death. However, there have now been several documented cases whereby clinically affected humans have survived following the rapid administration of PEP and/or intensive therapies, although, all but a few of these patients suffered substantial neurological sequelae (Willoughby 2009; Willoughby et al. 2005). There have also been a number of experimental studies in which clinically affected animals have been observed to recover and survive infection, without intervention, although recovery was accompanied by neurological sequelae (Jackson et al. 1989; Vos et al. 2004). A few controversial reports have also been published describing infected animals, with productive infections, showing no clinical signs, suggesting a carrier state (East et al. 2001; Veeraraghavan et al. 1970). These atypical outcomes can be difficult to investigate due to limitations in the diagnosis of rabies in a live animal (Jackson 2007b). It is currently unclear why these outcomes of infection occur, and further research is required to understand such instances. However, it is clear that the relative virulence of the infecting virus, viral load, site of wound, and immunological status of the infected host must all be critical to the outcome following exposure (Vos et al. 2004; Willoughby et al. 2005).

16.1.3 Lyssaviruses: Classification, Morphology, and Replication

The genus *Lyssavirus* belongs within the Order *Mononegavirales*, Family *Rhabdoviridae*. There are 12 established species within the Lyssavirus genus (ICTV 2011) and two recently identified viruses, namely Bokeloh bat lyssavirus (Freuling et al. 2010) and Ikoma lyssavirus (Marston et al. 2012) that are awaiting classification (Table 16.1). All lyssaviruses contain single-stranded, negative-sense RNA genomes with enveloped, bullet-shaped virions measuring approximately 75×180 nm (Warrell and Warrell 2004). Virions derive their envelope from the plasma membrane of the cell that they infect. The lyssavirus genomes are approximately 12,000 bp in length and contain genes that encode five proteins: the nucleoprotein (N); the phosphoprotein (P); the matrix protein (M); the glycoprotein (G), and the large polymerase protein (L) (Dietzschold et al. 2008). Of these proteins, the N protein encapsidates the negative-sense RNA genome within the virion forming a tight association with the RNA, which, along with P and L, forms the minimal replicative unit for these viruses: the ribonucleoprotein complex (RNP). This RNP structure is responsible for all elements of viral transcription and replication to generate viral proteins and nascent genomes, respectively (Schnell et al. 2010). The M protein plays a structural role between the RNP and the virion envelope (Schnell et al. 2010). The G protein is found throughout the virion envelope and is responsible for cell attachment and entry mechanisms (Rupprecht et al. 2002). This G protein is also the major antigenic determinant and is the major target for neutralizing antibodies following infection (Dietzschold et al. 2008).

TABLE 16.1

Classification of the Lyssaviruses

Species	Phylogroup	Geographical Range	Species from which Isolated	Human Deaths Reported
Rabies virus (RABV)	1	Worldwide	Wide range of mammals	Approx. 55,000 p.a.
Lagos bat virus (LBV)	2	Africa	Fruit bats, dogs, and cats	Unknown
Mokola virus (MOKV)	2	Africa	Shrews, cats, dogs, rodents, and humans	2
Duvenhage virus (DUVV)	1	Southern Africa	Insectivorous bats and humans	3
European bat lyssavirus 1 (EBLV-1)	1	Europe	Insectivorous bats, sheep, stone martens, and humans	2
European bat lyssavirus 2 (EBLV-2)	1	Europe	Insectivorous bats and humans	2
Australian bat lyssavirus (ABLV)	1	Australia	Fruit and insectivorous bats and humans	2
Aravan virus (ARAV)	1	Kyrgyzstan	Insectivorous bat	Unknown
Khujand virus (KHUV)	1	Tajikistan	Insectivorous bat	Unknown
Irkut virus (IRKV)	1	Eastern Siberia	Insectivorous bat	Unknown
West Caucasian bat virus (WCBV)	3	Caucasus	Insectivorous bat	Unknown
Shimoni bat virus (SHIBV)	2	Africa	Insectivorous bat	Unknown
Bokeloh bat lyssavirus (BBLV)	1?	Germany	Insectivorous bat	Unknown
Ikoma lyssavirus (IKOV)	3?	Tanzania	African civet	Unknown

Source: Freuling, C. et al., 2010, Discovery of a Lyssavirus in a Natterer's bat (Myotis nattereri) from Germany with unusual antigenic and molecular characteristics, in *Rabies in the Americas (RITA) XXI*, Guadalajara, Mexico; Healy, D. M., 2011, *Comparative Pathology of Lyssaviruses in a Murine Model*, School of Medicine, Dentistry and Biomedical Sciences, Centre for Infection and Immunity, Queen's University, Belfast, p. 261; ICTV, 2011, *ICTV Master Species List 2011 v2*, in *Viruses*, I.C.o.T.o. (Ed.), Virology Division, International Union of Microbiological Societies; Johnson, N. et al., 2006b, *Emerg. Infect. Dis.* 12, 1142–1144; Kuzmin, I. V. et al., 2010, *Virus Res.* 149, 197–210; Marston, D.A. et al., 2012, *Emerg. Infect. Dis.* 18, 664–667; Mensink, M. and Schaftenaar, W., 1998, When bad things happen to bats: the occurrence of a Lyssavirus in a closed population of Egyptian frugivorous bats (Rousettus aegyptiacus) at Rotterdam Zoo, European Association of Zoo and Wildlife Veterinarians (EAZWV) Second Scientific Meeting, pp. 147–151; Ronsholt, L. et al., 1998, *Vet. Rec.* 142, 519–520.

Lyssaviruses must gain entry into a host cell in order for replication to take place. The replication cycle of these viruses involves four main activities: uncoating, transcription, replication, and assembly (Figure 16.1) (Rupprecht et al. 2002). Initially, the viral G protein facilitates entry into the host cell by interacting with, and attaching to, cell surface receptors (Figure 16.1.1) (Lafon 2005). This leads to cell entry, either through direct fusion, whereby the viral envelope fuses with the host cell membrane, releasing the RNP into the cytoplasm of the cell or via receptor mediated endocytosis (RME), when the cell engulfs the viral particles through coated pits and uncoated vesicles on its surface (Wunner 2007). Following RME, virions are released from endosomal vesicles within the host cell, a process known as uncoating (Figure 16.1.2) (Schnell et al. 2010). Release is dependent on a reduction in endosomal pH that causes a conformational change in the viral G protein, resulting in membrane fusion and release of the RNP into the cell cytoplasm (Figure 16.1.3) (Gaudin et al. 1993).

Once in the cytoplasm of the infected cell, the virus genome initiates its replicative cycle commencing with the RNP acting as a transcriptase complex, capable of generating messenger RNA (mRNA) from the negative-sense RNA genome (Figure 16.1.4) (Schnell et al. 2010). These viral mRNAs are capped and polyadenylated by the host cellular machinery, and translated on free ribosomes within the cell (Figure 16.1.5) (Banerjee and Barik 1992). The exception to this is the G protein, which is moved to the rough endoplasmic reticulum (RER) and through the Golgi for translation and transport to the cell membrane (Figure 16.1.6) (Wunner 2007). A transcriptional gradient is generated where the transcriptase can only initiate the generation

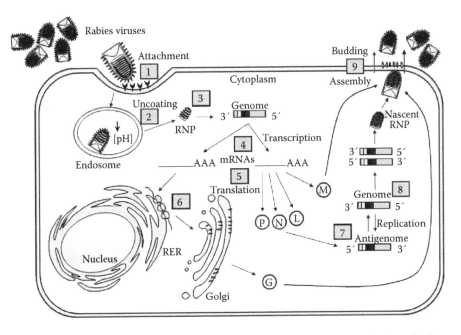

FIGURE 16.1 The intracellular life cycle of lyssaviruses following the infection of a host cell. All abbreviations are detailed in the text.

of transcripts from the 3' terminus of the genome, at the genome promoter (Banerjee and Barik 1992). As a result, 3' proximal genes are produced in abundance while those genes distal to the genome promoter are consecutively generated to lower levels (Schnell et al. 2010). At some point following infection, the RNP complex switches its function from that of a transcriptase complex, to a replicase complex, whereupon it subsequently generates full-length positive-sense RNA replicative intermediates (Figure 16.1.7) (Banerjee and Barik 1992). These positive-sense RNAs then act as the template for the generation of nascent negative-sense RNA genomes (Figure 16.1.8) (Banerjee and Barik 1992). Late on in the cycle, it is thought that interactions between nascent RNPs and the M protein enable movement of virus to the plasma membrane. It is at this site where interaction with G brings about assembly of a new virion, which then buds from the cell (Figure 16.1.9) (Schnell et al. 2010). The progeny virions are then capable of adhering to and infecting new host cells and the cycle is initiated once more.

16.2   PATHOGENESIS

The pathogenesis of rabies virus within a host follows a sequential pattern. This process is instigated by the entry of viral particles into the host, and is followed by the replication of the virus within the peripheral tissues, centripetal spread along the peripheral nerves to the CNS, dissemination within the spinal cord and brain, and centrifugal spread to the salivary glands and other organs (Figure 16.2) (Dietzschold et al. 2008). The duration of each step and pathology produced in disease progression are influenced by both host and viral factors, which are detailed below.

16.2.1   EXPOSURE

Lyssaviruses are unable to gain entry through intact skin, which acts as an effective defensive barrier. Virions must therefore enter where this barrier is broken, e.g., a wound or through mucous membranes, i.e., the eyes, nose, mouth. The mechanisms of exposure and viral entry into the host are often categorized into either "bite" or "nonbite" incidents. The vast majority of transmission occurs as a result of the bite of an infected animal, with transmission being facilitated by the presence of virus in the saliva (Figure 16.2.1) (Warrell and Warrell 2004). In contrast, "nonbite" exposures are far less common, but can occur through (i) the contamination of a preexisting open wound, (ii) scratches received from an infected host, (iii) inhalation of aerosolized virus, or (iv) through the transplantation of virus-infected organs, e.g., corneal transplants (Jackson 2007a; Johnson et al. 2006a). There are also reports of human-to-human transmission, which have included transplacental transmission, where virus was detected in both mother and baby postmortem (Sipahioglu and Alpaut 1985), and two cases where transmission is thought to have occurred between mother and child, one through a bite and the other through repeated oral contact (Fekadu et al. 1996). If transmission occurs, but a clear history of an exposure to rabies virus is not known or recalled (e.g., an unnoticed bite or scratch received from a bat), it is known as cryptic rabies. This inconspicuous transmission is a cause of human

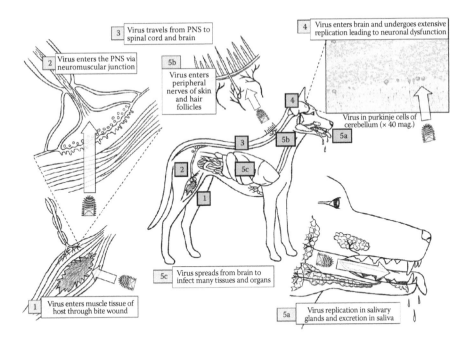

FIGURE 16.2   The sequential pattern of rabies pathogenesis occurring within a dog, following a bite wound (virions not to scale). PNS = peripheral nervous system.

fatalities in regions where effective medical intervention could have been sought had the individual been aware of their exposure (Messenger et al. 2002).

The lyssaviruses are maintained in a variety of reservoir hosts, which vary with viral species, strain, and location (Rupprecht et al. 2002). Rabies can follow urban (within domestic animal populations) or sylvatic (within wildlife species) transmission cycles. While the disease circulates within the reservoir host population, infected individuals come into contact with other species, allowing for spill-over events to occur. Transmission to humans occurs in this way (Banyard and Fooks 2011). All but two of the lyssavirus species have been isolated from members of the Order *Chiroptera* (bat species) (Table 16.1). However, members of the Family *Canidae*, particularly dogs, are the most important species as a source of human infection (Rupprecht et al. 2002).

Not all exposures to rabies virus through bite wounds received from rabid animals result in infection, clinical disease, and death (Cleaveland et al. 2002). It is thought that one of the major factors affecting the risk of developing rabies following a dog bite exposure is the location of the bite (Knobel et al. 2005). Estimates suggest that if no PEP is provided, the risk of developing rabies following a rabid dog bite is approximately 50%, depending on the severity and location of the wound received, with the risk increasing for head wounds and decreasing for bites sustained on extremities (Baltazard and Ghodssi 1954; Solomon et al. 2005). This should not preclude potentially exposed individuals from seeking immediate medical attention as the risk of developing rabies can be reduced through administration of rapid, effective PEP (Hampson et al. 2008; Jackson 2007a).

16.2.2 TRANSPORT OF RABIES VIRUS FROM THE BITE SITE TO THE CNS

For lyssaviruses to infect and successfully replicate, they must come into contact with a susceptible host cell. Virus initially enters the peripheral nerves at the inoculation site (Figure 16.2.2), then travels toward the CNS along peripheral motoneurons, replicating within neuronal cell bodies, before entering the spinal cord and brain (Figure 16.2.3) (Ugolini 2008).

The ability of the virus to enter a specific cell type is dictated by the viral G protein, which binds to specific receptors present on permissive cells (Lafon 2005). The viral G protein amino acid sequence is key to receptor utilization and pathogenesis, to the extent that a single amino acid substitution at position 333 in the G protein reduces neurovirulence dramatically, resulting in nonpathogenic variants (Dietzschold et al. 1983; Jackson 1991; Seif et al. 1985). The first substitution in G, combined with a second at position 330, prevents the virus from entering the nervous system (Coulon et al. 1998). A further substitution occurring at position 194 has also been identified (Faber et al. 2005), that is considered to be important for the development of safe live-attenuated vaccines because it prevented reversion to the natural virulent phenotype (Faber et al. 2009). Three specific host cell receptors have been implicated in virus entry. The nicotinic acetylcholine receptor (nAChR), present at neuromuscular junctions, and responsible for interneuronal communication (Lafon 2005); the neural cell adhesion molecule (NCAM) CD56, present at nerve termini and postsynaptic membranes, deep within neuromuscular junctions (Covault and Sanes 1986), and the low-affinity neurotrophin receptor (p75NTR), a nerve growth factor receptor (Dechant and Barde 2002) although the latter may not be necessary for lyssavirus–host cell interaction (Tuffereau et al. 2007). *In vitro*, lyssaviruses are able to replicate successfully in numerous different cell types (Reagan and Wunner 1985), and several cells that are susceptible to infection do not express the three currently implicated receptors, suggesting that further receptor molecules that are yet to be identified may enable virus entry (Tuffereau et al. 2007). Variations in the ability of viral strains to infect neuronal or nonneuronal cells have been observed (Thoulouze et al. 1997). Highly neurovirulent strains appear to have a narrow cell tropism, only infecting nervous tissue, whereas less-pathogenic attenuated strains have been shown to infect a range of cells, including neuronal and nonneuronal types (Thoulouze et al. 1997). It has also been suggested that differences in the structure, quantity, and availability of rabies receptors between different hosts may play a role in the variable susceptibility and pathogenesis observed between species. For example, it has been observed that there is a large quantity of nAChRs present in the muscles of red foxes (a highly susceptible species), compared with the relatively reduced quantity of these receptors in opossums (a highly resistant species) (Baer et al. 1990).

Once the virus has entered the peripheral nervous system, infection progresses by centripetal migration of virions from the periphery to the CNS. Migration occurs by retrograde axoplasmic flow. The virus has been reported to migrate in this way at a rate of 50–100 mm per day (Tsiang et al. 1991). It has been suggested that this movement is enabled through virus phosphoprotein interacting with actin- and microtubule-based motility networks within the nerves (i.e., dynein light chain 8) (Jacob et al. 2000; Raux et al. 2000). However, when deletions occur in the virus binding region for these networks, there appear to be only minor effects on virus motility. This suggests that other, as yet unidentified, interactions could be significant (Mebatsion 2001; Rasalingam et al. 2005). Once the virus reaches the dorsal root ganglia the virions undergo replication, before entering the neurons of the spinal cord, where further replication occurs. Upon entering the spinal cord, there is rapid centripetal dissemination, followed by extensive replication of the virus within the brain (Figure 16.2.4) (Jackson 2007b; Johnson et al. 2008b).

16.2.3 FROM THE CNS TO ONWARD TRANSMISSION

Following infection of the brain, there is centrifugal spread of the virions to other tissues and organs of the body via the peripheral nerves (Figure 16.2.5). Onward transmission is enabled at this stage as virus particles migrate along the nerves to the salivary glands, then replicate extensively within these glands, resulting in viral shedding in the saliva (Figure 16.2.5a) (Jackson 2007b). It is important to note that the virus always enters and replicates within the CNS before moving to the salivary glands. However, the pathology occurring within the CNS may not be very extensive by the time this movement has occurred, and viral shedding begins. Therefore, an infected host may be infectious before clinical signs are sufficient to indicate a specific diagnosis of rabies (Warrell and Warrell 2004). Neurons within the eyes, hair follicles (Figure 16.2.5b), and thoracic and abdominal organs (Figure 16.2.5c) have been shown to be infected at this centrifugal stage of disease progression. In addition, infection of nonneural tissue has been observed, including salivary gland acini, epithelial, and muscle cells (Jackson 2007b). The results of several studies suggest that viral spread at this stage is highly extensive. In one study, of two EBLV-2-positive bats, viral RNA was detected in brain, salivary glands, heart, tongue, stomach, lung, thyroid gland, intestine, liver, kidney, and bladder (Johnson et al. 2006b). Despite this broad tissue distribution, it is likely that the virus remains within highly innervated areas of these organs although spread into non-neuronal tissue, particularly in late stage disease, needs to be further investigated.

16.3 PATHOLOGY

Despite causing severe clinical deterioration, the pathological changes caused by rabies virus infection are predominantly noncytopathic in nature (Jackson 2007b). Even at a late stage in infection, where there is extensive infection of the host, the macroscopic structural changes observed, if present at all, can be mild and nonspecific (Dupont and Earle 1965). Changes seen may include inflammation of the spinal cord and brain, resulting in encephalomyelitis (Love and Wiley 2002) and ganglioneuritis in nerve centres (Banyard and Fooks 2011). Mild cerebral edema and congestion of some blood vessels has been observed, along with occasional focal changes in the parenchyma, perhaps related to prolonged clinical course (Rossiter and Jackson 2007; Rubin et al. 1970).

The histopathological changes are also mild and mostly related to inflammatory processes. Some degree of inflammatory cell infiltration is normally present, principally involving lymphocytes and monocytes, accompanied by some plasma cells. However, in cases with intense inflammation, the infiltrate is predominantly composed of neutrophils (Perl and Good 1991). In the majority of rabies cases, perivascular cuffing can be seen whereby mononuclear inflammatory cells form accumulations around vessels, mostly in the gray matter of the spinal cord and brain (Hicks et al. 2009). Excessive proliferation of the neuroglial supportive tissue (gliosis), along with accumulations of activated microglia (Babes' nodules) can also be seen in many infections (Rossiter and Jackson 2007). These pathological alterations are not unique for rabies and the occurrence, density, and distribution can be highly variable between the differing forms, and individual cases of disease (Rossiter and Jackson 2007). There have also been fatal cases of rabies where virtually no inflammatory changes were observed (Hicks et al. 2009). One change that is often observed, which distinguishes rabies infection from other viral encephalitides, is the intracytoplasmic inclusions named "Negri bodies." These are thought to be large aggregations of viral N and P proteins and have been implicated as possible specialized sites for viral transcription and replication (Lahaye et al. 2009). These markers of infection have been observed in many different regions of the CNS and their presence and distribution can be influenced by a range of host and virus factors including virus strain, host species, and the clinical phase of disease.

16.3.1 Cell Damage and Death

Within the affected neuronal tissue, in addition to abnormal accumulations of constituent cells and aberrant inclusions inside living cells, irreversible injury, degeneration, and cell death can occur. The damaged or dying cells can be highlighted in many cases by neuronophagia, whereby a microscopic pattern of accumulated phagocytic cells (microglia or macrophages) can be observed around the afflicted neurons (Rossiter and Jackson 2007). As with the other pathological changes, there is a high degree of variation in the extent of this cellular destruction. The neuroinvasiveness and replication of the virus is dependent upon the availability of intact neuronal cells. Therefore, in most naturally occurring infections, with high neuroinvasiveness, there tends to be minimal cell death compared with the less neuroinvasive fixed laboratory strains, which produce a greater extent of damage and degeneration (Dietzschold et al. 2008). It has been hypothesized that apoptotic cell death of neuronal tissue is a potential pathogenic mechanism of rabies virus (Jackson and Rossiter 1997). However, several studies have suggested that pathogenic strains of rabies virus do not induce apoptosis (Yan et al. 2001), while attenuated strains are proapoptotic (Morimoto et al. 1999), so the role of this process in rabies pathogenesis is currently unclear. It has also been proposed that degeneration of neuronal processes, with relative preservation of neuronal cell bodies, may be a major cause of neuronal dysfunction. This is due to the disruption of cytoskeletal integrity that has been observed in infections with pathogenic rabies strains (Li et al. 2005).

16.3.2 Functional Impairment

The dysfunction within the CNS of rabies virus infected individuals has been attributed to a number of causes. The results of several studies have suggested that functional impairment could partly be due to reduced neurotransmission capabilities of infected neurons. Decreased gene expression leading to inhibition of host cell protein synthesis has been reported (Fu et al. 1993). This has included a reduction in the binding ability of acetylcholine receptors (Tsiang 1982), and interference in the release and binding of neurotransmitters such as γ-amino-*n*-butyric acid (GABA) (Ladogana et al. 1994) and serotonin (Bouzamondo et al. 1993; Ceccaldi et al. 1993). Serotonin is of particular interest in rabies pathogenesis due to its possible involvement in the development of certain clinical signs characteristic of rabies (Jackson 2007b). In the healthy animal, this neurotransmitter is widely distributed in the brain, and is involved in the control of sleep, pain perception, and certain behaviors (Julius 1991). Another possible effect of rabies virus infection, which would lead to impairment and loss of neuronal function, is failure of the cells to produce effective action potentials through interference with ion channel function (Iwata et al. 1999, 2000). Additional studies are required to fully elucidate the direct causal mechanisms of these functional changes during infection (i.e., whether they are as a result of the direct interaction of viral particles or due to the stress or immune responses of the host).

16.4   IMMUNE RESPONSE

The first defense of virally infected cells is the innate immune response, which triggers the secretion of interferons (IFNs) (Schnell et al. 2010). Rabies virus phosphoprotein is thought to interfere with, and subvert, the innate immune response through the inhibition of a number of signaling molecules that up-regulate IFNs (Brzozka et al. 2005) and would normally be activated following recognition of viral infection (Schnell et al. 2010). However, in a murine model of rabies virus infection, the level of IFN-α, β, and γ transcripts, as well as some chemokine transcripts, were shown to be up-regulated in the brain (Johnson et al. 2008b). Despite the induction of these inflammatory and antiviral transcripts, the mice developed severe disease and it was hypothesized that the failure of innate immunity to prevent disease may be as a result of the virus replicating at such rapidity within the CNS that it overwhelms the host before the inflammatory and antiviral mechanisms can act (Johnson et al. 2008b).

The principal correlate of protection against rabies virus is neutralizing antibody (Hooper et al. 1998). However, during natural infection, the development of a neutralizing antibody response is rare until after the virus has reached the CNS, and disease has developed (Johnson et al. 2010a; Noah et al. 1998). The reason for this ineffective antibody response is not fully understood, but could be due to a number of virus and host factors. During the early stages of infection, there tends to be limited viral replication allowing the virus to bypass normal immune surveillance. The locations at which the majority of viral replication occurs—the dorsal root ganglia, the spinal cord, and the brain—are thought to be immunoprivileged sites in that they are not under the same level of immunosurveillance as other parts of the body (Johnson et al. 2010a). It has been reported that pathogenic strains of rabies virus replicate at a lower level while in the peripheral nervous system than attenuated variants (Faber et al. 2009), and that this reduction in replicative rate results in production of less viral antigen (Morimoto et al. 1999), and preservation of neuronal structures (Faber et al. 2009). Conversely, the attenuated viral strains, with high replication rates and large amounts of glycoprotein expressed are highly immunogenic, tending to induce strong adaptive immune responses, which allow infection to be cleared (Faber et al. 2009).

Once the virus has reached the brain, it is much more difficult for circulating antibodies to reach and neutralize infecting viral particles, as a result of the blood-brain barrier (BBB). Under normal conditions, the BBB restricts access of pro-inflammatory cytokines, chemokines, and immune cells in order to protect neuronal cells from damage caused by inflammation (Phares et al. 2006; Ruzek et al. 2011). When infection occurs with a pathogenic rabies virus, the permeability of the BBB does not increase (Faber et al. 2009; Ruzek et al. 2011; Schnell et al. 2010), whereas infection with an attenuated rabies virus leads to increased BBB permeability, allowing the immune response to clear the virus (Faber et al. 2009). T lymphocytes, which are capable of crossing the BBB and could therefore still clear the virally infected cells from the brain during a pathogenic infection, are unable to achieve this due to induced apoptosis of T cells as a result of the up-regulation of FasL in infected neurons (Baloul et al. 2004).

16.4.1 IMMUNITY TO INFECTION

Vaccination is highly effective at preventing disease when given preexposure or postexposure as it generates an adaptive immune response and triggers the production of neutralizing antibody. Preexposure vaccination with inactivated tissue culture-derived vaccine is recommended for veterinarians, those with occupational exposure to the virus, and travelers to rabies endemic areas. Current WHO recommendations are for administration of vaccine intramuscularly at days 0, 7, and 28. IgM is detectable within 4 days and IgG appears by day 7 (Johnson et al. 2010a). Postexposure vaccination is more intensive, with a series of inoculations (up to 4) given in protocols recommended by the WHO depending on the category of exposure. In the highest exposure risk category (category III), the initial postexposure vaccination should be accompanied by an injection of rabies immunoglobulin (RIG), which aims to neutralize any virus present at the site of introduction, in the lag period before the active immune system has responded to vaccination (WHO 2010).

16.4.2 THERAPY

Currently, thorough wound cleansing, postexposure vaccination, and administration of RIG are the only recommended interventions for rabies virus infection in humans. However, these procedures are not effective once symptoms develop and there is no antiviral therapy that directly inhibits rabies virus replication (Jackson et al. 2003). Palliative measures remain the principal option for care. Therapeutic coma has been proposed as a potential therapy after its success in saving the life of a teenager who developed rabies after being bitten by a bat in the United States (Willoughby et al. 2005). Several attempts to repeat this have unfortunately been unsuccessful (Hunter et al. 2010); however, there have been two further documented successes and a recent report of a human case in the United States where the patient successfully recovered (Pro-MED-mail 2011; Willoughby 2009).

16.5 STUDYING THE NEUROINVASIVENESS OF RABIES: EXPERIMENTAL MODELS OF INFECTION AND VACCINE DEVELOPMENT

A wide range of experimental models have been used to study rabies virus and to generate effective rabies virus vaccines. Louis Pasteur originally used rabbits to passage rabies virus, using the desiccated spinal cords removed from infected animals as the first vaccine. Mice were then developed as a simpler alternative although approaches to vaccine production using any animal material are now discouraged due to adverse immune reactions. The susceptibility of mice to infection has led to their use as a method of diagnosis and the use of inbred and knockout mouse strains is common to investigate rabies virus pathogenesis (Wang et al. 2005). Table 16.2 provides an overview of the animal models that have been used to study aspects of rabies virus biology. These models are divided into those studies that have used animals to assess susceptibility to infection or those that have investigated mechanisms of rabies pathogenesis. Alternatively, animals have provided models to assess vaccine

TABLE 16.2
Selected Examples of Animal Models Used to Investigate Rabies Pathogenesis

Animal	Reference	Comment
Mouse	(Wang et al. 2005)	Measure the up-regulation of innate immune transcripts using microarray analysis prepared from brain tissue
Rat	(Gillet et al. 1986)	Stereotactic inoculation enabled demonstration of axonal transport of RABV in rat brain
Dog	(Cho and Lawson 1989)	Demonstrate vaccine efficacy in an animal model
Fox	(Vos et al. 2001)	Efficacy studies of new rabies vaccines using a variety of inoculation routes
Ferret	(Niezgoda et al. 1997)	Demonstrate susceptibility of mustelids to rabies virus
Bat	(Johnson et al. 2008c) (Daubenton's bats)	Demonstrate susceptibility and experimentally investigate routes of transmission in Daubenton's bats (*Myotis daubentonii*)
	(Freuling et al. 2009) (Serotine bats)	Demonstrate susceptibility and experimentally investigate routes of transmission in serotine bats (*Eptesicus serotinus*)
	(Jackson et al. 2008) (Big brown bat)	Demonstrate susceptibility and seroconversion in the North American big brown bat (*Eptesicus fuscus*)
Syrian hamster	(Hanlon et al. 2001)	Used for protection studies for new rabies biologicals.
Guinea pig	(Hronovsky and Benda 1969)	Demonstration of aerosol transmission of rabies virus
Sheep	(Hanlon et al. 2001)	Susceptibility of sheep to infection

efficacy, which requires challenge with live virus. Rodents, including mice, rats, and guinea pigs have been used due to the ease of availability, and the relatively lower costs required for maintaining sufficient numbers to conduct statistically significant experiments. Larger mammals have been used where a specific need has been identified, such as determining the efficacy of an oral vaccine targeted at a particular species. One example of this is the determination of bait-acceptance and immunogenicity of oral rabies vaccine in the raccoon dog (*Nyctereutes procyonoides*) (Cliquet et al. 2006). On occasion, primates have been used as a surrogate for the effectiveness of experimental treatments in humans, for example, the use of monkeys to assess the ability of an attenuated strain of rabies to modify the course of lethal infection (Warrell et al. 1987). Another distinctive group of experimental animals are bats. These natural host species can help to answer key questions on the susceptibility and persistence of the lyssaviruses within bat populations (Fooks et al. 2009; Franka et al. 2006; Freuling et al. 2009; Johnson et al. 2008c).

In contrast, the neurotropic nature of rabies virus has led to the application of the virus to study neuronal pathways as a transneuronal tracer (Ugolini 1995). This use of the virus as a marker for neuronal networks has provided important information about viral pathogenesis. Specifically, the receptor locations, mechanisms, and neural pathways the virus uses to migrate from the periphery, to the CNS, have been studied in rodent and nonhuman primate models (Ugolini 2008).

16.6   FUTURE OUTLOOK

Rabies should be considered beside the major communicable disease threats to health. The high number of preventable injuries and deaths does not discriminate on age or gender, however, rabies should be considered as an important pediatric disease. It is evident that the global elimination of rabies requires an interdisciplinary control strategy. A realistic goal focused on the control of rabies in domestic dogs would result in a concomitant reduction of human mortality and would have a demonstrable impact on childhood mortality meeting one of the Millennium Development Goals to reduce child mortality.

The viruses that cause rabies belong to a large and complex group, and the continued study of these lyssaviruses, along with the effects they have on the broad range of host species they are able to infect, will enable us to further our understanding of the ways in which we can stop avoidable deaths from occurring. Current knowledge of these viruses has improved our understanding of rabies virus dynamics in the host.

The use of lyssaviruses as transneuronal tracers in future studies will allow further aspects of rabies neurovirulence and pathogenesis to be investigated and understood (Ugolini 2008). Further study and modeling of the virus-host interactions of both rabies and other neurotropic viral infections will help to clarify the subversion and avoidance mechanisms the virus uses to circumnavigate the hosts defenses. The continued use of technologies such as live-cell imaging in the future will enable the dynamics and spatiotemporal relationships in these interactions to be further analyzed (Chevalier et al. 2010). The development of safe, efficacious and affordable tools for preexposure and postexposure prophylaxis with simpler, single immunization regimens could lead to the elimination of rabies from areas of economic and political instability (Faber et al. 2009). Live-attenuated vaccines are also potential future candidates for treatment in the early stages of clinical human rabies as they are capable of inducing effective immune responses to clear virulent rabies virus from the CNS (Faber et al. 2009).

16.7 KEY POINTS

Lyssaviruses are neurovirulent, neurotropic viruses. They must enter a host and gain entry into a susceptible host cell in order for viral replication to take place and for a viable infection to be established. The factors that affect the ability of a virus population to infect the nervous system are numerous but include the neuroinvasiveness of the infecting viral strain and the susceptibility of the host species (i.e., the age, immune status and response produced upon infection). For a rabies virus population to be successful, it must be able to migrate from the site of infection, to the CNS, where efficient replication can occur, before moving to other organs of the body, particularly the salivary glands, to enable onward transmission to occur. Lyssaviruses are essentially noncytopathic, causing relatively minimal structural pathology, and appear to have evolved to preserve the integrity of the nervous system and perhaps maintain efficient viral spread. However, this does not prevent dysfunction of the nervous system occurring, which can be advantageous to the viral population where behavioral changes occur that improve transmission potential. The lyssaviruses have also evolved mechanisms to avoid, and subvert, the host immune response which could otherwise interfere with and potentially clear the infection.

ACKNOWLEDGEMENTS

This work was partially supported by Defra ROAME SV3500 and by funding from the European Commission Seventh Framework Programme under ANTIGONE (project number 278976).

REFERENCES

Asbury, A. K., and Cornblath, D. R. 1990. Assessment of current diagnostic criteria for Guillain-Barré syndrome. *Ann. Neurol.* 27 Suppl, S21–S24.

Baer, G. M. 2007. The history of rabies, In: Jackson, A. C., Wunner, W. H. (Eds.), *Rabies*, 2nd ed. Academic Press, Elsevier, pp. 1–22.

Baer, G. M., Shaddock, J. H., Quirion, R., Dam, T. V., and Lentz, T. L. 1990. Rabies susceptibility and acetylcholine receptor. *Lancet.* 335, 664–665.

Baloul, L., Camelo, S., and Lafon, M. 2004. Up-regulation of Fas ligand (FasL) in the central nervous system: A mechanism of immune evasion by rabies virus. *J. Neurovirol.* 10, 372–382.

Baltazard, M., and Ghodssi, M. 1954. Prevention of human rabies; treatment of persons bitten by rabid wolves in Iran. *Bull. World Health Organ.* 10, 797–803.

Banerjee, A. K., and Barik, S. 1992. Gene expression of vesicular stomatitis virus genome RNA. *Virology.* 188, 417–428.

Banyard, A. C., and Fooks, A. R. 2011. Rabies and rabies-related lyssaviruses, In: Palmer, S. R., Soulsby, L., Torgerson, P., Brown, D. W. G. (Eds.), *Oxford Textbook of Zoonoses: Biology, Clinical Practice, and Public Health Control*, 2nd ed. Oxford University Press, Oxford, pp. 398–422.

Bouzamondo, E., Ladogana, A., and Tsiang, H. 1993. Alteration of potassium-evoked 5-HT release from virus-infected rat cortical synaptosomes. *Neuroreport.* 4, 555–558.

Brzozka, K., Finke, S., and Conzelmann, K. K. 2005. Identification of the rabies virus alpha/beta interferon antagonist: Phosphoprotein P interferes with phosphorylation of interferon regulatory factor 3. *J. Virol.* 79, 7673–7681.

Ceccaldi, P. E., Fillion, M. P., Ermine, A., Tsiang, H., and Fillion, G. 1993. Rabies virus selectively alters 5-HT1 receptor subtypes in rat brain. *Eur. J. Pharmacol.* 245, 129–138.

Chevalier, G., Prat, C., Betourne, A., Szelechowski, M., Malnou, C. E., and Gonzalez-Dunia, D. 2010. Modeling virus-neuron interactions using borna disease virus, In: Garcin, D., Kolakofsky, D., Roux, L., and Whelan, S. (Eds.), *XIV International Conference on Negative Strand Viruses*, Brugge, Belgium, p. 160.

Cho, H. C., and Lawson, K. F. 1989. Protection of dogs against death from experimental rabies by postexposure administration of rabies vaccine and hyperimmune globulin (human). *Can. J. Vet. Res.* 53, 434–437.

Cleaveland, S., Fevre, E. M., Kaare, M., and Coleman, P. G. 2002. Estimating human rabies mortality in the United Republic of Tanzania from dog bite injuries. *Bull. World Health Organ.* 80, 304–310.

Cliquet, F., Guiot, A. L., Munier, A., Bailly, J., Rupprecht, C. E., and Barrat, J. 2006. Safety and efficacy of the oral rabies vaccine SAG2 in raccoon dogs. *Vaccine* 24, 4386–4392.

Coulon, P., Ternaux, J. P., Flamand, A., and Tuffereau, C. 1998. An avirulent mutant of rabies virus is unable to infect motoneurons *in vivo* and *in vitro*. *J. Virol.* 72, 273–278.

Covault, J., and Sanes, J. R. 1986. Distribution of N-CAM in synaptic and extrasynaptic portions of developing and adult skeletal muscle. *J. Cell Biol.* 102, 716–730.

Dacheux, L., Reynes, J. M., Buchy, P., Sivuth, O., Diop, B. M., Rousset, D., Rathat, C., Jolly, N., Dufourcq, J. B., Nareth, C., Diop, S., Iehle, C., Rajerison, R., Sadorge, C., and Bourhy, H. 2008. A reliable diagnosis of human rabies based on analysis of skin biopsy specimens. *Clin. Infect. Dis.* 47, 1410–1417.

Dechant, G., and Barde, Y. A. 2002. The neurotrophin receptor p75(NTR): Novel functions and implications for diseases of the nervous system. *Nat. Neurosci.* 5, 1131–1136.

Dietzschold, B., Li, J., Faber, M., and Schnell, M. 2008. Concepts in the pathogenesis of rabies. *Future Virol.* 3, 481–490.

Dietzschold, B., Wunner, W. H., Wiktor, T. J., Lopes, A. D., Lafon, M., Smith, C. L., and Koprowski, H. 1983. Characterization of an antigenic determinant of the glycoprotein that correlates with pathogenicity of rabies virus. *Proc. Natl. Acad. Sci. U S A* 80, 70–74.

Dupont, J. R., and Earle, K. M. 1965. Human rabies encephalitis. A study of forty-nine fatal cases with a review of the literature. *Neurology.* 15, 1023–1034.

East, M. L., Hofer, H., Cox, J. H., Wulle, U., Wiik, H., and Pitra, C. 2001. Regular exposure to rabies virus and lack of symptomatic disease in Serengeti spotted hyenas. *Proc. Natl. Acad. Sci. U S A*. 98, 15026–15031.

Faber, M., Faber, M. L., Papaneri, A., Bette, M., Weihe, E., Dietzschold, B., and Schnell, M. J. 2005. A single amino acid change in rabies virus glycoprotein increases virus spread and enhances virus pathogenicity. *J. Virol.* 79, 14141–14148.

Faber, M., Li, J., Kean, R. B., Hooper, D. C., Alugupalli, K. R., and Dietzschold, B. 2009. Effective preexposure and postexposure prophylaxis of rabies with a highly attenuated recombinant rabies virus. *Proc. Natl. Acad. Sci. U S A* 106, 11300–11305.

Fekadu, M., Endeshaw, T., Alemu, W., Bogale, Y., Teshager, T., and Olson, J. G. 1996. Possible human-to-human transmission of rabies in Ethiopia. *Ethiop. Med. J.* 34, 123–127.

Fooks, A. R. 2007. Rabies—the need for a 'one medicine' approach. *Vet. Rec.* 161, 289–290.

Fooks, A. R., Johnson, N., Muller, T., Vos, A., Mansfield, K., Hicks, D., Nunez, A., Freuling, C., Neubert, L., Kaipf, I., Denzinger, A., Franka, R., and Rupprecht, C. E. 2009. Detection of high levels of European bat lyssavirus type-1 viral RNA in the thyroid gland of experimentally-infected Eptesicus fuscus bats. *Zoonoses Public Health* 56, 270–277.

Franka, R., Constantine, D. G., Kuzmin, I., Velasco-Villa, A., Reeder, S. A., Streicker, D., Orciari, L. A., Wong, A. J., Blanton, J. D., and Rupprecht, C. E. 2006. A new phylogenetic lineage of rabies virus associated with western pipistrelle bats (Pipistrellus hesperus). *J. Gen. Virol.* 87, 2309–2321.

Freuling, C., Vos, A., Johnson, N., Kaipf, I., Denzinger, A., Neubert, L., Mansfield, K., Hicks, D., Nunez, A., Tordo, N., Rupprecht, C. E., Fooks, A. R., and Muller, T. 2009. Experimental infection of serotine bats (Eptesicus serotinus) with European bat lyssavirus type 1a. *J. Gen. Virol.* 90, 2493–2502.

Freuling, C., Wohlsein, P., Keller, B., Muhlback, E., Conraths, F. J., Teifke, J., Hoffman, B., Hoper, D., Korthase, C., Beer, M., Mettenleiter, T. C., and Muller, T. 2010. Discovery of a Lyssavirus in a Natterer's bat (Myotis nattereri) from Germany with unusual antigenic and molecular characteristics. In: *Rabies in the Americas (RITA) XXI*, Guadalajara, Mexico.

Fu, Z. F., Weihe, E., Zheng, Y. M., Schafer, M. K., Sheng, H., Corisdeo, S., Rauscher, F. J., 3rd, Koprowski, H., and Dietzschold, B. 1993. Differential effects of rabies and borna disease viruses on immediate-early- and late-response gene expression in brain tissues. *J. Virol.* 67, 6674–6681.

Gaudin, Y., Ruigrok, R. W., Knossow, M., and Flamand, A. 1993. Low-pH conformational changes of rabies virus glycoprotein and their role in membrane fusion. *J. Virol.* 67, 1365–1372.

Gillet, J. P., Derer, P., and Tsiang, H. 1986. Axonal transport of rabies virus in the central nervous system of the rat. *J. Neuropath. Exp. Neur.* 45, 619–634.

Hampson, K., Dobson, A., Kaare, M., Dushoff, J., Magoto, M., Sindoya, E., and Cleaveland, S. 2008. Rabies exposures, post-exposure prophylaxis and deaths in a region of endemic canine rabies. *Plos Neglect. Trop. Dis.* 2(11), e339, 1–9.

Hanlon, C. A., DeMattos, C. A., DeMattos, C. C., Niezgoda, M., Hooper, D. C., Koprowski, H., Notkins, A., and Rupprecht, C. E. 2001. Experimental utility of rabies virus-neutralizing human monoclonal antibodies in post-exposure prophylaxis. *Vaccine* 19, 3834–3842.

Healy, D. M. 2011. *Comparative Pathology of Lyssaviruses in a Murine Model*, School of Medicine, Dentistry and Biomedical Sciences, Centre for Infection and Immunity. Queen's University, Belfast, p. 261.

Hemachudha, T., Wacharapluesadee, S., Lumlertdaecha, B., Orciari, L. A., Rupprecht, C. E., La-ongpant, M., Juntrakul, S., and Denduangboripant, J. 2003. Sequence analysis of rabies virus in humans exhibiting encephalitic or paralytic rabies. *J. Infect. Dis.* 188, 960–966.

Hicks, D. J., Nunez, A., Healy, D. M., Brookes, S. M., Johnson, N., and Fooks, A. R. 2009. Comparative pathological study of the murine brain after experimental infection with classical rabies virus and European bat lyssaviruses. *J. Comp. Pathol.* 140, 113–126.

Hooper, D. C., Morimoto, K., Bette, M., Weihe, E., Koprowski, H., and Dietzschold, B. 1998. Collaboration of antibody and inflammation in clearance of rabies virus from the central nervous system. *J. Virol.* 72, 3711–3719.

Hronovsky, V., and Benda, R. 1969. Development of inhalation rabies infection in suckling guinea pigs. *Acta Virol.* 13, 198–202.

Hunter, M., Johnson, N., Hedderwick, S., McCaughey, C., Lowry, K., McConville, J., Herron, B., McQuaid, S., Marston, D., Goddard, T., Harkess, G., Goharriz, H., Voller, K., Solomon, T., Willoughby, R. E., and Fooks, A. R. 2010. Immunovirological correlates in human rabies treated with therapeutic coma. *J. Med. Virol.* 82, 1255–1265.

ICTV. 2011. *ICTV Master Species List 2011 v2*, In: Viruses, I.C.o.T.o. (Ed.). Virology Division, International Union of Microbiological Societies.

Iwata, M., Komori, S., Unno, T., Minamoto, N., and Ohashi, H. 1999. Modification of membrane currents in mouse neuroblastoma cells following infection with rabies virus. *Br. J. Pharmacol.* 126, 1691–1698.

Iwata, M., Unno, T., Minamoto, N., Ohashi, H., and Komori, S. 2000. Rabies virus infection prevents the modulation by alpha(2)-adrenoceptors, but not muscarinic receptors, of Ca2+ channels in NG108-15 cells. *Eur. J. Pharmacol.* 404, 79–88.

Jackson, A. C. 1991. Biological basis of rabies virus neurovirulence in mice: comparative pathogenesis study using the immunoperoxidase technique. *J. Virol.* 65, 537–540.

Jackson, A. C. 2007a. Human disease, In: Jackson, A. C., and Wunner, W. H. (Eds.), *Rabies*, 2nd ed. Academic Press, Elsevier, Amsterdam, pp. 309–340.

Jackson, A. C. 2007b. Pathogenesis, in: Jackson, A. C., and Wunner, W. H. (Eds.), *Rabies*, 2 ed. Academic Press, Elsevier, Amsterdam, pp. 341–381.

Jackson, A. C., Reimer, D. L., and Ludwin, S. K. 1989. Spontaneous-recovery from the encephalomyelitis in mice caused by street rabies virus. *Neuropathol. Appl. Neurobiol.* 15, 459–475.

Jackson, A. C., and Rossiter, J. P. 1997. Apoptosis plays an important role in experimental rabies virus infection. *J. Virol.* 71, 5603–5607.

Jackson, A. C., Warrell, M. J., Rupprecht, C. E., Ertl, H. C., Dietzschold, B., O'Reilly, M., Leach, R. P., Fu, Z. F., Wunner, W. H., Bleck, T. P., and Wilde, H. 2003. Management of rabies in humans. *Clin. Infect. Dis.* 36, 60–63.

Jackson, F. R., Turmelle, A. S., Farino, D. M., Franka, R., McCracken, G. F., and Rupprecht, C. E. 2008. Experimental rabies virus infection of big brown bats (Eeptesicus fuscus). *J. Wildl. Dis.* 44, 612–621.

Jacob, Y., Badrane, H., Ceccaldi, P. E., and Tordo, N. 2000. Cytoplasmic dynein LC8 interacts with lyssavirus phosphoprotein. *J. Virol.* 74, 10217–10222.

Johnson, N., Cunningham, A. F., and Fooks, A. R. 2010a. The immune response to rabies virus infection and vaccination. *Vaccine* 28, 3896–3901.

Johnson, N., Fooks, A., and McColl, K. 2008a. Reexamination of human rabies case with long incubation, Australia. *Emerg. Infect. Dis.* 14, 1950–1951.

Johnson, N., Mansfield, K. L., Hicks, D., Nunez, A., Healy, D. M., Brookes, S. M., McKimmie, C., Fazakerley, J. K., and Fooks, A. R. 2008b. Inflammatory responses in the nervous system of mice infected with a street isolate of rabies virus, In: Dodet, B., Fooks, A. R., Muller, T., and Tordo, N. (Eds.), *Towards the Elimination of Rabies in Eurasia. International Association for Biologicals (IABS)*, Paris, pp. 65–72.

Johnson, N., Phillpotts, R., and Fooks, A. R. 2006a. Airborne transmission of lyssaviruses. *J. Med. Microbiol.* 55, 785–790.

Johnson, N., Vos, A., Freuling, C., Tordo, N., Fooks, A. R., and Muller, T. 2010b. Human rabies due to lyssavirus infection of bat origin. *Vet. Microbiol.* 142, 151–159.

Johnson, N., Vos, A., Neubert, L., Freuling, C., Kaipf, I., Denzinger, A., Hicks, D., Núñez, A., Franka, R., Kuzmin, I., Rupprecht, C. E. and Fooks, A. R. 2008c. Experimental study of European bat lyssavirus type-2 infection in Daubenton's bats (*Myotis daubentonii*). *J. Gen. Virol.* 89, 2662–2672.

Johnson, N., Wakeley, P. R., Brookes, S. M., and Fooks, A. R. 2006b. European bat lyssavirus type 2 RNA in Myotis daubentonii. *Emerg. Infect. Dis.* 12, 1142–1144.

Julius, D. 1991. Molecular biology of serotonin receptors. *Annu. Rev. Neurosci.* 14, 335–360.

Knobel, D. L., Cleaveland, S., Coleman, P. G., Fevre, E. M., Meltzer, M. I., Miranda, M. E. G., Shaw, A., Zinsstag, J., and Meslin, F. X. 2005. Re-evaluating the burden of rabies in Africa and Asia. *Bull. World Health Organ.* 83, 360–368.

Kuzmin, I. V., Mayer, A. E., Niezgoda, M., Markotter, W., Agvvanda, B., Breiman, R. F., and Rupprecht, C. E. 2010. Shimoni bat virus, a new representative of the Lyssavirus genus. *Virus Res.* 149, 197–210.

Ladogana, A., Bouzamondo, E., Pocchiari, M., and Tsiang, H. 1994. Modification of tritiated gamma-amino-n-butyric acid transport in rabies virus-infected primary cortical cultures. *J. Gen. Virol.* 75(Pt 3), 623–627.

Lafon, M. 2005. Rabies virus receptors. *J. Neurovirol.* 11, 82–87.

Lahaye, X., Vidy, A., Pomier, C., Obiang, L., Harper, F., Gaudin, Y., and Blondel, D. 2009. Functional characterization of negri bodies (NBs) in rabies virus-infected cells: evidence that nbs are sites of viral transcription and replication. *J. Virol.* 83, 7948–7958.

Li, X. Q., Sarmento, L., and Fu, Z. F. 2005. Degeneration of neuronal processes after infection with pathogenic, but not attenuated, rabies viruses. *J. Virol.* 79, 10063–10068.

Love, S., and Wiley, C. A. 2002. Viral diseases, In: Graham, D. I., and Lantos, P. L. (Eds.), *Greenfield's Neuropathology*, 7th ed. Arnold, London, pp. 1–105.

Marston, D. A., Horton, D. L., Ngeleja, C., Hampson, K., McElhinney, L. M., Banyard, A. C., Haydon, D., Cleaveland, S., Rupprecht, C. E., Bigambo, M., Fooks, A. R., and Lembo, T. 2012. Ikoma lyssavirus: highly divergent novel lyssavirus in an African civet. *Emerg. Infect. Dis.* 18(4), 664–667.

Mebatsion, T. 2001. Extensive attenuation of rabies virus by simultaneously modifying the dynein light chain binding site in the P protein and replacing Arg333 in the G protein. *J. Virol.* 75, 11496–11502.

Mensink, M., and Schaftenaar, W. 1998. When bad things happen to bats: the occurrence of a Lyssavirus in a closed population of Egyptian frugivorous bats (Rousettus aegyptiacus) at Rotterdam Zoo, European Association of Zoo and Wildlife Veterinarians (EAZWV) Second Scientific Meeting, pp. 147–151.

Messenger, S. L., Smith, J. S., and Rupprecht, C. E. 2002. Emerging epidemiology of bat-associated cryptic cases of rabies in humans in the United States. *Clin. Infect. Dis.* 35, 738–747.

Morimoto, K., Hooper, D. C., Spitsin, S., Koprowski, H., and Dietzschold, B. 1999. Pathogenicity of different rabies virus variants inversely correlates with apoptosis and rabies virus glycoprotein expression in infected primary neuron cultures. *J. Virol.* 73, 510–518.

Neville, J. 2004. Rabies in the ancient world, In: King, A. A., Fooks, A. R., Aubert, M., and Wandeler, A. I. (Eds.), Historical *Perspective of Rabies in Europe and the Mediterranean Basin*. OIE (World Organization for Animal Health), Paris, pp. 1–13.

Nicholson, K. G. 1994. Human rabies, In: McKendall, R., and Stroop, W. (Eds.), *Handbook of Neurovirology*. M. Dekker, New York, pp. 463–480.

Niezgoda, M., Briggs, D. J., Shaddock, J., Dreesen, D. W., and Rupprecht, C. E. 1997. Pathogenesis of experimentally induced rabies in domestic ferrets. *Am. J. Vet. Res.* 58, 1327–1331.

Noah, D. L., Drenzek, C. L., Smith, J. S., Krebs, J. W., Orciari, L., Shaddock, J., Sanderlin, D., Whitfield, S., Fekadu, M., Olson, J. G., Rupprecht, C. E., and Childs, J. E. 1998. Epidemiology of human rabies in the United States, 1980 to 1996. *Ann. Intern. Med.* 128, 922–930.

Pasteur, L., 1885. Methode pour prevenir la rage apres morsure. Compte Rendue Academie *Science* 765–773.

Perl, D. P., and Good, P. F. 1991. The pathology of rabies in the central nervous system, In: Baer, G. M. (Ed.), *The Natural History of Rabies*, 2nd ed. CRC Press, Boca Raton, pp. 163–190.

Phares, T. W., Kean, R. B., Mikheeva, T., and Hooper, D. C. 2006. Regional differences in blood-brain barrier permeability changes and inflammation in the apathogenic clearance of virus from the central nervous system. *J. Immunol.* 176, 7666–7675.

Pro-MED-mail, 2011. Rabies—USA (04): Human Survival, 13-June-2011 ed. Pro-MED-mail.

Rasalingam, P., Rossiter, J. P., Mebatsion, T., and Jackson, A. C. 2005. Comparative pathogenesis of the SAD-L16 strain of rabies virus and a mutant modifying the dynein light chain binding site of the rabies virus phosphoprotein in young mice. *Virus Res.* 111, 55–60.

Raux, H., Flamand, A., and Blondel, D. 2000. Interaction of the rabies virus P protein with the LC8 dynein light chain. *J. Virol.* 74, 10212–10216.

Reagan, K. J., and Wunner, W. H. 1985. Rabies virus interaction with various cell lines is independent of the acetylcholine receptor. *Arch. Virol.* 84, 277–282.

Ronsholt, L., Sorensen, K. J., Bruschke, C. J. M., Wellenberg, G. J., van Oirschot, J. T., Johnstone, P., Whitby, J. E., and Bourhy, H. 1998. Clinically silent rabies infection in (zoo) bats. *Vet. Rec.* 142, 519–520.

Rossiter, J. P., Jackson, A. C. 2007. Pathology, In: Jackson, A. C., and Wunner, W. H. (Eds.), *Rabies*, 2nd ed. Academic Press, Elsevier, pp. 383–410.

Rubin, R. H., Sullivan, L., Summers, R., Gregg, M. B., and Sikes, R. K. 1970. A case of human rabies in Kansas: epidemiologic, clinical, and laboratory considerations. *J. Infect. Dis.* 122, 318–322.

Rupprecht, C. E., Hanlon, C. A., and Hemachudha, T. 2002. Rabies re-examined. *Lancet Infect. Dis.* 2, 327–343.

Ruzek, D., Salat, J., Singh, S. K., and Kopecky, J. 2011. Breakdown of the blood-brain barrier during tick-borne encephalitis in mice is not dependent on CD8(+) T-Cells. *PLoS One* 6(5), e20472, 1–9.

Schnell, M. J., McGettigan, J. P., Wirblich, C., and Papaneri, A. 2010. The cell biology of rabies virus: using stealth to reach the brain. *Nat. Rev. Microbiol.* 8, 51–61.

Seif, I., Coulon, P., Rollin, P. E., and Flamand, A. 1985. Rabies virulence: effect on pathogenicity and sequence characterization of rabies virus mutations affecting antigenic site III of the glycoprotein. *J. Virol.* 53, 926–934.

Sipahioglu, U., and Alpaut, S. 1985. Transplacental rabies in humans. *Mikrobiyol. Bul.* 19, 95–99.

Solomon, T., Marston, D., Mallewa, M., Felton, T., Shaw, S., McElhinney, L. M., Das, K., Mansfield, K., Wainwright, J., Kwong, G. N. M., and Fooks, A. R. 2005. Lesson of the week—paralytic rabies after a two week holiday in India. *Br. Med. J.* 331, 501–503.

Thoulouze, M. I., Lafage, M., MontanoHirose, J. A., and Lafon, M. 1997. Rabies virus infects mouse and human lymphocytes and induces apoptosis. *J. Virol.* 71, 7372–7380.

Tsiang, H. 1982. Neuronal function impairment in rabies-infected rat brain. *J. Gen. Virol.* 61(Pt 2), 277–281.

Tsiang, H., Ceccaldi, P. E., and Lycke, E. 1991. Rabies virus infection and transport in human sensory dorsal root ganglia neurons. *J. Gen. Virol.* 72(Pt 5), 1191–1194.

Tuffereau, C., Schmidt, K., Langevin, C., Lafay, F., Dechant, G., and Koltzenburg, M. 2007. The rabies virus glycoprotein receptor p75(NTR) is not essential for rabies virus infection. *J. Virol.* 81, 13622–13630.

Ugolini, G. 1995. Specificity of rabies virus as a transneuronal tracer of motor networks—transfer from hypoglossal motoneurons to connected 2nd-order and higher-order central-nervous-system cell groups. *J. Comp. Neurol.* 356, 457–480.

Ugolini, G. 2008. Use of rabies virus as a transneuronal tracer of neuronal connections: Implications for the understanding of rabies pathogenesis, In: Dodet, B., Fooks, A. R., Miller, T., Tordo, N. (Eds.), *Developments in Biologicals*, Karger, pp. 493–506.

Veeraraghavan, N., Gajanana, A., Rangasami, R., Connunni, P. T., Kumari, C., Saraswathi, K. C., Devaraj, R., and Hallan, K. M. 1970. Studies on the salivary excretion of rabies virus by the dog from Surandai., *Pasteur Institute Annual Report of the Director 1968 and Science Report 1969*. Pasteur Institute, Coonoor.

Vos, A., Muller, T., Neubert, L., Zurbriggen, A., Botteron, C., Pohle, D., Schoon, H., Haas, L., and Jackson, A. C. 2004. Rabies in red foxes (Vulpes vulpes) experimentally infected with European bat lyssavirus type 1. *J. Vet. Med. Ser. B—Infect. Dis. Vet. Public Health.* 51, 327–332.

Vos, A., Neubert, A., Pommerening, E., Muller, T., Dohner, L., Neubert, L., and Hughes, K. 2001. Immunogenicity of an E1-deleted recombinant human adenovirus against rabies by different routes of administration. *J. Gen. Virol.* 82, 2191–2197.

Wang, Z. W., Sarmento, L., Wang, Y. H., Li, X. Q., Dhingra, V., Tseggai, T., Jiang, B. M., and Fu, Z. F. 2005. Attenuated rabies virus activates, while pathogenic rabies virus evades, the host innate immune responses in the central nervous system. *J. Virol.* 79, 12554–12565.

Warrell, M. J., Ward, G. S., Elwell, M. R., and Tingpalapong, M. 1987. An attempt to treat rabies encephalitis in monkeys with intrathecal live rabies virus RV 675. Brief report. *Arch. Virol.* 96, 271–273.

Warrell, M. J., and Warrell, D. A. 2004. Rabies and other lyssavirus diseases. *Lancet.* 363, 959–969.

WHO. 2005. WHO expert consultation on rabies. World Health Organ Tech Rep Ser, 1–88.

WHO. 2010. Rabies, Fact Sheet No. 99. World Health Organization.

Willoughby, R. E., Jr. 2009. "Early death" and the contraindication of vaccine during treatment of rabies. *Vaccine* 27, 7173–7177.

Willoughby, R. E., Tieves, K. S., Hoffman, G. M., Ghanayem, N. S., Amlie-Lefond, C. M., Schwabe, M. J., Chusid, M. J., and Rupprecht, C. E. 2005. Brief report—Survival after treatment of rabies with induction of coma. *N. Engl. J. Med.* 352, 2508–2514.

Wunner, W. H. 2007. Rabies virus, In: Jackson, A. C., and Wunner, W. H. (Eds.), *Rabies*, 2nd ed. Academic Press, Elsevier, Amsterdam, pp. 23–68.

Yan, X., Prosniak, M., Curtis, M. T., Weiss, M. L., Faber, M., Dietzschold, B., and Fu, Z. F. 2001. Silver-haired bat rabies virus variant does not induce apoptosis in the brain of experimentally infected mice. *J. Neurovirol.* 7, 518–527.

17 Rubella Virus Infections

Jennifer M. Best, Susan Reef, and
Liliane Grangeot-Keros

CONTENTS

17.1 INTRODUCTION

Rubella, also known as German measles, is generally a mild disease and received lit-tle attention until 1941 when Norman McAlister Gregg, an Australian ophthalmolo-gist, demonstrated an association with congenital defects. He showed that congenital cataracts, cardiac defects, and deafness might result from maternal infection in early pregnancy. This constellation of defects later became known as congenital rubella syndrome (CRS). The frequency of defects was underestimated until the 1960s when there were extensive epidemics in Europe and the United States (Cooper 1975). The epidemic in the United States resulted in 12.5 million cases of rubella, approxi-mately 2000 of postinfectious encephalitis, and >20,000 cases of CRS. Both post-natal and congenital infection may produce neurological symptoms, but these are rare in postnatal infection; however, the rate of reported postnatal rubella encepha-litis has varied by geographical location with an increased rate seen in the Asia Pacific region. As no antiviral drugs are available to treat rubella or CRS, prevention of disease is a priority. Rubella vaccines were licensed in 1969 and 1970, allowing vaccination programs to be initiated in the United States, Europe, and Australia, with the aim of preventing infection in pregnancy and thereby congenital rubella. By 2010, 67% of the Member States of the World Health Organization included a rubella-containing vaccine in their national immunization programs (WHO 2011).

17.2 BIOLOGICAL PROPERTIES OF THE VIRUS

17.2.1 CLASSIFICATION AND VIRUS STRUCTURE

Electron microscopy shows that rubella virus (RV) is a pleomorphic virus, about 70 nm in diameter (Figure 17.1). RV is classified as a non-arthropod-borne *Togavirus* and is the only member of the *Rubivirus* genus. It is a single-stranded (SS) RNA virus with a lipoprotein envelope. RV genome structure and method of replication are similar to viruses of the *Alphavirus* genus of the Togaviridae, but RV antigens do not cross-react with other togaviruses. The SS RNA is contained in a protein capsid (C, 32 kDa), surrounded by the lipoprotein envelope containing two envelope proteins, E1 (58 kDa) and E2 (42–47 kDa). These envelope proteins induce the major immune responses. RV is a fragile virus and is easily destroyed by heat and extremes of pH.

There are no major antigenic differences between RV isolates, but at least 13 genotypes have been described. These are divided into two phylogenetic groups,

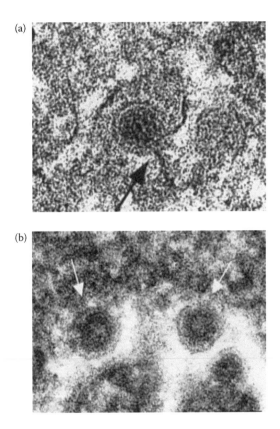

FIGURE 17.1 (a) Rubella virus polymorphism in the Golgi complex showing dense spherical particles (arrowheads) budding from Golgi membranes in infected Vero cells at 16 h post infection. (b) Viral particles (white arrows) with an annular-like morphology (dense periphery and less dense center) are seen budding from membranes. (Reprinted from *Virology*, 312, Risco, C., Carrascosa, J. L., and Frey, T. K., Structural maturation of rubella virus in the Golgi complex, 261–269, Copyright 2003, with permission from C. Risco and Elsevier.)

clades 1 and 2, which differ by 8%–10% at the nucleotide level (Abernathy et al. 2011; WHO 2007). Identification of genotypes is very important for tracking the spread of infection and characterizing the virus during elimination (see Prevention).

The genome of RV is a positive sense SS RNA, usually 9762 nucleotides in length, 5′ capped and 3′ polyadenylated. This RNA is infectious and serves as a messenger RNA during infection. The RV genome has a high G + C content (approximately 70%), which initially made sequencing difficult. The genome consists of a 40-nt 5′ untranslated region, a 5′ proximal 6351-nt open reading frame (ORF) coding for the nonstructural proteins (p150 and p90), a 3′ proximal 3192-nt ORF coding for the structural proteins, and a 59-nt 3′ untranslated region (Zhou et al. 2007). The order of genes is 5′-p150-p90-C-E2-E1-3′ (Figure 17.2).

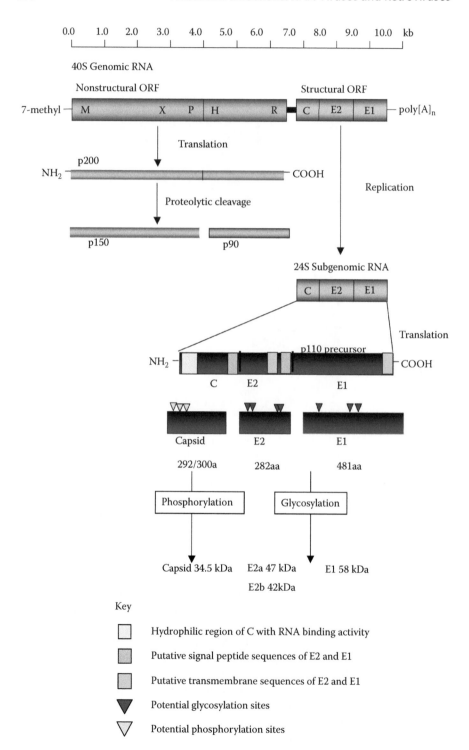

17.2.2 REPLICATION CYCLE

RV can infect a variety of cell lines. Virus replication takes place in the cytoplasm and is similar to the replication cycle of the alphaviruses (Best et al. 2009). Virus production reaches a peak at 24–48 h postinfection, and no effect on total cell RNA or protein synthesis has been noted.

The myelin oligodendrocyte glycoprotein (MOG) has recently been identified as a cell receptor for RV, although the use of other receptors has not been excluded (Cong et al. 2011). MOG is found mainly in the central nervous system (CNS), with lower levels in lymphoid and other tissues. The E1 protein binds to this receptor, RV enters the cytoplasm via the endocytic pathway, uncoating of the viral RNA occurs in the endosome, and viral RNA is released into the cytoplasm, where reproduction occurs.

Both 40S and 24S RNA are found in RV-infected cells. The 5′ 6351 nt nonstructural ORF of the 40S genomic RNA is translated to produce a 2116-amino acid polyprotein (p200; Figure 17.2). This polyprotein is cleaved by a host cell signal peptidase to give 2 nonstructural proteins, p150 and p90. The 24S subgenomic RNA produced from the 3′ structural ORF is translated to produce a 110-kDa polyprotein, which is cleaved by a host cell signalase to produce the three structural proteins (C, E2, and E1; Figure 17.2). These are transported to the Golgi complex where glycosylation and assembly of virus particles occurs (Risco et al. 2003). Virus particles are released by budding from the plasma membrane and intracellular membranes (Figure 17.1). The cytopathic effect induced by RV in some cell cultures is due to caspase-dependent apoptosis (Cooray et al. 2003).

The biological properties of RV have been reviewed in more detail by Chen and Icenogle (2007).

FIGURE 17.2 Schematic diagram of the replication, translation, and processing of RV nonstructural proteins and structural proteins. (Best, J. M., Cooray, S., and Banatvala, J. E.: Rubella, in *Topley & Wilson's Microbiology and Microbial Infections.* 2010. Copyright Wiley-VCH Verlag GmbH & Co. KGaA. Reproduced with permission.) The RV genome consists of two long nonoverlapping ORFs: the 5′ORF encodes the nonstructural proteins, and the 3′ORF encodes the structural proteins. The translation RV RNA produces the p200 precursor, which is cleaved to produce the p150 and p90 structural proteins. This initiates the synthesis of the full length negative strand RNA. The negative strand acts as a template for the synthesis of the full length positive strand RNA for new viral progeny and the 24S subgenomic RNA. The 24S subgenomic RNA is translated into the p110 polyprotein precursor, which is proteolytically cleaved and posttranslationally modified to produce the structural proteins C, E2, and E1. Within the 5′ nonstructural ORF are putative amino acid sequence motifs for methyltransferase (M), RNA-dependent RNA-polymerase (R), helicase (H), and papain-like cysteine protease (P) activity. The X motif indicates a region of unknown function, which has homology to alphaviruses, hepatitis E virus, and coronaviruses.

17.3 EPIDEMIOLOGY

RV is transmitted by aerosol via the respiratory route. Close contact is usually required for transmission to occur (e.g., within the family or at work), and it is therefore less infectious than measles, varicella, and influenza.

Before the introduction of rubella vaccination programs, rubella was a worldwide disease with epidemics occurring approximately every 5–9 years in the spring. In temperate climates RV was most frequently acquired in childhood. Serological studies showed that 50% of 9- to 11-year-old children had evidence of past infection, but 15%–20% of women of child-bearing age remained susceptible to rubella and therefore at risk of acquiring rubella when pregnant. In developing countries, there is considerable variation in the age of acquisition of rubella. Cutts et al. (1997) found that the proportion of susceptible women was 15%–20%, the same as in industrialized countries, with a higher rate of susceptibility in rural areas than in cities. It was estimated that 112,000 infants worldwide were born with CRS in 2008. (http://www.gavialliance.org/support/nvs/rubella/) (Cutts et al. 1997). The incidence of CRS was estimated as 0.8–4.0/100 live births during epidemics and 0.1–0.2/1000 live births during endemic periods. This burden of CRS justifies efforts to eradicate rubella (see Prevention).

Since the introduction of rubella vaccination programs (see Prevention) rubella has been eliminated from such countries as Sweden, Finland, and the WHO Region of the Americas.

Rubella incidence has decreased significantly in many other countries that introduced rubella vaccine through wide age-range campaigns or routine programs as used in the European region (Muscat et al. 2012; Zimmerman et al. 2011).

17.4 POSTNATALLY ACQUIRED INFECTION

17.4.1 CLINICAL PRESENTATION

Rubella is usually a mild disease in children, but may be more severe in adults, who may experience a prodrome with malaise and low-grade fever. Lymphadenopathy usually develops before the rash and may persist for 10–14 days after the rash has disappeared. The cervical, postauricular, and suboccipital lymph nodes are most frequently affected. The characteristic maculopapular rash appears after an incubation period of approximately 14 days (range 12–23 days) (Figures 17.3 and 17.4). A discrete rash appears first on the face and spreads quickly to the trunk and limbs. The rash may persist for 1–3 days or may be fleeting; lesions may coalesce. Cough, sore throat, conjunctivitis, and headache may also occur in adults. Occasionally, rubella presents with a more severe fever and constitutional symptoms similar to measles. Virus is excreted from about 7 days before the onset of rash and for 7–10 days thereafter, but patients are only infectious for about 10 days. Joint symptoms may occur, as described below (see Complications and Pathogenesis).

Laboratory diagnosis is required to confirm a diagnosis of rubella (see below), as clinical diagnosis is unreliable. Subclinical infection is common, and other virus infections present with similar symptoms. Measles, enteroviruses, and human herpes

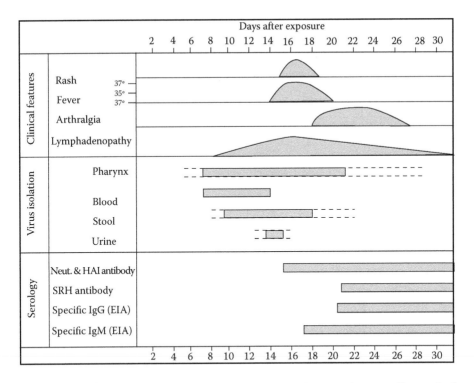

FIGURE 17.3 Relation between clinical and virological features of postnatally acquired rubella. (Best, J. M., Cooray, S., and Banatvala, J. E.: Rubella, in *Topley & Wilson's Microbiology and Microbial Infections.* 2010. Copyright Wiley-VCH Verlag GmbH & Co. KGaA. Reproduced with permission.)

FIGURE 17.4 (See color insert.) Macular–papular rash in postnatally acquired rubella infection. (Reproduced from Dr. D. Wallach and Editions De Boeck/Estem. With permission.)

TABLE 17.1
Differential Diagnosis of Postnatal Rubella in Different Geographical Regions

Virus Infection	Geographical Distribution								Key Features
	Africa	Asia	Australia	Europe	North America	Central America	South America	Pacific	
Rubella	+	+	+	+	+	+	+	+	
Parvovirus B19	+	+	+	+	+	+	+	+	Erythema infectiosum
Human herpes viruses 6 and 7	+	+	+	+	+	+	+	+	Exanthem subitum. Predominantly <2 years.
Measles	+	+	+	+	+	+	+	+	Prodrome with cough, conjunctivitis, coryza
Enteroviruses	+	+	+	+	+	+	+	+	Echovirus 9, coxsackie A9 most frequent.
Dengue	+	+	+	–	–	+	+	+	Joint and back pain, hemorrhagic complications in children.
West Nile fever	+	+	–	+	+	–	–	–	Joint pains
Chickungunya	+	+	–	–	–	–	–	–	Joint pains
Ross River	–	–	+	–	–	–	–	+	Joint pains
Sindbis	+	+	+	+	–	–	–	–	Joint pains

Source: Reprinted from *The Lancet,* 363, J. E. Banatvala and D. W. G. Brown, Rubella, pp. 1127–1137, Copyright (2004), with permission from J. E. Banatvala and Elsevier.

virus 6 and 7 may present with a similar rash, and parvovirus B19 and some arboviruses (e.g., Ross River, Dengue, Chikungunya) may present with both rash and
joint symptoms (Table 17.1).

17.4.2   Complications

17.4.2.1   Joint Symptoms

Joint symptoms are the most common complication of rubella. They may be
observed in ≤70% postpubertal females but are less common in prepubertal females
and males. These usually last for 3–4 days but occasionally persist for up to 1 month.
Symptoms vary from a transient stiffness of joints to arthritis with swelling, pain,
and limitation of movement. The joints most commonly affected are the fingers,
wrists, ankles, and knees. Joint symptoms are also observed in postpubertal females
after rubella vaccination (see below).

17.4.2.2   Postinfectious Encephalitis

Usually, it develops abruptly within a week of onset of rash and with recovery within
7–30 days. It may also occur in cases without rash. The prognosis is usually good
for survivors, but death rates reported vary from 0% to 30%. It has been reported
to occur in approximately 1 in 6000 cases. However, the incidence of encephalitis
was 1 in 1600 cases of rubella in a Japanese outbreak in 1987 (Moriuchi et al. 1990),
and recently in the South Pacific islands of Tonga and Samoa, the incidence was
estimated to be between 1 in 500 and 1 in 1000 cases (A. Ruben, personal communication). These cases occurred in children. Two of the eight cases of encephalitis
in Samoa died. In 2011, a rubella outbreak occurred in Tunisia, resulting in many
cases of encephalitis among children and adolescents, which are currently being
evaluated.

The most frequent symptoms of postinfectious encephalitis include headache,
vomiting, generalized convulsions, stiff neck, retroauricular lymphadenopathy, and
lethargy, often without fever (Dwyer et al. 1992). Nystagmus, diminished superficial
skin reflexes, and variable deep tendon reflexes may be detected on examination.
Those patients who die usually develop coma with normal fundi but fixed and dilated
pupils. Death occurs within 6–8 days of onset of neural symptoms. CSF is clear,
with an average cell count of $50/mm^3$, comprising mostly lymphocytes. CSF protein
levels are not usually elevated (reviewed by Chantler et al. 2001). EEG shows diffuse
or localized abnormalities, which may persist for a year or more. EEG and MRI are
probably more useful than CT scanning (Dwyer et al. 1992). Relapsing encephalitis
and polyradiculoneuritis are rare (Chang et al. 1997).

17.4.2.3   Other Complications

Other complications include bleeding disorders due to thrombocytopenia, which
occurs in about 1:3000 cases. Rare complications are Guillain-Barré syndrome,
bone marrow aplasia, autoimmune hemolytic anemia, hemophagocytic syndrome,
optic neuritis, and Fuchs heterochromic uveitis.

There is no specific or proven treatment for rubella. For persons infected with rubella, symptomatic treatment may be warranted for different manifestations such as arthralgias, myalgias, and fever.

17.4.2.4   Risks of Rubella Infection in Pregnancy

When rubella infection occurs in the first 10 weeks of pregnancy, RV will cross the placenta and cause a generalized and persistent infection of the fetus in about 90% of cases. After 10 weeks of gestation, the risks decline, with those infected at 13–16 weeks having an approximate 50% risk and only rare cases of deafness reported after infection at 17–18 weeks (reviewed by Best 2007). Infection prior to conception is not a risk to the fetus (Enders et al. 1988). Spontaneous abortion may occur in up to 20% of cases when infection occurs in the first 8 weeks of pregnancy. There is no treatment available to prevent transmission to the fetus, and termination of pregnancy (TOP) is usually offered when infection occurs in the first trimester. In those for whom TOP is not acceptable, normal human immunoglobulin or rubella hyperimmune globulin (if available) administered soon after exposure might reduce the amount of viremia and damage, although normal human immunoglobulin does not seem to reduce the incidence of fetal infection (Peckham 1974).

Following asymptomatic rubella reinfection in early pregnancy, RV may be transmitted to the fetus in about 10% of cases, and the risk of fetal damage is probably less than 5% (Best et al. 1989; Health Protection Agency 2011). The risk may be higher following symptomatic reinfection, but such cases are rare.

17.4.3   Immune Responses

Viremia is terminated by the development of antibodies. Serum antibodies may be detected by hemagglutination inhibition (HAI) 1–2 days after onset of rash, but antibodies are not detected by enzyme immunoassay (EIA) until 6–7 days (Figure 17.3). IgG antibodies usually persist for life but may sometimes decline to undetectable levels in older persons. Rubella IgM antibodies develop during the 5 days after onset of rash. These antibodies decline fairly quickly and are usually undetectable by 8 weeks postrash onset, although their detection depends on the sensitivity of the assay used. Antibodies may also be detected in oral fluid, urine, and nasopharyngeal secretions (WHO 2008). IgG, IgA, and IgM antibodies to the E1, E2, and C structural proteins have been detected.

The detection of rubella antibodies at levels >10 IU/mL is usually considered to provide evidence of immunity (Skendzel 1996; WHO 2008).

The cell-mediated immune response is also required to control infection and appears to persist for life. A mixed Th1/Th2 response is seen with serum interferon γ during acute rubella. An increase in serum interleukin 10 (IL-10) levels has been detected during the first 4 days of illness. Lymphoproliferative responses develop a few days after onset of rash and persist at low levels for many years; the strongest responses are against the E1 protein. MHC class II restricted CD4+ T helper and CD8+ cytotoxic T lymphocytes can be detected shortly after the antibody response and several antigenic domains recognized by these cells have been identified within the E1, E2, and C proteins (reviewed by WHO 2008).

17.4.4 LABORATORY DIAGNOSIS

A laboratory diagnosis is usually made by the detection of rubella IgM in serum (Thomas et al. 1992; Best et al. 2009). Oral fluid may be used instead of serum, but results should be confirmed with assays done on serum when testing a pregnant woman (Banatvala and Brown 2004; Manikkavasagan et al. 2010). EIA is the preferred assay for detection of both rubella IgG and IgM because it is sensitive and can be readily automated. Other assays, such as radial hemolysis and latex agglutination have been widely used in the past for the detection of rubella IgG and for screening purposes.

Laboratory diagnosis is particularly important in pregnant women with a rash or who have had contact with a rash illness, even if antibodies have been detected in the past or there is a history of immunization. Blood should be obtained as soon as possible after onset of rash, and serum tested for both rubella IgG and IgM. Rising IgG antibodies (using the same assay in one laboratory) and a positive IgM result confirm rubella infection. A positive IgM result alone should be confirmed by testing a second serum. The detection of rubella IgM in a woman without a rash or history of contact with a rash illness should be interpreted with caution (Thomas et al. 1992; Health Protection Agency 2011). Sometimes, the measurement of rubella-specific IgG avidity may help exclude or confirm recent primary infections (Best 2007; Thomas and Morgan-Capner 1991). Pregnant women who have had contact with a rubella-like illness and who are susceptible to rubella or are of unknown immune status, should be tested for rubella IgG and IgM as soon as possible. If shown to be susceptible, such women should be retested for up to 4 weeks after contact and offered a rubella-containing vaccine after delivery.

Antenatal screening programs for rubella antibody are available in some countries to identify women who are susceptible to rubella and should be offered immunization (see Prevention).

Laboratory diagnosis of rubella encephalitis is based either on the detection of rubella-specific IgM or the detection of viral RNA by reverse transcription polymerase chain reaction (RT-PCR) in cerebrospinal fluid (CSF). Viral isolation from CSF may be used for genotyping studies (Figueiredo et al. 2011). Intrathecal synthesis of rubella-specific IgG can also be investigated by calculation of the Goldmann-Witmer coefficient as follows: (CSF rubella-specific IgG/CSF total IgG)/(serum rubella-specific IgG/serum total IgG), but this procedure is not often used (Jacobi et al. 2007).

17.4.5 PATHOGENESIS

Humans are the only known host for rubella, although the virus can infect cell cultures derived from other animals. RV is spread via the respiratory route. Patients excrete the virus for ≤7 days before onset and 7–10 days after onset of rash (Figure 17.3). High titers may be excreted for about 10 days, when patients are infectious. Virus may also be detected for a shorter time in stools and urine. Virus particles transmitted by aerosol infect cells in the upper respiratory tract and spread to lymphoid tissue of the nasopharynx and upper respiratory tract. Replication of the virus in regional lymph nodes leads to lymphadenopathy. A viremia occurs for about 7 days before onset of rash, leading to systemic infection. Many tissues become infected, including the placenta in pregnant women. Mononuclear cells are probably involved in the spread of virus, but extracellular virus can also be detected in serum. Rubella induces a mild and transient immunosuppression, less pronounced than that observed with measles. A fall in total leukocytes, T cells, and neutrophils and a depression of lymphocyte responsiveness to mitogens and antigens are seen (reviewed in WHO 2008).

The mechanisms by which the rash and joint symptoms are induced by rubella are not fully understood. RV has been isolated from skin biopsies taken from skin with rash and skin from patients with subclinical rubella (Heggie 1978). Immune mechanisms may be involved. Administration of pooled human immunoglobulin has been shown to prevent rash, but not viremia. RV and rubella IgG antibodies can be detected in the synovial fluid and circulating immune complexes have been detected in serum, suggesting that immune complexes could be formed and these might cause joint symptoms. Hormonal factors may also play a role (reviewed by Best et al. 2005). Although RV has been isolated from synovial fluid from occasional patients with chronic inflammatory joint disease, there is no convincing evidence that rubella or rubella vaccination is associated with this condition. The pathogenesis of the encephalitis is also not understood. RV has been detected in brain tissue and RV has been detected in CSF by isolation and RT-PCR. Rubella-specific IgG and IgM antibodies can be detected in CSF. However, limited pathological data have not shown demyelination or inflammatory damage, which suggests that the encephalitis is not immune mediated.

17.5 CONGENITAL RUBELLA

17.5.1 CLINICAL PRESENTATION

The clinical features of congenital rubella infection (CRI) are variable, ranging from a wide spectrum to no anomalies. Severe anomalies are observed when fetal infection has occurred during the first trimester. Following infection between 13 and 16 weeks of gestation, hearing defects and retinopathy are the only defects that may be seen in up to 35% of infants, while after infection at 17–20 weeks, the risk of deafness is about 6% (Best et al. 2009). Symptoms may be present at birth or during the early months of life, but a few, such as hearing impairment and eye defects, are frequently delayed (see Delayed Manifestations). In addition, late-onset disorders such as type 1 diabetes mellitus may develop in the second decade of life.

There is no treatment available to prevent congenital rubella infection. When rubella is acquired in early pregnancy, almost every organ may be affected, but eye defects, cardiac defects, and hearing defects predominate. Congenital anomalies apparent at birth have been categorized as transient or permanent (Table 17.2). Some clinical features are used in the case definition used by WHO and for surveillance of CRI (Tables 17.2 and 17.3).

TABLE 17.2
Clinical Features of CRS

	Early Transient Features	Permanent Features, Some Recognized Late	Use in Surveillance[a]
Ocular defects			
Cataracts (unilateral/bilateral)		+	A
Glaucoma		+	A
Pigmentary retinopathy		+	A
Microphthalmia		+	
Iris hypoplasia		+	
Cloudy cornea	+		
Auditory defects			
Sensorineural deafness (unilateral/bilateral)		+	A
Cardiovascular defects			
Persistent ductus arteriosus		+	A
Pulmonary artery stenosis		+	A
Ventricular septal defect		+	A
Myocarditis	+		
Central nervous system			
Microcephaly		+	B
Pyschomotor retardation		+	
Meningoencephalitis	+		B
Behavioral disorders			
Speech disorders			
Intrauterine growth retardation	+		
Thrombocytopenia, with purpura	+		B
Hepatitis/ hepatosplenomegaly	+		B
Bone "lesions"	+		B
Pneumonitis	+		
Lymphadenopathy	+		
Diabetes mellitus		+	
Thyroid disorders		+	
Progressive rubella panencephalitis		+	

Source: Reprinted from *The Lancet*, 363, J. E. Banatvala and D. W. G. Brown, Rubella, pp. 1127–1137, Copyright (2004), with permission from J. E. Banatvala and Elsevier.

[a] For surveillance, a clinically confirmed case is defined as one in which two complications from group A or group B or one from group A or one from group B are present (WHO 1999).

TABLE 17.3
WHO Case Definition for CRS

Suspected Case

Any infant less than one year of age in whom a health worker suspects CRS. A health worker should suspect CRS when an infant aged 0–11 months presents with heart disease and/or suspicion of deafness and/or one or more of the following eye signs: white pupil (cataract), diminished vision, pendular movement of the eyes (nystagmus), squint, smaller eyeball (microphthalmus) or larger eye-ball (congenital glaucoma), or when an infant's mother has a history of suspected or confirmed rubella during pregnancy, even when the infant shows no signs of CRS.

Clinically Confirmed CRS Case

An infant in whom a qualified physician detects at least two of the complications in section A below or one from section A and one from section B:

A. Cataracts, congenital glaucoma, congenital heart disease, hearing impairment, pigmentary retinopathy.
B. Purpura, splenomegaly, microcephaly, mental retardation, meningoencephalitis, radiolucent bone disease, jaundice with onset within 24 hours after birth.

Laboratory-Confirmed CRS Case

An infant with clinically confirmed CRS who has a positive blood test for rubella-specific IgM. Where special laboratory resources are available the detection of RV in specimens from the pharynx or urine of an infant with suspected CRS provides laboratory confirmation of CRS.

Congenital Rubella Infection (CRI)

If a mother has suspected or confirmed rubella in pregnancy her infant should have a rubella-specific IgM test. An infant who does not have clinical signs of CRS but who has a positive rubella-specific IgM test is classified as having congenital rubella infection (CRI).

Source: Reproduced from the World Health Organization (2003). WHO standards for surveillance of selected vaccine-preventable diseases: Geneva, WHO/V&B/03.01. Available at: http://www .who.int/immunization/documents/WHO_VB_03.01/en/index.html. With permission.

17.5.2 TRANSIENT ABNORMALITIES

These are seen in the first few weeks of infancy and usually occur with permanent defects, such as those of the eye and heart. This combination of features reflects extensive infection and is associated with high perinatal mortality. Transient abnormalities include thrombocytopenic purpura (TCP) (Figure 17.5a), hepatosplenomegaly (Figure 17.5b), hemolytic anemia, and cloudy cornea (Table 17.2). Babies are often small-for-dates, with about 90% below the 50th growth percentile and 60% below the 10th percentile. TCP is associated with a reduced number of megakaryocytes in the bone marrow. A rare complication of TCP is intracranial hemorrhage. Radiolucencies of the long bones (Figure 17.5c) are seen in about 20% of infants and usually resolve within the first 1–2 months.

The CNS is involved in about 25% of infants who present with congenital abnormalities at birth. The most common manifestation is meningoencephalitis. Infants

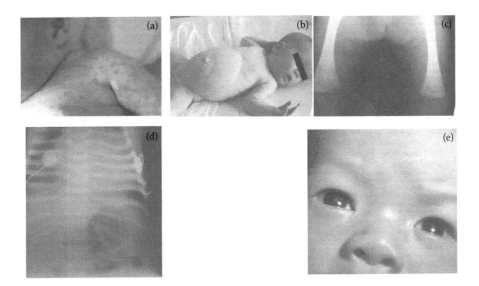

FIGURE 17.5 **(See color insert.)** Congenital anomalies in congenital rubella syndrome (CRS). (a) Case of CRS with maculo-papular rash and purpura; (b) case of CRS with hepatosplenomegaly; (c) case of CRS with radiolucencies of long bones; (d) case of CRS with cardiac dilatation; (e) cataracts (opacity of the lens). (Kindly provided by Dr. C. A. Bouhanna and Dr. J. C. Janaud, Hôpital intercommunal, Créteil, France, with permission from Dr. D. Wallach and Editions De Boeck/Estem.)

may be irritable or lethargic with a full fontanelle and consistent CSF changes. Some of those infants with severe meningoencephalitis will subsequently progress well neurologically, whereas others may be severely retarded and have ataxia, spastic diplegia, or communication problems.

17.5.3 Permanent Defects

17.5.3.1 Cardiac Defects

Cardiac defects are present in approximately 50% of infants whose mothers had rubella in the first 2 months of gestation (Reef et al. 2000). Patent ductus arteriosus and branch pulmonary artery stenosis are the most common cardiac defects and are responsible for much of the perinatal mortality seen with CRS (Oster et al. 2010). Less frequent abnormalities are ventricular septal defect, tetralogy of Fallot, aortic stenosis, transposition of the great vessels, and tricuspid atresia. With available treatment, including surgery, most cardiac defects can be corrected. A neonatal myocarditis may also occur in infants with these defects. Figure 17.5d shows an X-ray of cardiac dilation.

17.5.3.2 Eye Defects

The typical cataracts and pigmentary retinopathy seen in CRS were described by Gregg in 1941. The cataracts may consist of a central dense pearly white opacity (Figure 17.5e) or may be total with a more uniform density throughout the lens.

Bilateral cataracts are found in about 50% of affected infants; they are usually present at birth but may not be visible until several weeks later. Cataracts, which are often accompanied by microphthalmia (Figure 17.6a,b), are a useful marker for surveillance of CRS (Bloom et al. 2005; WHO 1999; Vijayalakshmi et al. 2007). Retinopathy is found in about 50% of affected infants. Hyperpigmented and hypopigmented areas of the retina give it a "salt and pepper" appearance, which can be a useful diagnostic indicator of CRS; however, because it does not cause any visual defects, it may not be suspected. Retinopathy is due to a defect in pigmentation and usually involves the macular areas. Glaucoma is less frequently observed than cataract. Other symptoms

(a)
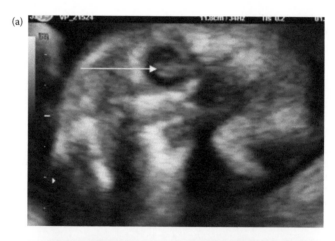

(b)
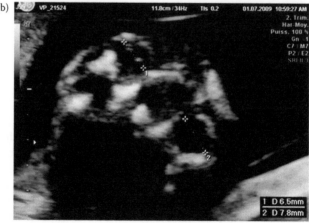

FIGURE 17.6 (a) Coronal view of fetal face at 19 weeks gestation by ultrasound. Microphthalmia and hyperechogenic lens (arrow). (b) Coronal view of fetal face at 19 weeks of gestation showing the ophthalmic asymmetry and microphthalmia. (Cordier, A. G., Vauloup-Fellous, C., Grangeot-Keros, L., Pinet, C., Benachi, A., Ayoubi, J. M., Picone, O.: Pitfalls in the diagnosis of congenital rubella syndrome in the first trimester of pregnancy. *Prenat Diagn.* 2012. 32(5), 496–7. Copyright Wiley-VCH Verlag GmbH & Co. KGaA. Reproduced with permission.)

are pupil rigidity, cloudy cornea, corneal opacity, microcornea, iris hypoplasia, optic atrophy, anophthalmos, chronic uveitis, corneal hydrops, choroidal neovascularization, and keratoconus (Arnold et al. 1994; Vijayalakshmi et al. 2007). Some of these ocular abnormalities may occur later in life (see below).

17.5.3.3   Hearing Defects

Hearing defects range from mild to severe. Sensorineural deafness occurs in ≥70% of infants with CRI, either in combination with other defects or it may be the only congenital defect, especially when maternal infection occurred after the first trimester. Deafness may be bilateral or unilateral with no characteristic audiometric pattern. The impact of congenital rubella deafness has been insufficiently appreciated in the past and continues to be difficult to assess in developing countries. In the early 1970s, before the widespread use of rubella immunization, a study in London estimated that 15% of all cases of sensorineural deafness were the result of CRI (Peckham et al. 1979); in many cases, rubella had not been diagnosed during pregnancy. Improvements in audiological methods and routine testing now help to detect hearing loss in early infancy.

17.5.3.4   CNS Abnormalities

It is estimated that as many as 80% of CRS patients exhibit neurological disorders. Lethargy, irritability, and motor disabilities are apparent in infancy (Frey 1997). Microcephaly may be present at birth or develop subsequently (Chang et al. 1996). As development progresses, infants affected by CRS may show mental retardation, motor disabilities, abnormal posture and movements, and seizures. The mental retardation may be associated with undetected hearing impairment.

17.5.4   Late-Onset Disease

This syndrome, consisting of chronic rubella-like rash, pneumonitis, failure to thrive, and persistent diarrhea, may develop between 3 and 12 months of age in infants with CRI. Mortality is high, but infants may recover if treated with corticosteroids. Hypogammaglobulinemia has also been reported. Hanshaw et al. (1985) suggested that this syndrome may be induced by circulating immune complexes.

17.5.5   Delayed Manifestations

Some defects may not be apparent for months or years and occur in >20% of children with CRS (Sever et al. 1985; Cooper and Alford 2006). This may be due to failure to recognize such defects as deafness, but sensorineural deafness and some CNS and ocular anomalies may develop later and progress in severity. In the eye, cataracts may develop after birth and resorption of the cataractous lens has also been reported. Glaucoma may develop between 3 and 22 years of age, and corneal hydrops, keratic precipitates, keratocornus, and spontaneous lens absorption have also been reported. Retinopathy has been associated with subretinal neovascularization leading to visual disturbance (Arnold et al. 1994). Vascular changes due to renal artery and aortic stenosis may also lead to hypertension.

Some CNS manifestations such as mental retardation and other behavioral dis-orders (autism, schizophrenia-like disease) may be delayed, and can be progressive. As many as 7% of CRS children may develop an autistic disorder (Chess et al. 1978; Hwang and Chen 2010). Some CRS patients develop schizophrenia-like disease (Lane et al. 1996; Lim et al. 1995). Exceptionally, progressive rubella encephalitis (PRP) may develop in children between the ages of 10 and 20 years. The main neu-rological features of PRP are dementia, cerebellar ataxia, and seizures. The course of this disease is slow and progressive, and death invariably occurs within a period of 1–10 years. Fortunately, PRP is a rare manifestation of CRS disorders (fewer than 50 cases have been described worldwide) (reviewed by Frey 1997). It is somewhat similar to subacute sclerosing panencephalitis due to chronic infection of the CNS with measles virus.

The most frequent endocrine abnormality is insulin-dependent diabetes mellitus (IDDM; juvenile-onset, type 1), which is seen in about 20% of adult CRS patients (Ginsberg-Fellner et al. 1985). About 5% of CRS patients develop thyroid dysfunc-tion, including hypothyroidism, hyperthyroidism, and thyroiditis, whereas 20%–40% have thyroid autoantibodies. In addition, growth hormone deficiency, poor growth, and early cessation of growth have been reported.

17.5.6 Clinical Diagnosis, Treatment, and Prognosis

Infants with CRS should be evaluated and treated by specialists for the different clinical manifestations associated with CRS. Infants with cardiac anomalies, hear-ing and visual impairments, as well as psychomotor difficulties, should be treated as soon as possible after birth but, as some of these defects may be progressive, repeated testing and continuing assessment of the therapeutic approach is required.

17.5.6.1 Clinical Diagnosis of Congenital Defects

17.5.6.1.1 Prenatal Diagnosis Using Imaging Techniques

Prenatal ultrasound descriptions of rubella congenital defects are relatively rare (Degani 2006). Recently, the use of ultrasound was assessed on a few cases of CRI (Migliucci et al. 2011): intrauterine growth retardation (IUGR), polyhydramnios, cardiomegaly, defects of atrial septum, hepatosplenomegaly, ascites, echogenic bowel, and placentomegaly were observed. However, as expected, ultrasound examination of cases with isolated deafness was normal. Microcephaly can also be observed. Ocular disorders are quite common following first-trimester infection, but only microphthal-mia and cataract are detectable on antenatal ultrasound scans (Figure 17.6a,b). Two clinical cases recently reported in France highlighted the limits and value of prenatal ultrasound examination: in the first case, a pregnant woman had had rubella testing at 7 weeks of gestation and was considered immune. When routine ultrasound scan was performed at 16 weeks, cerebral ventricle enlargement was observed without any other defect. At 17 weeks, ventricular enlargement was confirmed together with intra-hepatic calcifications and hyperechogenic bowel. At 19 weeks, femur length was at the 10th percentile. Because of these ultrasound anomalies, prenatal diagnosis of con-genital CMV, parvovirus B19, and toxoplasma infections were performed, but were all negative. Retrospective investigation retrieved a history of rash illness diagnosed as an allergy at 4 weeks of gestation. Considering the ultrasound anomalies and the history of rash, fetal blood was collected at 20 weeks. In this sample, interferon was detected at a high level (75 UI/mL, normal <2 UI/mL) together with rubella-specific IgM antibody, confirming the diagnosis of CRI (Furet et al. 2010). This case shows that ultrasound scans may help diagnose CRI in settings in which rubella cases are sporadic and very often misdiagnosed. In the second case, primary rubella infection with rash was described at around 5 weeks. The ultrasound examination at 16 weeks was normal, but RV RNA was detected by RT-nested PCR analysis of amniotic fluid obtained at 18 weeks, indicating CRI. The ultrasound scan performed at 19 weeks revealed IUGR, together with asymmetric bilateral microphthalmia (below the 5th percentile), opacity of the right lens, and an isolated hyperechogenic mitral focus. This latter case shows that a normal ultrasound scan does not exclude CRS, as abnormalities may be detected later in pregnancy and consequently points out the need of iterative ultrasound scans to check for fetal defects (Cordier et al. 2012). Although prenatal ultrasound results are nonspecific, they can help diagnose CRI and, in some cases, may be used as prognostic markers of the severity of CRS.

Computed tomography (CT) and fetal magnetic resonance imaging (MRI) can show abnormalities in the fetal brain of patients with CRI. The early detection of some brain abnormalities, such as microcephaly and cortical anomalies, may influence the prognosis of fetal infection. Upon examination of children with CRS, Yoshimura et al. (1996) observed a close relationship between ventricular dilatation and CNS sequelae (mental retardation, microcephaly, cerebral palsy) (Yoshimura et al. 1996). In this study, nine CRS patients were examined. Five patients without dilatation of the lateral ventricles had no sequelae except deafness, whereas among the 4 with dilatation, 3 had mental retardation, cerebral palsy, or microcephaly. By contrast, abnormal intensity areas in the white matter found by MRI were not strictly correlated with CNS sequelae. In the same way, Chang et al. (1996) obtained cranial ultrasound scans for 5 CRS infants whose ages ranged from 1 day to 2 months (Chang et al. 1996). Only 2 of these infants were small for their gestational age, and none of them were microcephalic at birth. Deafness and ocular lesions were found in 4 patients, and congenital heart disease was found in 3. All had abnormal ultrasound scans: linear-shaped hyperechogenicity over the basal ganglia or periventricular punctate hyper-echogenicity or subependymal cysts were observed. Follow-up ultrasonograms for 2 of the patients showed progressively enlarging hyperechogenic lesions. Calcification was found in both patients examined by means of CT. All patients became micro-cephalic with profound global developmental delay. Numazaki and Fujikawa (2003) described CT results in a CRS infant at 4 days of age (Numazaki and Fujikawa 2003). They noted several cortical low-density areas and calcifications of the periventricular area and basal ganglia. MRI performed at 4 weeks of age showed almost similar findings. At 2 months of age, the patient showed severe bilateral hearing loss. At 12 months of age, she had mild mental retardation and developmental delay.

17.5.6.1.2 Postnatal Clinical Diagnosis

The WHO has produced a case definition for CRS as shown in Table 17.3. The clinical diagnosis of congenital rubella should be confirmed by laboratory tests whenever possible.

17.5.6.1.3   Prognosis

The long-term prognosis for those infants with cardiac defects or profound deafness combined with cataracts and brain damage is extremely poor. Surviving children with severe CRS may have multiple congenital abnormalities and therefore require continuous and specialized medical care and education, and rehabilitation. However, many of those who were born in Australia in the early 1940s, when examined at 25 years of age, had developed far better than might have been expected, being of average intelligence, employed, and some were married and had normal children (Menser et al. 1967). Those born as a result of the 1964/1965 epidemic in the United States apparently had more problems, when studied in their twenties. One third required institutional care for severe handicaps, one third were still living with their parents, and a third were leading normal lives (Cooper and Alford 2006). The difference is probably due to the survival of more severely affected infants in the United States, due to improved medical care at that time. More recent studies of CRS patients have reported diabetes, thyroid disorders, early menopause, and osteoporosis at a higher prevalence than in the general population (Munroe 1999; Forrest et al. 2002).

17.5.6.1.4   Laboratory Diagnosis

Infants with CRI produce rubella IgG and IgM at birth, and high titers of RV may be excreted (Figure 17.7). The IgG response persists, but the IgM response declines and is seldom detectable after 18 months of age. The most convenient method for diagnosis is the detection of rubella IgM, by M-antibody capture EIA, in serum or oral fluid ideally taken before 3 months of age (Corcoran and Hardie 2005; Eckstein et al. 1996; Best and Enders 2007). A diagnosis can also be made by demonstrating the

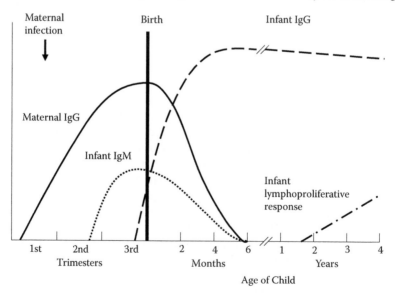

FIGURE 17.7   Serological markers for the diagnosis of congenital rubella. (Reproduced from Best and O'Shea, *Diagnostic Procedures for Viral, Rickettsial and Chlamydial Infections*, 7th edition, 1995. With permission from the American Public Health Association.)

TABLE 17.4
Laboratory Techniques for the Diagnosis of Congenital Rubella Infection

Established Methods	Prenatal Diagnosis	Diagnosis in Infancy
Rubella-specific IgM in serum	Yes	Birth–1 year
Rubella-specific IgM in oral fluid	No	Birth–1 year
Rubella-specific IgG	No	7 month–1 year
RV isolation in cell culture	Yes[a]	Birth–1 year
RT-PCR (RV RNA detection)	Yes	Birth–1 year

Source: Reprinted from *Rubella Viruses. Perspectives in Medical Virology Volume 15,* J. M. Best and G. Enders, Laboratory diagnosis of rubella and congenital rubella, pp. 39–77, Copyright (2007), with permission from Elsevier.

[a] Too slow to be useful.

persistence of rubella IgG in sera taken between 6 and 12 months of age (Table 17.4), when both IgM and IgG tests should be used. However, it is not possible to make a serological diagnosis after immunization with a rubella-containing vaccine.

A diagnosis can also be made by detection of RV in nasopharyngeal secretions (NPS), urine, oral fluid, lens aspirates, CSF, and EDTA-blood collected in the first 3 months (Table 17.4). As virus isolation is demanding and time consuming, RV is usually detected by RT-PCR (Bosma et al. 1995; Feng et al. 2011). RT-nested PCR has been used, but is currently being replaced by real-time PCR. It should be remembered that infants with CRS excrete high titers of RV, which is readily transmitted. Therefore isolation precautions should be employed and contact with pregnant women avoided.

Prenatal diagnosis of CRS is possible using amniotic fluid and/or fetal blood (Best 2007; Best and Enders 2007). Laboratory diagnosis has been reviewed in more detail by Best and Enders (2007) and Best et al. (2009).

17.5.7 PATHOLOGY AND PATHOGENESIS

The pathogenesis of CRS is not fully understood, as much of the work on CRI was done in the 1960s following extensive epidemics of rubella and before the introduction of vaccination. Recent studies have relied on work in cell cultures, as access to cases of CRS is limited due to the success of vaccination programs (see Prevention), and no reliable animal model has been established.

CRS is a progressive disease, due to the persistence of RV, which may continue to cause damage in later life. Structural defects result from defective organogenesis, tissue destruction, and scarring. When maternal infection occurs in the first trimester of pregnancy, at the time of organogenesis, every organ may be involved and RV can be isolated from all such organs (Rawls 1968; Thompson and Tobin 1970). RV is able to persist intracellularly in the presence of neutralizing antibodies. When infection occurs after the first trimester, RV may cross the placenta, but fetal immune responses, which will have by then developed, will terminate the infection and a persistent infection will not usually be established. Although the organ of Corti is susceptible to infection up to 16 weeks of gestation, other fetal damage is unlikely as organogenesis is complete by 8 weeks.

17.5.7.1 Histological Studies

In a classical histological study of fetuses obtained at TOP following maternal rubella in the first trimester, Töndury and Smith (1966) observed some damage in 68% of the 57 fetuses examined, but no gross external malformations were noted. Scattered foci of damage were seen in the chorion, and damaged endothelial cells from the blood vessels were seen to be desquamated into the blood vessels. Thus, during maternal viremia, infected cells may be transported into the fetal circulation to establish widespread infection of organs. In the heart, necrotic cellular damage was observed in the myocardium and the auricular wall was unusually thin in some specimens, which might lead to the septal defect of the heart. Obstructive lesions may occur in the pulmonary and renal arteries due to RV-induced damage to the intimal lining of the arteries. In the eye, fiber cells of the lens were damaged, and later, degenerative changes were seen in the lens, suggesting active disease leading to the characteristic cataracts observed by Gregg (1941). In the inner ear, foci of necrosis were noted in the epithelium of the cochlea and damage to the stria vascularis. Complete atrophy of the organ of Corti has been reported. This damage would lead to deafness. Sporadic foci of damage were also seen in the teeth and skeletal muscle. No inflammatory response was observed, because fetal immune responses have not developed in the first trimester.

17.5.7.2 Other Studies of the Eye

Ocular manifestations of CRS have been reviewed by Arnold et al. (1994) and Vijaylakshmi et al. (2002). Almost all ocular structures may be affected in CRS, and these authors suggested that ocular abnormalities are caused either by (1) direct disturbance of organogenesis due to inhibition of cell replication by RV or (2) tissue destruction and scarring caused by immune responses, which may progress throughout pregnancy. RV enters the lens before the development of the lens capsule. It may persist within the lens and has been isolated from cataracts from children up to the age of 3 years (Menser et al. 1967). Using RT-PCR, Rajasundari et al. (2008) detected RV RNA in 92% of lenses from confirmed cases of CRS aged 0–11 months. Cataract, microphthalmos, and glaucoma are probably caused by mitotic inhibition and slow growth of cells (Rajasundari et al. 2008). Retinopathy is reported in from 13.3% to 61% cases. Pigment deposits are seen throughout the retina and vary from fine powdery to granular shapes. Visual acuity is not affected by these pigmentory changes. Strabismus and nystagmus (disorders of motility) are frequent and likely to be the result of organic lesions in the eye.

17.5.7.3 Studies of the Brains from CRS Fetuses/Infants

Töndury and Smith (1966) saw no obvious damage in brain cells, but endothelial cell damage and small hemorrhages were seen in some cases, and the cortical width was abnormally small in 10 affected fetuses, when compared with normal fetuses. Peters and Davis (1966) reported areas of mineralization in the blood vessel walls in the putamen and other nuclei of the brain. *In vitro* studies in human fetal brain cells have shown that RV was found mainly in astrocytes, with oligodendrocytes and neurons only occasionally infected (Chantler et al. 1995). Infection of astrocytes may lead to focal areas of necrosis and the pattern of neurological deficit seen in CRS. The restricted replication in oligodendrocytes correlates with the lack of demyelination generally seen in CRS. The cell receptor for RV, MOG is a type I integral membrane protein and is expressed mainly in the CNS. Cong et al. have suggested that MOG is likely to facilitate the attachment of RV to brain cells, leading to cell damage (Cong et al. 2011).

17.5.7.4 Delayed CNS Disorders

Using MRI, Lim et al. (1995) compared brain morphology in adult patients with CRS who had schizophrenia-like symptoms with those of adult early-onset schizophrenic patients without CRS and healthy control subjects (Lim et al. 1995). CRS patients had smaller intracranial volumes than schizophrenic patients. In both affected groups, patients had smaller cortical gray matter volumes than the control group. In addition, they showed significant enlargement of the lateral ventricles. The observations in CRS patients are consistent with a developmental lesion that limits full brain growth, with the small intracranial volume due at least in part to reduced cortical gray matter. It is worth noting that nucleic acid from RV and other viruses was never detected in the brains of schizophrenia patients at autopsy (Taller et al. 1996).

Brain lesions associated with PRP include diffuse atrophy of the brain with ventricular dilatation (Kuroda and Matsui 1997) and alteration of the white matter (Weil et al. 1975). Extensive neuronal loss together with inflammatory damage can be observed.

The role of RV in the pathogenesis of PRP is not clear. RV has only been detected once in the brain of a CRS child with PRP using cocultivation techniques (Cremer et al. 1975). Martin et al. (1989) have suggested that virus-induced autoreactivity to brain antigens may be an important mechanism in chronic inflammatory disorders of the CNS. Circulating immune complexes may also play a role (see below).

17.5.7.5 Possible Mechanisms of Fetal Damage

Early *in vitro* studies suggested that RV may cause a retardation of cell division (Plotkin et al. 1965) and chromosomal damage (Nusbacher et al. 1967). Plotkin and Vaheri (1967) suggested that a specific protein found in RV-infected cells caused this slowing down of cell division, now recognized as mitotic inhibition. Recent work suggests that this may be due to disruption of actin filaments, which are an important component of the cytoskeleton (Lee and Bowden 2000). Naeye and Blanc (1965) showed that the organs of RV-infected fetuses were smaller and had fewer cells than those of uninfected fetuses of the same age (Naeye and Blanc 1965). Thus, mitotic inhibition during the period of organogenesis could result in congenital malformations. RV-induced fetal endothelial cell damage may cause hemorrhages in small blood vessels, leading to tissue necrosis and further damage to organs (e.g., liver, myocardium, organ of Corti) over a longer period.

Other suggested mechanisms of RV-induced fetal damage are RV-induced apoptosis of essential cells and viral interference with the cell cycle (Atreya et al. 2004; Cooray et al. 2005; Lee and Bowden 2000; Best et al. 2005). Caspase-dependent apoptosis is responsible for the cytopathogenicity induced by RV in cell cultures, and this is controlled by cell survival signaling pathways and by interferon (Adamo et al. 2008; Cooray et al. 2003, 2005; Duncan et al. 2000). Adamo et al. (2004) have shown that RV-infected fetal fibroblasts do not undergo apoptosis, although apoptosis does occur in RV-infected adult fibroblasts, as the background of gene expression is antagonistic to it in fetal fibroblasts (Adamo et al. 2008). This might help to explain the persistence of RV-infected fibroblasts in utero, although these findings do not exclude apoptosis in other cell types. In addition, the persisting virus may be able to disrupt normal cell growth. Thus, RV infection may interfere with the cell cycle, since the RV NSP p90 has been shown to interact with both the retinoblastoma protein (pRB), which is a cell cycle regulator, and the cytokinesis regulatory protein citron-K kinase (pCK) (Atreya et al. 2004). A strong interferon response and up-regulation of chemokines in RV-infected human embryonic fibroblasts also suggest that RV could disrupt growth and proliferation pathways (Adamo et al. 2008).

Following widespread infection of the fetus, the foci of infection may persist for some years, but only 1 in 10^3 to 1 in 10^5 fetal cells harbor RV (Rawls 1968). RV has been detected in NPS, CSF, and urine for up to 23 months (Best and Enders 2007), and RV has been isolated from lens aspirates from infants up to the age of 12 months, from a cataract from a 3-year-old child and the CSF of children with CNS involvement up to 18 months of age. Rubella antigen has been detected in the thyroid of a 5-year-old child, and RV was recovered from the brain of a 12-year-old child with PRP. Persisting RV would then be responsible for disruption of cell growth and differentiation, since viral proteins are known to bind to cell proteins involved in cell division and cellular proliferation pathways (see above). RV persistence in cell lines is more likely to be established at low multiplicities of infection, and virus replication may be limited by interferon production (Adamo et al. 2008) and defective interfering RNAs (Derdeyn and Frey 1995). Clones of infected cells may persist in such organs as the eye and brain for many years, as virus will not be exposed to the immune response. Defects of cell-mediated immunity would also help the persistence of RV. Defective lymphoproliferative responses may persist for 2–3 years (O'Shea et al. 1992), and other defective cell mediated immune responses may persist into the second decade of life (reviewed by Best et al. 2005). Mauracher et al. found that patients with CRS had significantly lower levels of antibodies to the RV E1 protein than rubella seropositive healthy controls when linearized E1 was used in Western blots under reducing conditions, and functional affinity of the E1-specific IgG was also significantly lower (Mauracher et al. 1993). As there was no difference in the levels of antibodies to the E2 and capsid proteins, selective immune tolerance to the E1 protein was suggested, which may be due to defects in cell-mediated immune responses.

Autoimmune mechanisms are thought to play a role in the pathogenesis of IDDM and other endocrine disorders, but the mechanisms are not fully understood. RV has been isolated from the pancreas of several infants who died from CRS (Sever et al. 1985). RV infection may damage islet cells and initiate a process that leads to

IDDM in later life. Rubella antigens have also been identified in the thyroid follicles of a patient with CRS and thyroid autoimmunity (Ziring et al. 1977). RV infection is not cytolytic in human fetal islet cells *in vitro*, but a depression of immunoreactive-secreted insulin has been observed (Numazaki et al. 1990). Immunoreactive epitopes in the RV capsid have been shown to share antigenicity with β-cell protein (Karounos et al. 1993). Autoantibodies to islet cells, which predict the onset of diabetes, have been detected in 20% of these patients. There may also be genetic susceptibility; the HLA types of patients with IDDM are typical of those with autoimmune disease, an increase of the haplotype HLA-A1, B8, DR3, and a decrease in the prevalence of HLA-DR2 (Forrest et al. 2002; Sever et al. 1985). Thus, CRI may increase the susceptibility to IDDM in these patients.

It has been suggested that circulating immune complexes (CICs) play an important role in "late-onset disease" and PRP. Coyle et al. (1992) reported rubella antibody-containing CICs in 21 of 63 (33%) patients with CRI (aged 5 months to 28 years), which were associated with late-onset clinical problems in 10 of the 21 positive subjects. Tardieu et al. (1980) studied eight boys with CRI, who developed severe clinical symptoms between 3 and 6 months of age—interstitial pneumonia, diarrhea, skins rash, hepatosplenomegaly, rapid neurological deterioration, and purpura, six of whom died (Tardieu et al. 1980). Rubella-specific CIC were detected in 4 patients in the acute phase of this illness. An initial disequilibrium of T and B lymphocytes was later corrected. Verder et al. (1986) studied an infant born to a mother who had laboratory-confirmed rubella at 13 weeks of gestation (Verder et al. 1986). The infant appeared well at birth, but failure to thrive and interstitial pneumonia were noted at 2 months of age. Other symptoms of late-onset disease developed including meningoencephalitis at 5½ months, which subsequently progressed with increasing lethargy, bulging fontanel, hydrocephalus, and hypodense areas on cerebral CT scan. Her condition improved on treatment with prednisone and plasma exchange transfusions. RV was isolated from PBL up to 8 months of age. High titers of rubella IgM, low rubella IgG, and an abnormally high total IgM were noted, and total lymphocyte counts were normal. Few CD8+ T cells were detected at 5 months of age, and there was only low activity of K and NK cells. Exchange transfusions at 9 months produced clinical improvement, cessation of viremia, and normalization of cytotoxic cell functions. These authors suggested that CIC were composed of rubella antigen and rubella IgM antibodies and that deficient cytotoxic lymphocyte functions were responsible for the failure to clear the CIC. CIC have also been found in the serum and occasionally in CSF from patients with PRP. These CIC contain rubella-specific IgG antibodies and rubella antigen (Coyle and Wolinsky 1981).

17.6 PREVENTION

17.6.1 Rubella Vaccines

The first live attenuated rubella vaccines were licensed in 1969–1970. Several vaccines were developed, but the RA27/3 strain is the most widely used, as it induces the best immune response (Reef and Plotkin 2007; WHO 2008). Rubella vaccine is generally administered in combination with measles (MR), measles and mumps

---

(MMR), or with the further addition of varicella (MMRV) (Centers for Disease Control and Prevention 2008).

Rubella vaccines cause few side effects in children, but rash, low-grade fever, irritability, lymphadenopathy, myalgia, paresthesia, and joint symptoms may occur 10–30 days after vaccination. Joint symptoms occur most frequently in postpubertal females (≤25%). Rubella vaccine is not associated with chronic joint disease. The first dose of MMRV may be associated with febrile seizures (Klein et al. 2010). Symptoms are rare after a second dose. MMR vaccines containing the Urabe strain of mumps have been associated with aseptic meningitis, but this is not found with the Jeryl Lynn strain of mumps (Department of Health 2010a).

In 1998, Wakefield et al. suggested an association between MMR vaccine and a "new syndrome" of autism and bowel disease, but subsequent epidemiological studies in several countries consistently failed to find evidence of a link between MMR vaccine and autism or inflammatory bowel disease (Honda et al. 2005; Pebody et al. 1998; Institute of Medicine 2001; WHO 2003; Department of Health 2010b). It is now accepted that Wakefield's paper was a small case series with no controls and relied on parental recall and beliefs. Ten of Wakefield's coauthors retracted the article's interpretation of a link with MMR vaccine (Murch et al. 2004), and the paper was finally retracted in 2010. It was recently suggested that Wakefield's article linking MMR vaccine and autism was not only wrong but fraudulent (Godlee et al. 2011). The consequences of Wakefield's paper were disastrous since MMR vaccination rates in the United Kingdom decreased sharply and were as low as 80% in 2003–2004, resulting in outbreaks of measles (Jansen et al. 2003).

17.6.1.1 Immune Responses

Rubella antibodies usually develop 10–28 days after vaccination. Only about 5% of vaccinees will fail to develop an immune response, which may be due to a concurrent infection or to maternal antibodies in infants or from blood transfusion or immunoglobulin. Some vaccinees will have preexisting low levels of antibodies detectable by alternative assays and may fail to develop higher concentrations of antibody. Vaccine-induced antibodies probably persist for life in most vaccinees, but it is advised to confirm immunity in women before pregnancy if they were vaccinated in childhood.

17.6.1.2 Contraindications

Pregnancy is a contraindication to vaccination with rubella-containing vaccines (RCV) and should be avoided for at least 1 month after vaccination (Centers for Disease Control and Prevention 2001; Department of Health 2010b). However, if a woman who is unknowingly pregnant is vaccinated, there is no indication for abortion or prenatal diagnosis, since no abnormalities compatible with CRS have been detected in infants after vaccination in pregnancy (Centers for Disease Control and Prevention 2001; Reef and Plotkin 2007; Castillo-Solorzano et al. 2011).

Other contraindications to vaccination with a RCV are severe immunodeficiency and intensive immune suppressive therapy, congenital immune disorders, a history of allergic reactions to components of the vaccine, and untreated active tuberculosis (WHO 2011). If MMR or other measles-containing vaccine is used, the contraindications to this vaccine should also be followed. Vaccination of persons who have received blood transfusion or other blood products should be delayed for at least 3 months. Administration of human anti-Rh (D) immunoglobulin is not a contraindication to postpartum vaccination. Vaccination should also be delayed in those who have a fever >38.5°C or other serious disease (Department of Health 2010b; WHO 2011). Neurological conditions are not normally a contraindication, unless there is current neurological deterioration, in which case vaccination should be delayed.

17.6.2 VACCINATION PROGRAMS

The aim of rubella vaccination programs is to prevent infection in pregnancy including CRS. Rubella vaccination programs were started in some countries in the early 1970s. Countries such as the United States introduced universal vaccination, where all children were offered vaccination to eliminate the disease. Other countries such as the United Kingdom introduced selective vaccination of prepubertal girls and susceptible adult women to protect the population at risk (i.e., pregnant women), but these programs were not entirely effective (Best et al. 2009; WHO 2011). Currently, most (92%) countries use two doses of MMR, with the first dose being administered between 12 and 24 months (WHO 2011). As of December 2010, a total of 130 WHO member states had introduced RCV, a 57% increase from 83 member states in 1996 (Figure 17.8). In addition, goals to eliminate rubella and CRS were established in the WHO Region of the Americas (by 2010), the WHO European Region (by 2015), and the WHO Western Pacific Region has established targets for accelerated rubella control and CRS prevention by 2015.

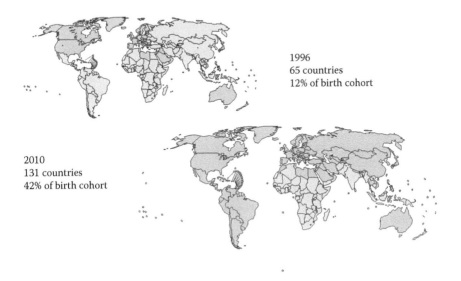

1996
65 countries
12% of birth cohort

2010
131 countries
42% of birth cohort

FIGURE 17.8 Countries using rubella vaccine in their national immunization system. (From WHO/IVB database and the "World Population Prospects: the 2010 Revision," New York, UN 193 WHO Member States. Date of Slide: 28 September 2011.)

In 2000, the first WHO rubella vaccine position paper was published, which placed an emphasis on direct protection of women of child-bearing age (WHO 2000). In 2011, the WHO guideline was updated and supports a paradigm shift in vaccination strategy for introduction of RCVs. The position paper recommends countries take advantage of the measles platform of two doses of measles vaccine to introduce MR or MMR vaccine using the strategy recommended (WHO 2011). This experience in part is based on country and regional experiences and focuses on the interruption of rubella transmission targeting children and adolescents. The recommended strategy includes: an initial catch-up campaign, followed immediately with introduction of the MR/MMR vaccine in the routine program. Vaccination of women of child-bearing age is now considered an additional strategy, as women were difficult to access in many settings, resulting in limited vaccine coverage, which allowed the continuing circulation of RV. Thus, susceptible pregnant women were at risk of exposure and subsequent rubella infection. In addition, since 2000, all countries have added delivery of a second dose of measles vaccine for all children either in campaigns or through the addition of a routine immunization visit. The second measles dose provides an opportunity to use combined MR/MMR vaccines that can reach 80% of all children, thereby effectively blocking rubella transmission and its associated risk of CRS.

REFERENCES

Abernathy, E. S., Hubschen, J. M., Muller, C. P., Jin, L., Brown, D., Komase, K., Mori, Y., Xu, W., Zhu, Z., Siqueira, M. M., Shulga, S., Tikhonova, N., Pattamadilok, S., Incomserb, P., Smit, S. B., Akoua-Koffi, C., Bwogi, J., Lim, W. W., Woo, G. K., Triki, H., Jee, Y., Mulders, M. N., de Filippis, A. M., Ahmed, H., Ramamurty, N., Featherstone, D., and Icenogle, J. P. (2011). Status of global virologic surveillance for rubella viruses. *J Infect Dis* 204 Suppl 1, S524–32.

Adamo, P., Asis, L., Silveyra, P., Cuffini, C., Pedranti, M., and Zapata, M. (2004). Rubella virus does not induce apoptosis in primary human embryo fibroblast cultures: a possible way of viral persistence in congenital infection. *Viral Immunol* 17(1), 87–100.

Adamo, M. P., Zapata, M., and Frey, T. K. (2008). Analysis of gene expression in fetal and adult cells infected with rubella virus. *Virology* 370(1), 1–11.

AP-HP, Gynecology-Obstetric Unit, Antoine Béclère Hospital, Clamart, France; UMR-S0782, Paris-Sud University, Clamart, France.

Arnold, J. J., McIntosh, E. D., Martin, F. J., and Menser, M. A. (1994). A fifty-year follow-up of ocular defects in congenital rubella: late ocular manifestations. *Aust N Z J Ophthalmol* 22(1), 1–6.

Atreya, C. D., Mohan, K. V., and Kulkarni, S. (2004). Rubella virus and birth defects: molecular insights into the viral teratogenesis at the cellular level. *Birth Defects Res A Clin Mol Teratol* 70(7), 431–7.

Banatvala, J. E., and Brown, D. W. (2004). Rubella. *Lancet* 363(9415), 1127–37.

Best, J. M. (2007). Rubella. *Semin Fetal Neonatal Med* 12(3), 182–92.

Best, J. M., Banatvala, J. E., Morgan-Capner, P., and Miller, E. (1989). Fetal infection after maternal reinfection with rubella: criteria for defining reinfection. *BMJ* 299(6702), 773–5.

Best, J. M., Cooray, S., and Banatvala, J. E. (2005). Rubella, in *Topley & Wilson's Microbiology and Microbial Infections. Virology, 10th edition, Volume 2* (Mahy, B. W. J., and ter Meulen, V., eds.), Edward Arnold, London, pp. 959–992.

Best, J. M., and Enders, G. (2007). Laboratory diagnosis of rubella and congenital rubella, in *Rubella Viruses. Perspectives in Medical Virology Volume 15* (Banatvala, J. E., and Peckham, C. eds.), Elsevier, London, pp. 39–77.

Best, J. M., Icenogle, J. P., and Brown, D. W. G. (2009). Rubella. In *Principles and Practice of Clinical Virology, 6th edition,* (Zuckerman, A. J., Banatvala, J. E., Schoub, B. D., Griffiths, P. D., and Mortimer, P. eds.) 561–92. Chichester: John Wiley & Sons, Ltd.

Best, J. M., and O'Shea, S. (1995). "Rubella Virus." In *Diagnostic Procedures for Viral, Rickettsial and Chlamydial Infections, 7th edition,* (Lennette, E. H., Lennette, D. A., and Lennette, E. T. eds.) 583–600. Washington, DC: American Public Health Association.

Bloom, S., Rguig, A., Berraho, A., Zniber, L., Bouazzaoui, N., Zaghloul, Z., Reef, S., Zidouh, A., Papania, M., and Seward, J. (2005). Congenital rubella syndrome burden in Morocco: a rapid retrospective assessment. *Lancet* 365(9454), 135–41.

Bosma, T. J., Corbett, K. M., Eckstein, M. B., O'Shea, S., Vijayalakshmi, P., Banatvala, J. E., Morton, K., and Best, J. M. (1995). Use of PCR for prenatal and postnatal diagnosis of congenital rubella. *J Clin Microbiol* 33(11), 2881–7.

Castillo-Solorzano, C., Reef, S. E., Morice, A., Vascones, N., Chevez, A. E., Castalia-Soares, R., Torres, C., Vizzotti, C., and Ruiz Matus, C. (2011). Rubella vaccination of unknowingly pregnant women during mass campaigns for rubella and congenital rubella syndrome elimination, the Americas 2001–2008. *J Infect Dis* 204 Suppl 2, S713–7.

Centers for Disease Control and Prevention. (2001). Revised ACIP recommendation for avoiding pregnancy after receiving a rubella-containing vaccine. *MMWR* 50 (No. 49): 1117.

Centers for Disease Control and Prevention. (2008). Update: Recommendations from the Advisory Committee on Immunization Practices (ACIP) regarding administration of Combination MMRV vaccine. *MMWR* 57 (No.10): 258–60.

Chang, D. I., Park, J. H., and Chung, K. C. (1997). Encephalitis and polyradiculoneuritis following rubella virus infection—a case report. *J Korean Med Sci* 12(2), 168–70.

Chang, Y. C., Huang, C. C., and Liu, C. C. (1996). Frequency of linear hyperechogenicity over the basal ganglia in young infants with congenital rubella syndrome. *Clin Infect Dis* 22(3), 569–71.

Chantler, J. K., Smyrnis, L., and Tai, G. (1995). Selective infection of astrocytes in human glial cell cultures by rubella virus. *Lab Invest* 72(3), 334–40.

Chantler, J., Wolinsky, J. S., and Tingle, A. (2001). Rubella virus, in *Fields Virology, 4th edition* (Knipe, D. M., Howley, P. M. et al. eds.), Lippincott, Williams & Wilkins, Philadelphia, pp. 963–90.

Chen, M.-H., and Icenogle, J. (2007). Molecular virology of rubella virus, in *Rubella Viruses, Perspectives in Medical Virology* (Banatvala, J., and Peckham, C. eds.), Elsevier, Amsterdam, pp. 1–18.

Chess, S., Fernandez, P., and Korn, S. (1978). Behavioral consequences of congenital rubella. *J Pediatr* 93(4), 699–703.

Cong, H., Jiang, Y., and Tien, P. (2011). Identification of the myelin oligodendrocyte glycoprotein as a cellular receptor for rubella virus. *J Virol* 85(21), 11038–47.

Cooper, L. Z. (1975). Congenital rubella in the United States, in *Infections of the Fetus and the Newborn Infant, Progress in Clinical and Biological Research, volume 3,* (Krugman, S., and Gershon, A. A. eds.), AR Liss, New York, pp. 1–21.

Cooper, L. Z., and Alford, C. A. (2006). Rubella, in *Infectious Diseases of the Fetus and Newborn Infant, 6th ed.* (Remington, J. S., Klein, J. O., Wilson, C. B., and Baker, C. J. eds.), Elsevier, WB Saunders, Philadelphia, pp. 894–926.

Cooray, S., Best, J. M., and Jin, L. (2003). Time-course induction of apoptosis by wild-type and attenuated strains of rubella virus. *J Gen Virol* 84(Pt 5), 1275–9.

Cooray, S., Jin, L., and Best, J. M. (2005). The involvement of survival signaling pathways in rubella-virus induced apoptosis. *Virol J* 2, 1.

Corcoran, C., and Hardie, D. R. (2005). Serologic diagnosis of congenital rubella: a cautionary tale. *Pediatr Infect Dis J* 24(3), 286–7.

Cordier, A. G., Vauloup-Fellous, C., Grangeot-Keros, L., Pinet, C., Benachi, A., Ayoubi, J. M., and Picone, O. (2012). Pitfalls in the diagnosis of congenital rubella syndrome in the first trimester of pregnancy. *Prenat Diagn.* 32(5), 496–497.

Coyle, P. K., and Wolinsky, J. S. (1981). Characterization of immune complexes in progressive rubella panencephalitis. *Ann Neurol* 9(6), 557–62.

Coyle, P. K., Wolinsky, J. S., Buimovici-Klein, E., Moucha, R., and Cooper, L. Z. (1992). Rubella-specific immune complexes after congenital infection and vaccination. *Infect Immun* 36: 498–503.

Cremer, N. E., Oshiro, L. S., Weil, M. L., Lennette, E. H., Itabashi, H. H., and Carnay, L. (1975). Isolation of rubella virus from brain in chronic progressive panencephalitis. *J Gen Virol* 29(2), 143–53.

Cutts, F. T., Robertson, S. E., Diaz-Ortega, J. L., and Samuel, R. (1997). Control of rubella and congenital rubella syndrome (CRS) in developing countries, Part 1: Burden of disease from CRS. *Bull World Health Organ* 75(1), 55–68.

Degani, S. (2006). Sonographic findings in fetal viral infections: a systematic review. *Obstet Gynecol Surv* 61(5), 329–36.

Department of Health. (2010a). Mumps. In: *Immunisation against Infectious Disease— "The Green Book."* Available at: http://www.dh.gov.uk/prod_consum_dh/groups/dh_digitalassets/@dh/@en/documents/digitalasset/dh_122638.pdf.

Department of Health. (2010b). Rubella. In: *Immunisation against Infectious Disease— "The Green Book."* Available at: http://www.dh.gov.uk/prod_consum_dh/groups/dh_digitalassets/@dh/@en/documents/digitalasset/dh_122641.pdf.

Derdyn, C. A., and Frey, T. K. (1995). Characterisations of defective-interfering RNAs of rubella virus generated during serial undiluted passage. *Virology* 206: 216–26.

Duncan, R., Esmaili, A., Law, L. M., Bertholet, S., Hough, C., Hobman, T. C., and Nakhasi, H. L. (2000). Rubella virus capsid protein induces apoptosis in transfected RK13 cells. *Virology* 275(1), 20–9.

Dwyer, D. E., Hueston, L., Field, P. R., Cunningham, A. L., and North, K. (1992). Acute encephalitis complicating rubella virus infection. *Pediatr Infect Dis J* 11(3), 238–40.

Eckstein, M. B., Brown, D. W., Foster, A., Richards, A. F., Gilbert, C. E., and Vijayalakshmi, P. (1996). Congenital rubella in south India: diagnosis using saliva from infants with cataract. *BMJ* 312(7024), 161.

Enders, G., Nickerl-Pacher, U., Miller, E., and Cradock-Watson, J. E. (1988). Outcome of confirmed periconceptional maternal rubella. *Lancet* 1(8600), 1445–7.

Feng, Y., Santibanez, S., Appleton, H., Lu, Y., and Jin, L. (2011). Application of new assays for rapid confirmation and genotyping of isolates of rubella virus. *J Med Virol* 83(1), 170–7.

Figueiredo, C. A., Oliveira, M. I., Afonso, A. M., Curti, S. P., and Durigon, E. L. (2011). Rubella encephalitis in a young adult male: isolation and genotype analysis. *Infection* 39(1), 73–5.

Forrest, J. M., Turnbull, F. M., Sholler, G. F., Hawker, R. E., Martin, F. J., Doran, T. T., and Burgess, M. A. (2002). Gregg's congenital rubella patients 60 years later. *Med J Aust* 177(11–12), 664–7.

Frey, T. K. (1997). Neurological aspects of rubella virus infection. *Intervirology* 40(2–3), 167–75.

Furet, E., Tassin, M., Anselem, O., Meritet, J. F., Floch, C., Blin, G., and Mandelbrot, L. (2010) Syndrome de rubéole congénitale à propos d'un cas. *Médecine Foetale et Echographie en Gynécologie* 83, 1–4.

Ginsberg-Fellner, F., Witt, M. E., Fedun, B., Taub, F., Dobersen, M. J., McEvoy, R. C., Cooper, L. Z., Notkins, A. L., and Rubinstein, P. (1985). Diabetes mellitus and autoimmunity in patients with the congenital rubella syndrome. *Rev Infect Dis* 7 Suppl 1, S170–6.

Godlee, F., Smith, J., and Marcovitch, H. (2011). Wakefield's article linking MMR vaccine and autism was fraudulent. *BMJ* 342, c7452.

Gregg, N.McA. (1941). Congenital cataract following German measles in mother. *Trans Ophthalmol Soc Aust* 3, 35–46.

Hanshaw, J. B., Dudgeon, J. A., and Marshall, W. C. (1985). *Viral Diseases of the Fetus and Newborn*, 2nd edition, W. B. Saunders, Philadelphia.

Heggie, A. D. (1978). Pathogenesis of the rubella exanthem: distribution of rubella virus in the skin during rubella with and without rash. *J Infect Dis* 137(1), 74–7.

Honda, H., Shimizu, Y., and Rutter, M. (2005). No effect of MMR withdrawal on the incidence of autism: a total population study. *J Child Psychol Psychiatry* 46(6), 572–9.

Health Protection Agency Rash Guidance Working Group. (2011). Guidance on viral rash in pregnancy: investigation, diagnosis and management of viral rash illness or exposure to viral rash illness in pregnancy. Available at: http://www.hpa.org.uk/web/HPAwebFile/ HPAweb_C/1294740918985.

Hwang, S. J., and Chen, Y. S. (2010). Congenital rubella syndrome with autistic disorder. *J Chin Med Assoc* 73(2), 104–7.

Institute of Medicine. (2001). *Immunization Safety Review: Measles-Mumps-Rubella Vaccine and Autism*. Available at: http://search.nap.edu/books/0309074479/html/.

Jacobi, C., Lange, P., and Reiber, H. (2007). Quantitation of intrathecal antibodies in cerebrospinal fluid of subacute sclerosing panencephalitis, herpes simplex encephalitis and multiple sclerosis: discrimination between microorganism-driven and polyspecific immune response. *J Neuroimmunol* 187(1–2), 139–46.

Jansen, V. A., Stollenwerk, N., Jensen, H. J., Ramsay, M. E., Edmunds, W. J., and Rhodes, C. J. (2003). Measles outbreaks in a population with declining vaccine uptake. *Science* 301(5634), 804.

Karounos, D. G., Wolinsky, J. S., and Thomas, J. W. (1993). Monoclonal antibody to rubella virus capsid protein recognizes a beta-cell antigen. *J Immunol* 150(7), 3080–5.

Klein, N. P., Fireman, B., Yih, W. K., Lewis, E., Kulldorff, M., Ray, P., Baxter, R., Hambidge, S., Nordin, J., Naleway, A., Belongia, E. A., Lieu, T., Baggs, J., and Weintraub, E. (2010). Measles-mumps-rubella-varicella combination vaccine and the risk of febrile seizures. *Pediatrics* 126(1), e1–8.

Kuroda, Y., and Matsui, M. (1997). [Progressive rubella panencephalitis]. *Nihon Rinsho* 55(4), 922–5.

Lane, B., Sullivan, E. V., Lim, K. O., Beal, D. M., Harvey, R. L., Jr., Meyers, T., Faustman, W. O., and Pfefferbaum, A. (1996). White matter MR hyperintensities in adult patients with congenital rubella. *AJNR Am J Neuroradiol* 17(1), 99–103.

Lee, J. Y., and Bowden, D. S. (2000). Rubella virus replication and links to teratogenicity. *Clin Microbiol Rev* 13(4), 571–87.

Lim, K. O., Beal, D. M., Harvey, R. L., Jr., Myers, T., Lane, B., Sullivan, E. V., Faustman, W. O., and Pfefferbaum, A. (1995). Brain dysmorphology in adults with congenital rubella plus schizophrenia-like symptoms. *Biol Psychiatry* 37(11), 764–76.

Manikkavasagan, G., Bukasa, A., Brown, K. E., Cohen, B. J., and Ramsay, M. E. (2010). Oral fluid testing during 10 years of rubella elimination, England and Wales. *Emerg Infect Dis* 16(10), 1532–8.

Martin, R., Marquardt, P., O'Shea, S., Borkenstein, M., and Kreth, H. W. (1989). Virus-specific and autoreactive T cell lines isolated from cerebrospinal fluid of a patient with chronic rubella panencephalitis. *J Neuroimmunol* 23(1), 1–10.

Mauracher, C. A., Mitchell, L. A., and Tingle, A. J. (1993). Selective tolerance to the E1 protein of rubella virus in congenital rubella syndrome. *J Immunol* 151(4), 2041–9.

Menser, M. A., Dods, L., and Harley, J. D. (1967). A twenty-five-year follow-up of congenital rubella. *Lancet* 2(7530), 1347–50.

Migliucci, A., Di Fraja, D., Sarno, L., Acampora, E., Mazzarelli, L. L., Quaglia, F., Mallia Milanes, G., Buffolano, W., Napolitano, R., Simioli, S., Maruotti, G. M., and Martinelli, P. (2011). Prenatal diagnosis of congenital rubella infection and ultrasonography: a preliminary study. *Minerva Ginecol* 63(6), 485–9.

Moriuchi, H., Yamasaki, S., Mori, K., Sakai, M., and Tsuji, Y. (1990). A rubella epidemic in Sasebo, Japan in 1987, with various complications. *Acta Paediatr Jpn* 32(1), 67–75.

Munroe, S. (1999). *A survey of late emerging manifestations of congenital rubella in Canada.* Canadian Deafblind and Rubella Association, Port Morien, Nova Scotia. Available at: http://www.cdbanational.com/rubellanews.html.

Murch, S. H., Anthony, A., Casson, D. H., Malik, M., Berelowitz, M., Dhillon, A. P., Thomson, M. A., Valentine, A., Davies, S. E., and Walker-Smith, J. A. (2004). Retraction of an interpretation. *Lancet* 363(9411), 750.

Muscat, M., Zimmerman, L., Bacci, S., Bang, H., Glismann, S., Molbak, K., and Reef, S. (2012). Toward rubella elimination in Europe: an epidemiological assessment. *Vaccine* 30(11), 1999–2007.

Naeye, R. L., and Blanc, W. (1965). Pathogenesis of congenital rubella. *JAMA* 194(12), 1277–83.

Numazaki, K., Goldman, H., Seemayer, T. A., Wong, I., and Wainberg, M. A. (1990). Infection by human cytomegalovirus and rubella virus of cultured human fetal islets of Langerhans. *In Vivo* 4(1), 49–54.

Numazaki, K., and Fujikawa, T. (2003). Intracranial calcification with congenital rubella syndrome in a mother with serologic immunity. *J Child Neurol* 18(4), 296–7.

Nusbacher, J., Hirschhorn, K., and Cooper, L. Z. (1967). Chromosomal abnormalities in congenital rubella. *N Engl J Med* 276(25), 1409–13.

O'Shea, S., Best, J., and Banatvala, J. E. (1992). A lymphocyte transformation assay for the diagnosis of congenital rubella. *J Virol Methods* 37(2), 139–47.

Oster, M. E., Riehle-Colarusso, T., and Correa, A. (2010). An update on cardiovascular malformations in congenital rubella syndrome. *Birth Defects Res A Clin Mol Teratol* 88(1), 1–8.

Peckham, C. S. (1974). Clinical and serological assessment of children exposed in utero to confirmed maternal rubella. *Br Med J* 1(5902), 259–61.

Pebody, R. G., Paunio, M., and Ruutu, P. (1998). Measles, measles vaccination, and Crohn's disease. Crohn's disease has not increased in Finland. *BMJ* 316(7146), 1745–6.

Peckham, C. S., Martin, J. A., Marshall, W. C., and Dudgeon, J. A. (1979). Congenital rubella deafness: a preventable disease. *Lancet* 1(8110), 258–61.

Peters, E. R., and Davis, R. L. (1966). Congenital rubella syndrome. Cerebral mineralizations and subperiosteal new bone formation as expressions of this disorder. *Clin Pediatr (Phila)* 5(12), 743–6.

Plotkin, S. A., Oski, F. A. et al. (1965). Some recently recognized manifestations of the rubella syndrome. *J Pediatr* 67, 182–91.

Plotkin, S. A., and Vaheri, A. (1967). Human fibroblasts infected with rubella virus produce a growth inhibitor. *Science* 156(3775), 659–61.

Rajasundari, T. A., Sundaresan, P., Vijayalakshmi, P., Brown, D. W., and Jin, L. (2008). Laboratory confirmation of congenital rubella syndrome in infants: an eye hospital based investigation. *J Med Virol* 80(3), 536–46.

Rawls, W. E. (1968). Congenital rubella: the significance of virus persistence. *Prog Med Virol* 10, 238–85.

Reef, S., and Plotkin, S. A. (2007). Rubella Vaccine, in *Rubella Viruses. Perspectives in Medical Virology Volume 15.* (Banatvala J. E. and Peckham, C. eds.), Elsevier, London, pp. 79–93.

Reef, S. E., Plotkin, S., Cordero, J. F., Katz, M., Cooper, L., Schwartz, B., Zimmerman-Swain, L., Danovaro-Holliday, M. C., and Wharton, M. (2000). Preparing for elimination of congenital rubella syndrome (CRS): summary of a workshop on CRS elimination in the United States. *Clin Infect Dis* 31(1), 85–95.

Risco, C., Carrascosa, J. L., and Frey, T. K. (2003). Structural maturation of rubella virus in the Golgi complex. *Virology* 312(2), 261–9.

Sever, J. L., South, M. A., and Shaver, K. A. (1985). Delayed manifestations of congenital rubella. *Rev Infect Dis* 7 Suppl 1, S164–9.

Skendzel, L. P. (1996). Rubella immunity. Defining the level of protective antibody. *Am J Clin Pathol* 106(2), 170–4.

Taller, A. M., Asher, D. M., Pomeroy, K. L., Eldadah, B. A., Godec, M. S., Falkai, P. G., Bogert, B., Kleinman, J. E., Stevens, J. R., and Torrey, E. F. (1996). Search for viral nucleic acid sequences in brain tissues of patients with schizophrenia using nested polymerase chain reaction. *Arch Gen Psychiatry* 53(1), 32–40.

Tardieu, M., Grospierre, B., Durandy, A., and Griscelli, C. (1980). Circulating immune complexes containing rubella antigens in late-onset rubella syndrome. *J Pediatr* 97(3), 370–3.

The editors of the *Lancet* (2010). Retraction—Ileal-lymphoid-nodular hyperplasia, non-specific colitis, and pervasive developmental disorder in children. *Lancet* 375, 445.

Thomas, H. I., and Morgan-Capner, P. (1991). Rubella-specific IgG1 avidity: a comparison of methods. *J Virol Methods* 31(2–3), 219–28.

Thomas, H. I., Morgan-Capner, P., Enders, G., O'Shea, S., Caldicott, D., and Best, J. M. (1992). Persistence of specific IgM and low avidity specific IgG1 following primary rubella. *J Virol Methods* 39(1–2), 149–55.

Thompson, K. M., and Tobin, J. O. (1970). Isolation of rubella virus from abortion material. *Br Med J* 2(5704), 264–6.

Töndury, G., and Smith, D. W. (1966). Fetal rubella pathology. *J Pediatr* 68(6), 867–79.

Verder, H., Dickmeiss, E., Haahr, S., Kappelgaard, E., Leerboy, J., Moller-Larsen, A., Nielsen, H., Platz, P., and Koch, C. (1986). Late-onset rubella syndrome: coexistence of immune complex disease and defective cytotoxic effector cell function. *Clin Exp Immunol* 63(2), 367–75.

Vijayalakshmi, P., Kakkar, G., Samprathi, A., and Banushree, R. (2002). Ocular manifestations of congenital rubella syndrome in a developing country. *Indian J Ophthalmol* 50(4), 307–11.

Vijayalakshmi, P., Rajasundari, T. A., Prasad, N. M. et al. (2007). Prevalence of eye signs in congenital rubella syndrome in South India: a role for population screening. *Brit J Ophthalmol* 91, 1467–70.

Wakefield, A. J., Murch, S. H., Anthony, A., Linnell, J., Casson, D. M., Malik, M., Berelowitz, M., Dhillon, A. P., Thomson, M. A., Harvey, P., Valentine, A., Davies, S. E., and Walker-Smith, J. A. (1998). Ileal-lymphoid-nodular hyperplasia, non-specific colitis, and pervasive developmental disorder in children. *Lancet* 351(9103), 637–41.

Weil, M. L., Itabashi, H., Cremer, N. E., Oshiro, L., Lennette, E. H., and Carnay, L. (1975). Chronic progressive panencephalitis due to rubella virus simulating subacute sclerosing panencephalitis. *N Engl J Med* 292(19), 994–8.

World Health Organization. (1999). Guidelines for surveillance of congenital rubella syndrome and rubella. Field test version. WHO/V&B/99.22. WHO, Geneva.

World Health Organization. (2000). Rubella vaccines: WHO position paper. *Weekly epidemiological record* 75, 161–9.

World Health Organization. (2003). WHO standards for surveillance of selected vaccine-preventable diseases: Geneva. (WHO/V&B/03.01). Available at: http://www.who.int/immunization/documents/WHO_VB_03.01/en/index.html.

World Health Organization. (2007). Update of standard nomenclature for wild-type rubella viruses. *Weekly epidemiological record* 82, 216–22.

World Health Organization. (2008). The immunological basis for immunization series, Module 11: rubella. WHO: Geneva. Available at: http://whqlibdoc.who.int/publications/2008/9789241596848_eng.pdf. Accessed October 2011.

World Health Organization. (2011). Rubella vaccines: WHO position paper. *Weekly epidemiological record* 86, 301–16.

Yoshimura, M., Tohyama, J., Maegaki, Y., Maeoka, Y., Koeda, T., Ohtani, K., and Ando, Y. (1996). [Computed tomography and magnetic resonance imaging of the brain in congenital rubella syndrome]. *No To Hattatsu* 28(5), 385–90.

Zhou, Y., Ushijima, H., and Frey, T. K. (2007). Genomic analysis of diverse rubella virus genotypes. *J Gen Virol* 88(Pt 3), 932–41.

Zimmerman, L., Rogalska, J., Wannemuehler, K. A., Haponiuk, M., Kosek, A., Pauch, E., Plonska, E., Veltze, D., Czarkowski, M. P., Buddh, N., Reef, S., and Stefanoff, P. (2011). Toward rubella elimination in Poland: need for supplemental immunization activities, enhanced surveillance, and further integration with measles elimination efforts. *J Infect Dis* 204 Suppl 1, S389–95.

Ziring, P. R., Gallo, G., Finegold, M., Buimovici-Klein, E., and Ogra, P. (1977). Chronic lymphocytic thyroiditis: identification of rubella virus antigen in the thyroid of a child with congenital rubella. *J Pediatr* 90(3), 419–20.

Section II

Retroviruses

18 Human T-Lymphotropic Virus

Motohiro Yukitake and Hideo Hara

CONTENTS

18.1 INTRODUCTION

In 1980, human T-lymphotropic virus type I (HTLV-I) was isolated from cultured CD4+ T-lymphocytes of a cutaneous T-cell lymphoma patient (Poiesz et al. 1980), who was later considered to have adult T-cell leukemia/lymphoma (ATL) (Poiesz et al. 1980; Uchiyama et al. 1977; Yoshida et al. 1984). In 1985, it was reported that 59% of patients with tropical spastic paraparesis (TSP) in Martinique were HTLV-I-seropositive (Gessain et al. 1985). Then, TSP patients in Jamaica and Colombia were also shown to have anti-HTLV-I antibodies in both serum and cerebrospinal fluid (CSF) (Rodgers-Johnson et al. 1985). Moreover, Osame et al. (1986) reported cases of HTLV-I-seropositive chronic progressive myelopathy in the south of Japan and named it HTLV-I-associated myelopathy (HAM). Soon after, HAM and HTLV-I-seropositive TSP were identified as the same disease, termed HAM/TSP (Osame 1990; Roman and Osame 1988). Epidemiological studies suggested that 10 to 20 million people worldwide are infected with HTLV-I (de The and Bomford 1993), but prevalence of HAM/TSP is only 0.1%–5% of HTLV-I-infected individuals (Hollsberg and Hafler 1993; Kaplan et al. 1990). In addition, there are some large endemic areas of HTLV-I infection in the south of Japan, Central and West Africa, the Caribbean, Central and South America, and the Middle East.

18.1.1 Structure and Biology of HTLV-I

HTLV-I has been classified into a type C oncovirus group (group VI; ssRNA-RT) by the International Committee on Taxonomy of Viruses and belonging to the family of Retroviridae. Unlike the human immunodeficiency virus (HIV), HTLV-I causes diseases, such as adult T-cell leukemia (ATL) and HAM/TSP, in less than 5% of infected individuals (Yamaguchi and Takatsuki 1993). In general, HTLV-I-related diseases (including not only HAM/TSP and ATL but also alveolitis, uveitis, polymyositis, and arthropathy) occur in around 10% of HTLV-I carriers. In other words, most people infected with HTLV-I are asymptomatic throughout their lives, whereas between 0.1% and 5% of HTLV-I carriers develop HAM/TSP (in comparison, lifetime risk of ATL ranges from 2% and 5%) (Kaplan et al. 1990).

HTLV-I is a round, enveloped virus of around 100 nm in diameter (Ohtsuki et al. 1982). The length of the HTLV-I genome has 9032 base pairs and encodes structural and enzymatic proteins similar to those of other retroviruses. The three typical structural and enzymatic genes, the group antigen (gag), polymerase (pol), and envelope antigen (env) genes, are flanked by long terminal repeats (LTRs) (Seiki et al. 1983). However, the HTLV-I genome has a unique region at the 3′ end called the pX region, which contains at least four partially overlapping reading frames (ORFs) encoding regulatory proteins such as the Tax transactivator (ORF4), the posttranscriptional regulator Rex (ORF3), and accessory proteins (p12, p13, p30) (Matsuura et al. 2010).

The full-length mRNA encodes both gag protein (p55) and pol protein. The gag protein is cleaved by the viral protease to yield the matrix (MA, p19), capsid (CA, P24), and nucleocapsid (NC, P15) proteins. The pol protein is synthesized by ribosomal frameshifting. In addition, a single-spliced mRNA encodes the env protein, and a double-spliced mRNA encodes the Tax and Rex proteins. Some other RNA frameshifts and transcript splicing patterns are also known. The LTRs located at the 5′ and 3′ ends of the viral genome are divided into U3, R, and U5 regions. The U3 region contains essential elements for control of proviral transcription, mRNA termination, and polyadenylation. The R region contains the Rex-responsive element (Ciminale et al. 1992). The functions of HTLV-I proteins and glycoproteins are listed in Table 18.1 (Albrecht and Lairmore 2002; Johnson et al. 2001; Lemasson et al. 2007; Satou et al. 2011).

HTLV-I has six subtypes: subtype A is also known as the cosmopolitan subtype sequenced from Japan (Seiki et al. 1982), which is found in many HTLV-I

TABLE 18.1
Functions of HTLV-I Proteins and Glycoproteins

HTLV-I Proteins and Glycoproteins	Functions
Envelope Proteins (Encoded by env)	
Surface glycoprotein (gp46)	Bind to host cell receptor
Transmembrane protein (gp21)	Anchors surface glycoproteins to virus
Structural Proteins (Encoded by gag)	
Matrix layer (p19)	Organize viral components at the inner cell membrane
Capsid (p24)	Protect viral RNA and proteins
Nucleocapsid (p15)	Nucleic acid-binding protein
Functional Proteins (Encoded by pol)	
Protease (p14)	Cleaves polyproteins into functional components
Reverse transcriptase (p95)	Converts single-stranded RNA to double-stranded DNA
Integrase	Facilitates insertion of provirus into host cell DNA
Regulatory Proteins	
Tax	Activates transcription provirus and host genes
	Transcriptional and posttranscriptional regulator
Rex	Modulates transport of viral RNA
	Posttranscriptional regulator of viral gene expression
HTLV-I bZIP factor	Down-regulates viral transcription
$p12^I$	Role in viral replication and T-cell activation
$pl3^{II}$	Targets mitochondria
$p30^{II}$	Modulates transcription

endemic areas worldwide; subtypes B, D, and F from Central Africa; subtype C from Melanesia, and subtype E from South and Central Africa (Proietti et al. 2005).

18.1.2 EPIDEMIOLOGY OF HTLV-I

Although it is difficult to estimate the exact global prevalence of HTLV-I because of limited population-based reports, it is estimated that approximately 10–20 million people are infected by HTLV-I globally (de The and Bomford 1993; de The and Kazanji 1996). There are some geographical clusters of HTLV-I in the south of Japan, Central and West Africa, the Caribbean, Central and South America, and the Middle East (Figure 18.1) (Levine et al. 1988; Mueller 1991; Proietti et al. 2005; Sonoda et al. 2011).

Japan is a key endemic area of HTLV-I infection. There are some endemic areas in the south of Japan, such as Kyusyu Island, Shikoku Island, and Okinawa Island (Yoshida et al. 1982). Although the prevalence in the general population varies from 0% to 37% (Yoshida et al. 1982), the migration of infected Japanese individuals has recently changed the prevalence throughout the whole of Japan. In the Caribbean islands, the rate of HTLV-I infection is observed to be high, and the prevalence is estimated with approximately 5% in Jamaica (Murphy et al. 1991). Africa is

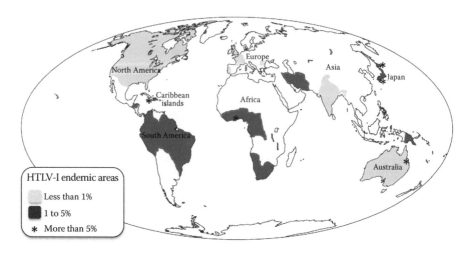

FIGURE 18.1   Worldwide distribution of HTLV-I. There are several high-prevalence areas: in the southern region of Japan, the Caribbean, the equatorial regions of Africa, South America, the Middle East, and Melanesia. It should be noted that HTLV-I endemic areas do not correspond exactly to the country boundaries.

estimated to be the origin of HTLV-I because all different primate T-lymphotropic viruses (PTLV) have been found there. Phylogenetic studies also suggest central Africa as the birthplace of PTLV. In Africa, although the study of the region is limited, the prevalence varies from 0.5% to around 5% (Dumas et al. 1991). In Brazil, the highest prevalence (1.35%) was reported for the central area and the coast, with the lowest (0.08%) in the north and south (Goncalves et al. 2010). In addition, there are smaller endemic foci in Australia (Aboriginal populations), Iran, and Papua New Guinea (Goncalves et al. 2010; Yoshida et al. 1982). In nonendemic areas such as Europe and North America, HTLV-I infection is mainly observed in immigrants from endemic areas, their offspring, and sexual contacts, as well as intravenous drug users and sex workers. From the data of blood donors in Europe and North America, the prevalence is quite low, for example, 0.0039% in France and 0.01%–0.03% in the United States and Canada (Biggar et al. 2006; Murphy et al. 1991).

18.1.3   TRANSMISSION

There are several routes of HTLV-I transmission. The main route from mother to child is through breastfeeding. The frequency of transmission through breastfeeding is estimated to be between 15% and 25%, and there are several factors that influence this, such as HTLV-I proviral load, mother-child HLA class I concordance, and the duration of breastfeeding (Biggar et al. 2006). Mother-to-child transmission during the gestation period also occurs, but the frequency is less than 5%. As HTLV-I is present in the genital secretions of infected individuals, sexual transmission of HTLV-I is the other main route. In sexual transmission, higher transmission efficiency from men to women than from women to men has been suggested (Murphy et al. 1996). Intravenous exposure to blood is also an important route of HTLV-I transmission. Transfusion of HTLV-I-infected cellular blood components results in seroconversion in more than 40% of recipients (Murphy et al. 1996). Compared with that for cellular blood component transfusion, plasma products and cold storage of blood transfusion result in a lower rate of transmission, presumably due to the absence and/or death of HTLV-I-infected lymphocytes (Donegan et al. 1990). The use of contaminated needles and syringes among the drug users is another route of HTLV-I transmission (Feigal et al. 1991).

18.1.4 PREVENTION

Considering the poor prognosis of ATL and HAM/TSP, prevention of HTLV-I infection is important. For HAM/TSP, patients experience long-lasting progressive physical impairments. Thus, public health interventions such as counseling and education of high-risk individuals and populations are indispensable. Since the implementation of a program to prevent intravenous exposure to HTLV-I in Japan in 1986, many countries, especially those with endemic areas (United States, Canada, Brazil, and several European countries), started to implement systematic and permanent screening of all blood donors (Osame et al. 1990). This important public health intervention has been shown to be effective in preventing HTLV-I transmission, and, as a result, this intervention succeeds in decreasing the number of new infections in the overall population. For HTLV-I-seropositive individuals, it is advisable not to donate blood, organs, semen, or milk (Goncalves et al. 2010). As mother-to-child transmission is the other important problem, prenatal screening for HTLV-I should be carried out, especially in endemic areas (Carneiro-Proietti et al. 2002). It is well recognized that neonatal infection with HTLV-I is preventable through short-term breastfeeding for less than 3 months after birth and/or bottle-feeding (Takahashi et al. 1991). Cesarean delivery should also be considered to minimize the risk of perinatal transmission (Goncalves et al. 2010).

Counseling and education for HTLV-I-infected individuals, as well as the general public in endemic areas, are important not only to prevent HTLV-I infection but also to provide psychological and social support. In addition, access to correct information about HTLV-I infection is very important (Guiltinan et al. 1998).

18.2 HAM/TSP

18.2.1 PATHOLOGY

Macroscopically, the spinal cord shows mild to severe atrophy with thickening of the leptomeninges. Spinal cord atrophy is symmetric and can occur throughout the entire spinal cord, especially the thoracic cord. In general, representative pathological findings in HAM/TSP are inflammatory infiltration and diffuse loss of myelin and axons (Figure 18.2) (Akizuki et al. 1988; Iwasaki 1990; Izumo 2010). Microscopic pathological findings can be divided into two phases depending on the duration of the disease. In patients with a relatively short clinical course, for example, a few years or shorter, infiltration of mononuclear cells and degeneration of both myelin and axons are the main findings. Inflammatory lesions continuously extend to the entire spinal cord but are the most severe in the middle to lower thoracic spinal cord. Inflammation is observed in both gray and white matter with inflammatory lymphocyte infiltration. In addition, lymphocyte

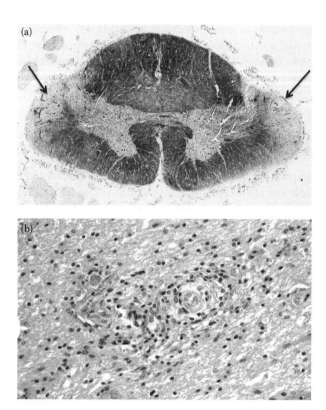

FIGURE 18.2 Pathological features of HAM/TSP patient. (a) Macroscopic findings of thoracic spinal cord. Arrows show the symmetrical degeneration in the lateral column (Klüver–Barrera stain). (b) Microscopic findings of thoracic spinal cord. Perivascular and parenchymal infiltration of mononuclear cells was observed (hematoxylin–eosin stain). These pictures were kindly provided by Dr. Izumo, Molecular Pathology, Center for Chronic Viral Diseases, Graduate School of Medical and Dental Sciences, Kagoshima University, Kagoshima, Japan.

infiltration is observed more frequently in the deeper portion of the cord than in the surface areas, and more severe in the anteriolateral column than in the posterior column (Izumo 2010). On the other hand, patients with a longer clinical course show less inflammatory change in the spinal cord, and both myelin and axon are degenerated monotonically. Tissue in the spinal cord shows gliosis with foamy cells, microglial cells, and a small number of lymphocytes. Fibrous thickening of the vessel wall and pia mater is also observed. Inflammatory changes and gliosis are also present in the gray matter, but neuronal cells are relatively well preserved in the spinal cord. Although the tissue damage is most severe in the thoracic cord, corticospinal damage is also observed as ascending to the cervical spinal cord and brainstem. These types of damage are recognized as a result of Wallerian degeneration. In the brain, similar inflammatory changes are also observed to milder degrees (Aye et al. 2000).

The predominance of inflammation in the middle to lower thoracic cord is explained by the assertion that an anatomical site with slow blood flow, namely, the

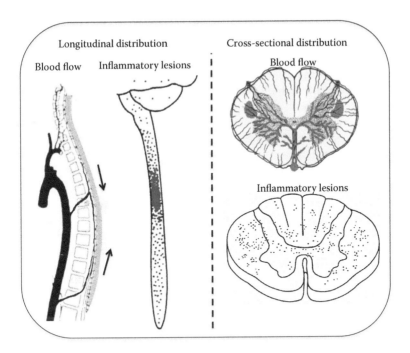

FIGURE 18.3 Distribution of inflammatory lesions and blood supply of the spinal cord. Longitudinal and cross-sectional distribution of inflammatory lesions of HAM/TSP seemed to be identical with slow blood flow area. (Modified from Aye, M.M. et al. 2000, *Acta Neuropathol.* 100, 245–252; Izumo, S. 2010, *Neuropathology* 30, 480–485.)

area of endings of central and peripheral spinal arteries, may be associated with the distribution of pathological changes (Figure 18.3) (Aye et al. 2000). Similar findings are also observed in the brain.

18.3 IMMUNOPATHOLOGY

18.3.1 T-Cell-Mediated Immune Responses in the Spinal Cord

In patients with a relatively short clinical course, there are many inflammatory cells including CD4+ T cells, CD8+ T cells, and macrophages in affected spinal cord parenchyma (Umehara et al. 1993). B cells are also observed in the affected lesion but are mainly located in perivascular spaces. Proinflammatory cytokines such as interleukin (IL)-1β, (TNF)-α, and interferon (IFN)-γ were detected in perivascular infiltrating cells including macrophages, astrocytes, and microglia at the active inflammatory lesions (Umehara et al. 1994). Expression of myeloid-related protein (MRP) 14 and MRP-8, essential proteins in Ca^{2+}-dependent functions during inflammation, has been observed in infiltrating/activated macrophages and microglia (Abe et al. 1999). Among various adhesion molecules, high expression of vascular cell adhesion molecule 1 (VCAM-1) on the endothelium (Umehara et al. 1996), and up-regulation of very late antigen 4 (VLA-4) and monocyte chemoattractant protein 1

(MCP-1) in the infiltrating cells, has been observed. Intracellular adhesion molecule 1 (ICAM-1) and lymphocyte function-associated antigen 1 (LFA-1) are also considered as being related to lymphocyte infiltration (Cabre et al. 1999). The immunoreactivity for HLA class I and up-regulation of HLA class II are found on various cells such as endothelial cells, microglia, and infiltrating mononuclear cells in the lesions. On the other hand, patients with a longer clinical course show CD8+ T-cell predominance with down-regulation of proinflammatory cytokine expression in the affected lesions (Matsuura et al. 2010). Although macrophages are also detectable in the affected lesions, down-regulation of activated markers such as MRP-14 or MRP-8 has been observed (Umehara et al. 1994). Even in cases with a long clinical course, active inflammatory pathological change has been reported in some cases (Iwasaki et al. 2004). Thus, the disease progression of HAM/TSP is different among individuals. In the brain, perivascular inflammatory infiltration was observed in deep white matter and in the marginal area of cortex and white matter with similar types of infiltrating cells. Taken together, these findings strongly suggest that immune responses, especially T-cell-mediated immune responses, play a critical role in the pathogenesis of HAM/TSP.

18.3.2 DETECTION OF HTLV-I-INFECTED CELLS AND HTLV-I PROVIRUS IN SPINAL CORD LESIONS

In general, strong HTLV-I-specific antibody response with high titer is correlated with proviral load, and an increased number of HTLV-I-specific HLA class I-restricted CD8+ cytotoxic T lymphocytes (CTLs) is one of the characteristic features of HAM/TSP. These observations support the presence of persistent HTLV-I proviral expression *in vivo*. In addition, CD4+ T cells are recognized as a predominant target of HTLV-I infection. In PBMC of patients with HAM/TSP, despite high HTLV-I proviral loads being observed at higher levels than in asymptomatic carriers, HTLV-I tax-expressing cells are hardly detected. As HTLV-I tax has functions to activate cellular genes including inflammatory cytokines, HTLV-I tax-expressing cells are believed to play important roles in the pathogenesis of HAM/TSP. On the other hand, tax includes a dominant epitope recognized by HTLV-I-specific CD8+ CTLs. These findings have suggested that strong HTLV-I tax expression is necessary to increase the number of HTLV-I-specific CD8+ CTLs. In the CSF of patients with HAM/TSP, HTLV-I proviral load and HTLV-I tax expression were reported more frequently than in the PBMC. It is noteworthy that HTLV-I proviral load has been shown to have a significant association with clinical progression and with recent onset of HAM/TSP. In the spinal cord lesions of patients with HAM/TSP, pathological studies have revealed that HTLV-I DNA was localized to inflammatory infiltrating UCHL-1-positive cells (suggestive of T cells) but not in CD68+ cells (suggestive of macrophages) around the perivascular areas in the affected lesions by PCR *in situ* hybridization (PCR-ISH) (Matsuoka et al. 1998). The percentage of PCR-ISH-positive T cells was estimated at about 10% of infiltrated T cells in active chronic lesions. Another study showed that Tax mRNA expression was detected in infiltrating CD4+ T cells in active lesions by PCR-ISH (Moritoyo et al. 1996). Among the CD4+ T cells, CD45RO+helper/inducer T cells were reported as major HTLV-I-harboring cells *in vivo*. Furthermore, quantitative PCR analysis showed that the

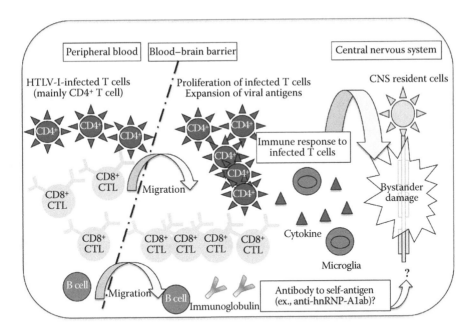

FIGURE 18.4 Hypothesis on the pathogenesis of HAM/TSP. Immune responses of CD8[+] CTL to HTLV-I-infected T cells (mainly CD4; T cells) produce cytokines, which would damage bystander neuronal cells. Autoimmunity to self-antigen on the neuronal cells (for example, antibodies to hnRNP-A1 cross-reacted with HTLV-1-tax) is still uncertain. ab, antibody; CNS, central nervous system; CTL, cytotoxic T lymphocytes; hnRNP-A1, heterogeneous nuclear ribonuclear protein A1.

amount of HTLV-I DNA decreased in parallel with the number of infiltrating CD4[+] T cells in the affected spinal cord. These findings suggest that infiltrating CD4[+] T cells, especially those with HTLV-I tax expression, should be a preferential viral reservoir in the CSF. Although humoral immunity might also play a role in the development of HAM/TSP, definitive pathological data have not been reported (Levin et al. 1998; Yukitake et al. 2008a). Taken together, these data strongly indicate that T-cell-mediated immune responses against HTLV-I-infected cells (mainly CD4[+] T cells) play a main role in the pathogenic mechanism of spinal cord injury in HAM/TSP patients. Furthermore, because there is no evidence that HTLV-I infects neuronal cells, neuronal cell damage is interpreted as a bystander effect (Figure 18.4).

18.3.3 CLINICAL FEATURES OF HAM/TSP

It should be helpful to understand the history of HAM/TSP discovery to shed light on the clinical features of HAM/TSP. In Japan, HAM/TSP was established from disease entities such as primary lateral sclerosis and spinal spastic paraparesis (Osame and Igata 1989), which show gait disturbance with upper motor symptoms and pathological reflexes. Therefore, clinical features of HAM/TSP resemble those of such neurodegenerative diseases to some degree.

HAM/TSP is characterized by spastic paraparesis with the presence of anti-HTLV-I antibodies in both serum and CSF (Table 18.2) (Osame 1990). The weakness of lower extremities is symmetric, and disease progression usually occurs slowly. In addition, in some cases, symptoms are static after initial progression. In over 60% of patients with HAM/TSP, weakness of the lower limbs is the first symptom. In contrast, weakness in the arms is rarely present. Almost all patients show spastic weakness

---

TABLE 18.2
Diagnostic Guidelines for HAM/TSP

I. Clinical criteria

The florid clinical picture of chronic spastic paraparesis is not always seen when the patient first presents. A single symptom or physical sign may be the only evidence of early HAM/TSP.

A. Age and sex incidence

Mostly sporadic and adult, but sometimes familial, occasionally seen in childhood; females predominant

B. Onset

This is usually insidious but may be sudden

C. Main neurological manifestations

1. Chronic spastic paraparesis, which usually progresses slowly, sometimes remains static after initial progression
2. Weakness of the lower limbs more marked proximally
3. Bladder disturbance usually an early feature. Constipation usually occurs later; impotence or decreased libido is common
4. Sensory symptoms such as tingling, pins and needles, burning, etc., are more prominent than objective physical signs
5. Low lumbar pain with radiation to the legs is common
6. Vibration sense is usually impaired; proprioception is less often affected
7. Hyperreflexia of the lower limbs, often with clonus and Babinski sign
8. Hyperreflexia of upper limbs; positive Hoffmann and Trömner signs are common; weakness may be absent
9. Exaggerated jaw jerk in some patients

D. Less frequent neurological findings

Cerebellar signs, optic atrophy, deafness, nystagmus, other cranial nerve deficits, hand tremor, absent, or depressed ankle jerk. Convulsions, cognitive impairment, dementia, or impaired consciousness are rare

E. Other neurological manifestations that may be associated with HAM/TSP:

Muscular atrophy, fasciculations (rare), polymyositis, peripheral neuropathy, polyradiculopathy, cranial neuropathy, meningitis, encephalopathy

F. Systemic nonneurological manifestations that may be associated with HAM/TSP:

Pulmonary alveolitis, uveitis, Sjören syndrome, arthropathy, vasculitis, ichthyosis, cryoglobulinemia, monoclonal gammopathy, adult T-cell leukemia/lymphoma

II. Laboratory diagnosis

A. Presence of HTLV-1 antibodies or antigens in blood and cerebrospinal fluid (CSF)
B. CSF may show mild lymphocyte pleocytosis
C. Lobulated lymphocyte may be present in blood and/or CSF
D. Mild to moderate increase of protein may be present in CSF
E. Viral isolation when possible from blood and/or CSF

in the lower extremities, hyperreflexia, and extensor plantar responses. Although the strength of the arms is usually preserved, brisk deep tendon reflexes tend to develop in the upper extremities (Nakagawa et al. 1995). Bladder dysfunction is the other common symptom in HAM/TSP patients. Patients often experience urinary frequency, urgency, or incontinence (Oliveira et al. 2007). Coexistence of irritative and obstructive urinary dysfunction is characteristic of HAM/TSP, and urinary symptoms sometimes occur before the development of weakness of the lower extremities. Urodynamic studies usually reveal an overactive bladder, and detrusor sphincter dyssynergia (DDS) is also common. Constipation, back pain, and sensory disturbance/numbness in the lower limbs are also common symptoms. Numbness in the lower limbs is usually mild. In patients with a longer clinical course, autonomic dysfunctions such as dyshidrosis, orthostatic hypotension, and impotence are also observed. In addition, small numbers of patients show finger tremor, cerebellar signs, and mild cognitive impairment.

The main laboratory finding is high antibody titers against HTLV-I in both serum and CSF (Osame 1990). Atypical lymphocytes called "flower cells" are sometimes observed in peripheral blood and CSF (Figure 18.5) (Osame and Igata 1989). Various systemic laboratory abnormalities are also found in HAM/TSP patients. Hypergammaglobulinemia and increased $\beta2$-microglobulin are also found in the serum. In the CSF, pleocytosis and elevation of protein concentration are common abnormal findings. Increased neopterin concentration in CSF is also observed (Nakagawa et al. 1995; Nomoto et al. 1991). The presence of oligoclonal IgG bands, elevated concentrations of various cytokines such as TNF-α and IL-6, and increased intrathecal antibody synthesis specific for HTLV-I have also been reported (Hollsberg and Hafler 1993; Link et al. 1989; Osame et al. 1987).

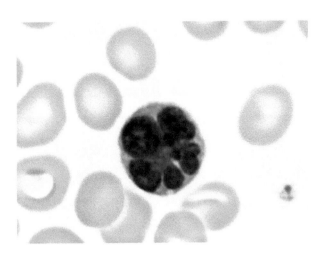

FIGURE 18.5 "Flower cell" in the peripheral blood. Flower cells are atypical lymphoid cells with lobulated nuclei. They are commonly observed in the peripheral blood of HTLV-1 infected individuals, but less common in the CSF of HAM/TP patients. (Courtesy of Dr. Fukushima, Division of Hematology, Department of Internal Medicine, Faculty of Medicine, Saga University, Saga, Japan.)

On neuroradiological aspects, thoracic cord atrophy without signal intensity changes on magnetic resonance images (MRI) is accepted to be characteristic of HAM/TSP, but its incidence is varied, ranging from 20% to 74% (Alcindor et al. 1992; Bagnato et al. 2005; Ferraz et al. 1997). In addition, reports of HAM/TSP patients with signal intensity changes on MRI have been reported (Shakudo et al. 1999; Umehara et al. 2006; Watanabe et al. 2001). In our study, the MRI findings of the spinal cord can be classified into three types: "normal" (57.9%), "atrophy" (34.2%), and "T2 hyperintensity" (7.9%) (Figure 18.6). Spinal cord atrophy on

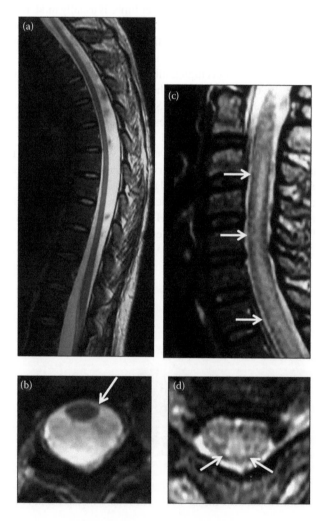

FIGURE 18.6 Spinal cord MR images in the atrophy, and T2 hyperintensity type of HAM/TSP patients. Diffuse spinal cord atrophy (arrow in panel b) was observed on T2WI in the atrophy type (a, sagittal image; b, axial image of the thoracic cord at the Th7 spine level). Diffuse hyperintensity areas (arrows in panels c and d) were observed on T2WI (c, sagittal image at the cervical spine; d, axial image of the cervical cord at the C7 spine level).

MRI was shown to have little value for the prediction of prognosis of disability or responsiveness to interferon α therapy. In contrast, HAM/TSP patients showing T2 hyperintensity tend to show subacute onset and rapid progression of severe paraparesis of lower extremities (Yukitake et al. 2008b). Chronic progressive HAM/TPS patients with T2 hyperintensity in the cervical cord were also reported (Umehara et al. 2004).

A subacute progressive form of HAM/TSP, which progresses to a severe stage within a few months, is also known (Lima et al. 2007; Nakagawa et al. 1995; Yukitake et al. 2008b). Nakagawa et al. (1995) found 14 patients (9.2%) showing rapid progression of motor impairments within two years among 153 HAM/TSP patients. As mentioned above, the subacute progressive form of HAM/TSP sometimes shows T2 hyperintensity on spinal MRI. Furthermore, the incidence of the subacute progressive form of HAM/TSP (9.2%) is similar to that of T2 hyperintensity on spinal MRI (7.9%). Taking these finding together, the incidence of a clinically malignant form of HAM/TSP, which usually shows T2 hyperintensity on spinal MRI, is estimated to be less than 10%. In laboratory findings, the subacute progressive form of HAM/TSP tends to show increased CSF IgG levels, high CSF anti-HTLV-I antibody titers, and increased CSF neopterin concentration (Kuroda et al. 1991; Nakagawa et al. 1995). For the treatment of such rapid progression, high doses of methylprednisolone are sometimes given intravenously, but the efficacy is limited. HAM/TSP patients with suspected HTLV-I infection via blood transfusion or organ transplantation also show relatively fast progression in some cases (Kuroda et al. 1992). Summarized clinical features of HAM/TSP are shown in Table 18.3.

TABLE 18.3
Summarized Clinical Features of HAM/TSP

	Neurological Manifestations	Laboratory/MRI Findings
Main findings	Spastic paraparesis	Presence of HTLV-I antibody in both
	Neurogenic bladder	serum and CSF
Common	Hyperreflexia of upper limbs	Mild pleocytosis in CSF
	Impaired vibration sense	Elevation of protein in CSF
	Sensory disturbance of lower limbs	
	Low lumbar pain	Normal spinal MRI findings (around 60%)
Less common	Hand tremor	Flower cells in CSF
	Cerebellar sign	
	Peripheral neuropathy	Spinal cord atrophy on MRI (over 30%)
Rare	Subacute progressive myelopathy	T2 hyperintensity on spinal MRI
	Dementia	(less than 10%)
	Leukoencephalopathy	
	ALS-like manifestation	

Note: CSF, cerebrospinal fluid; ALS: amyotrophic lateral sclerosis.

18.4 RISK FACTORS FOR HAM/TSP

The prevalence of HAM/TSP is only 0.1%–5% in HTLV-I-infected individuals, and the remaining individuals spend their lifetime as asymptomatic carriers. The lifetime risk of developing HAM/TSP among carriers is estimated to be 0.23% in Japan. Therefore, HTLV-I is necessary but not sufficient to develop HAM/TSP. Although the crucial risk factors for the development of HAM/TSP among HTLV-I carriers are still unknown, several factors have been considered. Female predominance (female/male, 2–2.3:1) has been reported. Although HAM/TSP can develop at all ages, many HAM/TSP patients notice the neurological impairments at middle age. HTLV-I PVL is considered as an important risk factor for the development of HAM/TSP. Several studies have shown that HTLV-I PVL in PBMCs of HAM/TSP patients is about five to sixteen fold higher than that of asymptomatic carriers (Hashimoto et al. 1998; Kubota et al. 1993; Nagai et al. 1998). It has also been reported that the prevalence of HAM/TSP increased as HTLV-I PVL exceeded 1% in PBMCs. In CSF, HTLV-I PVL of HAM/TSP patients also increased compared with that in the PBMCs. In particular, it is noteworthy that the ratio of HTLV-I PVL in CSF cells to that in PBMCs was significantly associated with clinical progression of HAM/TSP and with recent onset of HAM/TSP (Takenouchi et al. 2003). These observations strongly suggest that increased HTLV-I PVL is a strong risk factor associated with clinical progression of HAM/TSP. HTLV-I tax expression is also considered to be a risk factor for HAM/TSP. The level of HTLV-I tax mRNA expression in HTLV-I-infected cells was significantly higher in HAM/TSP patients than in asymptomatic carriers (Yamano et al. 2002), and this finding correlated with the HTLV-I proviral load, Tax-specific CD8[+] T-cell frequency, and disease severity. It has also been shown that persistent HTLV-I gene expression *in vivo* was necessary for the maintenance of HTLV-I PVL (Asquith et al. 2007). In the view of genomic integrations, it was reported that transcriptionally active genomic regions in HTLV-I determine the rate of HTLV-I proviral expression (Meekings et al. 2008). It has been suspected that the genomic integration of HTLV-I to certain regions may induce high HTLV-I tax expression, and subsequent tax-induced proliferation that defines HTLV-I PVL. Thus, both HTLV-I tax expression and HTLV-I PVL may drive the expansion of HTLV-I-specific CTLs (Bangham et al. 2009).

Although HTLV-I tax expression is thought to be a risk factor, HTLV-I tax expression in PBMCs of HAM/TSP is less frequent. Recently, HBZ has also been considered as not only part of the pathogenesis of HAM/TSP but also having a correlation with disease severity, with much higher expression than HTLV-I tax (Saito et al. 2009; Satou et al. 2011). It has been reported that HTLV-I HBZ mRNA load in PBMCs was significantly correlated with HTLV-I PVL, neopterin concentrations in CSF, and motor disability in HAM/TSP patients (Saito et al. 2009).

Although HTLV-I PVL is an important risk factor for HAM/TSP, HTLV-I PVL observed in both HAM/TSP patients and asymptomatic carriers is varied and overlapping (Nagai et al. 1998). Interestingly, HTLV-I PVL in asymptomatic carriers with HAM/TSP in their families was higher than in asymptomatic carriers without HAM/TSP in their families. On the other hand, it has been thought that the sequence of HTLV-I varies little other than in terms of the tax gene within or between hosts.

These data suggest that genetic factors in hosts cause variation in HTLV-I PVL among HTLV-I-infected individuals. In human leukocyte antigen (HLA) class I, HLA-A*02 and Cw*08 were found to be independently associated with a lower risk of developing HAM/TSP. The association between these two class I alleles and low HTLV-I PVL was observed in an asymptomatic carrier group (Jeffery et al. 2000; Vine et al. 2002). On the other hand, HLA-B*5401 was associated with higher HTLV-I PVL and an increased risk of developing HAM/TSP (Vine et al. 2002). These results suggest that HLA class I-restricted immune responses influence HTLV-I PVL. In HLA class I, HLA-DRB1*0101 increased the risk of HAM/TSP (Jeffery et al. 2000). Interestingly, these associations between HLA genotypes and susceptibility to HAM/TSP sometimes show different results among ethnic groups. Other genetic factors have also been reported. Polymorphisms of TNF-α, stromal-cell-derived factor 1, and IL-15 were shown to influence the outcome of HTLV-I infection (Vine et al. 2002). Polymorphism in the IL-10 promoter was also reported to affect both HTLV-I PVL and risk of developing HAM/TSP (Sabouri et al. 2004). On the viral side, an association between HTLV-I tax gene sequence variation and the risk of HAM/TSP was reported. This previous study demonstrated that the HTLV-I tax subgroup A was more frequently observed in HAM/TSP than in asymptomatic carriers (Furukawa et al. 2000).

18.5   TREATMENT OF HAM/TSP

Although numerous therapeutic trials have been reported, there is no definitive treatment for HAM/TSP (Izumo et al. 1996; Nagai and Osame 2002; Nakagawa et al. 1996; Nakamura 2009). On the basis of the pathogenesis of HAM/TSP as mentioned above, two main strategies should be considered: immunomodulatory therapy and antiviral therapy. The strategies of immunomodulatory therapies for the suppression of chronic inflammatory status with immune activation can be characterized as follows: suppression of immune activation, especially that caused by HTLV-I-infected cells, inhibition of the transmigration of HTLV-I-infected cells into the spinal cord, and reduction of chronic inflammation in the spinal cord via the down-regulation of proinflammatory cytokines and/or adhesion molecule expression. On the other hand, the therapies focusing on antiviral effects are divided mainly into three parts: suppression of HTLV-I expression and/or replication, inhibition of the proliferation of HTLV-I-infected cells, and elimination of HTLV-I-infected cells.

18.5.1   Immunomodulatory Therapy for the Treatment of HAM/TSP

18.5.1.1   Interferon α and β

IFN-α and IFN-β are classified as type I IFNs and have various biological functions including immunomodulation and antiviral effects. Among various therapeutic agents for HAM/TSP, IFN-α is the only agent to have been proven as effective in multiple, randomized, double-blind, and controlled trials (Izumo et al. 1996). Therapeutic effects were observed in a dose-dependent manner, and significant improvements of motor and urinary dysfunctions were observed in about 70% of HAM/TSP patients treated with 3.0 MU of IFN-α. Therapeutic benefits continued for 4 weeks after the trial without serious adverse effects. Significant decrease of spontaneous PBL proliferation *in vitro* was observed. HTLV-I proviral loads in the peripheral blood were significantly decreased in combination with the reduction of memory T cells among CD8^{high+} T cells. These observations suggested that the reduction of HTLV-I proviral loads or HTLV-I tax mRNA expression in the peripheral blood occurred under IFN-α therapy for HAM/TSP. These findings probably show that one of the immune mechanisms of IFN-α therapy for HAM/TSP is a correction of Th1/Th2 imbalance, which is thought to deviate toward Th1 in HAM/TSP.

IFN-β has also been reported for the treatment of HAM/TSP (Oh et al. 2005). As well as the improvements of motor dysfunctions, reductions of HTLV-I tax mRNA load and the frequency of HTLV-I-specific CD8$^+$ T cells were observed in the peripheral blood. Significant decrease of spontaneous PBL proliferation *in vitro* was also observed. Interestingly, HTLV-I proviral loads in the peripheral blood remained unchanged.

Although the effects of HTLV-I proviral loads were different, both IFN-α and IFN-β have been thought to have efficacy for the treatment of HAM/TSP via immuno-modulatory mechanisms such as correction of Th1/Th2 imbalance.

18.5.1.2 Corticosteroid Hormone

Corticosteroid has been shown to be an efficient agent for various inflammatory and autoimmune diseases. As HAM/TSP is a chronic inflammatory disease in spinal cord showing immunopathological features, corticosteroid has been one of the most popular agents for the treatment of HAM/TSP. Although high doses of methylprednisolone are sometimes given intravenously, oral prednisolone (PSL) has been the most popular treatment for HAM/TSP. Short-term efficacy of PSL treatment for HAM/TSP has been reported (Nakagawa et al. 1996). In this study, 107 of 131 HAM/TSP patients (81.7%) showed improvement of motor functions. On the other hand, data showing nonefficient or transient benefit of PSL treatment for HAM/TSP have also been reported. In addition, the long-term efficacy of PSL treatment for HAM/TSP is unclear because of several adverse effects such as opportunistic infections, gastric ulcer, glucose intolerance, hypertension, and osteoporosis. Although the efficacy of PSL treatment for HAM/TSP seems to be limited, it has to be mentioned that HTLV-I proviral loads in PBMCs of HAM/TSP patients were significantly decreased in PSL treatment over 5 years.

18.5.1.3 Other Immunomodulatory Agents for the Treatment of HAM/TSP

Blood purification (plasmapheresis and lymphocytapheresis), oral administration of pentoxifylline, intravenous heparin administration, high-dose intravenous gamma-globulin administration, intermittent high-dose oral administration of vitamin C, intravenous administration of fosfomycin followed by oral administration of erythromycin, and fermented milk drink were applied in attempts to treat HAM/TSP (Nakagawa et al. 1996; Nakamura et al. 2009). In general, these agents had less adverse effects, but the efficacy for HAM/TSP tended to be limited and transient.

18.5.1.4 Antiviral Therapy for the Treatment of HAM/TSP

As mentioned above, IFN-α and IFN-β are considered as having both antiviral effects and immunomodulatory effects.

Some nucleoside reverse-transcriptase inhibitors, such as zidovudine, lamivudine, tenofovir, abacavir, zalcitabine, and stavudine, have successfully inhibited HTLV-I replication (Hill et al. 2003). Treatment with zidovudine, a thymidine analogue, at a high dose in 10 HAM/TSP patients for 24 weeks showed clinical benefits in some patients without referring to the changes of HTLV-I proviral loads. In a lamivudine therapeutic trial on 5 HAM/TSP patients, significant reduction of HTLV-I proviral loads in the PBMCs was observed in all 5 patients, but clinical improvements were observed in only 1 patient. However, a clinical trial with combination therapy by zidovudine and lamivudine in a randomized, double-blind, placebo-controlled study showed no significant results in terms of both clinical features and laboratory findings (Taylor et al. 2006).

The use of anti-Tac, an antibody to the IL-2 receptor (IL-2R), was also attempted for the treatment of HAM/TSP patients. Productions of IL-2 and IL-2R by HTLV-I tax transactivation in HTLV-I-infected cells are thought to dysregulate cellular gene expression by HTLV-I tax, and this dysregulation is believed to initiate a process of T-cell activation and proliferation by autocrine or paracrine loop. Thus, IL-2 and/or IL-2R blockage might decrease HTLV-I-infected cells through apoptosis of HTLV-I-infected cells by IL-2 deprivation. Treatment for HAM/TSP patients using daclizumab, humanized anti-Tac antibody, showed mild improvement of motor disability in three of nine patients without serious adverse effects (Lehky et al. 1998). In terms of anti-HTLV-I effects, selective down-regulation of activated T cells expressing IL-2R receptor in the PBMCs and a decrease of spontaneous proliferation of PBMCs were observed. In addition, HTLV-I proviral load in the PBMCs was markedly reduced after the treatment. These results suggest that humanized anti-Tac antibody has the efficacy to reduce IL-2R-presenting HTLV-I-infected cells in the peripheral blood of HAM/TSP patients.

Anti-CC chemokine receptor 4 (CCR4) antibodies, which is another humanized antibody, might also be considered for use in the treatment of HAM/TSP in future. Anti-CCR4 antibody has a strong antibody-dependent cellular cytotoxic effect, and favorable results in a phase I study of anti-CCR4 antibody focused on the treatment of relapsed CCR4-positive ATL and peripheral T-cell lymphoma have been presented (Yamamoto et al. 2010).

Some favorable anti-HTLV-I results for histone deacetylase enzyme inhibitor and prosultiamine have also been reported in the treatment of HAM/TSP (Nakamura 2009; Nakamura et al. 2009).

18.5.2 Symptomatic Treatment

Symptomatic treatment is still an important arm of HAM/TSP therapy because many of these therapies are tolerable in the long term (Araujo and Silva 2006; Goncalves et al. 2010). Antispastic drugs are used to reduce spasticity, but the efficacy is usually limited. Rehabilitation programs are also useful for HAM/TSP patients. In progressive cases of HAM/TSP, patients often use a cane and/or a wheelchair. For neurological bladder, the best bladder management is intermittent cleaning catheterization associated with an anticholinergic drug and an antispastic muscle agent. Because urinary tract infections, such as cystitis and pyelonephritis, are common in HAM/

TSP patients, antibiotic agents are used when the active infections are observed. Renal and ureteral lithiasis, vesicoureteral reflux, and chronic renal failure sometimes coexist with HAM/TSP. Analgesics are also used for the treatment of pain and dysesthesia associated with myelopathy, elevated muscle tones, and joint contractures. Constipation is a very common bowel dysfunction. Not only the use of laxative products, but also adequate and timely food and fluid intake, should be considered.

18.6 OTHER NEUROMUSCULAR DISORDERS ASSOCIATED WITH HTLV-I INFECTION

It is also known that people with HTLV-I infection sometimes develop not only HAM/TSP and ATL but also other nonneuromuscular or neuromuscular disorders. The same as for HAM/TSP, the pathogenic association between these disorders and HTLV-I infection is still unclear.

In nonneuromuscular disorders, uveitis, alveolitis, arthritis, dermatitis, opportunistic infections, Sjögren syndrome, and SLE have been reported as possibly associated with HTLV-I infection (Goncalves et al. 2010; Verdonck et al. 2007).

In neuromuscular disorders, the following disorders have been discussed (Araujo and Silva 2006; Goncalves et al. 2010; Verdonck et al. 2007). Inflammatory muscle disorders in HTLV-I-infected individuals with and without myelopathy have been reported. Pathological studies have demonstrated that HTLV-I proviral DNA and HTLV-I tax expression were observed in the infiltrating cells but not in muscle fibers in patients with HTLV-I-seropositive polymyositis (Higuchi et al. 1995). In inclusion body myositis (IBM), which is also common in elderly people, it has also been observed that HTLV-I proviral DNA and HTLV-I tax mRNA were present in the infiltrating cells (Matsuura et al. 2008). Although peripheral neuropathies sometimes coexist in HAM/TSP, those in HTLV-I-infected individuals without myelopathy have also been reported (Kiwaki et al. 2003). The incidence of peripheral neuropathies in HTLV-I-seropositive individuals is reportedly higher (8.6%) than that in HTLV-I-seronegative individuals (2.6%). Other neurological impairments such as amyotrophic lateral sclerosis-like syndrome, cognitive deficits, depression, dysautonomia, leukoencephalopathy, cerebellar ataxia, ophthalmological diseases, and meningitis are reported in HTLV-I-seropositive individuals (Araujo and Silva 2006; Goncalves et al. 2010; Verdonck et al. 2007). It is important that we consider the difficulty in proving a true association between HTLV-I infection and these neurological manifestations. Unlike for HAM/TSP, we have limited data to prove strong associations between HTLV-I infection and these neurological manifestations.

18.7 HTLV-II AND NEUROLOGICAL DISEASES

HTLV-II is closely related to HTLV-I with approximately 70% genomic homology. HTLV-II is endemic in Native Americans and epidemic in injecting drug abusers worldwide. The mode of transmission of HTLV-II is similar to that of HTLV-I. Breastfeeding, sexual transmission, contaminated blood products, and intravenous drug abuse are established modes of transmission. Clinical features of HTLV-II-associated neurological diseases are also similar to those of HAM/TSP (Araujo and Hall 2004). Although HTLV-II-associated diseases have been reported less frequently than HAM/TSP, the main neurological feature is chronic progressive myelopathy resembling HAM/TSP, but with much lower frequency. Spinal cord atrophy has been the most common abnormal feature on spinal MRI. Abnormal T2 high intensities with or without cord swelling have also been reported on spinal MRI. On head MRI, high-intensity signals in the periventricular and subcortical white matter on T2-weighted images are frequent abnormal features. In contrast with HTLV-I, the role of HTLV-II in the development of neurological disorders has been much less clear. In addition, concomitant HIV infection makes its difficult to prove the exact association between HTLV-II and such neurological diseases.

REFERENCES

Abe, M., Umehara, F., Kubota, R., Moritoyo, T., Izumo, S., and Osame, M. 1999. Activation of macrophages/microglia with the calcium-binding proteins MRP14 and MRP8 is related to the lesional activities in the spinal cord of HTLV-I associated myelopathy. *J. Neurol.* 246, 358–364.

Akizuki, S., Setoguchi, M., Nakazato, O., Yoshida, S., Higuchi, Y., Yamamoto, S., and Okajima, T. 1988. An autopsy case of human T-lymphotropic virus type I-associated myelopathy. *Hum. Pathol.* 19, 988–990.

Albrecht, B., and Lairmore, M. D. 2002. Critical role of human T-lymphotropic virus type 1 accessory proteins in viral replication and pathogenesis. *Microbiol. Mol. Biol. Rev.* 66, 396–406.

Alcindor, F., Valderrama, R., Canavaggio, M., Lee, H., Katz, A., Montesinos, C., Madrid, R. E., Merino, R. R., and Pipia, P. A. 1992. Imaging of human T-lymphotropic virus type I-associated chronic progressive myeloneuropathies. *Neuroradiology* 35, 69–74.

Araujo, A., and Hall, W. W. 2004. Human T-lymphotropic virus type II and neurological disease. *Ann. Neurol.* 56, 10–19.

Araujo, A. Q., and Silva, M. T. 2006. The HTLV-1 neurological complex. *Lancet Neurol.* 5, 1068–1076.

Asquith, B., Zhang, Y., Mosley, A. J., de Lara, C. M., Wallace, D. L., Worth, A., Kaftantzi, L., Meekings, K., Griffin, G. E., Tanaka, Y., Tough, D. F., Beverley, P. C., Taylor, G. P., Macallan, D. C., and Bangham, C. R. 2007. *In vivo* T lymphocyte dynamics in humans and the impact of human T-lymphotropic virus 1 infection. *Proc. Natl. Acad. Sci. U S A* 104, 8035–8040.

Aye, M. M., Matsuoka, E., Moritoyo, T., Umehara, F., Suehara, M., Hokezu, Y., Yamanaka, H., Isashiki, Y., Osame, M., and Izumo, S. 2000. Histopathological analysis of four autopsy cases of HTLV-I-associated myelopathy/tropical spastic paraparesis: inflammatory changes occur simultaneously in the entire central nervous system. *Acta Neuropathol.* 100, 245–252.

Bagnato, F., Butman, J. A., Mora, C. A., Gupta, S., Yamano, Y., Tasciyan, T. A., Solomon, J. M., Santos, W. J., Stone, R. D., McFarland, H. F., and Jacobson, S. 2005. Conventional magnetic resonance imaging features in patients with tropical spastic paraparesis. *J. Neurovirol.* 11, 525–534.

Bangham, C. R., Meekings, K., Toulza, F., Nejmeddine, M., Majorovits, E., Asquith, B., and Taylor, G. P. 2009. The immune control of HTLV-1 infection: selection forces and dynamics. *Front Biosci.* 14, 2889–2903.

Biggar, R. J., Ng, J., Kim, N., Hisada, M., Li, H. C., Cranston, B., Hanchard, B., and Maloney, E. M. 2006. Human leukocyte antigen concordance and the transmission risk via breast-feeding of human T cell lymphotropic virus type I. *J. Infect Dis.* 193, 277–282.

Cabre, P., al-Fahim, A., and Oger, J. 1999. Enhanced adherence of endothelial cells blood mononuclear cells in HAM/TSP. *Rev. Neurol. (Paris)* 155, 273–279.

Carneiro-Proietti, A. B., Catalan-Soares, B., and Proietti, F. A. 2002. Human T cell lymphotropic viruses (HTLV-I/II) in South America: should it be a public health concern? *J. Biomed. Sci.* 9, 587–595.

Ciminale, V., Pavlakis, G. N., Derse, D., Cunningham, C. P., and Felber, B. K. 1992. Complex splicing in the human T-cell leukemia virus (HTLV) family of retroviruses: novel mRNAs and proteins produced by HTLV type I. *J. Virol.* 66, 1737–1745.

de The, G., and Bomford, R. 1993. An HTLV-I vaccine: why, how, for whom? *AIDS Res Hum. Retroviruses* 9, 381–386.

de The, G., and Kazanji, M. 1996. An HTLV-I/II vaccine: from animal model to clinical trials? *J. Acquir. Immune Defic. Syndr. Hum. Retrovirol.* 13(Suppl 1), S191–S198.

Donegan, E., Busch, M. P., Galleshaw, J. A., Shaw, G. M., and Mosley, J. W. 1990. Transfusion of blood components from a donor with human T-lymphotropic virus type II (HTLV-II) infection. The Transfusion Safety Study Group. *Ann. Intern. Med.* 113, 555–556.

Dumas, M., Houinato, D., Verdier, M., Zohoun, T., Josse, R., Bonis, J., Zohoun, I., Massougbodji, A., and Denis, F. 1991. Seroepidemiology of human T-cell lymphotropic virus type I/II in Benin (West Africa). *AIDS Res. Hum. Retroviruses* 7, 447–451.

Feigal, E., Murphy, E., Vranizan, K., Bacchetti, P., Chaisson, R., Drummond, J. E., Blattner, W., McGrath, M., Greenspan, J., and Moss, A. 1991. Human T cell lymphotropic virus types I and II in intravenous drug users in San Francisco: risk factors associated with seropositivity. *J. Infect Dis.* 164, 36–42.

Ferraz, A. C., Gabbai, A. A., Abdala, N., and Nogueira, R. G. 1997. [Magnetic resonance in HTL-I associated myelopathy. Leukoencephalopathy and spinal cord atrophy]. *Arq. Neuropsiquiatr.* 55, 728–736.

Furukawa, Y., Yamashita, M., Usuku, K., Izumo, S., Nakagawa, M., and Osame, M. 2000. Phylogenetic subgroups of human T cell lymphotropic virus (HTLV) type I in the tax gene and their association with different risks for HTLV-I-associated myelopathy/tropical spastic paraparesis. *J. Infect Dis.* 182, 1343–1349.

Gessain, A., Barin, F., Vernant, J. C., Gout, O., Maurs, L., Calender, A., and de The, G. 1985. Antibodies to human T-lymphotropic virus type-I in patients with tropical spastic paraparesis. *Lancet* 2, 407–410.

Goncalves, D. U., Proietti, F. A., Ribas, J. G., Araujo, M. G., Pinheiro, S. R., Guedes, A. C., and Carneiro-Proietti, A. B. 2010. Epidemiology, treatment, and prevention of human T-cell leukemia virus type 1-associated diseases. *Clin. Microbiol. Rev.* 23, 577–589.

Guiltinan, A. M., Murphy, E. L., Horton, J. A., Nass, C. C., McEntire, R. L., and Watanabe, K. 1998. Psychological distress in blood donors notified of HTLV-I/II infection. Retrovirus Epidemiology Donor Study. *Transfusion* 38, 1056–1062.

Hashimoto, K., Higuchi, I., Osame, M., and Izumo, S. 1998. Quantitative *in situ* PCR assay of HTLV-1 infected cells in peripheral blood lymphocytes of patients with ATL, HAM/TSP and asymptomatic carriers. *J. Neurol. Sci.* 159, 67–72.

Higuchi, I., Hashimoto, K., Kashio, N., Izumo, S., Inose, M., Izumi, K., Ohkubo, R., Nakagawa, M., Arimura, K., and Osame, M. 1995. Detection of HTLV-I provirus by *in situ* polymerase chain reaction in mononuclear inflammatory cells in skeletal muscle of viral carriers with polymyositis. *Muscle Nerve* 18, 854–858.

Hill, S. A., Lloyd, P. A., McDonald, S., Wykoff, J., and Derse, D. 2003. Susceptibility of human T cell leukemia virus type I to nucleoside reverse transcriptase inhibitors. *J. Infect Dis.* 188, 424–427.

Hollsberg, P., and Hafler, D. A. 1993. Seminars in medicine of the Beth Israel Hospital, Boston. Pathogenesis of diseases induced by human lymphotropic virus type I infection. *N. Engl. J. Med.* 328, 1173–1182.

Iwasaki, Y. 1990. Pathology of chronic myelopathy associated with HTLV-Iinfection (HAM/TSP). *J. Neurol. Sci.* 96, 103–123.

Iwasaki, Y., Sawada, K., Aiba, I., Mukai, E., Yoshida, M., Hashizume, Y., and Sobue, G. 2004. Widespread active inflammatory lesions in a case of HTLV-I-associated myelopathy lasting 29 years. *Acta Neuropathol.* 108, 546–551.

Izumo, S. 2010. Neuropathology of HTLV-1-associated myelopathy (HAM/TSP). *Neuropathology* 30, 480–485.

Izumo, S., Goto, I., Itoyama, Y., Okajima, T., Watanabe, S., Kuroda, Y., Araki, S., Mori, M., Nagataki, S., Matsukura, S., Akamine, T., Nakagawa, M., Yamamoto, I., and Osame, M. 1996. Interferon-alpha is effective in HTLV-I-associated myelopathy: a multicenter, randomized, double-blind, controlled trial. *Neurology* 46, 1016–1021.

Jeffery, K. J., Siddiqui, A. A., Bunce, M., Lloyd, A. L., Vine, A. M., Witkover, A. D., Izumo, S., Usuku, K., Welsh, K. I., Osame, M., and Bangham, C. R. 2000. The influence of HLA class I alleles and heterozygosity on the outcome of human T cell lymphotropic virus type I infection. *J. Immunol.* 165, 7278–7284.

Johnson, J. M., Harrod, R., and Franchini, G. 2001. Molecular biology and pathogenesis of the human T-cell leukaemia/lymphotropic virus type-1 (HTLV-1). *Int. J. Exp. Pathol.* 82, 135–147.

Kaplan, J. E., Osame, M., Kubota, H., Igata, A., Nishitani, H., Maeda, Y., Khabbaz, R. F., and Janssen, R. S. 1990. The risk of development of HTLV-I-associated myelopathy/tropical spastic paraparesis among persons infected with HTLV-I. *J. Acquir. Immune Defic. Syndr.* 3, 1096–1101.

Kiwaki, T., Umehara, F., Arimura, Y., Izumo, S., Arimura, K., Itoh, K., and Osame, M. 2003. The clinical and pathological features of peripheral neuropathy accompanied with HTLV-I associated myelopathy. *J. Neurol. Sci.* 206, 17–21.

Kubota, R., Fujiyoshi, T., Izumo, S., Yashiki, S., Maruyama, I., Osame, M., and Sonoda, S. 1993. Fluctuation of HTLV-I proviral DNA in peripheral blood mononuclear cells of HTLV-I-associated myelopathy. *J. Neuroimmunol.* 42, 147–154.

Kuroda, Y., Fujiyama, F., and Nagumo, F. 1991. Analysis of factors of relevance to rapid clinical progression in HTLV-I-associated myelopathy. *J. Neurol. Sci.* 105, 61–66.

Kuroda, Y., Takashima, H., Yukitake, M., and Sakemi, T. 1992. Development of HTLV-I-associated myelopathy after blood transfusion in a patient with aplastic anemia and a recipient of a renal transplant. *J. Neurol. Sci.* 109, 196–199.

Lehky, T. J., Levin, M. C., Kubota, R., Bamford, R. N., Flerlage, A. N., Soldan, S. S. Leist, T. P., Xavier, A., White, J. D., Brown, M., Fleisher, T. A., Top, L. E., Light, S., McFarland, H. F., Waldmann, T. A., and Jacobson, S. 1998. Reduction in HTLV-I proviral load and spontaneous lymphoproliferation in HTLV-I-associated myelopathy/tropical spastic paraparesis patients treated with humanized anti-Tac. *Ann. Neurol.* 44, 942–947.

Lemasson, I., Lewis, M. R., Polakowski, N., Hivin, P., Cavanagh, M. H., Thebault, S., Barbeau, B., Nyborg, J. K., and Mesnard, J. M. 2007. Human T-cell leukemia virus type 1 (HTLV-1) bZIP protein interacts with the cellular transcription factor CREB to inhibit HTLV-1 transcription. *J. Virol.* 81, 1543–1553.

Levin, M. C., Krichavsky, M., Berk, J., Foley, S., Rosenfeld, M., Dalmau, J., Chang, G., Posner, J. B., and Jacobson, S. 1998. Neuronal molecular mimicry in immune-mediated neurologic disease. *Ann. Neurol.* 44, 87–98.

Levine, P. H., Blattner, W. A., Clark, J., Tarone, R., Maloney, E. M., Murphy, E. M., Gallo, R. C., Robert-Guroff, M., and Saxinger, W. C. 1988. Geographic distribution of HTLV-I and identification of a new high-risk population. *Int. J. Cancer.* 42, 7–12.

Lima, M. A., Harab, R. C., Schor, D., Andrada-Serpa, M. J., and Araujo, A. Q. 2007. Subacute progression of human T-lymphotropic virus type I-associated myelopathy/tropical spastic paraparesis. *J. Neurovirol.* 13, 468–473.

Link, H., Cruz, M., Gessain, A., Gout, O., de The, G., and Kam-Hansen, S. 1989. Chronic progressive myelopathy associated with HTLV-I: oligoclonal IgG and anti-HTLV-I IgG antibodies in cerebrospinal fluid and serum. *Neurology* 39, 1566–1572.

Matsuoka, E., Takenouchi, N., Hashimoto, K., Kashio, N., Moritoyo, T., Higuchi, I., Isashiki, Y., Sato, E., Osame, M., and Izumo, S. 1998. Perivascular T cells are infected with HTLV-I in the spinal cord lesions with HTLV-I-associated myelopathy/tropical spastic paraparesis: double staining of immunohistochemistry and polymerase chain reaction *in situ* hybridization. *Acta Neuropathol.* 96, 340–346.

Matsuura, E., Umehara, F., Nose, H., Higuchi, I., Matsuoka, E., Izumi, K., Kubota, R., Saito, M., Izumo, S., Arimura, K., and Osame, M. 2008. Inclusion body myositis associated with human T-lymphotropic virus-type I infection: eleven patients from an endemic area in Japan. *J. Neuropathol. Exp. Neurol.* 67, 41–49.

Matsuura, E., Yamano, Y., and Jacobson, S. 2010. Neuroimmunity of HTLV-I Infection. *J. Neuroimmune Pharmacol.* 5, 310–325.

Meekings, K. N., Leipzig, J., Bushman, F. D., Taylor, G. P., and Bangham, C. R. 2008. HTLV-1 integration into transcriptionally active genomic regions is associated with proviral expression and with HAM/TSP. *PLoS Pathog.* 4, e1000027.

Moritoyo, T., Reinhart, T. A., Moritoyo, H., Sato, E., Izumo, S., Osame, M., and Haase, A. T. 1996. Human T-lymphotropic virus type I-associated myelopathy and tax gene expression in CD4+ T lymphocytes. *Ann. Neurol.* 40, 84–90.

Mueller, N. 1991. The epidemiology of HTLV-I infection. *Cancer Causes Control* 2, 37–52.

Murphy, E. L., Figueroa, J. P., Gibbs, W. N., Holding-Cobham, M., Cranston, B., Malley, K., Bodner, A. J., Alexander, S. S., and Blattner, W. A. 1991. Human T-lymphotropic virus type I (HTLV-I) seroprevalence in Jamaica. I. Demographic determinants. *Am. J. Epidemiol.* 133, 1114–1124.

Murphy, E. L., Wilks, R., Hanchard, B., Cranston, B., Figueroa, J. P., Gibbs, W. N., Murphy, J., and Blattner, W. A. 1996. A case-control study of risk factors for seropositivity to human T-lymphotropic virus type I (HTLV-I) in Jamaica. *Int. J. Epidemiol.* 25, 1083–1089.

Nagai, M., and Osame, M. 2002. Pathogenesis and treatment of human T-cell lymphotropic virus Type I-associated myelopathy. *Expert. Rev. Neurother.* 2, 891–899.

Nagai, M., Usuku, K., Matsumoto, W., Kodama, D., Takenouchi, N., Moritoyo, T., Hashiguchi, S., Ichinose, M., Bangham, C. R., Izumo, S., and Osame, M. 1998. Analysis of HTLV-I proviral load in 202 HAM/TSP patients and 243 asymptomatic HTLV-I carriers: high proviral load strongly predisposes to HAM/TSP. *J. Neurovirol.* 4, 586–593.

Nakagawa, M., Izumo, S., Ijichi, S., Kubota, H., Arimura, K., Kawabata, M., and Osame, M. 1995. HTLV-I-associated myelopathy: analysis of 213 patients based on clinical features and laboratory findings. *J. Neurovirol.* 1, 50–61.

Nakagawa, M., Nakahara, K., Maruyama, Y., Kawabata, M., Higuchi, I., Kubota, H., Izumo, S., Arimura, K., and Osame, M. 1996. Therapeutic trials in 200 patients with HTLV-I-associated myelopathy/tropical spastic paraparesis. *J. Neurovirol.* 2, 345–355.

Nakamura, T. 2009. HTLV-I-associated myelopathy/tropical spastic paraparesis (HAM/TSP): the role of HTLV-I-infected Th1 cells in the pathogenesis, and therapeutic strategy. *Folia Neuropathol.* 47, 182–194.

Nakamura, T., Nishiura, Y., and Eguchi, K. 2009. Therapeutic strategies in HTLV-I-associated myelopathy/tropical spastic paraparesis (HAM/TSP). *Cent. Nerv. Syst. Agents Med. Chem.* 9, 137–149.

Nomoto, M., Utatsu, Y., Soejima, Y., and Osame, M. 1991. Neopterin in cerebrospinal fluid: a useful marker for diagnosis of HTLV-I-associated myelopathy/tropical spastic paraparesis. *Neurology* 41, 457.

Oh, U., Yamano, Y., Mora, C. A., Ohayon, J., Bagnato, F., Butman, J. A., Dambrosia, J., Leist, T. P., McFarland, H., and Jacobson, S. 2005. Interferon-beta1a therapy in human T-lymphotropic virus type I-associated neurologic disease. *Ann. Neurol.* 57, 526–534.

Ohtsuki, Y., Akagi, T., Takahashi, K., and Miyoshi, I. 1982. Ultrastructural study on type C virus particles in a human cord T-cell line established by co-cultivation with adult T-cell leukemia cells. *Arch. Virol.* 73, 69–73.

Oliveira, P., Castro, N. M., and Carvalho, E. M. 2007. Urinary and sexual manifestations of patients infected by HTLV-I. *Clinics (Sao Paulo)* 62, 191–196.

Osame, M. 1990. Review of WHO Kagoshima meeting and diagnostic guidelines for HAM/TSP, In: *Human Retrovirology HTLV*. Raven Press, New York, pp. 191–197.

Osame, M., and Igata, A. 1989. The history of discovery and clinico-epidemiology of HTLV-I-associated myelopathy(HAM). *Jpn. J. Med.* 28, 412–414.

Osame, M., Janssen, R., Kubota, H., Nishitani, H., Igata, A., Nagataki, S., Mori, M., Goto, I., Shimabukuro, H., Khabbaz, R. et al. 1990. Nationwide survey of HTLV-I-associated myelopathy in Japan: association with blood transfusion. *Ann. Neurol.* 28, 50–56.

Osame, M., Matsumoto, M., Usuku, K., Izumo, S., Ijichi, N., Amitani, H., Tara, M., and Igata, A. 1987. Chronic progressive myelopathy associated with elevated antibodies to human T-lymphotropic virus type I and adult T-cell leukemialike cells. *Ann. Neurol.* 21, 117–122.

Osame, M., Usuku, K., Izumo, S., Ijichi, N., Amitani, H., Igata, A., Matsumoto, M., and Tara, M. 1986. HTLV-I associated myelopathy, a new clinical entity. *Lancet* 1, 1031–1032.

Poiesz, B. J., Ruscetti, F. W., Gazdar, A. F., Bunn, P. A., Minna, J. D., and Gallo, R. C. 1980. Detection and isolation of type C retrovirus particles from fresh and cultured lymphocytes of a patient with cutaneous T-cell lymphoma. *Proc. Natl. Acad. Sci. U S A* 77, 7415–7419.

Proietti, F. A., Carneiro-Proietti, A. B., Catalan-Soares, B. C., and Murphy, E. L. 2005. Global epidemiology of HTLV-I infection and associated diseases. *Oncogene* 24, 6058–6068.

Rodgers-Johnson, P., Gajdusek, D. C., Morgan, O. S., Zaninovic, V., Sarin, P. S., and Graham, D. S. 1985. HTLV-I and HTLV-III antibodies and tropical spastic paraparesis. *Lancet* 2, 1247–1248.

Roman, G. C., and Osame, M. 1988. Identity of HTLV-I-associated tropical spasticparaparesis and HTLV-I-associated myelopathy. *Lancet* 1, 651.

Sabouri, A. H., Saito, M., Lloyd, A. L., Vine, A. M., Witkover, A. W., Furukawa, Y., Izumo, S., Arimura, K., Marshall, S. E., Usuku, K., Bangham, C. R., and Osame, M. 2004. Polymorphism in the interleukin-10 promoter affects both provirus load and the risk of human T lymphotropic virus type I-associated myelopathy/tropical spastic paraparesis. *J. Infect Dis.* 190, 1279–1285.

Saito, M., Matsuzaki, T., Satou, Y., Yasunaga, J., Saito, K., Arimura, K., Matsuoka, M., and Ohara, Y. 2009. *In vivo* expression of the HBZ gene of HTLV-1 correlates with proviral load, inflammatory markers and disease severity in HTLV-1 associated myelopathy/tropical spastic paraparesis (HAM/TSP). *Retrovirology* 6, 19.

Satou, Y., Yasunaga, J., Zhao, T., Yoshida, M., Miyazato, P., Takai, K., Shimizu, K., Ohshima, K., Green, P. L., Ohkura, N., Yamaguchi, T., Ono, M., Sakaguchi, S., and Matsuoka, M. 2011. HTLV-1 bZIP factor induces T-cell lymphoma and systemic inflammation *in vivo*. *PLoS Pathog.* 7, e1001274.

Seiki, M., Hattori, S., Hirayama, Y., and Yoshida, M. 1983. Human adult T-cell leukemiavirus: complete nucleotide sequence of the provirus genome integrated in leukemia cell DNA. *Proc. Natl. Acad. Sci. U S A* 80, 3618–3622.

Seiki, M., Hattori, S., and Yoshida, M. 1982. Human adult T-cell leukemia virus: molecular cloning of the provirus DNA and the unique terminal structure. *Proc. Natl. Acad. Sci. U S A* 79, 6899–6902.

Shakudo, M., Inoue, Y., and Tsutada, T. 1999. HTLV-I-associated myelopathy: acuteprogression and atypical MR findings. *AJNR Am. J. Neuroradiol.* 20, 1417–1421.

Sonoda, S., Li, H. C., and Tajima, K. 2011. Ethnoepidemiology of HTLV-1 related diseases: ethnic determinants of HTLV-1 susceptibility and its worldwide dispersal. *Cancer Sci.* 102, 295–301.

Takahashi, K., Takezaki, T., Oki, T., Kawakami, K., Yashiki, S., Fujiyoshi, T., Usuku, K., Mueller, N., Osame, M., Miyata, K. et al. 1991. Inhibitory effect of maternal antibody on mother-to-child transmission of human T-lymphotropic virus type I. The Mother-to-Child Transmission Study Group. *Int. J. Cancer* 49, 673–677.

Takenouchi, N., Yamano, Y., Usuku, K., Osame, M., and Izumo, S. 2003. Usefulness of proviral load measurement for monitoring of disease activity in individual patients with human T-lymphotropic virus type I-associated myelopathy/tropical spastic paraparesis. *J. Neurovirol.* 9, 29–35.

Taylor, G. P., Goon, P., Furukawa, Y., Green, H., Barfield, A., Mosley, A., Nose, H., Babiker, A., Rudge, P., Usuku, K., Osame, M., Bangham, C. R., and Weber, J. N. 2006. Zidovudine plus lamivudine in Human T-Lymphotropic Virus type-I-associated myelopathy: a randomised trial. *Retrovirology* 3, 63.

Uchiyama, T., Yodoi, J., Sagawa, K., Takatsuki, K., and Uchino, H. 1977. Adult T-cell leukemia: clinical and hematologic features of 16 cases. *Blood* 50, 481–492.

Umehara, F., Izumo, S., Nakagawa, M., Ronquillo, A. T., Takahashi, K., Matsumuro, K., Sato, E., and Osame, M. 1993. Immunocytochemical analysis of the cellular infiltrate in the spinal cord lesions in HTLV-I-associated myelopathy. *J. Neuropathol. Exp. Neurol.* 52, 424–430.

Umehara, F., Izumo, S., Ronquillo, A. T., Matsumuro, K., Sato, E., and Osame, M. 1994. Cytokine expression in the spinal cord lesions in HTLV-I-associated myelopathy. *J. Neuropathol. Exp. Neurol.* 53, 72–77.

Umehara, F., Izumo, S., Takeya, M., Takahashi, K., Sato, E., and Osame, M. 1996. Expression of adhesion molecules and monocyte chemoattractant protein–1 (MCP-1) in the spinal cord lesions in HTLV-I-associated myelopathy. *Acta Neuropathol.* 91, 343–350.

Umehara, F., Nagatomo, S., Yoshishige, K., Saito, M., Furukawa, Y., Usuku, K., and Osame, M. 2004. Chronic progressive cervical myelopathy with HTLV-I infection: variant form of HAM/TSP? *Neurology* 63, 1276–1280.

Umehara, F., Tokunaga, N., Hokezu, Y., Hokonohara, E., Yoshishige, K., Shiraishi, T., Okubo, R., and Osame, M. 2006. Relapsing cervical cord lesions on MRI in patients with HTLV-I-associated myelopathy. *Neurology* 66, 289.

Verdonck, K., Gonzalez, E., Van Dooren, S., Vandamme, A. M., Vanham, G., and Gotuzzo, E. 2007. Human T-lymphotropic virus 1: recent knowledge about an ancient infection. *Lancet Infect. Dis.* 7, 266–281.

Vine, A. M., Witkover, A. D., Lloyd, A. L., Jeffery, K. J., Siddiqui, A., Marshall, S. E., Bunce, M., Eiraku, N., Izumo, S., Usuku, K., Osame, M., and Bangham, C. R. 2002. Polygenic control of human T lymphotropic virus type I (HTLV-I) provirus load and the risk of HTLV-I-associated myelopathy/tropical spastic paraparesis. *J. Infect Dis.* 186, 932–939.

Watanabe, M., Yamashita, T., Hara, A., Murakami, T., Ando, Y., Uyama, E., Mita, S., and Uchino, M. 2001. High signal in the spinal cord on T2-weighted images in rapidly progressive tropical spastic paraparesis. *Neuroradiology* 43, 231–233.

Yamaguchi, K., and Takatsuki, K. 1993. Adult T cell leukaemia-lymphoma. *Baillieres Clin. Haematol.* 6, 899–915.

Yamamoto, K., Utsunomiya, A., Tobinai, K., Tsukasaki, K., Uike, N., Uozumi, K., Yamaguchi, K., Yamada, Y., Hanada, S., Tamura, K., Nakamura, S., Inagaki, H., Ohshima, K., Kiyoi, H., Ishida, T., Matsushima, K., Akinaga, S., Ogura, M., Tomonaga, M., and Ueda, R. 2010. Phase I study of KW-0761, a defucosylated humanized anti-CCR4 antibody, in relapsed patients with adult T-cell leukemia-lymphoma and peripheral T-cell lymphoma. *J. Clin. Oncol.* 28, 1591–1598.

Yamano, Y., Nagai, M., Brennan, M., Mora, C. A., Soldan, S. S., Tomaru, U., Takenouchi, N., Izumo, S., Osame, M., and Jacobson, S. 2002. Correlation of human T-cell lymphotropic virus type 1 (HTLV-1) mRNA with proviral DNA load, virus-specific CD8(+) T cells, and disease severity in HTLV-1-associated myelopathy (HAM/TSP). *Blood* 99, 88–94.

Yoshida, M., Miyoshi, I., and Hinuma, Y. 1982. Isolation and characterization of retrovirus from cell lines of human adult T-cell leukemia and its implication in the disease. *Proc. Natl. Acad. Sci. U S A* 79, 2031–2035.

Yoshida, M., Seiki, M., Yamaguchi, K., and Takatsuki, K. 1984. Monoclonal integration of human T-cell leukemia provirus in all primary tumors of adult T-cell leukemia suggests causative role of human T-cell leukemia virus in the disease. *Proc. Natl. Acad. Sci. U S A* 81, 2534–2537.

Yukitake, M., Sueoka, E., Sueoka-Aragane, N., Sato, A., Ohashi, H., Yakushiji, Y., Saito, M., Osame, M., Izumo, S., and Kuroda, Y. 2008a. Significantly increased antibody response to heterogeneous nuclear ribonucleoproteins in cerebrospinal fluid of multiple sclerosis patients but not in patients with human T-lymphotropic virus type I-associated myelopathy/tropical spastic paraparesis. *J. Neurovirol.* 14, 130–135.

Yukitake, M., Takase, Y., Nanri, Y., Kosugi, M., Eriguchi, M., Yakushiji, Y., Okada, R., Mizuta, H., and Kuroda, Y. 2008b. Incidence and clinical significances of human T-cell lymphotropic virus type I-associated myelopathy with T2 hyperintensity on spinal magnetic resonance images. *Int. Med.* 47, 1881–1886.

19 Human Immunodeficiency Virus Neuropathogenesis

Ritu Mishra and Sunit K. Singh

CONTENTS

19.1 INTRODUCTION

Inflammation encompassing the brain tissues as a result of virus infection is known as viral encephalitis. There are many viruses responsible for viral encephalitis, and it is one of the emerging health issues worldwide (Shoji et al. 2002). To combat against viral encephalitis, a better understanding of events that occur within the central nervous system (CNS) after viral exposure is needed. Viral infections immensely activate the host immune responses at periphery and in CNS, results in neuroinflammation and acts as a key process in the viral neuropathogenesis. Human immunodeficiency virus 1 (HIV-1) is well studied (Wang, Rumbaugh, and Nath 2006) among other viruses responsible for encephalitis or dementia. Within the retrovirus family, HIV belongs to subgroup known as lentiviruses (Worlein et al. 2005) and responsible for acquired

457

immunodeficiency syndrome (AIDS). HIV has two copies of single-stranded RNA in its genome. The transcript produced from the viral promoter is approximately 10 kb long. This transcript contains seven structured subdomains throughout its length, namely long terminal repeats (LTR), transactivating region (TAR), rev responsive element (RRE), psi elements (PE), a TTTTTT slippery site (SLIP), *cis*-acting repressive sequences (CRS), and inhibitory/instability RNA sequences (INS). The ends of each strand of HIV RNA contain an RNA sequence called LTR. LTR regions are reported to have promoter sequences. The HIV genome encodes nine open reading frames (ORFs), namely group specific antigen (gag), polymerase (pol), envelope (env), transactivator of transcription (tat), regulator of virion protein expression (rev), negative effector (nef), viral infectivity factor (vif), viral protein R (vpr), and viral protein U (vpu) (Johri et al. 2011). Broadly, these genes can be categorized into two categories, structural and nonstructural genes. The gag, pol, and env genes are structural genes in HIV genome, which contain information to make the structural proteins for new virus particles. Gag, Pol, and Env are synthesized as polyproteins, which subsequently get proteolyzed into individual proteins (Frankel and Young 1998). Nonstructural genes can be further classified as accessory and regulatory proteins. Accessory proteins include Vif, Vpr, Vpu, and Nef, which are unique to primate lentiviruses (Johri et al. 2011). Whereas, HIV Rev and Tat proteins are designated as HIV regulatory proteins. HIV is known to infect cells of the host's immune system, causing persistent and chronic infection (Narayan and Clements 1989). HIV is neurovirulent and manifests neurological complications (Williams et al. 2008). More than 65 million people globally have been infected with the HIV since its discovery in the early 1980s (Power et al. 2009). Neurological disorders caused by HIV infection covers both the central and the peripheral nervous systems (McArthur et al. 2005). Neurological complications relevant to CNS have been reported in more than 50% of untreated HIV patients (Clifford 2008). In addition to dementia symptoms, AIDS patients show some common viremia-related symptoms such as fever, skin rash, oral ulcers, and lymphadenopathy after 2–3 weeks of primary HIV infection (Pope and Haase 2003). However, HIV can enter into nervous suystem at any stage of infection and can have adverse effects on overall quality of life (Power et al. 2009). The neuropathology of primary HIV-1-associated CNS disorders, characterized as HIV-1-associated neurocognitive disorders (HANDs) (Antinori et al. 2007) and that can be distinguished from secondary processes such as opportunistic infections or malignancies.

The development of HIV-associated dementia (HAD) or AIDS dementia complex (ADC) is a unique syndrome and is characterized by clinical manifestations such as neurocognitive impairment (forgetfulness, poor concentration and comprehension, slowed mental processing), accompanied by emotional disturbances (agitation, apathy), and followed by motor dysfunctions (tremor, bradykinesia, ataxia, and spasticity) (Power et al. 2009).

19.2 BRAIN CELLS: AS HIV RESERVOIR AND EXECUTOR OF THE NEUROINFLAMMATION

HIV is known to enter the brain soon after infection (Figure 19.1). The appearance of meningitis (Carne et al. 1985; Hoffmann et al. 2001) and intrathecal synthesis

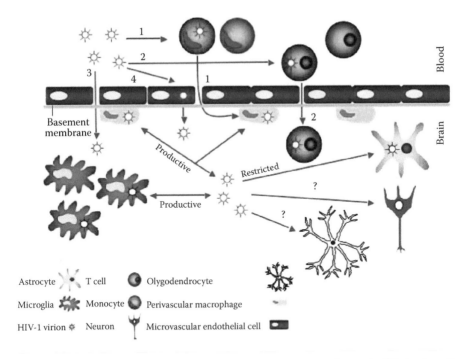

FIGURE 19.1 **(See color insert.)** HIV-1 neuroinvasion. (1) According to the "Trojan horse" hypothesis, the entry of HIV-1 into the brain takes place by the migration of infected monocytes, which differentiate into perivascular macrophage. (2) The passage of infected CD4+ T cells can be another source of infection in the brain. Other probable causes of CNS infection might be (3) the direct entrance of the virus or (4) entrance of HIV-1 by transcytosis of brain microvascular endothelial cells. Once the virus is in the brain, it productively infects macrophages and microglia. Astrocyte infection is known to be restricted. The infection of oligodendrocytes, especially neurons, is questionable. (Reproduced from Ghafouri, M. et al., 2006, *Retrovirology* 3, 28. With permission.)

of HIV-1 antibody (Carter et al. 1988) are among the evidence of HIV infection in brain. HIV-DNA has been detected in the postmortem brain samples of patients who died with HIV infection (Davis et al. 1992). Many groups have revealed a condition of immune activation in the brain, with enhanced levels of cytokines and other proinflammatory factors. Astrocytes and microglia have been primarily reported to be productively infected by HIV (An et al. 1999). The increased expression of adhesion molecules (Seilhean et al. 1997), an enhanced astrocyte activation (Geiger et al. 2006), and loss of astrocytic functions have been reported to attribute to HIV-associated neuropathology (Saito et al. 1994; Tornatore et al. 1994; Vallat et al. 1998).

The most accepted mechanism of HIV entry into the brain is the "Trojan horse" mechanism. The mechanism postulates the role of HIV-infected monocytes/macrophages crossing the blood–brain barrier (BBB) and disseminating the virus (Meltzer and Gendelman 1992; Vazeux et al. 1987). Many studies have found the evidence of HIV infection in astrocytes (Tornatore et al. 1994; Wiley et al. 1986). It is not well understood whether neuroectodermal cells, particularly neurons, get infected by HIV. There are few reports stating HIV-1 infection in cerebral endothelial cells (An et al. 1999; Tornatore et al. 1994). Endothelial cell loss can take place with apoptosis through the HIV proteins secreted out extracellularly from the HIV infected cells (Acheampong et al. 2005). The microglial cells and monocytes can be called as a long term reservoir and source of transmission of HIV infection in the CNS. HIV RNA has been detected in a variety of cell types such as macrophage/microglial cells and multinucleated giant cells (Stoler et al. 1986). Microglial physiology is the main focus for a cascade of events, which can lead to neuronal dysfunction and death. Several molecular mediators of neuronal injury in HAD originate from microglia (Garden 2002). HIV-1 infection in the CNS is centered around viral replication in cells of glial and macrophage lineage (Gendelman et al. 1994b), which has been found to be correlated with development of dementia. Microglial nodules develop much before the onset of AIDS or HIV induced viral encephalitis (HIVE) and are known as the hallmark of neuro-AIDS (Kibayashi et al. 1996).

The detailed role of macrophages/microglia in the pathogenesis of HIV-1-associated neurocognitive impairment has been reviewed extensively elsewhere (Yadav and Collman 2009). In general, HIV-1 infection and immunopositivity is restricted to the perivascular compartment, as shown by widespread staining of the parenchymal microglia (Morris et al. 1999). The privileged areas of CNS act as a sanctuary site for the persistence of HIV-1, which again turns into a challenging task from a treatment point of view.

HIV infection and the complexity of disease progression focus on the cytopathic effects of the infection first in CD4$^+$ T cells, and then later, in the cells of macrophage lineage (Pantaleo et al. 1993; Rosenberg and Fauci 1991). The rapid loss in the number of the CD4$^+$ T-cells in peripheral blood is the reflection of highly productive infection of HIV in CD4$^+$ T-cells. Such productive HIV infection leads to a loss of cell-mediated immune (CMI) responses and suppression of Th1 cytokines, such as *Interleukin-2 (IL-2)* and Interferon-gamma (IFN-γ) (Dalgleish 1995). This lays the foundation for the development of state of immunodeficiency in the host and manifests itself in two ways: first, development of selected tumors and turning the host favorable for various types of opportunistic pathogens (Liu et al. 1999); second, support the progressive virus replication in the brain (Gendelman et al. 1994a).

Infiltration of infected macrophages into the brain is accompanied by massive cytokine/chemokine induction (Della Chiara et al. 2010). Pathological changes of HIV induced neuroinflammation include perivascular accumulations of mononuclear cells (Bell 1998; Gendelman et al. 1994b). The mechanism of the neurological complications in HIV-infected individuals is not well understood. How does HIV enter into the CNS early during infection and remain slow/silent for such a long period? It is not well understood whether heightened neurological complications in final AIDS are due to virus reactivation or due to a renewed phase of viral neuroinvasion. However, many groups support the notion that the virus replicates continuously in the CNS at low levels (Williams et al. 2008).

19.3 ROLE OF HIV PROTEINS IN NEUROPATHOGENESIS

The HIV-1-encoded small nuclear transcriptional activator protein, Tat (trans-activator of transcription), is the first protein to be expressed in the virus life cycle (Li et al. 2009). Tat is a virally encoded protein that can be released by HIV-1-infected cells and can activate HIV-infected and/or uninfected cells to release potentially neurotoxic substances. Tat has been detected in the extracellular space and sera of infected individuals (Hudson et al. 2000; Wiley et al. 1996) and may directly interact with surrounding neurons (Cheng et al. 1998; Tardieu et al. 1992). Anti-tat antibodies have been reported in the brains of patients with HIV encephalitis (Del Valle et al. 2000). The source of Tat proteins in the CNS is still confusing—whether the Tat protein is released by infected cells of the brain or transported across the BBB from peripheral viral sources (Banks et al. 2005).

Tat can contribute to neuropathogenesis through various mechanisms. It can stimulate proinflammatory responses through production of several cytokines including Interleukin-1 beta (IL-1β), Tumor necrosis factor-alpha (TNF-α), Interleukin-6 (IL-6), and transforming growth factor beta (TGF-β) (Zauli et al. 1992). Tat induces TNF-α production, activation of different G proteins, and followed by Ca^{2+} mobilization and activation of the protein kinase C pathway, which might result in downstream activation of NF-kB (Contreras et al. 2005). In addition, Tat stimulates the p38 MAPK and the JAK/STAT pathways, which activate Interferon gamma-induced protein 10 (IP-10) production. Tat induces host-soluble factors such as IFN-γ, which, in turn, induces the chemokines as IP-10 production by macrophages (Dhillon et al. 2008). These effects of Tat and other HIV proteins on macrophage/microglia suggest that viral proteins are important contributors to the activation events leading to HIV-induced neuroinflammation.

Tat exerts a toxic effect on neurons via cytokines, chemokines, and nitric oxide (NO) released by microglia (Thomas et al. 2009), which in turn leads to the apoptosis.

Astrocytes, neurons, and endothelial cells are equally prone to Tat-induced inflammatory responses, which can further augment the infiltration of monocytes into the brain (Pu et al. 2003). Tat is known to significantly contribute in the disruption of the BBB by altering the distribution of endothelial cell-tight junction proteins such as claudin 1, claudin 5, ZO-1, and ZO-2, which ultimately leads to enhanced transmigration of monocytes and lymphocytes (Andras et al. 2003; Toborek et al. 2003) in the brain.

Another HIV-1 protein, gp120, can also be directly neurotoxic by inducing neuronal apoptosis, mainly through interactions with the chemokine receptor CXCR4. Recombinant gp120 from the R5 strains of HIV-1 is known to induce apoptosis in a human neuronal cell line. These receptors are expressed on neurons, suggesting the role of CCR5 in neuronal activation and damage (Xu et al. 2004). gp120 disrupts calcium homeostasis in neurons, which triggers mitochondrial membrane disruption and activation of caspases and endonucleases via the intrinsic pathway leading to apoptosis (Mattson et al. 2005). The extrinsic pathway, which involves the up-regulation of the death receptor Fas, has also been demonstrated to be a mechanism for gp120-induced neuronal apoptosis (Thomas et al. 2009).

Vpr is a 96-amino acid HIV-1-encoded virion-incorporated protein and essential for HIV-1 replication in macrophages (Subbramanian et al. 1998). Vpr has been recently reported in sustantial amounts in both the basal ganglia and the frontal cortex of HIVE patients. It was mainly found in the resident macrophages and neurons (Wheeler et al. 2006). Soluble HIV-1 Vpr protein is reported in the serum of HIV-infected patients with neurological disorders (Levy et al. 1994). In the mouse model, the expression of HIV-1 Vpr in brain monocytoid cells has been implicated in neuronal injury and other motor dysfunctions (Jones et al. 2007). Exogenous treatment of soluble Vpr also perturbs the neuronal membrane potentials, leading to apoptosis (Patel et al. 2000). Vpr directly exert cytotoxic effects on neurons by activating the glia, which results into the release of neurotoxic substances. Vpr can also alter the expression of various important cytokines and inflammatory proteins in infected as well as uninfected cells (Mukerjee et al. 2011). Vpr is known to be taken up by neurons and leads to the deregulation of calcium homeostasis. Vpr can also activate the oxidative stress pathway involving mitochondrial dysfunction (Mukerjee et al. 2011).

Neuronal injuries by various viral proteins, including Tat, Nef, Vpr, and the Env proteins gp120 have been explained by multiple theories. HIV envelope proteins, such as gp120 as well as Tat, have been reported to mimic of many chemokines; therefore, HIV-induced neuronal injury can be mediated by chemokine receptor signaling. Various experiments showed that blocking of chemokine receptor signaling can prevent HIV/gp120-induced neuronal apoptosis (Meucci et al. 2000; Zheng et al. 1999), and Stromal cell-derived factor-1 (SDF-1) directly exerts neurotoxic effects through the stimulation of chemokine receptors (Kaul and Lipton 1999). Various reports demonstrate the different mechanisms of neuroinflammation through various HIV proteins and differential clinical picture by different HIV clades. Models of HIV infection, including simian and feline immunodeficiency virus infection, have shown the role of individual viral strains and the specific viral proteins in contributing to neuroinflammation (van Marle and Power 2005). Differences in genetic susceptibility at the individual or population level might play an important role because clinically evident disease affects only a subset of HIV-infected patients, although HIV-1 neuroinvasion and neurotropism occur in most of the HIV-infected patients (van Marle and Power 2005). HIV-associated neurological disorders (HANDs) have also been reported among patients having higher CD4+ T-cell levels, which were earlier believed to show up among HIV patients having CD4+ T-cell counts below 200 cells/μL of blood (Power et al. 2009).

19.4 CYTOKINES: ADDITIVE ROLE IN NEUROPATHOGENESIS

Microglia and macrophages within the brain release both α- and β-chemokines in response to HIV infection of the CNS (Lindl et al. 2010). These chemokines and cytokines can bind to neurons because neurons express chemokine receptors (Rottman et al. 1997). This bystander way of HIV-induced inflammatory response might play a critical role in HIV infection in the brain. There is experimental evidence showing the elevated levels of the α-chemokines, CXCL10/IP-10 and CXCL12/SDF-1α, in the brains and CSF of HAD patients (Cinque et al. 2005). α-chemokines are expressed in many types of CNS cells constitutively and can have both neuroprotective and neurotoxic effects (Khan et al. 2008). It can also bind CXCR chemokine receptors and thereby increases intracellular calcium in G protein-dependent signaling. During HIV infection, the major chemoattractants, i.e., CCL3, CCL4, CCL5, CCL2, and CX3CL1, have been implicated in increased trafficking of monocytes into the brain. Brain autopsy samples of patients having HAD symptoms died with HIV infection (diagnosed with HAD) have been reported to have infected monocytes (Kanmogne et al. 2007; Mukhtar and Pomerantz 2000).

In the peripheral circulation, chronic immune activation takes place due to immune responses against HIV, and extracellularly secreted HIV proteins such as gp120 and Tat. Immune activation results into the activation of monocytes, which acquire invasive phenotype by induced expression CD16 and CD163. These activated monocytes have enhanced migratory capacity and cross through the blood brain barrier, whose integrity is comprised by HIV proteins and other pro-inflammatory mediators generated by activated cells ("push" mechanism). In the CNS, monocytes differentiate into macrophages and release infectious viruses, which in turn infect other cells through the CD4/CCR5 receptor complex. The infected cells release viral proteins (i.e., gp120 & Tat), express cytokines, chemokines and other proinflammatory factors, which activate neighbouring uninfected and/or infected cells in bystander fashion. Chemokines such as monocyte chemoattractant protein-1 (MCP-1) and SDF-1α further recruit monocytes into the CNS ("pull" mechanism). Some of these factors also activate the brain microvascular endothelial cells (BMVECs), which results into induced expression of adhesion molecules such as intercellular adhesion molecule-1 (ICAM-1) and vascular cell adhesion molecule-1 (VCAM-1) on BMVECs, which helps in the entry of inflammatory cells in brain. These two mechanisms, "push" and "pull," to contribute to monocytes/macrophage accumulation and activation inside CNS (Yadav and Collman 2009). HIV is believed to cross the BBB via the transport of infected CD4+ T cells and/or monocytes. However, free HIV particles can also enter the CNS through transcytosis of the BBB, which is not believed to be a major route.

19.5 NEURONAL DAMAGE

19.5.1 Excitotoxicity and Oxidative Stress

Despite the lack of data supporting widespread productive neuronal infection, it is clear that neuronal loss occurs in the brain of HIV-infected persons (Adle-Biassette et al. 1995; Dunfee et al. 2006; Gray et al. 2000). Neuronal damage can happen by various direct and indirect pathways, induced by viral infection or after exposure to viral toxic proteins. Both virus and glial cell-derived proteins may contribute to neuronal damage (Nath et al. 1999) (Figure 19.2). Infected macrophages and microglial cells are believed to contribute to pathological changes in the neurons through the secretion of viral (gp120, Tat, and Nef) and cellular (cytokines, chemokines, and nitric oxide) products (Kolson and Pomerantz 1996; Lipton and Gendelman 1995). Viral proteins, particularly gp120, gp41, tat, nef, and cytokines, prostaglandins, proteases, arachidonic acid, or quinolinic acid metabolites produced by activated brain resident cells are attributed to neuroinflammation (Everall et al. 1993).

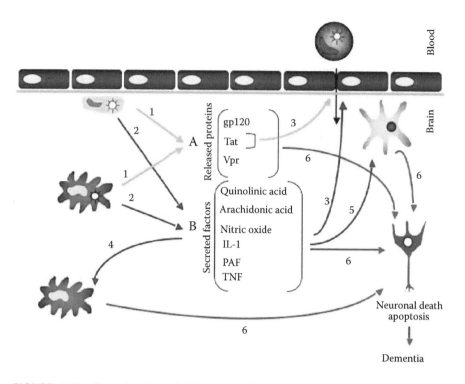

FIGURE 19.2 **(See color insert.)** Mechanism of neuropathogenesis. Two components of this mechanism are (A) the direct effect of the HIV-1 infection, including HIV-1 proteins, and (B) the indirect consequence of infection comprising the secretion of cytokines and neurotoxins. The infected macrophages and microglia participate actively in the neurodegeneration by (1) shedding viral proteins and (2) releasing a significant amount of cytokines and neurotoxins into the CNS. (3) Tat and TNF-α contribute to the disruption of the BBB, which in turn become more permeable to infected monocytes and cytokines present in the periphery. The secreted proinflammatory cytokines activates (4) microglia and (5) astrocytes, which in turn secrete neurotoxins; moreover, the alteration of astrocytes function results in an increase in the level of neurotoxicity in the brain. (6) Multifactorial neuronal injury: neurotoxins released from several sources, as the direct and indirect consequences of HIV-1 infection lead to neuronal injury. (Reproduced from Ghafouri, M. et al., 2006, *Retrovirology* 3, 28. With permission.)

In particular, HIV Tat protein is known to be transported along neural pathways and is well described as the cause of neurotoxic damage at remote sites (Bruce-Keller et al. 2003). These reports emphasized that each of these toxins can damage nerve cells, but severity increases manifold for neuronal apoptosis in a combination of both cellular and viral factors (Xu et al. 2004). Many *in vitro* studies also confirmed the glutamate-mediated excitotoxicity as a factor of neuroinflammation. Glutamate, an excitatory neurotransmitter (Fonnum 1984), is known to be involved in HIV-induced neurotoxicity (Jiang et al. 2001; Zhao et al. 2004). Many studies demonstrated that astrocytes normally take up glutamate, keeping extracellular glutamate concentration low in the brain, and thus astrocytes display their neuroprotective role

(Fonnum 1984). In astrocytes, the glutamate gets converted into glutamine via mitochondrial glutamine synthetase and transported to neurons for synthesis of GABA (γ-amino butyric acid), a neurotransmitter (Porcheray et al. 2006). This is known as the glutamine–glutamate cycle between astrocytes and neurons, which establishes the brain nitrogen homeostasis. This action is inhibited in HIV infection, probably due to cellular inflammatory mediators and viral proteins. An increase in extracellular glutamate concentration contributes to neuronal death through hyperactivation of N-methyl-D-aspartate receptors (NMDAR), a mechanism addressed as excitotoxicity. Excitatory amino acid transporters (EAAT), are mainly expressed on glial cells, which ensures the clearance of extracellular glutamate (Gegelashvili and Schousboe 1997). EAAT-1 and EAAT-2 genes are reported to be expressed on glia (Chaudhry et al. 1995; Danbolt et al. 1992; Lehre et al. 1995) and provide *in vivo* protection against glutamate toxicity (Rothstein 1996). Astrocytes play a key role as a neuroprotector against glutamate stress in the course of HIV infection. In a study, the 6-h exposure of either HIV-1 gp120 or Tat to astrocytes resulted in a 60% reduction in glutamate uptake by astrocytes and reduction in EAAT-2 expression but not EAAT-1 (Fallarino et al. 2003; Kort 1998). Considerable loss in EAAT expression in perineuronal microglia in HIV infection has been reported in cases of HIVE (Vallat-Decouvelaere et al. 2003).

Tat activates the neuronal excitatory NMDAR, leading to excitotoxicity and consequent apoptosis of neurons (Li et al. 2008; Song et al. 2003; Kaul et al. 2001). *In vivo* studies showed that production of super oxide anion and nitric oxide is significantly increased in *demented*, compared with AIDS patients without dementia (Boven et al. 1999).

Tat has been shown to depolarize neurons through direct interaction with neuronal membranes and may act as substrate to increase the aggregation of neural cultures (Nath 2002). A minor exposure ranging in nanomolar concentrations of gp120 can hyperactivate the NMDAR by binding through the glycine-binding sites of the NMDAR (Fontana et al. 1997). This is another mechanism by which HIV/gp120 or Tat may exert an adverse effect on neuronal cells. Another HIV-1 protein Vpr is also now shown to affect cultured hippocampal neurons through formation of a cation-permeable channel (Piller et al. 1998).

Hyperactivation of the NMDAR provokes intracellular signals leading to apoptosis or necrosis of neuronal cells (Bonfoco et al. 1995). In the case of severe excitotoxic insults, the cells die early through the process of necrosis/apoptosis (Bonfoco et al. 1995). Molecular mechanism imparting neuronal apoptosis due to excitotoxicity is diversified involving Ca^{2+} overload, p38 MAPK activation, release of cytochrome c from mitochondria, activation of caspases, free radical formation, lipid peroxidation, and chromatin condensation (Budd et al. 2000; Ghatan et al. 2000).

Oxidative stress alters the cellular lipid metabolism, producing harmful molecules, such as ceramide, sphingomyelin, hydroxynonenal, etc., which are observed in patients with HAND (Sacktor et al. 2004). Detection of oxidized proteins in the CSF also confirms the role of oxidative stress in HAND (Turchan et al. 2003). Tat and Vpr are reported to increase oxidative stress in neurons due to mitochondrial dysfunction. These reports suggest that oxidative stress is an important mode of neuronal death and subsequent neurodegeneration (Lindl et al. 2010). Neuroprotective potentials of many antioxidants have been demonstrated *in vitro*, which establishes that oxidative stress is an important factor in neurodegeneration (Turchan et al. 2003).

19.5.2 Impairment of Neurogenesis

Adult neurogenesis (ANG) was initially thought to occur only in rodents. Recent findings show that ANG also takes place in humans and other primates (Eriksson et al. 1998). ANG is important for maintaining the homeostatic state of CNS and is involved in learning, memory, olfaction, and anxiety-related behaviors (Revest et al. 2009). ANG has been reported to get perturbed in HAND (Rodriguez et al. 2008; Taupin 2009). Astrocytes provide trophic support to both mature and immature neurons, but this support gets impaired in cases of HIV infection in the brain and that restricts the proliferation and migration of Neural Progenitor Cells (NPCs) (Eriksson et al. 1998). Maturation and differentiation of NPCs are dependent on cell cycle regulation (Herrup and Yang 2007). Disruption at the level of cell cycle proteins such as the transcription factor, E2F1, and its regulator, the retinoblastoma gene, are reported to be dysregulated in patients having HAND (Hoglinger et al. 2007). Another cell cycle protein *doublecortin (dcx)* (microtubule protein) expressed in immature neurons was shown to be disrupted in HAND (Herrup and Yang 2007). Dysregulated expression of E2F1 disrupts the *dcx*, which ultimately leads to the disruption in ANG. Disruption of ANG and its molecular regulation trims down the plasticity of the CNS, which leads to devastating consequences in brain regions assaulted by HIV-induced toxicity (Karl et al. 2005).

19.6 HIV-ASSOCIATED NEUROLOGICAL DISORDERS

In 1983, Snider et al. reported for the first time that the underlying pathogen in AIDS likely affect the CNS. In 1982, the first descriptive report appeared explaining about the damage to the nervous system due to AIDS (Scaravilli et al. 2007). However, Snider et al. (1983) are credited with the first systematic description of the CNS complications of AIDS in a case series of 50 patients. The existence of neurocognitive impairment directly attributable to HIV was not well understood until 1987 (Woods et al. 2009). It is a relatively recent event revealing involvement of the CNS in AIDS (Snider et al. 1983; Vivithanaporn et al. 2010). In the last three decades, numerous experimental studies contributed to a better understanding of the HIV neuropathogenesis.

The neurological complications in AIDS patients are mostly due to HIV infection in the CNS, and it is also confirmed by viral detection within brain tissues (Shaw et al. 1985), together with the observation of multinucleated giant cells (MGC). These cells are considered unique to AIDS and considered as a hallmark of the syndrome (Budka 1986). The neuropathological abnormalities are collectively called HIV-associated neurological disorders (HAND). Although the severe form of HAND is typically ascertained during the late stages of infection. It was later found that moderate neuropsychological, neurophysiological, and neuroimaging abnormalities can occur well before the advanced stages of AIDS (Heaton et al. 1995). This suggests that HIV neuropathogenesis is a gradual process and HIV-induced neuroinflammation may begin at any time in the course of infection and can act as a trigger for the development of HAND.

19.7 GENERAL SYMPTOMS AND CLASSIFICATION OF NEURO-AIDS

HAND is a broad term given to describe the cumulative anomalies observed and best correlated with the altered CNS structure and function in HIV-infected individuals. Based on the stage of infection and AIDS development, the severity of these disorders varies. Among AIDS patients, about half are symptomatic for neurological disorders and a few of them fit in the research classification of dementia (Hogan and Wilkins 2011). Variability can be attributed to disease stage, treatment, and the techniques and diagnostic tools used to detect the impairment (Hogan and Wilkins 2011).

Patients should fulfill certain criteria to be considered as a subject of HAND. The affected person should demonstrate an acquired deficiency in at least two neurocognitive domains and show impairment in work or activities of daily living (ADLs), and an abnormality in motor abilities or specified neuropsychiatric functions (e.g., motivation, liability, and social behavior) (Woods et al. 2009). However, Grant and Atkinson elaborated the definitions of the American Academy of Neurology (AAN) in 1995 and included an additional diagnosis of "subsyndromic neurocognitive impairment." The neuro-AIDS patients falling in this category demonstrate mild neurocognitive deficits that do not interfere with ADLs (Woods et al. 2009).

HAND defines three categories of disorders according to the extent and severity of dysfunctions (Ghafouri et al. 2006; Valcour et al. 2011) (Table 19.1):

1. Asymptomatic neurocognitive impairment (ANI)
2. Mild neurocognitive disorder (MND)
3. HIV-associated dementia (HAD)

TABLE 19.1
Research Criteria for HIV-Associated Neurocognitive Disorders

Diagnosis Entity	Cognitive Performance	Functional Performance
Normal cognition	Normal	Normal
Asymptomatic neurocognitive impairment	Acquired impairment in at least two cognitive domains (<1 SD)	Does not impact daily functions
Mild neurocognitive disorder	Acquired impairment in at least two cognitive domains (<1 SD)	Interferes with daily function to at least a mild degree (eg, work inefficiency, reduced mental acuity)
HIV-associated dementia	Acquired impairment in at least 2 domains, typically in multiple domains with at least 2 domains with severe impairment (<2 SD)	Marked impact on daily functions

Source: Reproduced from Valcour, V., Sithinamsuwan, P., Letendre, S., and Ances, B. (2011). *Curr HIV/AIDS Rep* 8(1), 54–61. With permission.

19.7.1 ASYMPTOMATIC NEUROCOGNITIVE IMPAIRMENT

ANI does not affect everyday functioning among patients. It was added as a diagnosis for the initial and mild cases of HAND, also referred to as subsyndromic neurocognitive impairment (Grant et al. 1995). This class of neurological impairments represents over 50% of diagnosed cases, including around 21%–30% of the asymptomatic HIV-infected individuals (Robertson et al. 2007). These abnormalities, while mild, are demonstrable, neurocognitive impairment.

It is very important to preidentify those at risk for more significant cognitive as well as functional deficits. This can be regarded as a window for foreseeing the patterns of individual susceptibility for neurological impairments and make judicial decisions for further treatment before severe cognitive deficits start affecting the everyday functioning with detrimental consequences (Woods et al. 2009). In other words, detection and treatment of patients at this earliest stage of HAND actually provide the best chance to prevent further progression of disease.

19.7.2 MILD NEUROCOGNITIVE DISORDER

MND subjects show an advanced and severe form of impairment, which involve difficulties in pursuing daily activities. About 20%–40% of HAND cases are encountered with MND, which comprises 5%–20% of the HIV population overall (Woods et al. 2009; Grant et al. 1999).

This category of subjects should meet at least two of the following criteria:

1. Decline in more than two instrumental activities of daily living (ADLs) (e.g., financial management).
2. Reduced cognitive abilities, followed by significant reduction in job responsibilities and unemployment.
3. Decline in vocational skills, e.g., frequent errors, decreased productivity, and difficulty in achieving prior levels of skill and performance.
4. Self- or proxy-report of increased problems in areas of day-to-day life activities (this criterion should exclude self-report of current depression because depression itself is a kind of biased self-report).
5. Inabilities of subject for everyday functioning (e.g., medication management).

19.7.3 HIV-ASSOCIATED DEMENTIA

HIV dementia is a result of multifactorial events, and it is difficult to name any single cellular or viral factor alone as a causative factor. There are many gaps in understanding the exact correlation between the cognitive disorders and the different HIV-induced changes. HAD represents the most severe form of HAND. It includes all the terms and criteria listed for MND in terms of its functional impact, but all symptoms are given in their more severe form and chronic disabilities found in AIDS patients. It also demonstrates a decline in two or more of the cognitive domains accompanied with marked decline in ADL. In the early 1990s, HAD was thought to be faced by an extremely wide range (6%–30%) of HIV-infected individuals after onset of AIDS (Maj et al. 1994; McArthur et al. 1993).

The use of combined antiretroviral therapy (cART) improved the circumstances by lowering the incidences of HAD, but approximately 4%–7% of persons with AIDS still experience HAD (Grant et al. 1999). Recent assessments suggest that only 1%–2% of HIV persons actually meet the criteria for HAD (Grant et al. 2005).

Other neurocognitive impairments such as severe movement abnormalities, i.e., chorea, myoclonus, dyskinesia, and dystonia, are not very common in HIV infection but can be observed in individuals with HAD (Mirsattari et al. 1999). However, slowed movement (bradykinesia) and slowed information processing (bradyphrenia) are the commonly observed features among neuro-AIDS patients (Woods et al. 2009).

Learning and memory dysfunctions are known to be highly prevalent in HIV infection and reported in almost 40%–60% of AIDS patients (Rippeth et al. 2004). The level of impairment ranges from mild to moderate but may increase from moderate to severe among patients in advanced stages of AIDS (Reger et al. 2002). The severity of AIDS affects the attention and memory of patients. During early stages of HIV infection, basic attention/concentration skills appear relatively unaffected (Reger et al. 2002). Neuroimaging studies have suggested that increased attention load increases the frontoparietal activation, leading to impairment in attention and working memory recollection (Chang et al. 2004). Visuoperception/visuospatial functioning are very important aspects of cognitive health. These are reported to be generally unaffected in HIV infection, as the occipital and parietal cortices are generally not affected very badly in neuro-AIDS. Cognitive and visual impairments, language impairments, and particularly speech difficulties are also frequently challenged cognitive features among HIV-infected children (Wolters et al. 1997), compared to adults. Language and speech irregularities appear more frequently in HIV patients with CNS opportunistic infection (e.g., in progressive multifocal leukoencephalopathy). Thorough investigations of spatial cognition are needed to characterize the nature and origin of various neurological impairments in HIV-infected patients.

19.8 DIAGNOSIS OF HIV-ASSOCIATED NEUROLOGICAL DISORDERS (HAND)

Dementia is initiated through substantial immune deficiency caused by HIV and consequent systemic opportunistic infections and complications of AIDS. HIV-associated dementia is characterized by some clinical features such as cerebral and basal ganglia atrophy and diffuse periventricular white matter hyperintensities, which can be visualized through magnetic resonance imaging (Dal Pan et al. 1992; Simpson and Tagliati 1994). Diminished levels of neuronal metabolite N-acetyl-aspartate levels are also used to diagnose dementia by magnetic resonance spectroscopy (Sacktor et al. 2005). Elevated levels of choline are used as an indicator of inflammation (Ernst et al. 2003). Serological investigations show high protein and IgG levels with an accompanying pleocytosis in the cerebrospinal fluid of 66% of HAD patients. HIV is known to preferentially infect the basal ganglia and deep white matter, thereby displaying the cardinal features of a "subcortical dementia." This makes HAD not readily detected by the routine mental status examination such as Folstein Mini, unless the patient is critically demented (Skinner et al. 2009). Nevertheless, background correction caused by substance abuse is essential to be taken into consideration, helping the exclusion of residual neuropsychiatric deficits, especially evident with long-standing crack/ cocaine use. These neuroimaging techniques as well as cerebrospinal fluid analyses are sufficient to exclude other factors causing similar images in the brain. However, paradoxes exist, and deterioration in neurological status after initiation of highly active antiretroviral therapy (HAART) has been reported and is termed as neurological immune reconstitution inflammatory syndrome (neuro-IRIS) and requires careful analysis of disease history and neuroimaging as well (Power et al. 2009).

19.9 HIV-ASSOCIATED NEUROPATHOLOGIES AND ASSOCIATION OF OPPORTUNISTIC INFECTIONS

Autopsy and other histological studies suggest the neuropathological changes in more than 90% of HIV/AIDS patients (Johnson 1998). The changes in brain tissues of HIV-1-infected patients are very evident, and some of them have been found to be unique to HIV infection. The pathobiology of primary HIV-related neurological disorders are generally defined by neuroinflammation and neuronal injury (Jones and Power 2006). There are multiple histopathological hallmarks of HIV-1-associated neuropathologies. Significant infiltration and accumulation of macrophages in brain tissues, the appearance of microglial nodules, and specially multinucleated giant cells (MGCs) become prominent in the central white matter and deep gray matter in HIV dementia (Budka 1986). These MGCs are actually virus-induced fusion of microglia and/or macrophages. The neuropathological hallmarks such as appearance of MGCs, perivascular cuffs comprised of macrophages and lymphocytes, and diffuse white matter pallor are now confirmed with magnetic resonance imaging and spectroscopy findings (Sharer 1992). Viral antigens particularly viral proteins have been detected and well correlated with the state of HIVE in the CNS. Enhanced astrogliosis, indicative of astrocyte activation and damage as well as the loss of specific neuron subpopulations, particularly those in hippocampus and basal ganglia, are very frequently seen in cognition and motor dysfunction. The loss is also evident at synaptic connections and myelin pallor accompanied with the loss of myelin and oligodendrocytes surrounding neuronal axons (Gendelman et al. 1994b; Lawrence and Major 2002). Neuronal apoptosis along with other forms of cell deaths, autophagy, and necrosis can likely contribute to reduced neural cell survival and health (Jones and Power 2006).

Three main types of changes have been reported in brain tissue of patients with HAD (Scaravilli et al. 2007). First, the presence of disseminated foci or more diffuse lesions including myelin loss, reactive astrocytosis, and microglial activation displayed as microglial nodules, macrophages, and accumulation of MGCs during high viral load. Second, diffuse myelin pallor, particularly the severe form in the centrum semiovale, is frequently associated with HIV leukoencephalopathy. In the case of extreme HIV-induced pathology, these kinds of lesions are regarded as very common and may overlap in one third of cases (Budka et al. 1991). In addition to these characterized lesions, axonal damage has also been reported by immunocytochemistry studies, which reveal the extremely frequent deposition of the beta-amyloid protein precursor in neurons of AIDS patients (Giometto et al. 1997).

In other cases of noninfectious neurodegenerative disorders, focal CNS involvement is more prominent in the early stages of the disease (Seeley et al. 2009), whereas in HIV induced neurodegeneration shows a broader CNS impact; mainly focused on the deep gray matter structures and subcortical regions. This explains the clinical manifestations that revolve around cognitive, motor, and behavioral dysfunctions. Other frequent CNS associated changes include apathy and depression in HAD (Hoare et al. 2010; Sharer 1992; Warriner et al. 2010).

When HIV directly infects the cells of CNS, it causes HAD, which falls under the category of progressive subcortical dementia. However, HIV infection of the peripheral nervous system results in a painful sensory neuropathy termed as distal sensory polyneuropathy. These sensory neuropathies were shown to be exacerbated by several antiretroviral drugs (Power et al. 2009).

HIV-induced neurological manifestations can also be categorized in two major groups. The first group includes the neurological syndromes that are directly caused by HIV-1 infection and more frequently encountered in AIDS patients. The second group of neurological syndromes includes opportunistic infections and consequent neurological perturbations. HIV infection exacerbates the opportunistic infections in the brain, and enhances the coexistence of morbid illnesses (Valcour et al. 2011). Secondary infections make the treatment of HAND a harder goal to achieve despite the availability of HAART. The CNS environment is reported to be more discordant than in the lymphoid system, and it is evident that the CNS can harbor virus, very different from virus in plasma (Valcour et al. 2011).

Opportunistic infections take place as a consequence of HIV-induced immunosuppression. Opportunistic infection in the central and peripheral nervous system consists of toxoplasmic encephalitis, cryptococcal meningitis, progressive multifocal leukoencephalopathy (PML), primary CNS lymphoma, CNS tuberculosis, cytomegalovirus encephalitis and radiculitis, or multidermatomal herpes zoster (Mamidi et al. 2002; Roullet 1999).

19.10 TREATMENT: CNS COMPLICATIONS AND HAART

Currently, highly active antiretroviral therapy (HAART) is the most effective treatment for controlling HIV replication in patients and thereby avoiding the early onset of the AIDS. Therefore, HAART also seems promising in controlling HAND. The usual HAART regimen combines three or more different drugs such as two nucleoside reverse transcriptase inhibitors (NRTIs) and a protease inhibitor (PI), two NRTIs and a non-nucleoside reverse transcriptase inhibitor (NNRTI) or other such combinations. Treatment with either two nucleoside analogue reverse transcriptase inhibitors and the nonnucleoside analogue reverse transcriptase inhibitor, nevirapine, has been shown to improve neuropsychological performance in HIV/AIDS patients (Price et al. 1999). Improvement in neuropsychological performance has also been reported with two nucleoside analogue reverse transcriptase inhibitors and a protease inhibitor (Langford et al. 2006; Sacktor et al. 1999; von Giesen et al. 2002).

HAART has shown convincing benefit in turning back deteriorative HIV-associated dementia (Anthony and Bell 2008; Boisse et al. 2008; Brew et al. 2009), but poor drug penetrance into the CNS still restrains the efficacy of HAART (Langford et al. 2006). The therapy became ineffective in those cases, where patients were exhibiting a plateau or "burnt-out" phase of HIV-associated dementia. Even the subjects receiving HAART showed continued neuropsychiatric disease progression (Brew et al. 2007). Other than HAART, there are several drugs reported to be neuroprotective and have been employed for treating HIV-associated dementia (McArthur et al. 2005). Amantidine has shown protective effect in HAD patients, especially in improving motor disabilities. Matrix metalloproteinase (MMP) inhibitors have also shown promising results against HIV-induced neurotoxicity (Zhang et al. 2003). Minocycline, a broad-spectrum antibiotic, has been found to be useful in suppressing microglia/macrophage activation and can control the severity of neuroinflammation (Zink et al. 2005). Valproic acid, a well-known antidepressant, has also been used in treating dementia (Schifitto et al. 2006).

According to WHO and the Joint United Nations Programme on HIV/AIDS (2004), HAART therapy has been significantly helpful in increasing the life expectancy of AIDS patients. Surprisingly, neuroinflammation still persists even after the use of HAART in AIDS patients. Age has been consistently identified as a risk factor for cognitive impairment in HIV-infected patients (Valcour et al. 2011).

Successive reports after the introduction of HAART has shown two most peculiar effects: first, being effective in suppressing HIV replication, which in turn reduces both the morbidity and neurobehavioral disorders. Second, it modifies the pathological pattern of neuro-AIDS HAART is successful in suppressing HIV replication (Pakker et al. 1997) and improving cellular immunity (Autran et al. 1997) and provides a wide range of protection against opportunistic infections (Jellinger et al. 2000; Maschke et al. 2000; Chiappini et al. 2007). A decrease in immune activation has also been observed compared with the pre-HAART era. HAART therapy suppresses the level of HIV RNA in plasma but has shown high levels of microglial/macrophage activation in the basal ganglia and hippocampus region (Anthony et al. 2005). The prevalence of severe forms of dementia can be minimized by the use of HAART, but the occurrence of HIV dementia is increasing with the increased chronicity of HIV-1 infection and prolonged survival of HIV-infected individuals carrying on HAART therapy (Dore et al. 2003; McArthur et al. 2003; Neuenburg et al. 2002). About 25% of patients under treatment show intolerance to the drugs, which manifests as nausea, anorexia, skin rash, hepatitis, and neuropsychiatric disorders. The appearance of dementia mostly starts during the advanced stages of AIDS. These observations suggest that CNS does not get complete therapeutic effects of HAART compared to the effects at periphery.

In conclusion, the introduction of HAART has dramatically modified the course and prognosis of HIV infection and is helpful in increasing the life expectancy of patients. Therefore, it is crucial to understand the multidimensional course of HAND, which differs from normal pathological manifestations of AIDS and thus need different approaches to deal with HIV induced neuroinflammation and neuro-degeneration effectively.

ACKNOWLEDGEMENT

Authors thankfully acknowledge the financial support provided by "Indo-Swiss Grant" DST/INT/SWISS/P-44/2012, through Dept. of Science and Technology, Govt. of India, New Delhi.

REFERENCES

Acheampong, E. A., Parveen, Z., Muthoga, L. W., Kalayeh, M., Mukhtar, M., and Pomerantz, R. J. (2005). Human Immunodeficiency virus type 1 Nef potently induces apoptosis in primary human brain microvascular endothelial cells via the activation of caspases. *J Virol* 79(7), 4257–69.

Adle-Biassette, H., Levy, Y., Colombel, M., Poron, F., Natchev, S., Keohane, C., and Gray, F. (1995). Neuronal apoptosis in HIV infection in adults. *Neuropathol Appl Neurobiol* 21(3), 218–27.

An, S. F., Groves, M., Giometto, B., Beckett, A. A., and Scaravilli, F. (1999). Detection and localisation of HIV-1 DNA and RNA in fixed adult AIDS brain by polymerase chain reaction/*in situ* hybridisation technique. *Acta Neuropathol* 98(5), 481–7.

Andras, I. E., Pu, H., Deli, M. A., Nath, A., Hennig, B., and Toborek, M. (2003). HIV-1 Tat protein alters tight junction protein expression and distribution in cultured brain endo-thelial cells. *J Neurosci Res* 74(2), 255–65.

Anthony, I. C., and Bell, J. E. (2008). The Neuropathology of HIV/AIDS. *Int Rev Psychiatry* 20(1), 15–24.

Anthony, I. C., Ramage, S. N., Carnie, F. W., Simmonds, P., and Bell, J. E. (2005). Influence of HAART on HIV-related CNS disease and neuroinflammation. *J Neuropathol Exp Neurol* 64(6), 529–36.

Antinori, A., Arendt, G., Becker, J. T., Brew, B. J., Byrd, D. A., Cherner, M., Clifford, D. B., Cinque, P., Epstein, L. G., Goodkin, K., Gisslen, M., Grant, I., Heaton, R. K., Joseph, J., Marder, K., Marra, C. M., McArthur, J. C., Nunn, M., Price, R. W., Pulliam, L., Robertson, K. R., Sacktor, N., Valcour, V., and Wojna, V. E. (2007). Updated research nosology for HIV-associated neurocognitive disorders. *Neurology* 69(18), 1789–99.

Autran, B., Carcelain, G., Li, T. S., Blanc, C., Mathez, D., Tubiana, R., Katlama, C., Debre, P., and Leibowitch, J. (1997). Positive effects of combined antiretroviral therapy on CD4+ T cell homeostasis and function in advanced HIV disease. *Science* 277(5322), 112–6.

Banks, W. A., Robinson, S. M., and Nath, A. (2005). Permeability of the blood–brain barrier to HIV-1 Tat. *Exp Neurol* 193(1), 218–27.

Bell, J. E. (1998). The neuropathology of adult HIV infection. *Rev Neurol (Paris)* 154(12), 816–29.

Boisse, L., Gill, M. J., and Power, C. (2008). HIV infection of the central nervous system: clinical features and neuropathogenesis. *Neurol Clin* 26(3), 799–819, x.

Bonfoco, E., Krainc, D., Ankarcrona, M., Nicotera, P., and Lipton, S. A. (1995). Apoptosis and necrosis: two distinct events induced, respectively, by mild and intense insults with N-methyl-D-aspartate or nitric oxide/superoxide in cortical cell cultures. *Proc Natl Acad Sci U S A* 92(16), 7162–6.

Boven, L. A., Gomes, L., Hery, C., Gray, F., Verhoef, J., Portegies, P., Tardieu, M., and Nottet, H. S. (1999). Increased peroxynitrite activity in AIDS dementia complex: implications for the neuropathogenesis of HIV-1 infection. *J Immunol* 162(7), 4319–27.

Brew, B. J., Crowe, S. M., Landay, A., Cysique, L. A., and Guillemin, G. (2009). Neurodegeneration and ageing in the HAART era. *J Neuroimmune Pharmacol* 4(2), 163–74.

Brew, B. J., Halman, M., Catalan, J., Sacktor, N., Price, R. W., Brown, S., Atkinson, H., Clifford, D. B., Simpson, D., Torres, G., Hall, C., Power, C., Marder, K., Mc Arthur, J. C., Symonds, W., and Romero, C. (2007). Factors in AIDS dementia complex trial design: results and lessons from the abacavir trial. *PLoS Clin Trials* 2(3), e13.

Bruce-Keller, A. J., Chauhan, A., Dimayuga, F. O., Gee, J., Keller, J. N., and Nath, A. (2003). Synaptic transport of human immunodeficiency virus-Tat protein causes neurotoxicity and gliosis in rat brain. *J Neurosci* 23(23), 8417–22.

Budd, S. L., Tenneti, L., Lishnak, T., and Lipton, S. A. (2000). Mitochondrial and extramitochondrial apoptotic signaling pathways in cerebrocortical neurons. *Proc Natl Acad Sci U S A* 97(11), 6161–6.

Budka, H. (1986). Multinucleated giant cells in brain: a hallmark of the acquired immune deficiency syndrome (AIDS). *Acta Neuropathol* 69(3–4), 253–8.

Budka, H., Wiley, C. A., Kleihues, P., Artigas, J., Asbury, A. K., Cho, E. S., Cornblath, D. R., Dal Canto, M. C., DeGirolami, U., Dickson, D. et al. (1991). HIV-associated disease of the nervous system: review of nomenclature and proposal for neuropathology-based terminology. *Brain Pathol* 1(3), 143–52.

Carne, C. A., Tedder, R. S., Smith, A., Sutherland, S., Elkington, S. G., Daly, H. M., Preston, F. E., and Craske, J. (1985). Acute encephalopathy coincident with seroconversion for anti-HTLV-III. *Lancet* 2(8466), 1206–8.

Carter, J. L., Hafler, D. A., Dawson, D. M., Orav, J., and Weiner, H. L. (1988). Immunosuppression with high-dose i.v. cyclophosphamide and ACTH in progressive multiple sclerosis: cumulative 6-year experience in 164 patients. *Neurology* 38(7 Suppl 2), 9–14.

Chang, L., Tomasi, D., Yakupov, R., Lozar, C., Arnold, S., Caparelli, E., and Ernst, T. (2004). Adaptation of the attention network in human immunodeficiency virus brain injury. *Ann Neurol* 56(2), 259–72.

Chaudhry, F. A., Lehre, K. P., van Lookeren Campagne, M., Ottersen, O. P., Danbolt, N. C., and Storm-Mathisen, J. (1995). Glutamate transporters in glial plasma membranes: highly differentiated localizations revealed by quantitative ultrastructural immunocytochemistry. *Neuron* 15(3), 711–20.

Cheng, J., Nath, A., Knudsen, B., Hochman, S., Geiger, J. D., Ma, M., and Magnuson, D. S. (1998). Neuronal excitatory properties of human immunodeficiency virus type 1 Tat protein. *Neuroscience* 82(1), 97–106.

Chiappini, E., Galli, L., Tovo, P. A., Gabiano, C., Lisi, C., Gattinara, G. C., Esposito, S., Vigano, A., Giaquinto, C., Rosso, R., Guarino, A., and de Martino, M. (2007). Changing patterns of clinical events in perinatally HIV-1-infected children during the era of HAART. *AIDS* 21(12), 1607–15.

Cinque, P., Bestetti, A., Marenzi, R., Sala, S., Gisslen, M., Hagberg, L., and Price, R. W. (2005). Cerebrospinal fluid interferon-gamma-inducible protein 10 (IP-10, CXCL10) in HIV-1 infection. *J Neuroimmunol* 168(1–2), 154–63.

Clifford, D. B. (2008). HIV-associated neurocognitive disease continues in the antiretroviral era. *Top HIV Med* 16(2), 94–8.

Contreras, X., Bennasser, Y., Chazal, N., Moreau, M., Leclerc, C., Tkaczuk, J., and Bahraoui, E. (2005). Human immunodeficiency virus type 1 Tat protein induces an intracellular calcium increase in human monocytes that requires DHP receptors: involvement in TNF-alpha production. *Virology* 332(1), 316–28.

Dal Pan, G. J., McArthur, J. H., Aylward, E., Selnes, O. A., Nance-Sproson, T. E., Kumar, A. J., Mellits, E. D., and McArthur, J. C. (1992). Patterns of cerebral atrophy in HIV-1-infected individuals: results of a quantitative MRI analysis. *Neurology* 42(11), 2125–30.

Dalgleish, A. G. (1995). Autoimmune mechanisms of depletion of CD4 cells in HIV infection. *Br J Haematol* 91(3), 525–34.

Danbolt, N. C., Storm-Mathisen, J., and Kanner, B. I. (1992). An [Na++ K+]coupled L-glutamate transporter purified from rat brain is located in glial cell processes. *Neuroscience* 51(2), 295–310.

Davis, L. E., Hjelle, B. L., Miller, V. E., Palmer, D. L., Llewellyn, A. L., Merlin, T. L., Young, S. A., Mills, R. G., Wachsman, W., and Wiley, C. A. (1992). Early viral brain invasion in iatrogenic human immunodeficiency virus infection. *Neurology* 42(9), 1736–9.

Del Valle, L., Croul, S., Morgello, S., Amini, S., Rappaport, J., and Khalili, K. (2000). Detection of HIV-1 Tat and JCV capsid protein, VP1, in AIDS brain with progressive multifocal leukoencephalopathy. *J Neurovirol* 6(3), 221–8.

Della Chiara, G., Fortis, C., Tambussi, G., and Poli, G. (2010). The rise and fall of intermittent interleukin-2 therapy in HIV infection. *Eur Cytokine Netw* 21(3), 197–201.

Dhillon, N., Zhu, X., Peng, F., Yao, H., Williams, R., Qiu, J., Callen, S., Ladner, A. O., and Buch, S. (2008). Molecular mechanism(s) involved in the synergistic induction of CXCL10 by human immunodeficiency virus type 1 Tat and interferon-gamma in macrophages. *J Neurovirol* 14(3), 196–204.

Dore, G. J., McDonald, A., Li, Y., Kaldor, J. M., and Brew, B. J. (2003). Marked improvement in survival following AIDS dementia complex in the era of highly active antiretroviral therapy. *AIDS* 17(10), 1539–45.

Dunfee, R., Thomas, E. R., Gorry, P. R., Wang, J., Ancuta, P., and Gabuzda, D. (2006). Mechanisms of HIV-1 neurotropism. *Curr HIV Res* 4(3), 267–78.

Eriksson, P. S., Perfilieva, E., Bjork-Eriksson, T., Alborn, A. M., Nordborg, C., Peterson, D. A., and Gage, F. H. (1998). Neurogenesis in the adult human hippocampus. *Nat Med* 4(11), 1313–7.

Ernst, T., Chang, L., and Arnold, S. (2003). Increased glial metabolites predict increased working memory network activation in HIV brain injury. *Neuroimage* 19(4), 1686–93.

Everall, I., Luthert, P., and Lantos, P. (1993). A review of neuronal damage in human immunodeficiency virus infection: its assessment, possible mechanism and relationship to dementia. *J Neuropathol Exp Neurol* 52(6), 561–6.

Fallarino, F., Grohmann, U., Hwang, K. W., Orabona, C., Vacca, C., Bianchi, R., Belladonna, M. L., Fioretti, M. C., Alegre, M. L., and Puccetti, P. (2003). Modulation of tryptophan catabolism by regulatory T cells. *Nat Immunol* 4(12), 1206–12.

Fonnum, F. (1984). Glutamate: a neurotransmitter in mammalian brain. *J Neurochem* 42(1), 1–11.

Fontana, G., Valenti, L., and Raiteri, M. (1997). Gp120 can revert antagonism at the glycine site of NMDA receptors mediating GABA release from cultured hippocampal neurons. *J Neurosci Res* 49(6), 732–8.

Frankel, A. D., and Young, J. A. (1998). HIV-1: fifteen proteins and an RNA. *Annu Rev Biochem* 67, 1–25.

Garden, G. A. (2002). Microglia in human immunodeficiency virus-associated neurodegeneration. *Glia* 40(2), 240–51.

Gegelashvili, G., and Schousboe, A. (1997). High affinity glutamate transporters: regulation of expression and activity. *Mol Pharmacol* 52(1), 6–15.

Geiger, K. D., Stoldt, P., Schlote, W., and Derouiche, A. (2006). Ezrin immunoreactivity reveals specific astrocyte activation in cerebral HIV. *J Neuropathol Exp Neurol* 65(1), 87–96.

Gendelman, H. E., Baldwin, T., Baca-Regen, L., Swindells, S., Loomis, L., and Skurkovich, S. (1994a). Regulation of HIV1 replication by interferon alpha: from laboratory bench to bedside. *Res Immunol* 145(8–9), 679–84; discussion 684–5.

Gendelman, H. E., Lipton, S. A., Tardieu, M., Bukrinsky, M. I., and Nottet, H. S. (1994b). The neuropathogenesis of HIV-1 infection. *J Leukoc Biol* 56(3), 389–98.

Ghafouri, M., Amini, S., Khalili, K., and Sawaya, B. E. (2006). HIV-1 associated dementia: symptoms and causes. *Retrovirology* 3, 28.

Ghatan, S., Larner, S., Kinoshita, Y., Hetman, M., Patel, L., Xia, Z., Youle, R. J., and Morrison, R. S. (2000). p38 MAP kinase mediates bax translocation in nitric oxide-induced apoptosis in neurons. *J Cell Biol* 150(2), 335–47.

Giometto, B., An, S. F., Groves, M., Scaravilli, T., Geddes, J. F., Miller, R., Tavolato, B., Beckett, A. A., and Scaravilli, F. (1997). Accumulation of beta-amyloid precursor protein in HIV encephalitis: relationship with neuropsychological abnormalities. *Ann Neurol* 42(1), 34–40.

Grant, I., and Atkinson, J. H. (1995). Psychiatric aspects of acquired immune deficiency syndrome. In H. I. Kaplan and B. J. Sadock (Eds.), Comprehensive textbook of psychiatry Baltimore: Williams and Wilkins (Vol. 2, pp. 1644–1669).

Grant, I., and Atkinson, J. H. (1999). Neuropsychiatric aspects of HIV infection and AIDS. In B. J. Sadock and V. A. Sadock (Eds.), Kaplan and Sadock's comprehensive textbook of psychiatry, Baltimore: Williams and Wilkins vii (pp. 308–335).

Grant, I., Sacktor, N., and McArthur, J. C. (2005). HIV neurocognitive disorders. In H. E. Gendelman, I. Grant, I. Everall, S. A. Liptonv and S. Swindells (Eds.), The neurology of AIDS, New York: Oxford University (2nd ed., pp. 359–373).

Gray, F., Adle-Biassette, H., Brion, F., Ereau, T., le Maner, I., Levy, V., and Corcket, G. (2000). Neuronal apoptosis in human immunodeficiency virus infection. *J Neurovirol* 6 Suppl 1, S38–S43.

Heaton, R. K., Grant, I., Butters, N., White, D. A., Kirson, D., Atkinson, J. H., McCutchan, J. A., Taylor, M. J., Kelly, M. D., Ellis, R. J. et al. (1995). The HNRC 500—neuropsychology of HIV infection at different disease stages. HIV Neurobehavioral Research Center. *J Int Neuropsychol Soc* 1(3), 231–51.

Herrup, K., and Yang, Y. (2007). Cell cycle regulation in the postmitotic neuron: oxymoron or new biology? *Nat Rev Neurosci* 8(5), 368–78.

Hoare, J., Fouche, J. P., Spottiswoode, B., Joska, J. A., Schoeman, R., Stein, D. J., and Carey, P. D. (2010). White matter correlates of apathy in HIV-positive subjects: a diffusion tensor imaging study. *J Neuropsychiatry Clin Neurosci* 22(3), 313–20.

Hoffmann, C., Tabrizian, S., Wolf, E., Eggers, C., Stoehr, A., Plettenberg, A., Buhk, T., Stellbrink, H. J., Horst, H. A., Jager, H., and Rosenkranz, T. (2001). Survival of AIDS patients with primary central nervous system lymphoma is dramatically improved by HAART-induced immune recovery. *AIDS* 15(16), 2119–27.

Hogan, C., and Wilkins, E. (2011). Neurological complications in HIV. *Clin Med* 11(6), 571–5.

Hoglinger, G. U., Breunig, J. J., Depboylu, C., Rouaux, C., Michel, P. P., Alvarez-Fischer, D., Boutillier, A. L., Degregori, J., Oertel, W. H., Rakic, P., Hirsch, E. C., and Hunot, S. (2007). The pRb/E2F cell-cycle pathway mediates cell death in Parkinson's disease. *Proc Natl Acad Sci U S A* 104(9), 3585–90.

Hudson, L., Liu, J., Nath, A., Jones, M., Raghavan, R., Narayan, O., Male, D., and Everall, I. (2000). Detection of the human immunodeficiency virus regulatory protein tat in CNS tissues. *J Neurovirol* 6(2), 145–55.

Jellinger, K. A., Setinek, U., Drlicek, M., Bohm, G., Steurer, A., and Lintner, F. (2000). Neuropathology and general autopsy findings in AIDS during the last 15 years. *Acta Neuropathol* 100(2), 213–20.

Jiang, Z. G., Piggee, C., Heyes, M. P., Murphy, C., Quearry, B., Bauer, M., Zheng, J., Gendelman, H. E., and Markey, S. P. (2001). Glutamate is a mediator of neurotoxicity in secretions of activated HIV-1-infected macrophages. *J Neuroimmunol* 117(1–2), 97–107.

Johnson, R. T. (1998). Viral infections of the nervous system. 2nd ed. Philadelphia: Lippincott-Raven Publishers.

Johri, M. K., Mishra, R., Chhatbar, C., Unni, S. K., and Singh, S. K. (2011). Tits and bits of HIV Tat protein. *Expert Opin Biol Ther* 11(3), 269–83.

Jones, G., and Power, C. (2006). Regulation of neural cell survival by HIV-1 infection. *Neurobiol Dis* 21(1), 1–17.

Jones, G. J., Barsby, N. L., Cohen, E. A., Holden, J., Harris, K., Dickie, P., Jhamandas, J., and Power, C. (2007). HIV-1 Vpr causes neuronal apoptosis and *in vivo* neurodegeneration. *J Neurosci* 27(14), 3703–11.

Kanmogne, G. D., Schall, K., Leibhart, J., Knipe, B., Gendelman, H. E., and Persidsky, Y. (2007). HIV-1 gp120 compromises blood-brain barrier integrity and enhances monocyte migration across blood-brain barrier: implication for viral neuropathogenesis. *J Cereb Blood Flow Metab* 27(1), 123–34.

Karl, C., Couillard-Despres, S., Prang, P., Munding, M., Kilb, W., Brigadski, T., Plotz, S., Mages, W., Luhmann, H., Winkler, J., Bogdahn, U., and Aigner, L. (2005). Neuronal precursor-specific activity of a human doublecortin regulatory sequence. *J Neurochem* 92(2), 264–82.

Kaul, M., Garden, G. A., and Lipton, S. A. (2001). Pathways to neuronal injury and apoptosis in HIV-associated dementia. *Nature* 410(6831), 988–94.

Kaul, M., and Lipton, S. A. (1999). Chemokines and activated macrophages in HIV gp120-induced neuronal apoptosis. *Proc Natl Acad Sci U S A* 96(14), 8212–6.

Khan, M. Z., Brandimarti, R., Shimizu, S., Nicolai, J., Crowe, E., and Meucci, O. (2008). The chemokine CXCL12 promotes survival of postmitotic neurons by regulating Rb protein. *Cell Death Differ* 15(10), 1663–72.

Kibayashi, K., Mastri, A. R., and Hirsch, C. S. (1996). Neuropathology of human immunodeficiency virus infection at different disease stages. *Hum Pathol* 27(7), 637–42.

Kolson, D. L., and Pomerantz, R. J. (1996). AIDS Dementia and HIV-1-induced neurotoxicity: possible pathogenic associations and mechanisms. *J Biomed Sci* 3(6), 389–414.

Kort, J. J. (1998). Impairment of excitatory amino acid transport in astroglial cells infected with the human immunodeficiency virus type 1. *AIDS Res Hum Retroviruses* 14(15), 1329–39.

Langford, D., Marquie-Beck, J., de Almeida, S., Lazzaretto, D., Letendre, S., Grant, I., McCutchan, J. A., Masliah, E., and Ellis, R. J. (2006). Relationship of antiretroviral treatment to postmortem brain tissue viral load in human immunodeficiency virus-infected patients. *J Neurovirol* 12(2), 100–7.

Lawrence, D. M., and Major, E. O. (2002). HIV-1 and the brain: connections between HIV-1-associated dementia, neuropathology and neuroimmunology. *Microbes Infect* 4(3), 301–8.

Lehre, K. P., Levy, L. M., Ottersen, O. P., Storm-Mathisen, J., and Danbolt, N. C. (1995). Differential expression of two glial glutamate transporters in the rat brain: quantitative and immunocytochemical observations. *J Neurosci* 15(3 Pt 1), 1835–53.

Levy, D. N., Refaeli, Y., MacGregor, R. R., and Weiner, D. B. (1994). Serum Vpr regulates productive infection and latency of human immunodeficiency virus type 1. *Proc Natl Acad Sci U S A* 91(23), 10873–7.

Li, W., Huang, Y., Reid, R., Steiner, J., Malpica-Llanos, T., Darden, T. A., Shankar, S. K., Mahadevan, A., Satishchandra, P., and Nath, A. (2008). NMDA receptor activation by HIV-Tat protein is clade dependent. *J Neurosci* 28(47), 12190–8.

Li, W., Li, G., Steiner, J., and Nath, A. (2009). Role of Tat protein in HIV neuropathogenesis. *Neurotox Res* 16(3), 205–20.

Lindl, K. A., Marks, D. R., Kolson, D. L., and Jordan-Sciutto, K. L. (2010). HIV-associated neurocognitive disorder: pathogenesis and therapeutic opportunities. *J Neuroimmune Pharmacol* 5(3), 294–309.

Lipton, S. A., and Gendelman, H. E. (1995). Seminars in medicine of the Beth Israel Hospital, Boston. Dementia associated with the acquired immunodeficiency syndrome. *N Engl J Med* 332(14), 934–40.

Liu, Z. Q., Muhkerjee, S., Sahni, M., McCormick-Davis, C., Leung, K., Li, Z., Gattone, V. H., 2nd, Tian, C., Doms, R. W., Hoffman, T. L., Raghavan, R., Narayan, O., and Stephens, E. B. (1999). Derivation and biological characterization of a molecular clone of SHIV(KU-2) that causes AIDS, neurological disease, and renal disease in rhesus macaques. *Virology* 260(2), 295–307.

Maj, M., Satz, P., Janssen, R., Zaudig, M., Starace, F., D'Elia, L., Sughondhabirom, B., Mussa, M., Naber, D., Ndetei, D. et al. (1994). WHO Neuropsychiatric AIDS study, cross-sectional phase II. Neuropsychological and neurological findings. *Arch Gen Psychiatry* 51(1), 51–61.

Mamidi, A., DeSimone, J. A., and Pomerantz, R. J. (2002). Central nervous system infections in individuals with HIV-1 infection. *J Neurovirol* 8(3), 158–67.

Maschke, M., Kastrup, O., Esser, S., Ross, B., Hengge, U., and Hufnagel, A. (2000). Incidence and prevalence of neurological disorders associated with HIV since the introduction of highly active antiretroviral therapy (HAART). *J Neurol Neurosurg Psychiatry* 69(3), 376–80.

Mattson, M. P., Haughey, N. J., and Nath, A. (2005). Cell death in HIV dementia. *Cell Death Differ* 12 Suppl 1, 893–904.

McArthur, J. C., Brew, B. J., and Nath, A. (2005). Neurological complications of HIV infection. *Lancet Neurol* 4(9), 543–55.

McArthur, J. C., Haughey, N., Gartner, S., Conant, K., Pardo, C., Nath, A., and Sacktor, N. (2003). Human immunodeficiency virus-associated dementia: an evolving disease. *J Neurovirol* 9(2), 205–21.

McArthur, J. C., Hoover, D. R., Bacellar, H., Miller, E. N., Cohen, B. A., Becker, J. T., Graham, N. M., McArthur, J. H., Selnes, O. A., Jacobson, L. P. et al. (1993). Dementia in AIDS patients: incidence and risk factors. Multicenter AIDS Cohort Study. *Neurology* 43(11), 2245–52.

Meltzer, M. S., and Gendelman, H. E. (1992). Mononuclear phagocytes as targets, tissue reservoirs, and immunoregulatory cells in human immunodeficiency virus disease. *Curr Top Microbiol Immunol* 181, 239–63.

Meucci, O., Fatatis, A., Simen, A. A., and Miller, R. J. (2000). Expression of CX3CR1 chemokine receptors on neurons and their role in neuronal survival. *Proc Natl Acad Sci U S A* 97(14), 8075–80.

Mirsattari, S. M., Berry, M. E., Holden, J. K., Ni, W., Nath, A., and Power, C. (1999). Paroxysmal dyskinesias in patients with HIV infection. *Neurology* 52(1), 109–14.

Morris, A., Marsden, M., Halcrow, K., Hughes, E. S., Brettle, R. P., Bell, J. E., and Simmonds, P. (1999). Mosaic structure of the human immunodeficiency virus type 1 genome infecting lymphoid cells and the brain: evidence for frequent *in vivo* recombination events in the evolution of regional populations. *J Virol* 73(10), 8720–31.

Mukerjee, R., Chang, J. R., Del Valle, L., Bagashev, A., Gayed, M. M., Lyde, R. B., Hawkins, B. J., Brailoiu, E., Cohen, E., Power, C., Azizi, S. A., Gelman, B. B., and Sawaya, B. E.

(2011). Deregulation of microRNAs by HIV-1 Vpr protein leads to the development of neurocognitive disorders. *J Biol Chem* 286(40), 34976–85.

Mukhtar, M., and Pomerantz, R. J. (2000). Development of an *in vitro* blood-brain barrier model to study molecular neuropathogenesis and neurovirologic disorders induced by human immunodeficiency virus type 1 infection. *J Hum Virol* 3(6), 324–34.

Narayan, O., and Clements, J. E. (1989). Biology and pathogenesis of lentiviruses. *J Gen Virol* 70 (Pt 7), 1617–39.

Nath, A. (2002). Human immunodeficiency virus (HIV) proteins in neuropathogenesis of HIV dementia. *J Infect Dis* 186 Suppl 2, S193–8.

Nath, A., Conant, K., Chen, P., Scott, C., and Major, E. O. (1999). Transient exposure to HIV-1 Tat protein results in cytokine production in macrophages and astrocytes. A hit and run phenomenon. *J Biol Chem* 274(24), 17098–102.

Neuenburg, J. K., Brodt, H. R., Herndier, B. G., Bickel, M., Bacchetti, P., Price, R. W., Grant, R. M., and Schlote, W. (2002). HIV-related neuropathology 1985 to 1999: rising prevalence of HIV encephalopathy in the era of highly active antiretroviral therapy. *J Acquir Immune Defic Syndr* 31(2), 171–7.

Pakker, N. G., Roos, M. T., van Leeuwen, R., de Jong, M. D., Koot, M., Reiss, P., Lange, J. M., Miedema, F., Danner, S. A., and Schellekens, P. T. (1997). Patterns of T-cell repopulation, virus load reduction, and restoration of T-cell function in HIV-infected persons during therapy with different antiretroviral agents. *J Acquir Immune Defic Syndr Hum Retrovirol* 16(5), 318–26.

Pantaleo, G., Graziosi, C., and Fauci, A. S. (1993). New concepts in the immunopathogenesis of human immunodeficiency virus infection. *N Engl J Med* 328(5), 327–35.

Patel, C. A., Mukhtar, M., and Pomerantz, R. J. (2000). Human immunodeficiency virus type 1 Vpr induces apoptosis in human neuronal cells. *J Virol* 74(20), 9717–26.

Piller, S. C., Jans, P., Gage, P. W., and Jans, D. A. (1998). Extracellular HIV-1 virus protein R causes a large inward current and cell death in cultured hippocampal neurons: implications for AIDS pathology. *Proc Natl Acad Sci U S A* 95(8), 4595–600.

Pope, M., and Haase, A. T. (2003). Transmission, acute HIV-1 infection and the quest for strategies to prevent infection. *Nat Med* 9(7), 847–52.

Porcheray, F., Leone, C., Samah, B., Rimaniol, A. C., Dereuddre-Bosquet, N., and Gras, G. (2006). Glutamate metabolism in HIV-infected macrophages: implications for the CNS. *Am J Physiol Cell Physiol* 291(4), C618–26.

Power, C., Boisse, L., Rourke, S., and Gill, M. J. (2009). NeuroAIDS: an evolving epidemic. *Can J Neurol Sci* 36(3), 285–95.

Power, C., Kong, P. A., Crawford, T. O., Wesselingh, S., Glass, J. D., McArthur, J. C., and Trapp, B. D. (1993). Cerebral white matter changes in acquired immunodeficiency syndrome dementia: alterations of the blood-brain barrier. *Ann Neurol* 34(3), 339–50.

Price, R. W., Yiannoutsos, C. T., Clifford, D. B., Zaborski, L., Tselis, A., Sidtis, J. J., Cohen, B., Hall, C. D., Erice, A., and Henry, K. (1999). Neurological outcomes in late HIV infection: adverse impact of neurological impairment on survival and protective effect of antiviral therapy. AIDS Clinical Trial Group and Neurological AIDS Research Consortium study team. *AIDS* 13(13), 1677–85.

Pu, H., Tian, J., Flora, G., Lee, Y. W., Nath, A., Hennig, B., and Toborek, M. (2003). HIV-1 Tat protein upregulates inflammatory mediators and induces monocyte invasion into the brain. *Mol Cell Neurosci* 24(1), 224–37.

Reger, M., Welsh, R., Razani, J., Martin, D. J., and Boone, K. B. (2002). A meta-analysis of the neuropsychological sequelae of HIV infection. *J Int Neuropsychol Soc* 8(3), 410–24.

Revest, J. M., Dupret, D., Koehl, M., Funk-Reiter, C., Grosjean, N., Piazza, P. V., and Abrous, D. N. (2009). Adult hippocampal neurogenesis is involved in anxiety-related behaviors. *Mol Psychiatry* 14(10), 959–67.

Rippeth, J. D., Heaton, R. K., Carey, C. L., Marcotte, T. D., Moore, D. J., Gonzalez, R., Wolfson, T., and Grant, I. (2004). Methamphetamine dependence increases risk of neuropsychological impairment in HIV infected persons. *J Int Neuropsychol Soc* 10(1), 1–14.

Robertson, K. R., Smurzynski, M., Parsons, T. D., Wu, K., Bosch, R. J., Wu, J., McArthur, J. C., Collier, A. C., Evans, S. R., and Ellis, R. J. (2007). The prevalence and incidence of neurocognitive impairment in the HAART era. *AIDS* 21(14), 1915–21.

Rodriguez, J. J., Jones, V. C., Tabuchi, M., Allan, S. M., Knight, E. M., LaFerla, F. M., Oddo, S., and Verkhratsky, A. (2008). Impaired adult neurogenesis in the dentate gyrus of a triple transgenic mouse model of Alzheimer's disease. *PLoS One* 3(8), e2935.

Rosenberg, Z. F., and Fauci, A. S. (1991). Immunopathology and pathogenesis of human immunodeficiency virus infection. *Pediatr Infect Dis J* 10(3), 230–8.

Rothstein, J. D. (1996). Excitotoxicity hypothesis. *Neurology* 47(4 Suppl 2), S19–25; discussion S26.

Rottman, J. B., Ganley, K. P., Williams, K., Wu, L., Mackay, C. R., and Ringler, D. J. (1997). Cellular localization of the chemokine receptor CCR5. Correlation to cellular targets of HIV-1 infection. *Am J Pathol* 151(5), 1341–51.

Roullet, E. (1999). Opportunistic infections of the central nervous system during HIV-1 infection (emphasis on cytomegalovirus disease). *J Neurol* 246(4), 237–43.

Sacktor, N., Haughey, N., Cutler, R., Tamara, A., Turchan, J., Pardo, C., Vargas, D., and Nath, A. (2004). Novel markers of oxidative stress in actively progressive HIV dementia. *J Neuroimmunol* 157(1–2), 176–84.

Sacktor, N., Skolasky, R. L., Ernst, T., Mao, X., Selnes, O., Pomper, M. G., Chang, L., Zhong, K., Shungu, D. C., Marder, K., Shibata, D., Schifitto, G., Bobo, L., and Barker, P. B. (2005). A multicenter study of two magnetic resonance spectroscopy techniques in individuals with HIV dementia. *J Magn Reson Imaging* 21(4), 325–33.

Sacktor, N. C., Lyles, R. H., Skolasky, R. L., Anderson, D. E., McArthur, J. C., McFarlane, G., Selnes, O. A., Becker, J. T., Cohen, B., Wesch, J., and Miller, E. N. (1999). Combination antiretroviral therapy improves psychomotor speed performance in HIV-seropositive homosexual men. Multicenter AIDS Cohort Study (MACS). *Neurology* 52(8), 1640–7.

Saito, Y., Sharer, L. R., Epstein, L. G., Michaels, J., Mintz, M., Louder, M., Golding, K., Cvetkovich, T. A., and Blumberg, B. M. (1994). Overexpression of nef as a marker for restricted HIV-1 infection of astrocytes in postmortem pediatric central nervous tissues. *Neurology* 44(3 Pt 1), 474–81.

Scaravilli, F., Bazille, C., and Gray, F. (2007). Neuropathologic contributions to understanding AIDS and the central nervous system. *Brain Pathol* 17(2), 197–208.

Schifitto, G., Peterson, D. R., Zhong, J., Ni, H., Cruttenden, K., Gaugh, M., Gendelman, H. E., Boska, M., and Gelbard, H. (2006). Valproic acid adjunctive therapy for HIV-associated cognitive impairment: a first report. *Neurology* 66(6), 919–21.

Seeley, W. W., Crawford, R. K., Zhou, J., Miller, B. L., and Greicius, M. D. (2009). Neurodegenerative diseases target large-scale human brain networks. *Neuron* 62(1), 42–52.

Seilhean, D., Dzia-Lepfoundzou, A., Sazdovitch, V., Cannella, B., Raine, C. S., Katlama, C., Bricaire, F., Duyckaerts, C., and Hauw, J. J. (1997). Astrocytic adhesion molecules are increased in HIV-1-associated cognitive/motor complex. *Neuropathol Appl Neurobiol* 23(2), 83–92.

Sharer, L. R. (1992). Pathology of HIV-1 infection of the central nervous system. A review. *J Neuropathol Exp Neurol* 51(1), 3–11.

Shaw, G. M., Harper, M. E., Hahn, B. H., Epstein, L. G., Gajdusek, D. C., Price, R. W., Navia, B. A., Petito, C. K., O'Hara, C. J., Groopman, J. E. et al. (1985). HTLV-III infection in brains of children and adults with AIDS encephalopathy. *Science* 227(4683), 177–82.

Shoji, H., Azuma, K., Nishimura, Y., Fujimoto, H., Sugita, Y., and Eizuru, Y. (2002). Acute viral encephalitis: the recent progress. *Intern Med* 41(6), 420–8.

Simpson, D. M., and Tagliati, M. (1994). Neurologic manifestations of HIV infection. *Ann Intern Med* 121(10), 769–85.

Skinner, S., Adewale, A. J., DeBlock, L., Gill, M. J., and Power, C. (2009). Neurocognitive screening tools in HIV/AIDS: comparative performance among patients exposed to anti-retroviral therapy. *HIV Med* 10(4), 246–52.

Snider, W. D., Simpson, D. M., Nielsen, S., Gold, J. W., Metroka, C. E., and Posner, J. B. (1983). Neurological complications of acquired immune deficiency syndrome: analysis of 50 patients. *Ann Neurol* 14(4), 403–18.

Song, L., Nath, A., Geiger, J. D., Moore, A., and Hochman, S. (2003). Human immunodeficiency virus type 1 Tat protein directly activates neuronal N-methyl-D-aspartate receptors at an allosteric zinc-sensitive site. *J Neurovirol* 9(3), 399–403.

Stoler, M. H., Eskin, T. A., Benn, S., Angerer, R. C., and Angerer, L. M. (1986). Human T-cell lymphotropic virus type III infection of the central nervous system. A preliminary *in situ* analysis. *JAMA* 256(17), 2360–4.

Subbramanian, R. A., Kessous-Elbaz, A., Lodge, R., Forget, J., Yao, X. J., Bergeron, D., and Cohen, E. A. (1998). Human immunodeficiency virus type 1 Vpr is a positive regulator of viral transcription and infectivity in primary human macrophages. *J Exp Med* 187(7), 1103–11.

Tardieu, M., Hery, C., Peudenier, S., Boespflug, O., and Montagnier, L. (1992). Human immunodeficiency virus type 1-infected monocytic cells can destroy human neural cells after cell-to-cell adhesion. *Ann Neurol* 32(1), 11–7.

Taupin, P. (2009). Adult neurogenesis and the pathogenesis of Alzheimer's disease. *Med Sci Monit* 15(3), LE1.

Thomas, S., Mayer, L., and Sperber, K. (2009). Mitochondria influence Fas expression in gp120-induced apoptosis of neuronal cells. *Int J Neurosci* 119(2), 157–65.

Toborek, M., Lee, Y. W., Pu, H., Malecki, A., Flora, G., Garrido, R., Hennig, B., Bauer, H. C., and Nath, A. (2003). HIV-Tat protein induces oxidative and inflammatory pathways in brain endothelium. *J Neurochem* 84(1), 169–79.

Tornatore, C., Chandra, R., Berger, J. R., and Major, E. O. (1994). HIV-1 infection of subcortical astrocytes in the pediatric central nervous system. *Neurology* 44(3 Pt 1), 481–7.

Turchan, J., Pocernich, C. B., Gairola, C., Chauhan, A., Schifitto, G., Butterfield, D. A., Buch, S., Narayan, O., Sinai, A., Geiger, J., Berger, J. R., Elford, H., and Nath, A. (2003). Oxidative stress in HIV demented patients and protection ex vivo with novel antioxidants. *Neurology* 60(2), 307–14.

Valcour, V., Sithinamsuwan, P., Letendre, S., and Ances, B. (2011). Pathogenesis of HIV in the central nervous system. *Curr HIV/AIDS Rep* 8(1), 54–61.

Vallat-Decouvelaere, A. V., Chretien, F., Gras, G., Le Pavec, G., Dormont, D., and Gray, F. (2003). Expression of excitatory amino acid transporter-1 in brain macrophages and microglia of HIV-infected patients. A neuroprotective role for activated microglia? *J Neuropathol Exp Neurol* 62(5), 475–85.

Vallat, A. V., De Girolami, U., He, J., Mhashilkar, A., Marasco, W., Shi, B., Gray, F., Bell, J., Keohane, C., Smith, T. W., and Gabuzda, D. (1998). Localization of HIV-1 co-receptors CCR5 and CXCR4 in the brain of children with AIDS. *Am J Pathol* 152(1), 167–78.

van Marle, G., and Power, C. (2005). Human immunodeficiency virus type 1 genetic diversity in the nervous system: evolutionary epiphenomenon or disease determinant? *J Neurovirol* 11(2), 107–28.

Vazeux, R., Brousse, N., Jarry, A., Henin, D., Marche, C., Vedrenne, C., Mikol, J., Wolff, M., Michon, C., Rozenbaum, W. et al. (1987). AIDS subacute encephalitis. Identification of HIV-infected cells. *Am J Pathol* 126(3), 403–10.

Vivithanaporn, P., Heo, G., Gamble, J., Krentz, H. B., Hoke, A., Gill, M. J., and Power, C. (2010). Neurologic disease burden in treated HIV/AIDS predicts survival: a population-based study. *Neurology* 75(13), 1150–8.

von Giesen, H. J., Koller, H., Theisen, A., and Arendt, G. (2002). Therapeutic effects of non-nucleoside reverse transcriptase inhibitors on the central nervous system in HIV-1-infected patients. *J Acquir Immune Defic Syndr* 29(4), 363–7.

Wang, T., Rumbaugh, J. A., and Nath, A. (2006). Viruses and the brain: from inflammation to dementia. *Clin Sci (Lond)* 110(4), 393–407.

Warriner, E. M., Rourke, S. B., Rourke, B. P., Rubenstein, S., Millikin, C., Buchanan, L., Connelly, P., Hyrcza, M., Ostrowski, M., Der, S., and Gough, K. (2010). Immune activation and neuropsychiatric symptoms in HIV infection. *J Neuropsychiatry Clin Neurosci* 22(3), 321–8.

Wheeler, E. D., Achim, C. L., and Ayyavoo, V. (2006). Immunodetection of human immunodeficiency virus type 1 (HIV-1) Vpr in brain tissue of HIV-1 encephalitic patients. *J Neurovirol* 12(3), 200–10.

Wiley, C. A., Baldwin, M., and Achim, C. L. (1996). Expression of HIV regulatory and structural mRNA in the central nervous system. *AIDS* 10(8), 843–7.

Wiley, C. A., Schrier, R. D., Nelson, J. A., Lampert, P. W., and Oldstone, M. B. (1986). Cellular localization of human immunodeficiency virus infection within the brains of acquired immune deficiency syndrome patients. *Proc Natl Acad Sci U S A* 83(18), 7089–93.

Williams, R., Bokhari, S., Silverstein, P., Pinson, D., Kumar, A., and Buch, S. (2008). Nonhuman primate models of neuroAIDS. *J Neurovirol* 14(4), 292–300.

Wolters, P. L., Brouwers, P., Civitello, L., and Moss, H. A. (1997). Receptive and expressive language function of children with symptomatic HIV infection and relationship with disease parameters: a longitudinal 24-month follow-up study. *AIDS* 11(9), 1135–44.

Woods, S. P., Moore, D. J., Weber, E., and Grant, I. (2009). Cognitive neuropsychology of HIV-associated neurocognitive disorders. *Neuropsychol Rev* 19(2), 152–68.

Worlein, J. M., Leigh, J., Larsen, K., Kinman, L., Schmidt, A., Ochs, H., and Ho, R. J. (2005). Cognitive and motor deficits associated with HIV-2(287) infection in infant pigtailed macaques: a nonhuman primate model of pediatric neuro-AIDS. *J Neurovirol* 11(1), 34–45.

Xu, Y., Kulkosky, J., Acheampong, E., Nunnari, G., Sullivan, J., and Pomerantz, R. J. (2004). HIV-1-mediated apoptosis of neuronal cells: Proximal molecular mechanisms of HIV-1-induced encephalopathy. *Proc Natl Acad Sci U S A* 101(18), 7070–5.

Yadav, A., and Collman, R. G. (2009). CNS inflammation and macrophage/microglial biology associated with HIV-1 infection. *J Neuroimmune Pharmacol* 4(4), 430–47.

Zauli, G., Davis, B. R., Re, M. C., Visani, G., Furlini, G., and La Placa, M. (1992). TAT protein stimulates production of transforming growth factor-beta 1 by marrow macrophages: a potential mechanism for human immunodeficiency virus-1-induced hematopoietic suppression. *Blood* 80(12), 3036–43.

Zhang, K., McQuibban, G. A., Silva, C., Butler, G. S., Johnston, J. B., Holden, J., Clark-Lewis, I., Overall, C. M., and Power, C. (2003). HIV-induced metalloproteinase processing of the chemokine stromal cell derived factor-1 causes neurodegeneration. *Nat Neurosci* 6(10), 1064–71.

Zhao, J., Lopez, A. L., Erichsen, D., Herek, S., Cotter, R. L., Curthoys, N. P., and Zheng, J. (2004). Mitochondrial glutaminase enhances extracellular glutamate production in HIV-1-infected macrophages: linkage to HIV-1 associated dementia. *J Neurochem* 88(1), 169–80.

Zheng, J., Thylin, M. R., Ghorpade, A., Xiong, H., Persidsky, Y., Cotter, R., Niemann, D., Che, M., Zeng, Y. C., Gelbard, H. A., Shepard, R. B., Swartz, J. M., and Gendelman, H. E. (1999). Intracellular CXCR4 signaling, neuronal apoptosis and neuropathogenic mechanisms of HIV-1-associated dementia. *J Neuroimmunol* 98(2), 185–200.

Zink, M. C., Uhrlaub, J., DeWitt, J., Voelker, T., Bullock, B., Mankowski, J., Tarwater, P., Clements, J., and Barber, S. (2005). Neuroprotective and anti-human immunodeficiency virus activity of minocycline. *JAMA* 293(16), 2003–11.

Index

Page numbers followed by *f* and *t* indicate figures and tables, respectively.

T - #0213 - 111024 - C0 - 234/156/24 - PB - 9780367576530 - Gloss Lamination